# The Founders of Operative Surgery

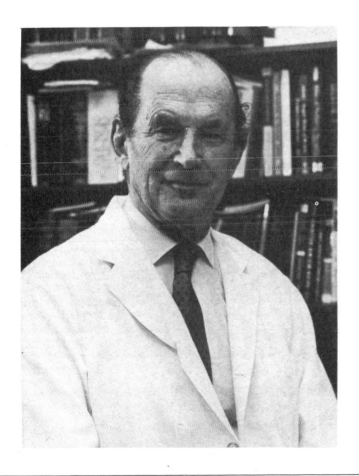

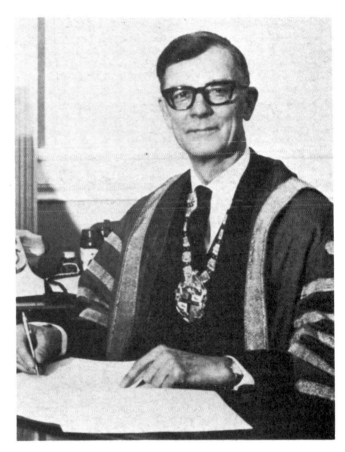

**Charles Granville Rob** MC, MChir, FRCS, FACS
Professor of Surgery, Uniformed Services University of the
Health Sciences, E Edward Hébert School of Medicine,
Bethesda, Maryland
Quondam: Professor of Surgery, St Mary's Hospital Medical
School, London 1950–1960;
Professor and Chairman, Department of Surgery, University of
Rochester, New York, 1960–1978
Professor of Surgery, East Carolina University, 1978–1983

**Lord Smith of Marlow** KBE, MS, FRCS, Hon DSc
(Exeter and Leeds), Hon MD (Zurich), Hon FRACS,
Hon FRCS(Ed.), Hon FACS, Hon FRCS(Can.), Hon FRCSI,
Hon FRCS(SA), Hon FDS
Honorary Consulting Surgeon, St George's Hospital, London
Quondam: Surgeon, St George's Hospital, London,
1946–1978;
President of the Royal College of Surgeons of England,
1973–1977

Rob & Smith's

# Operative Surgery

# Paediatric Surgery

**Fourth Edition**

# Rob & Smith's
# Operative Surgery

General Editors

**Hugh Dudley** ChM, FRCS(Ed.), FRACS, FRCS
Professor of Surgery, St Mary's Hospital, London, UK

**David C. Carter** MD, FRCS(Ed.), FRCS(Glas.)
St Mungo Professor of Surgery, University of Glasgow;
Honorary Consultant Surgeon, Royal Infirmary, Glasgow, UK

**R. C. G. Russell** MS, FRCS
Consultant Surgeon, Middlesex Hospital, St John's Hospital for Diseases of the Skin, and Royal National Nose, Throat and Ear Hospital, London, UK

Rob & Smith's
# Operative Surgery

# Paediatric Surgery

## Fourth Edition

Edited by

**Lewis Spitz** MB, ChB, PhD, FRCS(Ed), FRCS(Eng), FAAP(Hon)
Nuffield Professor of Paediatric Surgery, Institute of Child Health, University of London; Consultant Paediatric Surgeon, Hospital for Sick Children, Great Ormond Street, London, UK

**H. Homewood Nixon** MA, MB, BChir, FRCS(Eng), FRCSI(Hon), FACS(Hon), FAAP(Hon)
Consulting Paediatric Surgeon, The Hospital for Sick Children, Great Ormond Street and St. Mary's Hospital, Paddington, London, UK

**Butterworths**
London   Boston   Durban   Singapore   Sydney   Toronto   Wellington

© Butterworth and Co. (Publishers) Ltd, 1988

First edition published in eight volumes 1956–1958
Second edition published in fourteen volumes 1968–1971
Third edition published in nineteen volumes 1976–1981
Fourth edition published 1983–

---

**British Library Cataloguing in Publication Data**
Rob, Charles, *1913–*
    Rob & Smith's operative surgery. — 4th ed.
    Paediatric surgery
    1. Medicine surgery
    I. Title    II. Smith, Rodney Smith, *Baron,*
    *1914–*    III. Spitz, Lewis    IV. Nixon, H. H.
    (Harold Homewood)    V. Dudley, Hugh, *1926*
    VI. Carter, David C. (David Craig), *1940–*
    VII. Russell, R. C. G. (Ronald Christopher
    Gordon)    VIII. Operative surgery
    617

    ISBN 0-407-00666-4

---

**Library of Congress Cataloging in Publication Data**
(Revised for Vol. 10)

Rob & Smith's operative surgery.

    Rev. ed. of: Operative surgery. 3rd ed. 1976–
    Includes bibliographies and index.
    Contents: [1] Alimentary tract and abdominal wall.
1. General principles, oesophagus, stomach, duodenum,
small intestine, abdominal wall, hernia/edited by
Hugh Dudley – [10] Paediatric surgery.
    1. Surgery, Operative    2. Surgery, Operative ·
I. Rob, Charles    II. Smith of Marlow, Rodney Smith,
Baron, 1914–    .    III. Dudley, Hugh A. F. (Hugh
Arnold Freeman)    IV. Pories, Walter J. V.    Carter,
David C. (David Craig)    VI. Operative surgery.
[DNLM: 1. Surgery, Operative.    W0 500 061 1982]
RD32.06    1983        617'.91        83-14465
ISBN 0-407-00651-6 (v. 1)

Photoset by Butterworths Litho Preparation Department
Printed by Anchor Brendon Ltd, Tiptree, Essex.
Bound by Robert Hartnoll Ltd, Bodmin, Cornwall.

# Volumes and Editors

## Alimentary Tract and Abdominal Wall

1 **General Principles · Oesophagus · Stomach · Duodenum · Small Intestine · Abdominal Wall · Hernia**

**Hugh Dudley ChM, FRCS(Ed.), FRACS, FRCS**
Professor of Surgery, St Mary's Hospital, London, UK

2 **Liver · Portal Hypertension · Spleen · Biliary Tract · Pancreas**

**Hugh Dudley ChM, FRCS(Ed.), FRACS, FRCS**
Professor of Surgery, St Mary's Hospital, London, UK

3 **Colon, Rectum and Anus**

**Ian P. Todd MS, MD(Tor), FRCS, DCH**
Consulting Surgeon, St Bartholomew's Hospital, London;
Consultant Surgeon, St Mark's Hospital and
King Edward VII Hospital for Officers, London, UK

**L. P. Fielding MB, FRCS**
Chief of Surgery, St Mary's Hospital, Waterbury, Connecticut, USA;
Associate Professor of Surgery, Yale University, Connecticut, USA

## Cardiac Surgery

**Stuart W. Jamieson MB, FRCS, FACS**
Professor and Head, Cardiothoracic Surgery,
University of Minnesota, Minneapolis, Minnesota, USA

**Norman E. Schumway MD, PhD, FRCS**
Professor and Chairman, Department of Cardiovascular Surgery,
Stanford University School of Medicine, California, USA

## The Ear

**John C. Ballantyne FRCS, HonFRCSI, DLO**
Consultant Ear, Nose and Throat Surgeon,
Royal Free and King Edward VII Hospital for Officers, London, UK
Honorary Consultant in Otolaryngology to the Army

**Andrew Morrison FRCS, DLO**
Senior Consultant Otolaryngologist, The London Hospital, UK

## General Principles, Breast and Extracranial Endocrines

**Hugh Dudley ChM, FRCS(Ed.), FRACS, FRCS**
Professor of Surgery, St Mary's Hospital, London, UK

**Walter J. Pories MD, FACS**
Professor and Chairman, Department of Surgery, School of Medicine,
East Carolina University, Greenville, North Carolina, USA

## Gynaecology and Obstetrics

**J. M. Monaghan MBChB, FRCS(Ed.), FRCOG**
Consultant Gynaecological Surgeon, Head of the Regional Department of
Gynaecological Oncology, Queen Elizabeth Hospital, Gateshead, Tyne and
Wear, UK

## The Hand

**Rolfe Birch FRCS**
Consultant Orthopaedic Surgeon, PNI Unit and Hand Clinic,
Royal National Orthopaedic Hospital, London and
St Mary's Hospital, London, UK

**Donal Brooks MA, MB, FRCS, FRSCI**
Consulting Orthopaedic Surgeon, University College Hospital
and Royal National Orthopaedic Hospital, London, UK;
Civilian Consultant in Hand Surgery to the Royal Navy and
Royal Air Force, UK

## Neurosurgery

**Lindsay Symon TD, FRCS, FRCS(Ed.)**
Professor of Neurological Surgery, Institute of Neurology,
The National Hospital, Queen Square, London, UK

**David G. T. Thomas MRCP, FRCSE**
Senior Lecturer and Consultant Neurosurgeon,
Institute of Neurology, The National Hospital,
Queen Square, London, UK

**Kemp Clarke MD**
Professor and Chairman, Division of Neurological Surgery,
Southwestern Medical School, Dallas, Texas, USA

## Nose and Throat

**John C. Ballantyne FRCS, HonFRCSI, DLO**
Consultant Ear, Nose and Throat Surgeon,
Royal Free and King Edward VII Hospital for Officers, London, UK;
Honorary Consultant in Otolaryngology to the Army

**D. F. N. Harrison MD, MS, FRCS, FRACS**
Professor of Laryngology and Otology,
Royal National Throat, Nose and Ear Hospital, London, UK

## Ophthalmic Surgery

**Thomas A. Rice MD**
Assistant Clinical Professor of Ophthalmology,
Case Western Reserve University School of Medicine,
Cleveland, Ohio, USA;
formerly of the Wilmer Ophthalmological Institute

**Ronald G. Michels MD**
Professor of Ophthalmology, The Wilmer Ophthalmological Institute,
The Johns Hopkins University School of Medicine,
Maryland, USA

**Walter W. J. Stark MD**
Professor of Ophthalmology, The Wilmer Ophthalmological Institute,
The Johns Hopkins University School of Medicine,
Maryland, USA

## Orthopaedics (in 2 volumes)

**George Bentley ChM, FRCS**
Professor of Orthopaedic Surgery, Institute of Orthopaedics,
Royal National Orthopaedic Hospital, London, UK

**Robert B. Greer III MD, FACS**
Professor of Orthopedic Surgery, The Milton S. Hershey Medical
Center and College of Medicine of the Pennsylvania State University,
Hershey, Pennsylvania, USA

## Paediatric Surgery

**L. Spitz MB, ChB, PhD, FRCS(Ed.), FRCS(Eng.), FAAP(Hon)**
Nuffield Professor of Paediatric Surgery, Institute of Child Health,
University of London; Consultant Paediatric Surgeon, London, UK

**H. Homewood Nixon MA, MB, BChir, FRCS(Eng.), FRCSI(Hon.), FACS(Hon.), FAAP(Hon)**
Consultant Paediatric Surgeon, The Hospital for Sick Children,
Great Ormond Street, London and St Mary's Hospital, Paddington,
London, UK

**Plastic Surgery**

**T. L. Barclay ChM, FRCS**
Consultant Plastic Surgeon, St Luke's Hospital,
Bradford, West Yorkshire, UK

**Desmond A. Kernahan, MD**
Chief, Division of Plastic Surgery,
The Children's Memorial Hospital, Chicago, Illinois, USA

**Thoracic Surgery**

**J. W. Jackson MCh, FRCS**
(Late) Consultant Thoracic Surgeon, Harefield Hospital, Middlesex,
UK

**D. K. C. Cooper MD, PhD, FRCS**
Department of Cardiac Surgery, University of Cape Town
Medical School, Cape Town, South Africa

**Trauma**

**John V. Robbs FRCS**
Associate Professor of Surgery,
Department of Surgery, University of Natal, South Africa

**Howard R. Champion FRCS**
Chief, Trauma Service;
Director, Surgery Critical Care Services,
The Washington Hospital Center, Washington, DC, USA

**Donald Trunkey MD**
San Francisco General Hospital, San Francisco, California, USA

**Urology**

**W. Scott McDougal MD**
Professor and Chairman, Department of Urology,
Vanderbilt University Medical Center, Nashville, Tennessee, USA

**Vascular Surgery**

**James A. DeWeese MD**
Professor and Chairman, Division of Cardiothoracic Surgery,
University of Rochester Medical Center, Rochester, New York, USA

**Head and Neck**

**Ian McGregor ChM, FRCS**
Formerly Director, Plastic and Oral Surgery Unit, Canniesburn
Hospital, Glasgow, UK

**David J. Howard FRCS, FRCS(Ed.)**
Deputy Director, Professorial Unit, Institute of Laryngology and
Otology, London and the Royal National Throat, Nose and Ear
Hospital, London, UK

# Contributors

**I. Aaronson** MA, MB, BChir, FRCS
Professor of Urology, Medical University of South Carolina, Charleston, South Carolina, USA

**R. Peter Altman** MD
Professor of Surgery and Pediatrics, Columbia University College of Physicians and Surgeons, and Director, Pediatric Surgery, Babies Hospital, Columbia-Presbyterian Medical Center, New York, New York, USA

**J. D. Atwell** FRCS
Consultant Paediatric Surgeon, Wessex Regional Centre for Paediatric Surgery, The General Hospital, Southampton, UK

**Edward Austin** MD
Attending in Surgery (Pediatric), Cedars Sinai Medical Center; Consultant in Pediatric Surgery, Olive View Medical Center, Los Angeles, California, USA

**John F. R. Bentley** FRCS, FRCS(Ed.), FRCS(Glas.)
Formerly Consultant Surgeon, Royal Hospital for Sick Children, Glasgow, UK

**Harry C. Bishop** AB, MD, FACS, FAAP
Senior Surgeon, The Children's Hospital of Philadelphia; Associate Professor of Pediatric Surgery, University of Pennsylvania School of Medicine, Pennsylvania, USA

**E. Thomas Boles Jr.** MD
Professor and Director, Division of Pediatric Surgery, Department of Surgery, Ohio State University College of Medicine, and Chief, Department of Pediatric Surgery, Children's Hospital, Columbus, Ohio, USA

**Scott J. Boley** MD, FAAP, FACS
Professor of Surgery and Pediatrics and Chief of Pediatric Surgical Services, Albert Einstein College of Medicine, New York, New York, USA

**R. J. Brereton** MB, ChB, FRCS(Ed.), FRCS(Eng.)
Senior Lecturer in Paediatric Surgery, Institute of Child Health, University of London, London, UK

**I. W. Broomhead** MA, MB, MChir, FRCS
Consultant Plastic Surgeon, Guy's Hospital, London and The Hospital for Sick Children, Great Ormond Street, London, UK

**M. Carcassonne**
Professor of Paediatric Surgery, Surgeon in Chief, Department of Paediatric Surgery, School of Medicine, Marseille, France

**S. Joseph Cohen** MB, BCh, MRCP, FRCS
Consultant Paediatric Surgeon, Booth Hall Children's Hospital, Royal Manchester Children's Hospital, St Mary's Hospital, Manchester; Lecturer in Paediatric Surgery, University of Manchester, Manchester, UK

**R. C. M. Cook** FRCS
Consultant Paediatric Surgeon, Alder Hey Children's Hospital, Liverpool, UK

**D. K. C. Cooper** MA, MD, PhD, FRCS
Cardiothoracic Surgeon, Oklahoma Transplantation Institute, Oklahoma City, Oklahoma, USA; formerly Associate Professor of Cardiothoracic Surgery, University of Cape Town Medical School, Cape Town, South Africa

**S. Cywes** MMed(Surg), FACS, FRCS(Eng)
Professor of Paediatric Surgery, University of Cape Town; Chief Surgeon, Red Cross War Memorial Children's Hospital, Cape Town, South Africa

**A. Delarue**
Senior Registrar, Department of Paediatric Surgery, School of Medicine, Marseille, France

**Marc De Leval** MD
Consultant Cardiothoracic Surgeon, The Hospital for Sick Children, Great Ormond Street, London, UK

**J. A. S. Dickson** FRCS(Ed.), FRCS
Consultant Paediatric Surgeon, Children's Hospital, Sheffield, UK

**Patricia K. Donahoe** MD
Chief of Pediatric Surgery, Massachusetts General Hospital; Professor of Surgery, Harvard Medical School, Boston, Massachusetts, USA

**J. W. Duckett** MD
Director of Pediatric Urology, Children's Hospital, Philadelphia, Pennsylvania, USA

**Patrick G. Duffy** FRCS
Consultant Urological Surgeon, Hospital for Sick Children, Great Ormond Street; Senior Lecturer in Paediatric Urology, Institute of Urology, University of London, London, UK

**H. B. Eckstein** MD, MChir, FRCS
(Late) Consultant Paediatric Surgeon, The Hospital for Sick Children, Great Ormond Street, London and Queen Mary's Hospital for Children, Carshalton, Surrey, UK

**David M. Evans** FRCS
Consultant Plastic Surgeon, Wexham Park Hospital, Slough, UK

**John N. G. Evans** MB, BS, DLO, FRCS
Consultant Ear, Nose and Throat Surgeon, The Hospital for Sick Children, Great Ormond Street and St Thomas's Hospital London, UK

**J. A. Fixsen** MChir, FRCS
Consultant Orthopaedic Surgeon, The Hospital for Sick Children, Great Ormond Street, London, UK

**E. Fonkalsrud** MD
Professor and Chief of Pediatric Surgery, and Vice-Chairman, Department of Surgery, University of California, Los Angeles School of Medicine, Los Angeles, California, USA

**J. D. Frank** LRCP(Lond.), MRCS(Eng.), FRCS(Eng.)
Consultant Paediatric Surgeon and Urologist, Royal Hospital for Sick Children, Bristol, UK

**Stephen L. Gans** MD
Clinical Professor of Surgery (Pediatric), University of California, Los Angeles; Chairman, Subdivision of Pediatric Surgery, Cedars Sinai Medical Center, Los Angeles, California, USA

**D. N. Grant** FRCS
Consultant Neurosurgeon, National Hospital for Nervous Diseases, London and The Hospital for Sick Children, Great Ormond Street, London, UK

**Jay L. Grosfeld** MD
Professor and Chairman Department of Surgery, Indiana University School of Medicine; Surgeon in Chief, James Whitcomb Riley Hospital for Children, Indianapolis, Indiana, USA

**J. Alex Haller** MD
Robert Garrett Professor of Surgery, Department of Pediatric Surgery, The Johns Hopkins Hospital, Baltimore, USA

**W. H. Hendren** MD, FACS
Chief of Surgery, The Children's Hospital, Boston; Visiting Surgeon, Massachusetts General Hospital; Robert E. Gross Professor of Surgery, Harvard Medical School, Boston, USA

**Edward R. Howard** MS, FRCS
Consultant Surgeon, King's College Hospital, London, UK

**Ambrose Jolleys** MD, FRCS
Paediatric Surgeon, Royal Manchester Children's Hospital and St Mary's Hospital, Manchester, UK

**Peter G. Jones** MS(Melb.), FRCS(Eng.), FRACS, FACS, FAAP(Hon)
Surgeon, Royal Children's Hospital, Melbourne, Victoria, Australia

**T. R. Karl** MD
Kaiser Permanente Medical Center, San Francisco, California, USA

**E. M. St. G. Kiely** FRCS, FRCSI
Consultant Paediatric Surgeon, The Hospital for Sick Children, Great Ormond Street, London, UK

**S. H. Kim** MD
Clinical Associate Professor of Surgery, Harvard Medical School; Visiting Surgeon, Massachusetts General Hospital, Boston, Massachusetts, USA

**I. S. Kirkland** FRCS(Ed.), FRCS(Glas.)
Consultant Paediatric Surgeon, Western General Hospital, Edinburgh, UK

**J. R. Lilly** MD
Professor and Chief of Pediatric Surgery, University of Colorado School of Medicine, Denver, Colorado, USA

**James Lister** MD, FRCS(Ed.), FRCS(Glas.), FRCS(Eng.), FAAP(Hon)
Formerly Professor of Paediatric Surgery, University of Liverpool; Consultant Paediatric Surgeon, Alder Hey Children's Hospital, Liverpool, UK

**David A. Lloyd** MD, FRCS
Associate Professor of Pediatric Surgery, University of Pittsburgh School of Medicine, and The Children's Hospital, Pittsburgh, Pennsylvania, USA

**J. C. Molenaar** MD
Professor, Erasmus University, Rotterdam, The Netherlands

**N. A. Myers** AM, FRCS, FRACS
Senior Surgeon, Royal Children's Hospital, Melbourne; Professorial Associate, University of Melbourne, Victoria, Australia

**H. Homewood Nixon** MA, MB, BChir, FRCS(Eng.), FRCSI(Hon), FACS(Hon), FAAP(Hon)
Consulting Paediatric Surgeon, The Hospital for Sick Children, Great Ormond Street, London and St Mary's Hospital, Paddington, London, UK

**Barry O'Donnell** MCh, FRCS, FRCS(I), Hon FAAP
Professor of Paediatric Surgery, Royal College of Surgeons in Ireland; Consultant Paediatric Surgeon, Children's Research Centre, Our Lady's Hospital for Sick Children, Dublin, Ireland

**Prem Puri** MS, FACS
Associate Paediatric Surgeon, Our Lady's Hospital for Sick Children; Consultant Paediatric Surgeon, National Children's Hospital, Dublin, Ireland

**John G. Raffensperger** MD
Surgeon, The Children's Memorial Hospital, Chicago, USA

**Philip G. Ransley** FRCS
Consultant Urological Surgeon, The Hospital for Sick Children, Great Ormond Street, London; Senior Lecturer in Paediatric Urology, Institute of Urology and Institute of Child Health, University of London, UK

**Marleta Reynolds** MD
Children's Memorial Hospital, Northwestern University Medical School, Chicago, Illinois, USA

**Marc I. Rowe** MD
Professor of Pediatric Surgery, University of Pittsburgh School of Medicine, and The Children's Hospital, Pittsburgh, Pennsylvania, USA

**John E. S. Scott** MD, FRCS, FAAP
Senior Lecturer in Paediatric Surgery, University of Newcastle upon Tyne; Consulting Paediatric Surgeon, Newcastle Area Health Authority (Teaching), UK

**J. Siebert** MD
Resident in Surgery, Massachusetts General Hospital, Boston, Massachusetts, USA

**Lewis Spitz** MB, ChB, PhD, FRCS(Ed), FRCS(Eng), FAAP(I Ion)
Nuffield Professor of Paediatric Surgery, Institute of Child Health, University of London, and The Hospital for Sick Children, Great Ormond St, London, UK

**J. Stark** MD, FRCS
Consultant Cardiothoracic Surgeon, Hospital for Sick Children, Great Ormond Street, London, UK

**U. G. Stauffer** MD
Director, Department of Surgery, University Children's Hospital, Zürich; Professor of Paediatric Surgery, University of Zürich, Switzerland

**Gianna P. Stellin** MD
Assistant Professor of Surgery, University of California at Irvine, Orange, California, USA

**Edward Sumner** MA, BM, BCh, FFARCS
Consultant Anaesthetist, The Hospital for Sick Children, Great Ormond Street, London, UK

**D. F. M. Thomas** MRCP, FRCS
Consultant Paediatric Surgeon, St. James's University Hospital, and The General Infirmary, Leeds, UK

**P. Upadhyaya** MS, FRCS(Eng), FAMS
Professor of Paediatric Surgery, King Faisal University, Dammam – 31451, Saudi Arabia

**George C. Vaos** MD
Formerly Research Fellow, Department of Paediatric Surgery, University of Liverpool; Alder Hey Children's Hospital, Liverpool, UK

**Robert H. Whitaker** FRCS
Consultant Paediatric Urologist, Addenbrooke's Hospital, Cambridge; Associate Lecturer, University of Cambridge, Cambridge, UK

**C. B. Williams** BM, BCh, FRCP
Consultant Physician, St Mark's Hospital for Diseases of the Rectum and Colon and St Bartholomew's Hospital, London, UK

**Vanessa M. Wright** FRCS
Consultant Paediatric Surgeon, Queen Elizabeth Hospital for Children, and University College Hospital, London, UK

**Daniel G. Young** MB, ChB, FRCS(Glas.), FRCS(Ed.), DTM&H
Reader in Paediatric Surgery and Honorary Consultant Paediatric Surgeon, Royal Hospital for Sick Children, Glasgow, UK

# Contributing Medical Artists

**Paul Andriesse**
28 Lloyd St, Winchester, Massachusetts 01890, USA

**Angela Christie**
130 The Heights, Northolt Park, Middlesex, UK

**Kevin Marks** MMAA BA(Hons)
53 Rookwood Avenue, Wallington, Surrey SM6 8HQ, UK

**John E. Nixon**
Medical Illustration Department, Emerson Hall 102, 545 Barnhill Drive, Indiana University Medical Center, Indianapolis, Indiana 46223, USA

**Gillian Oliver**
71 Crawford Road, Hatfield, Hertfordshire AL10 0PF, UK

**Jean Perry**
3 Southern Crescent, Bramhall, Cheshire SK7 3AQ, UK

**Philip Wilson**
23 Normanhurst Road, St Paul's Cray, Orpington, Kent BR5 3AL, UK

# Contents

# Preface

This is only the second edition of a separate volume devoted to Paediatric Surgery in the series of Operative Surgery. The scope and extent of subject matter has been enlarged in accordance with the increasing sophistication of the specialty. New chapters include transport of the surgical neonate, pre- and postoperative management, anaesthesiology and various endoscopic diagnostic and therapeutic procedures. In addition to the indications for the operation, contributors have been encouraged to include where relevant the postoperative complications, and mortality and morbidity statistics. The illustrations have been largely deputed to three artists to give a more consistent style.

The number of contributors has increased to 65, and we were fortunate in obtaining contributions from leading authorities in the specialty from most parts of the world. The volume has had a prolonged gestational period and we are particularly grateful for the patience of those authors who submitted their chapters on schedule and also to those authors whose contributions were only requested at very short notice in order to maintain coverage of this rapidly developing specialty.

L. Spitz
H. H. Nixon

Illustrations by Kevin Marks

# Transfer for surgery

**D. F. M. Thomas**   MRCP, FRCS
Consultant Paediatric Surgeon, St James's University Hospital and The General Infirmary, Leeds, UK

Neonatal and specialized paediatric surgery should ideally be performed in regional or national centres. This arrangement ensures the most rational use of resources and surgical expertise, but has the disadvantage that patients and their parents may have to travel considerable distances to benefit from this specialized care. Fortunately, newborn infants can withstand long journeys with relative impunity, provided that they are protected against the threats of hypothermia, aspiration pneumonia, hypoxia and hypoglycaemia. Speed of transfer is rarely the prime consideration. Adequate resuscitation prior to transfer and attention to certain details during the journey are of greater importance. The most suitable form of transport (e.g. adequately equipped ambulances, fixed-wing aircraft, helicopters) varies from country to country, depending on financial and geographical considerations. Ideally a team consisting of a neonatal surgical resident and an intensive care nurse should travel out from the regional centre to the referring hospital to collect the baby. If this is not possible, it should be the responsibility of the specialist centre to advise the referring hospital by telephone of what is needed. The transfer of older children poses fewer problems and can more reasonably be undertaken by staff from the referring hospital.

# Principles of transfer

## Correction and prevention of hypothermia

### 1

Hypothermia is best corrected at the referring hospital unless there are pressing indications for immediate transfer. Radiant overhead heaters are more effective than incubators for this purpose. While no absolute figure can be given, a minimum core temperature of 35°C (monitored with a rectal thermocouple probe rather than a mercury thermometer) is desirable. A portable incubator is essential to maintain a neutral thermal environment (32°–34°C) throughout the journey. As an additional precaution against heat loss, the infant can be wrapped in a metal foil swaddler. A range of portable transport incubators is now available and it is important to check that the incubator in use can be fixed securely to the structure of the ambulance or aircraft and that the electrical power supplies are compatible.

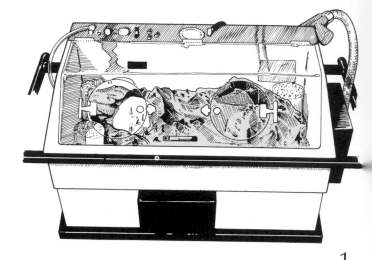

1

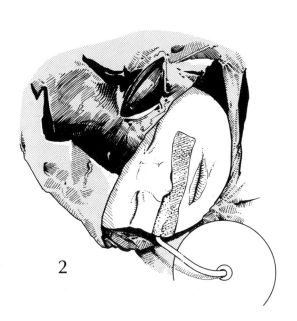

2

## Nasogastric intubation

### 2

In general, no infant should be transferred without a nasogastric tube *in situ*. This applies also to infants who are not thought to be suffering from intestinal obstruction. Fine-bore tubes have a tendency to kink or curl up and are less effective in decompressing the stomach. For these reasons, a size 8-Fr tube or larger should be used for term neonates, while a size 6-Fr nasogastric tube is appropriate for preterm infants. If introduction via the nose proves difficult, the tube may be passed via the mouth. Once in position, the nasogastric tube should be aspirated with a syringe at regular intervals (e.g. every 15–20 minutes) and *left open on free drainage* at all other times.

In addition to gastric content, saliva and pharyngeal secretions may also be inhaled so that oropharyngeal suction will also be required throughout the journey. Infants with oesophageal atresia are at particular risk in this respect. Over-enthusiastic oropharyngeal suction should be avoided, as this can cause retching and hence risk of vomiting if the stomach is not aspirated first. As a precaution against the failure of portable mechanical suction devices, it is wise to include a simple disposable mucus extractor with the equipment for the journey.

## Position of infant during transfer

The prone position, in which gastro-oesophageal reflux is least likely to occur, is suitable for most patients, especially those with lesions involving the back, such as meningomyelocele and· sacrococcygeal teratoma. The lateral position should be adopted for infants with anomalies of the anterior abdominal wall, i.e. exomphalos, gastroschisis, ectopia vesicae. Infants requiring ventilatory support and those with significant abdominal distension are best nursed in the supine position. An infant with oesophageal atresia may be transported either in the 45° upright supine position (which is difficult to achieve in currently available portable incubators) or in the prone position. In either case, meticulous suction of the oropharynx is essential to prevent aspiration.

Regardless of the position of the infant within the incubator, it is important that additional padding is used to minimize movement and possible trauma during the journey.

## Intravenous infusion

A term infant who has no exceptional fluid losses has only minimal fluid requirements for the first 24 hours of life. Intravenous infusion need not be established as a routine and should be reserved for infants in whom there is a specific indication. These include *abnormal losses*, e.g. evaporative loss from exposed intestine (gastroschisis, ruptured exomphalos) and significant aspirate or vomitus in intestinal obstruction, *hypovolaemia, acidosis* and *hypoglycaemia*. Fine plastic infusion cannulae are preferred to metal needles since the latter tend to 'cut out' of peripheral veins during transfer. Infusion by gravity drip is difficult to regulate during an ambulance journey – portable syringe pumps are more suitable for accurate administration of small-volume infusions.

## Ventilatory support

Unlike premature babies (who are often transferred for the management of respiratory distress), most 'surgical' neonates do not require ventilatory support in transit. Congenital diaphragmatic hernia is the most frequent indication for ventilation, but some infants with oesophageal atresia and those with cystic hygroma or micrognathia and a compromised airway may also benefit from endotracheal intubation. The decision whether or not to intubate should be made before the outset of the journey, as the procedure is difficult to carry out in a moving vehicle. Nasotracheal intubation requires additional expertise but has the advantage that the tube can be fixed with greater security and is less likely to become dislodged during the journey. Mechanical ventilators are now incorporated into transport incubators and it is important that the medical member of the transport team is fully conversant with the functioning of this equipment. If there are any doubts about the mechanical ventilator, it is safer to hand-ventilate throughout the journey. *Ventilation by face mask is to be discouraged:* not only is it an ineffective means of assisting respiration, but some of the ventilating gas is invariably introduced into the stomach, resulting in abdominal distension and thus further aggravating respiratory embarrassment.

## Additional precautions

1. Vitamin K 1 mg should be given by intramuscular injection.
2. Since the preparation of blood for transfusion in the neonatal period is complicated by the presence of passively acquired maternal antibodies, a maternal specimen (10 ml of clotted blood is usually sufficient) will be required by the haematologist.
3. A legally valid consent form authorizing operation should be signed by one or both parents.

Exceptional precautions are required in the following conditions.

### Gastroschisis and ruptured exomphalos

The exposed viscera are a potent source of heat and fluid loss and, in addition, traction on unsupported loops of bowel may result in intestinal ischaemia. The bowel should be supported, but not covered, by one or two warm saline packs and the entire abdomen enclosed by wrapping it in several layers of clingfilm or polythene. Intravenous infusion with plasma should be commenced to counteract hypovolaemia and the blood glucose level checked at frequent intervals.

### Meningomyelocele

The exposed neural tissue should be protected by a moist saline swab held in position by clingfilm wrapped around the trunk.

### Neonatal necrotizing enterocolitis

Affected neonates are usually premature and often in poor general condition. Assisted ventilation helps to ensure good tissue oxygenation, and intravenous infusion will be required before transfer for the correction of acidosis or hypoglycaemia and for the administration of broad spectrum antibiotics.

### Further reading

Blake, A. M., McIntosh, N., Reynolds, E. O. R., St. Andrew, D. (1975) Transport of newborn infants for intensive care. British Medical Journal, 4, 13–17

Bishop, H. C. (1957) Safe transportation of newborn infants for emergency surgery. Journal of the American Medical Association, 165, 1230–1233

Chance, G. W., Matthew, J. D., Gash, J., Williams, G., Cunningham, K. (1978) Neonatal transport: a controlled study of skilled assistance. Mortality and morbidity of neonates <1.5 kg birth weight. Journal of Paediatrics, 93, 662–666

Spitz, L., Wallis, M., Graves, H. F. (1984) Transport of the surgical neonate. Archives of Disease in Childhood, 59, 284–288

Thomas, D. F. M. (1982) Transfer of neonates for surgery. Hospital Update, 8, 955–963

# Preoperative and postoperative management

**Marc I. Rowe** MD
Professor of Surgery, Division of Pediatric Surgery, University of Pittsburgh School of Medicine, and Children's Hospital of Pittsburgh, Pittsburgh, Pennsylvania, USA

**David A. Lloyd** MD, FRCS
Associate Professor of Surgery, Division of Pediatric Surgery, University of Pittsburgh School of Medicine, and Children's Hospital of Pittsburgh, Pittsburgh, Pennsylvania, USA

## Variations in individual children

The neonate, infant, child and adolescent differ significantly from each other and from the adult. The most distinctive and rapidly changing physiological characteristics occur during the neonatal period, due to the newborn infant's adaptation to the extrauterine environment, differences in the physiological maturity of individual newborn infants, the small size of these patients, and the demands of growth and development. For these reasons this chapter will emphasize the management of the newborn infant.

## Low-birth-weight (LBW) baby

The normal full-term infant has a gestational age of 38 weeks or more, and a body weight greater than 2500 g. Most babies who weigh less than 2500 g are born prematurely, but at least one-third of LBW babies are more than 38 weeks gestational age, and are small because of intrauterine abnormalities affecting growth. There are important physiological differences between small for gestational age infants and premature infants.

### PREMATURE INFANT

Premature infants are those born before 38 weeks gestational age, regardless of birth weight. When the gestational age is not accurately known, prematurity can be confirmed by physical examination. The principal features of prematurity are a head circumference below the 50th percentile, a thin, semi-transparent skin, absence of plantar creases, soft malleable ears, absence of breast tissue, undescended testicles with a flat scrotum and, in females, relatively enlarged labia minora.

Apnoeic episodes are common and may occur spontaneously or as non-specific signs of problems such as sepsis or hypothermia. Prolonged apnoea with significant hypoxia leads to bradycardia and ultimately to cardiac arrest. All premature infants should therefore have electrocardiographic pulse monitoring with the alarm set at a minimum pulse rate of 90 beats per minute. In the infant with respiratory difficulties, chest radiographs are important to detect hyaline membrane disease (which is common in premature infants), and congestive cardiac failure. The lungs and retinae of preterm infants are very susceptible to high oxygen levels, and even relatively brief exposures may result in permanent blindness. Infants receiving oxygen therapy therefore require arterial blood $P_{O_2}$ monitoring. Because of the high incidence in premature infants of patent ductus arteriosus with right-to-left shunting, blood gases should be measured from the upper limbs or head.

The small premature infant may be unable to tolerate oral feeding, and gastric-tube feeds or total parenteral nutrition may be required. Bilirubin metabolism may be impaired, therefore the serum bilirubin should be monitored for rising levels of unconjugated bilirubin.

### SMALL FOR GESTATIONAL AGE (SGA) INFANT

Although body weight is low, the body length and head circumference of the SGA infant approach that of an infant of normal weight for age. Compared with a premature infant of equivalent weight, the SGA infant is older and more mature, and faces different physiological problems.

The metabolic rate is higher and fluid and caloric requirements are increased. In addition, the relative lack of body fat and limited liver glycogen stores predispose to thermal instability and hypoglycaemia. Close monitoring of the blood sugar is therefore essential, particularly after operation. Polycythaemia is common and the haematocrit should be monitored. Persistently high haematocrits may necessitate plasma exchange transfusions to avoid the potential risks of hyperviscosity. SGA infants also have an increased risk of meconium aspiration syndrome.

# Metabolic considerations in the care of the newborn infant

## TEMPERATURE CONTROL

Newborn infants are susceptible to heat loss because of their large surface area, low body fat relative to body weight, and high thermoneutral temperature zone. Newborn babies generate heat not by shivering but by metabolizing their brown fat reserve. When an infant is exposed to a cold environment metabolic work increases above basal levels and calories are consumed to maintain body temperature. If prolonged, this leads to depletion of the limited energy reserves, and predisposes to hypothermia and increased mortality.

The environmental temperature must be maintained near the appropriate thermoneutral zone for each individual patient. This is 34–35°C for LBW infants up to 12 days of age and 31–32°C at 6 weeks of age. Infants weighing 2000–3000 g have a thermoneutral zone of 31–34°C at birth and 29–31°C at 12 days. The environmental temperature is best controlled by placing the infant in an incubator. Either the ambient temperature of the incubator can be monitored and maintained at thermoneutrality, or a servo system can be used. The latter regulates the incubator temperature according to the patient's skin temperature, which is monitored by means of a skin probe on the infant. The normal skin temperature for a full-term infant is 36.2°C and for an LBW infant is 36.5°C. Increased metabolic activity can be detected by comparing skin and rectal temperatures, which normally differ by 1.5°C. A decrease in skin temperature while the rectal temperature remains constant, suggests that the metabolic rate has increased to maintain the core temperature.

In a cold environment such as in the Operating Room or X-ray department, heat loss may be reduced by wrapping the head, extremities, and as much of the trunk as possible in wadding, plastic sheets or aluminium foil. Stockingette alone does not prevent evaporative heat and water loss and should be lined with plastic. On the operating table a plastic sheet is placed beneath the infant. After draping, the infant is covered by a large adhesive plastic sheet: this retains evaporative heat and water and also prevents the infant from becoming wet during the operation. Any exposed intestine should be wrapped in plastic. An overhead infrared heating lamp is focused on the baby during induction of anaesthesia and preparation for operation, and again at the termination of the operation. Solutions used for skin cleansing should be warmed.

## GLUCOSE HOMEOSTASIS

Fetal glucose requirements are obtained almost entirely from the mother by transplacental diffusion, with very little derived from fetal gluconeogenesis. Following delivery, the limited liver glycogen stores are rapidly depleted and the blood glucose level then depends on the infant's capacity for gluconeogenesis, the adequacy of substrate stores, and energy requirements. Infants at high risk of developing hypoglycaemia include LBW (especially SGA) infants, infants of toxaemic or diabetic mothers, and infants requiring surgery who are unable to take oral nutrition and who have the additional metabolic stresses of their disease and the surgical procedure.

The clinical features of hypoglycaemia are non-specific and include a weak or high-pitched cry, cyanosis, apnoea, jitteriness or trembling, apathy, and seizures. The differential diagnosis includes other metabolic disturbances or sepsis. Over 50 per cent of infants with symptomatic hypoglycaemia suffer significant neurological damage. Neonatal hypoglycaemia is defined as a serum glucose level less than 1.66 mmol/l in the full term infant, and less than 1.11 mmol/l in the LBW infant. However, neurological abnormalities have been reported with higher blood glucose levels. Older children, particularly those with depleted stores and severe metabolic demands, are also at risk of hypoglycaemia.

All paediatric surgical patients, particularly neonates, are therefore monitored for hypoglycaemia. Blood glucose level is measured by Dextrostix every two hours, and this is correlated at intervals with serum glucose determinations, the frequency depending on the stability of the infant. Intravenous fluids should contain a minimum of 10 per cent dextrose, and if non-dextrose-containing solutions such as blood or plasma are being administered, close monitoring of the blood glucose level is essential. The symptomatic infant should be treated urgently with 50 per cent dextrose, 1–2 ml/kg intravenously, and maintenance intravenous dextrose 10–15 per cent at 80–100 ml/kg per 24 hours.

## CALCIUM AND MAGNESIUM HOMEOSTASIS

The fetus receives calcium by active transport across the placenta, 75 per cent of the total requirement being transferred after the 28th week of gestation. Hypocalcaemia, defined as serum calcium less than 1.75 mmol/l, is most likely to occur 24–48 hours after delivery. The causes include decreased calcium stores, decreased renal phosphate excretion and relative hypoparathyroidism. LBW infants are at greatest risk, particularly if they are premature, associated with a complicated pregnancy or delivery, or receiving bicarbonate infusions. The symptoms of hypocalcaemia are non-specific as with hypoglycaemia, and include jitteriness, high-pitched crying, cyanosis, vomiting, twitching, or seizures. The diagnosis is confirmed by determining the serum calcium level. However, the ionized fraction of the serum calcium may be low, resulting in clinical hypocalcaemia without a great reduction of the total serum calcium level; this may occur in surgical babies receiving sodium bicarbonate or undergoing exchange transfusion.

Hypocalcaemia is prevented by adding calcium gluconate to daily maintenance therapy, either 1–2 g/24 hours intravenously or 2 g/24 hours by mouth. Symptomatic hypocalcaemia is treated by intravenous administration of 10 per cent calcium gluconate in a dose of 6 ml for an LBW baby and 10 ml for a full-term infant; the rate should not exceed 1 ml/min.

Magnesium and calcium metabolism are closely related, and hypomagnesaemia may coexist with hypocalcaemia. If there is no response to correction of calcium deficiency, a serum magnesium level should be obtained. Hypomagnesaemia is corrected by administering 50 per cent magnesium sulphate, 0.2 ml/kg every four hours, followed by oral magnesium sulphate 30 mEq/day.

Although most seizures occurring in the newborn period have a cerebral cause and are not secondary to hypoglycaemia or hypocalcaemia, the latter should be suspected in high-risk infants, particularly after operation. A jittery baby should therefore have an immediate Dextrostix determination as well as serum glucose and calcium measurements. Treatment should be prompt, glucose being given intravenously when hypoglycaemia is suspected, followed by intravenous calcium if symptoms persist.

## BLOOD VOLUME

Total blood, plasma, and red cell volumes are higher during the first few postnatal hours than at any other time in an individual's life. These elevated levels may be further increased if a significant placental transfusion takes place at delivery. Several hours after birth, plasma shifts out of the circulation, and total blood and plasma volumes decrease. The high red blood cell volume persists, decreasing slowly to reach adult levels by the seventh postnatal week. In infants over two months of age the blood volume is approximately 75–80 ml/kg.

In the newborn infant polycythaemia is defined as a venous haematocrit greater than 65 per cent. This may be associated with high blood viscosity, which is further increased by a fall in body temperature. Haemodilution may be indicated, since hyperviscosity may be an aetiological factor in several disorders, for example central nervous system dysfunction or necrotizing enterocolitis.

## JAUNDICE

Haempigments, notably haemoglobin, are catabolized in the spleen and liver to produce bilirubin. The bilirubin is conjugated with glucuronic acid in the liver, forming a water-soluble substance which is excreted via the biliary system into the intestine. In the fetus, the lipid-soluble, unconjugated (indirect) bilirubin is cleared across the placenta. In the fetal intestine beta-glucuronidase hydrolyses conjugated bilirubin which is then reabsorbed for transplacental clearance. Circulating bilirubin is bound to albumin.

In the newborn the capacity for conjugating bilirubin is not fully developed and may be exceeded by the bilirubin load. This results in transient physiological jaundice which reaches a maximum at the age of four days but returns to normal levels by the sixth day. Usually the maximum

bilirubin level does not exceed 170 μmol/l. Physiological jaundice is particularly likely to occur with SGA and premature infants, in whom higher and more prolonged hyperbilirubinaemia may be encountered.

High serum levels of unconjugated bilirubin in the newborn can result in brain damage (kernicterus). Predisposing factors are hypoalbuminaemia, acidosis, cold stress, hypoglycaemia, caloric deprivation, hypoxia, and competition for bilirubin-binding sites by drugs (e.g. frusemide, digoxin, or gentamicin) or free fatty acids. Persistence of intestinal beta-glucuronidase, particularly with intestinal obstruction, increases the bilirubin load.

Clinical jaundice is apparent at serum bilirubin levels of 120–135 μmol/l. A rapid rise early in the newborn period suggests haemolysis, secondary either to inherited enzyme defects or to maternal–newborn blood-group incompatibilities. Prolonged hyperbilirubinaemia is often associated with an increase in conjugated bilirubin due to biliary obstruction or hepatocellular dysfunction. Breast-milk jaundice commonly appears between 1 and 8 weeks of age. Intestinal obstruction can intensify jaundice by increasing the enterohepatic circulation of bilirubin. Finally, jaundice is an early and important sign of septicaemia.

If haemolysis is suspected, serial haematocrit estimations, reticulocyte counts, peripheral blood smears, and a Coombs' test are appropriate. Evaluation of neonatal sepsis includes haematocrit, white cell count and differential, platelet count, chest radiograph and cultures of blood, urine, and CSF.

Phototherapy is widely used prophylactically in high-risk infants to decrease the serum bilirubin by photo-degradation of bilirubin in the skin to water-soluble products. It is continued until the total serum bilirubin is less than 170 μmol/l and falling. Exchange transfusion is indicated when the indirect bilirubin level exceeds 340 μmol/l. The precise indications vary according to the individual patient, and in very low-birth-weight infants exchange transfusion is indicated at much lower levels of serum bilirubin. Factors increasing the risk of kernicterus, mentioned above, also influence the indications for exchange transfusion.

## VITAMIN K

The routine administration of vitamin K to all newborn infants to prevent hypoprothrombinaemia and haemorrhagic disease of the newborn is established practice. This may be overlooked during the activities attendant on the birth of an infant with major congenital anomalies. When in doubt, 1 mg vitamin K should be administered by intramuscular or intravenous injection.

## CALORIC REQUIREMENTS

The paediatric patient requires a relatively large caloric intake because of the high basal metabolic rate, caloric requirements for growth and development, energy needs to maintain body heat, and the limited energy reserves. These requirements vary according to age and environmental factors, and are significantly increased by cold stress, surgical operations, infections and injuries, particularly burns. Calorie requirements are increased 10–25 per cent by surgical operations, more than 50 per cent by infection, and 150 per cent by burns. Energy reserves are limited in the newborn infant, whose liver glycogen stores are consumed in the first three hours of life, and to an even greater extent in the preterm and SGA infant.

The caloric needs of an infant are calculated according to the requirements for basal metabolism plus growth (Table 1). Consideration must also be given to the adequacy of energy reserves and the presence of stress factors such as cold, infection, and trauma, including surgery.

**Table 1 Calorie requirements of various age groups**

| Age | Cal/kg per 24 hours |
| --- | --- |
| *Basal metabolism: Full-term infant* | |
| Birth | 32 |
| 2 weeks | 48 |
| 1 year | 40 |
| Teen | 23 |
| *Growth calories* | |
| Birth | 33 |
| 3 months | 18 |
| 6 months | 12 |
| 1 year | 12 |
| Teen | 18 |
| *Total calories (maintenance + growth)* | |
| Newborn term (0–4 days) | 110–120 |
| Low birth weight | 120–130 |
| 3–4 months | 100–106 |
| 5–12 months | 100 |
| 1–7 years | 90–75 |
| 7–12 years | 75–60 |
| 12–18 years | 60–30 |

## FLUID AND ELECTROLYTE MANAGEMENT

Effective fluid and electrolyte management involves, initially, calculating the water and electrolyte requirements for maintaining metabolic functions, plus the replacement of estimated fluid and electrolyte deficits and continuing losses. Taking these factors into consideration, a tentative programme is devised for fluid and electrolyte administration. Orders are written for a finite period of time, usually 8 hours, but shorter intervals are necessary for critically ill patients. The patient's response is monitored and the programme adjusted accordingly, taking into account ongoing losses.

## Calculating maintenance needs

In the newborn infant, the basic maintenance requirement of water is the volume required for growth, renal excretion (renal water), and replacement of losses from the skin, lungs, and stools. Stool water loss has been estimated at 5–10 ml/100 calories expended, the lower figure applying to infants not being fed. In the surgical patient with postoperative ileus there is usually no significant stool water loss. Growth is inhibited during periods of severe stress and is also not a major factor under these conditions. The basal fluid maintenance requirement is therefore renal water plus insensible loss.

### Renal water

The volume of water required for excretion by the kidney depends on the renal solute load and the renal concentrating ability of the infant. The solute load that the kidneys must excrete is derived from endogenous tissue catabolism and exogenous protein and electrolyte intake. The osmolar load is thus reduced by growth and increased by tissue necrosis, high osmolar feeds, and infusions. The volume of fluid administered should be sufficient to allow excretion of the solute load at a urine osmolality between 250 and 290 mOsm/kg water. We found that during the first three postoperative days the osmolar load in newborn infants ranged between 8.8 and 33.4 mOsm/kg per 24 hours (mean 16.47). The calculated ideal urine output, representing the renal water required to excrete this load, averaged 62.6 ml/kg per 24 hours, with a wide range from 33.6 to 132 ml/kg per 24 hours.

### Insensible loss

Invisible continuing loss of water occurs from the lungs (respiratory water loss) and through the skin (transepithelial water loss), and constitutes the insensible water loss (IWL). Respiratory water loss (RWL) accounts for approximately one third of IWL in infants older than 32 weeks gestational age and is approximately 5 ml/kg body weight per 24 hours at a relative humidity of 50 per cent. Transepithelial water loss (TEWL) for a full-term infant in a thermoneutral environment is approximately 7 ml/kg body weight. The insensible water loss, therefore, for a full-term infant in a thermoneutral environment at 50 per cent relative humidity is 12 ml/kg per 24 hours.

Chief among the factors that affect IWL are the gestational age of the infant and the relative humidity of the environment. For infants of 25–27 weeks gestation TEWL has been estimated at 128 ml/kg per 24 hours in 50 per cent relative humidity. The relative humidity has a marked effect on TEWL, which decreases to almost zero as the relative humidity approaches 100 per cent, and increases progressively as the relative humidity falls. With the use of plastic sheets the relative humidity around the infant can be increased, and TEWL reduced by 50–70 per cent. Conversely, radiant warmers and phototherapy lights increase IWL by 50 per cent in infants less than 1500 g and by 80 per cent in infants larger than 1500 g.

## Management programme

The most commonly used method of calculating fluid requirements is based on body weight. However, because of the many factors affecting maintenance requirements, there is no close or constant relationship between body weight and fluid and electrolyte needs. Nevertheless, in the older child, fluid calculations based on body weight

(Table 2) may be helpful as a guide to initial maintenance requirements, which are then adjusted as the patient is monitored.

**Table 2 Calculation of maintenance fluid requirements**

| Body weight | Fluid volume/24 hours |
|---|---|
| 1–10 kg | 100 ml/kg |
| 11–20 kg | 1000 ml + 50 ml/each kg over 10 kg |
| >20 kg | 1500 ml + 20 ml/each kg over 20 kg |

The greatest variations occur in the newborn period, particularly in LBW infants. In the neonate, basal requirements are more accurately calculated by estimating the renal water needs and insensible water loss of the individual infant. We found that the mean osmolar load in the postoperative neonate is approximately $16.5\pm6$ mOsm/kg per 24 hours, and the volume of water needed to excrete this is $63\pm28$ ml/kg per 24 hours.

TEWL is derived from a Table we have adapted from Hammarlund *et al.* (Table 3). Respiratory water loss is approximately 5 ml/kg per 24 hours, and is negligible when infants are intubated and on a ventilator. The basal requirement, therefore, for a 3-day-old, 31-week gestational age infant is 63 ml/kg per 24 hours renal water, plus 5 ml/kg per 24 hours respiratory water loss, plus 12 ml/kg per 24 hours TEWL, a total of 80 ml/kg per 24 hours. Adjustments are made according to the infant's special needs; for example, following major abdominal surgery, fluid and calorie requirements may be increased by 25–50 per cent. Further adjustments are made according to the patient's response to the fluid programme. Neonates weighing less than 1000 g may need 160 ml/kg per 24 hours, and those over 1000 g may require 110–130 ml/kg per 24 hours. With premature infants a fluid intake greater than 170 ml/kg per 24 hours is associated with an increased risk of congestive cardiac failure, patent ductus arteriosus and necrotizing enterocolitis.

Requirements during the first day of life are unique (a) because of the greatly expanded extracellular fluid volume in the newly born baby, which decreases after 24 hours, and (b) because newborn infants with intestinal obstruction are not hypovolaemic, as a result of intrauterine adjustments across the placenta. During the first 24 hours basic maintenance fluid should not exceed 90 ml/kg per 24 hours in preterm infants weighing less than 1000 g or less than 32 weeks gestational age, or 75 ml/kg per 24 hours in larger infants.

The basic electrolyte and energy requirements are provided by sodium chloride 34 mEq/l in 5 or 10 per cent dextrose, with the addition of potassium 20 or 30 mEq/l once urine production has been established.

## Calculation of additional losses

External losses from the intestinal tract (nasogastric drainage and fistulae) and drainage tubes are directly measured and replaced volume for volume with sodium chloride 77 mEq/l and potassium 2 DmEq/l. Protein-rich losses (e.g. from chest tubes) are replaced with albumin solution or fresh frozen plasma. When losses are large or prolonged or if renal function is compromised, the electrolyte content of these fluids should be analysed to allow precise replacement. Internal losses into body cavities or tissues (third-space losses) cannot be measured, and adequate replacement of these losses depends on careful monitoring of the patient's response.

## MONITORING THE FLUID AND ELECTROLYTE PROGRAMME

### Clinical features

Severe isotonic and hypovolaemic dehydration results in poor capillary filling and collapse of peripheral veins. The skin is cool and mottled, with reduced turgor; the mucous membranes are dry and the anterior fontanelle is sunken. These findings occur with 10 per cent body fluid losses in a child and 15 per cent in an infant. Hypertonic dehydration is more difficult to detect clinically since the decrease in circulating blood volume is considerably less than the total loss of body fluids. Signs of shock occur late and central nervous system signs, including lethargy, stupor and seizures, predominate.

**Table 3 Transepithelial water loss in newborns***

| Postnatal age (days) | Gestational age (and mean birth weight) | | | |
|---|---|---|---|---|
| | 25–27 weeks ($0.869 \pm 0.100\,kg$) | 28–30 weeks ($1.340 \pm 0.240\,kg$) | 31–36 weeks ($2.110 \pm 0.300\,kg$) | 37–41 weeks ($3.600 \pm 0.390\,kg$) |
| <1 | $129 \pm 39$ | $42 \pm 13$ | $12 \pm 5$ | $7 \pm 2$ |
| 1 | $110 \pm 27$ | $39 \pm 11$ | $11 \pm 5$ | $6 \pm 1$ |
| 3 | $71 \pm 9$ | $32 \pm 9$ | $12 \pm 4$ | $6 \pm 1$ |
| 5 | $51 \pm 7$ | $27 \pm 7$ | $12 \pm 4$ | $6 \pm 1$ |
| 7 | $43 \pm 9$ | $24 \pm 7$ | $12 \pm 4$ | $6 \pm 1$ |
| 14 | $32 \pm 10$ | $18 \pm 6$ | $9 \pm 3$ | $6 \pm 1$ |
| 21 | $28 \pm 10$ | $15 \pm 6$ | $8 \pm 2$ | $6 \pm 0$ |
| 28 | $24 \pm 11$ | $15 \pm 6$ | $7 \pm 1$ | $7 \pm 1$ |

* g/kg per 24 hours
Modified from Hammarlund *et al.*

## Body weight

Serial measurements of the body weight are a useful guide to total body water in the infant. Fluctuations over a 24-hour period are primarily related to loss or gain of fluid, 1 g body weight being approximately equal to 1 ml water. Errors will occur if changes in clothing, dressings and tubes are not accounted for and if scales are not regularly calibrated.

## Urine volume and composition

If the volume of fluid administered is inadequate, urine volume falls and concentration increases. With excess fluid administration the opposite occurs. We aim to achieve a urine output which will maintain a urine osmolality of 250–290 mOsm/kg (specific gravity: 1009–1012) in newborn infants, usually 2 ml/kg per hour. For older infants and children hydration is adequate if the urine output is 1–2 ml/kg per hour with an osmolality between 280 and 300 mOsm/kg.

When the osmolar load is large, for example with extensive tissue destruction or with infusion of high osmolar solutions, urine flow may have to be increased to provide adequate renal clearance. Accurate measurements of urine flow and concentration are fundamental to the management of critically ill infants and children, and in this situation we recommend insertion of a urethral catheter.

The urine specific gravity is a reliable indicator of hypertonicity (s.g.>1012) and hypotonicity (s.g.<1008) but is unreliable when urine is in the isotonic range (s.g. 1009–1001). When fluid monitoring is critical, as in the severely ill infant, urine osmolarity rather than specific gravity estimations provide more precise information.

A rising blood urea nitrogen level and falling urine output may be due to either acute renal failure or prerenal oliguria with azotaemia resulting from hypovolaemia. The distinction between these two states is important for appropriate treatment. Initially, the response to a fluid challenge of 20 ml/kg of 5 per cent dextrose and sodium chloride 34 mEq/l over 1 or 2 hours is monitored. If the urine output does not increase, mannitol 1 g/kg or frusemide 2–3 mg/kg is given intravenously. If oliguria persists, the sodium and creatinine levels in the blood and urine are estimated and the fractional sodium excretion calculated, using the formula:

$$Fe_{Na} = \frac{urine\ sodium/serum\ sodium}{urine\ creatinine/serum\ creatinine} \times 100$$

An $Fe_{Na}$ greater than 2.5–3 per cent suggests acute renal failure.

## Haematocrit and refractometer total protein

Serial haematocrit and refractometer total protein measurements are simple, rapid techniques for estimating plasma water changes with dehydration and rehydration. Serial changes in haematocrit over a 24-hour period in the absence of haemolysis or bleeding suggest a loss or gain of plasma water. Changes in the total protein, as measured by refractometer in the absence of massive protein loss, are usually directly related to changes in serum water and can confirm the changes of the haematocrit.

## Serum electrolytes, blood urea nitrogen and sugar, and serum osmolality

The haematocrit and refractometer measurements serve principally as a guide to the adequacy of the volume of fluid administered to the patient. Measurements of serum electrolytes, blood urea nitrogen, blood sugar, and serum osmolality are helpful in planning the programme that will replace ongoing losses and deficits of electrolytes. Once a tentative programme has been initiated and the fluid orders have been written, the responses of the patient can then be simply monitored by measuring serum osmolality.

An increase in osmolality suggests that too little water or too great a quantity of electrolytes, usually sodium, has been given. A fall in osmolality suggests that sodium replacement is inadequate or that too great a quantity of water is being administered. An unexpected change in osmolality, particularly an increase, requires immediate determination of serum electrolytes, blood urea nitrogen and sugar values and a calculation of the osmolality. Serum osmolality can be measured directly or calculated by the following formula:

$$Osmolality = serum\ sodium \times 1.86 + \frac{Blood\ urea\ nitrogen}{2.8} + \frac{glucose}{18} + 5$$

It is then possible to determine whether the rise in osmolality is due to an increase in serum sodium, the development of hyperglycaemia, or a high blood urea nitrogen. Occasionally the measured serum osmolality is higher than calculated osmolality. This suggests that the increase in serum osmolality is due to some unidentified osmolar active substance such as a metabolic by-product resulting from sepsis, shock or radio-opaque contrast material.

# Perioperative management

In the surgical patient, fluid, serum electrolyte and acid–base abnormalities are corrected before operation except in the case of immediate emergency surgery. Intraoperative fluid requirements consist of the estimated maintenance requirement, plus replacement of pre-existing deficits (if uncorrected), plus replacement of estimated intraoperative and electrolyte losses, including blood. The need for intraoperative blood transfusion is determined by the child's clinical condition (pulse, blood pressure, haematocrit, urine output) in relation to measured losses in sponges and suction bottles. A transfusion of 20 ml/kg whole blood or 10 ml/kg packed cells will be tolerated by infants with normal cardiovascular function.

# General considerations

## Gastrointestinal decompression

The importance of gastric decompression in the surgical newborn infant cannot be over-emphasized. The distended stomach carries the risk of aspiration and pneumonia, and may also impair diaphragmatic excursions, resulting in respiratory distress. With diaphragmatic hernia, ventilation is progressively impaired as the herniated intestine becomes distended with air and fluid. With gastroschisis, omphalocele, and diaphragmatic hernia the ability to reduce the prolapsed intestine into the abdominal cavity is impaired by intestinal distension.

All these situations can be alleviated by adequate orogastric or nasogastric tube decompression. If a single-lumen tube is used, intermittent aspiration by syringe or machine is required. With a double-lumen sump tube, such as the Replogle tube, continuous suction may be used with a negative pressure of 40–60 mmHg. The correct position of the tube in the stomach is confirmed by carefully measuring the tube prior to insertion, by noting the nature of the aspirate, and by radiographs. Careful and adequate taping of the tube is essential to avoid displacement. The use of gastrostomy tubes for postoperative gastric decompression is decreasing in popularity, but should be considered when prolonged postoperative gastric or intestinal stasis is anticipated.

## Antimicrobial therapy

Deficiencies in the immune system of the newborn infant render it vulnerable to major bacterial insults. Low levels of IgM reduce humoral resistance to Gram-negative organisms. Prophylactic antimicrobial therapy is advised for infants undergoing major surgery, particularly of the gastrointestinal tract or genitourinary system. Adequate cover is provided by combining a penicillin (e.g. ampicillin) or first-generation cephalosporin (e.g. cefazolin) with an aminoglycoside (usually gentamicin or tobramycin). Metronidazole or clindamicin is added when anaerobic infection is suspected. Alternatively, single-drug therapy using a broad-spectrum cephalosporin (e.g. cefotaxime) may be appropriate. Antibiotics are commenced prior to operation and may be discontinued after two or three days if there is no evidence of infection.

# Diagnostic studies

Most tests pose an additional burden to the already stressed infant, and diagnostic studies should be restricted to those essential for diagnosis and proper management. The volume of blood drawn for laboratory tests should be documented as these small volumes cumulatively represent significant blood loss in a small infant. All studies should be done with minimal disturbance of the infant, taking steps to prevent heat loss. When the infant is transferred to other departments for investigational procedures, monitoring and resuscitation equipment should be available with a surgeon in attendance. Prior to using hyperosmolar radio-opaque contrast materials, intravenous fluids must be administered and fluid deficits corrected. This applies whether the material is given by the intravascular or gastrointestinal route. To counteract the osmotic effect of the contrast medium, an intravenous infusion of sodium chloride 34 mEq/l at twice maintenance rate is maintained during the radiographic study and continued afterwards for 2–4 hours. During this period the infant is carefully monitored as described above.

# Transport

Whenever possible, a trained transport team, which includes a nurse and physician with the necessary expertise for intubation and respiratory support, should transport newborn infants. A portable incubator is used. Vital functions are monitored throughout. When intestinal obstruction is present, intravenous fluids and continuous gastric decompression must be provided. Unless fluid losses have been high, intravenous fluids may not be required for newborn infants during shorter journeys, but an intravenous infusion may be needed to provide glucose requirements.

## Further reading

Bell, E. F., Oh, W. (1979) Fluid and electrolyte balance in very low birth weight infants. Clinical Perinatology, 6, 139–150

Hammarlund, K., Sedin, G., Stromberg, B. (1983) Transepidermal water loss in newborn infants. Acta Paediatrica Scandinavica, 72, 721–728

Krummel, T. M., Lloyd, D. A., Rowe, M. I. (1985) The postoperative response of the term and preterm newborn infant to sodium administration. Journal of Pediatric Surgery, 20, 803–809

Oh, W. (1982) Symposium on the newborn. Pediatric Clinics of North America, 29, 1055–1298

Rowe, M. I. (1986) Fluid and electrolyte management. In Pediatric Surgery, Vol. 4, K. J. Welch, J. G. Randolph, M. M. Ravitch, J. A. O'Neill, M. I. Rowe (eds.). Chicago, Year Book Medical Publishers

Rowe, M. I., Pettit, B. J. (1986) Management of the critically ill patient. In Pediatric Surgery, Vol. 4, K. J. Welch, J. G. Randolph, M. M. Ravitch, J. A. O'Neill, M. I. Rowe (eds.). Chicago, Year Book Medical Publishers

Smith, C. A., Nelson, M. N. (1976) (eds.) The Physiology of newborn infants, 4th edn. Springfield, Charles C. Thomas

Illustrations by Kevin Marks

# Paediatric anaesthesia

**Edward Sumner**   MA, BM, BCh, FFARCS
Consultant Anaesthetist, The Hospital for Sick Children, London, UK

## Introduction

Paediatric anaesthesia is recognized as an independent specialized subject. It is generally accepted that the term applies to infants and children up to the age of 3 years[1].

The biochemical, physiological and psychological needs peculiar to young children are best met in a children's environment. The policy in the UK is to concentrate paediatric surgery and intensive care in children's departments and children's hospitals, so that each centre for neonatal surgery serves a population of about 2 million. This is now feasible because transport of sick babies, even over very large distances, by surface or air, is now completely routine and safe even for intubated and ventilated patients. At the Hospital for Sick Children, Great Ormond Street, London, we believe this to be the right approach so that inexperienced anaesthetists will not be faced with difficult paediatric emergencies such as intussusception or bronchoscopy for foreign body. We administer 450 neonatal anaesthetics per year for all types of surgery out of an annual total of 10 000, and about 700 patients per year undergo mechanical ventilation in our intensive care units. The demand for this type of treatment is increasing.

The differences between adult and paediatric anaesthesia are related to differences in anatomy and physiology – differences which are most marked in the very young. Nowadays babies with a gestational age as low as 26 weeks with weights of 600 g are surviving so that the implications of the traditional neonatal period of 28 days of life in terms of development have become meaningless. The weight of the baby and an assessment of function of its various bodily systems are more important guides than the age

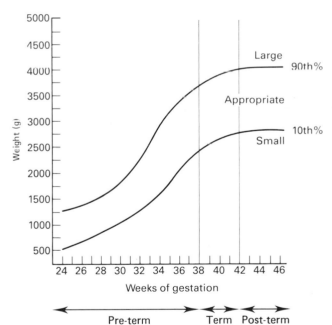

*Figure 1*   Percentile chart showing appropriate weight for gestational age

from birth. For a given gestational age the morbidity and mortality are greater the lower the birth weight (*Figure 1*)[2]. Thus all children should be accurately weighed on admission to hospital. Much surgery in children up to 3 years is done for congenital defects and it is as well to remember that such defects are often multiple. For example, a cleft palate or tracheo-oesophageal fistula is very often associated with a cardiac defect.

# Physiological differences between neonates and older children

Infants have poor respiratory reserve and respiratory failure is a common sequel to pathology in any system[3].

Total pulmonary resistance at 25 cm $H_2O \cdot l^{-1} \cdot s^{-1}$ is five times that of the adult.

Lung compliance is very low (6 ml/cmH$_2$O compared to 160 ml/cmH$_2$O in the adult) but the infant chest wall is an amazingly compliant structure so that small babies have great difficulty in maintaining a normal functional residual capacity (FRC) in states where pulmonary compliance is further reduced. The chest wall provides no counter-resistance to the collapsing forces of the lungs as it will do later in life. Hence the response to constant distending pressure in the form of positive end-expiratory pressure (PEEP) or continuous positive airway pressure (CPAP) is strikingly beneficial in this age group.

After birth an eight-fold increase in alveoli occurs and the adult number is reached by the age of 6 years. The airways resistance (and thus the work of breathing) remains high, until finally the airways begin to enlarge from about the same time as the full complement of alveoli are present.

Closing volume occurs within tidal breathing until 6 years of life so that there is an increase in physiological right-to-left (R – L) shunt during this period and an even greater effect on oxygenation should the FRC fall, as it does with pulmonary disease or during anaesthesia.

The resistance of the nasal passages in newborn babies is relatively great (45 per cent of the total). They are obligatory nose breathers, so respiratory obstruction may occur if the nares are blocked, e.g. by choanal atresia or by too large a nasogastric tube[4]. We use this facility of nose breathing with great effect to apply distending pressure in the form of CPAP using one nasal prong.

Alveolar ventilation and oxygen consumption per body weight are twice that of the adult, as manifest by the alarming rate at which cyanosis appears if ventilatory problems arise.

Respiration during the early months of life is purely diaphragmatic (the bucket-handle effect of ribs becomes operational towards the end of the first year of life) so that respiratory failure may ensue if the diaphragm is splinted, e.g. by abdominal distension or with phrenic palsy. Attempts to increase alveolar ventilation can be made only by increasing the respiratory rate, which explains why a rising respiratory rate is such a good sign of increased respiratory distress in infants. Phrenic palsy may occur as part of a birth injury, but is more commonly associated with damage to the phrenic nerve during thoracic or cardiac surgery.

# 1

The circulation of the neonate is labile and may revert to the fetal pattern with blood flowing from right to left through a patent ductus (DA) and/or through the foramen ovale (FO) if subject to conditions which promote pulmonary vasoconstriction – a state known as transitional circulation[5]. This state, previously known as persistent fetal circulation, is a transitional state between the fetal circulation including the placenta and that of the adult when the right and left sides are quite separate. The duct may reopen with exposure to hypoxia or fluid overload until it is firmly closed by fibrosis after 3–4 weeks. Attempts can be made to close the duct pharmacologically, using small doses of a prostaglandin synthetase inhibitor such as salicylate or, more commonly, indomethacin, with a fair chance of success. Conversely, prostaglandin $E_2$ may be infused to maintain ductal patency where this is essential, for example in severely cyanosed infants with pulmonary artery atresia, until a systemic-pulmonary shunt of the Blalock type may be created surgically[6].

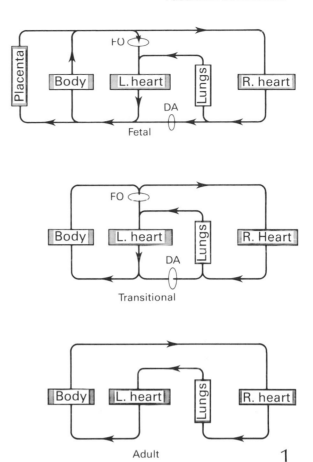

The lability of the pulmonary vasculature is caused by abundant arteriolar smooth muscle, extending more peripherally than in later life (due to a failure of normal regression of the muscle in the first few hours of life). These arterioles constrict in response to hypoxia, hypercapnia or acidosis via an adrenergic mechanism (this response is abolished after sympathectomy[7]). Some infants develop this state of transitional circulation following a rise in pulmonary vascular resistance (PVR) and a R–L shunt through the ductus or patent foramen ovale. Such critical hypoxaemia with a shunt of 80 per cent occurs commonly in hyaline membrane disease, congenital diaphragmatic hernia and meconium aspiration, but often there is no recognizable cause. If left untreated these babies will die in a vicious cycle of cyanosis, acidosis and falling cardiac output. Steps must be taken to reverse the high PVR. A high inspiratory oxygen concentration ($FiO_2$), hyperventilation if possible, a pH greater than 7.4 and the pulmonary vasodilating drug tolazoline may all be necessary to achieve this reduction[8].

Neonates do attempt to maintain core temperature at 37°C but may not succeed because of an initial low basic metabolic rate, a large surface-to-weight ratio, immature sweat function and also the inability to move from adverse conditions[9]. Superficial thermoreceptors exist in the trigeminal area of the face; hence a cold stimulus causes an increase in metabolic heat production from hydrolysis of triglycerides in brown fat, causing a great increase in oxygen consumption which may make existing hypoxia worse. Brown fat is distributed over the back and provides thermal lagging for the major intrathoracic vessels. The metabolic response to cold is inhibited by general anaesthesia, hypoxia, hypoglycaemia and prematurity. Babies are nursed in the neutral thermal environment at which their oxygen demands are minimal – as low as 31°C for a 3 kg term baby and up to 36°C for those with low birth weight (Figure 2). If preterm babies are allowed to cool there is increased mortality and morbidity. They are more likely to develop hyaline membrane disease, acidosis, hypoxia, coagulopathy, intraventricular haemorrhage and a subsequent slower rate of brain growth.

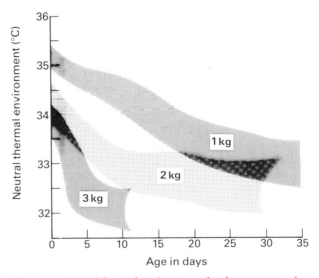

*Figure 2*   Neutral thermal environment for three groups of infants of differing birth weights

2

Some heat loss is inevitable in the operating theatre, but this can be minimized by using warm wrappings, aluminium swaddlers, aluminium foil to the head and limbs to reflect radiant heat, a heated mattress, an overhead heater during induction of anaesthesia, and by maintaining an ambient temperature of 24°C without draughts and using heated, humidified anaesthetic gases[10,11]. A thermostatically controlled hot-air mattress (Howarth Air Engineering Ltd.) is particularly effective in maintaining the temperature of small patients and is routinely used for patients under 1 year of age.

The mean cord haemoglobin concentration is approximately 18 g/dl at birth and rises by 1–2 g/dl in the first days of life because of low fluid intake and a decrease in extracellular fluid volume. After that, the level declines (*Figure 3*) and causes the physiological anaemia of infancy. Premature babies have a greater fall because of lower red cell production and survival[12]. At birth 70 per cent of the haemoglobin is HbF, which has a greater affinity for oxygen, possibly because of a relative insensitivity to 2–3 diphosphoglycerate which itself lowers the oxygen affinity of the haemoglobin molecule. HbF is replaced by HbA by 3 months of age, at which time sickle tests are needed in susceptible children. A haemoglobin concentration below 10 g/dl is always abnormal and should be investigated. Non-emergency surgery should be delayed pending investigation of severe anaemias.

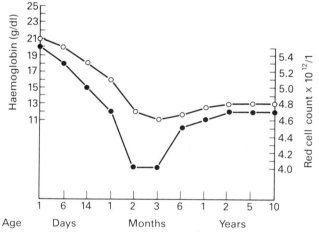

*Figure 3* Changes in haemoglobin concentration and red cell count in the first 10 years of life. ○—○ Haemoglobin; ●—● red cell count

The blood volume of an infant with a normal Hb is estimated to be 80–85 ml/kg. In premature babies it is greater, perhaps as much as 100 ml/kg. The blood volume of the newborn baby is more variable than that of the older infant and depends on the magnitude of the placental transfusion. Difficulties may arise if blood replacement is based on a percentage of the estimated blood volume.

Carbohydrate reserves of the normal newborn are relatively low and, as most glycogen is synthesized after 36 weeks' gestation, those of the preterm baby may be very low. Blood sugar levels should average 2.7–3.3 mmol/l (50–60 mg/dl) and hypoglycaemia of less than 1.6 mmol/l (30 mg/dl) is treated by infusion of 10 per cent dextrose, or a bolus of 1 ml/kg 25 per cent dextrose if urgent correction

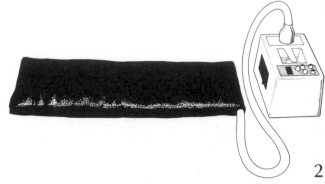

2

of hypoglycaemia is indicated. Four-hourly testing with Dextrostix is mandatory, as only very severe hypoglycaemia is symptomatic. There is no agreement as to the hypoglycaemic effect of preoperative starvation, but *4 hours* between induction of anaesthesia and the last feed is the maximum desirable, and small children should be woken for a drink of 5 per cent dextrose solution if they are first on a morning list. Children below 15 kg weight are at the greatest risk from hypoglycaemia.

Maturity of liver enzyme systems is complete by 2 months of age. Synthesis of the vitamin K dependent clotting factors II, VII, IX and X is suboptimal until then. Minimal levels of clotting factors occur on the second or third day of life and this is partially prevented by routine intramuscular administration of vitamin $K_1$ to all newborn babies.

Hepatic immaturity also means that drugs detoxicated in the liver, e.g. barbiturates and opiates, should be used with extreme caution. The conjugation of bilirubin is very inefficient and uncoupling of at least one of the two molecules occurs at times of stress such as hypoxia or acidosis. After liver maturity is reached most drugs are well tolerated because of the high metabolic rate of the young child – this may mean that techniques of intravenous anaesthesia become unstable and difficult to manage with altered pharmacokinetics.

The newborn baby has no diuretic response to a water load for the first 48 hours of life. By the end of the first week dilute urine can be produced, but the output falls before the full load has been excreted.

**Table 1 Basic fluid requirements of neonates 7 days after birth**

| Birthweight | Volume/24 hours |
| --- | --- |
| <1000 g | 180 ml/kg |
| 1000–2500 g | 150 ml/kg |
| >2500 g | 120 ml/kg |

Fluid maintenance requirements for full-term newborn babies start at 20–40 ml/kg per 24 hours on day one, increasing by 20 ml/kg each day until the levels shown in the table are reached by the end of the first week of life[13]. Fluid retention associated with surgery is usually severe and restriction to the requirements suggested for the neonatal period is necessary during and after operation. All intravenous fluids for maintenance in infancy should contain dextrose 4 per cent or 10 per cent depending on blood sugar, usually in combination with one-fifth normal (0.18 per cent) saline solution.

# Preoperative

## Assessment of patient

Fitness for general anaesthesia and surgery must be assessed in the light of the urgency of surgery. It frequently involves weighing up the risks related to an associated medical problem against the benefits of surgery. This requires cooperation between the anaesthetist and the surgeon. Many centres run preoperative clinics in which medical problems can be identified and appropriate investigations (X-rays, etc.) performed and treatment instituted. The parents and patients can be given the necessary instructions for admission to hospital, which is especially important for day-stay patients.

No cold surgery should be undertaken on any patient with an acute intercurrent illness[14]. Operation should be deferred until one month after the last symptoms of respiratory tract infection, croup or the acute exanthems have subsided. After bronchiolitis, pulmonary abnormalities of increased resistance and reduced compliance may persist for as long as one year. In patients with chronic respiratory disease lung function is assessed by measuring airway resistance, compliance and lung volumes, and by ventilation:perfusion scans. Baseline blood gas estimations may show a metabolic alkalosis compensating for respiratory acidosis, or a raised $Paco_2$ if there is incipient respiratory failure.

Patients with values 50 per cent of the predicted normal may be expected to develop respiratory problems postoperatively and those with only 30 per cent of predicted values with a resting $Paco_2$ above 40 mmHg (5.2 kPa) will undoubtedly need postoperative respiratory support.

Preoperative antibiotic prophylaxis against subacute bacterial endocarditis is usually necessary in patients with corrected or uncorrected congenital heart disease, particularly if they are to be intubated[15]. Benzylpenicillin 1 mega unit intravenously with induction of anaesthesia, or amoxicillin 1–3 g orally one hour before operation may be given. For Gram-negative organisms associated with intestinal and genitourinary surgery, gentamicin 2 mg/kg combined with metronidazole 7.5 mg/kg intravenously is more appropriate.

The history, including exercise tolerance, and physical examination should reveal any problems such as respiratory obstruction or failure, and alert the anaesthetist to the possibility of technical problems such as difficult intubation, for example in patients with Pierre-Robin syndrome or Still's disease.

Many paediatric centres perform minor surgery of all specialities (up to 15 per cent of cases) on a day-stay basis. This arrangement is more cost-effective, more convenient for the parents and has obvious psychological advantages for the child[16]. Anaesthetic techniques of premedication, intubation, inhalational or intravenous anaesthesia, local blocks and postoperative analgesia are the same as for hospitalized patients. However, facilities must be available to admit the child overnight if the anaesthesia or surgery has not been straightforward or if the parents feel they cannot manage the child at home.

Infants and small children are vulnerable to the psychological stress of being in hospital and undergoing surgery. They are totally dependent on their parents, and prolonged separation in the early months of life may cause problems with maternal bonding. Children between 2 and 4 years of age are especially vulnerable as they may have unreasonable fears about hospitals and surgery but may not yet have developed the intellectual mechanisms to deal with these fears[17]. Full preparation with a kindly and sympathetic approach is therefore required. In most children over 6 kg in weight this should be supplemented by preoperative sedation.

## Premedication

There is no ideal agent for premedication. The aim is to achieve only *mild* sedation since the doses required to produce sleep in most will cause oversedation in a few.

The following basic regimens are used for premedications at the Hospital for Sick Children in London:

*Children weighing less than 6 kg:* atropine only.
*Children weighing less than 15 kg:* trimeprazine 3–4 mg/ kg by mouth 2 hours before operation, or pethidine compound 0.075 ml/kg intramuscularly 1 hour before operation.
*Children weighing more than 15 kg:* papaveretum 0.4 mg/kg plus hyoscine 0.08 mg/kg intramuscularly 1 hour before operation.

## Special equipment

Specialized apparatus with *low resistance to breathing* (less than $30\,cmH_2O\cdot l^{-1}\cdot s^{-1}$ during quiet breathing) and *minimal dead space* is necessary as babies already have a high airway resistance and a rather higher ratio of dead space to tidal volume than adults[18].

# 3

Ayres T-piece with Jackson Rees' modification has almost universal approval for small baby anaesthesia. The T-piece has been extensively studied and no rebreathing with spontaneous or controlled ventilation occurs unless the fresh gas flow (FGF) is reduced below 220 ml/kg per minute[19]. No circuit should be used at the limit of its function, so in practice at least 4 litres FGF are used.

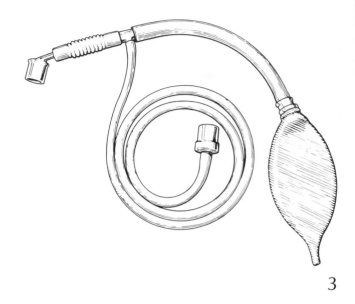

3

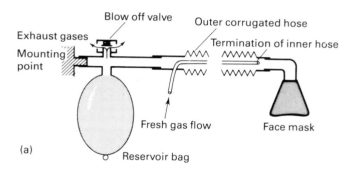

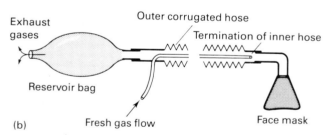

(a) The Bain circuit. (b) Paediatric modification of the Bain circuit

4

# 4

Scavenging of polluting expired gases is most safely achieved by an indirect, active system, with nothing directly connected to the expiratory limb of the T-piece. The Bain coaxial circuit is also very useful for many paediatric procedures, particularly those involving the head and neck. Both the Bain circuit (a) and its paediatric modification (b) are shown.

We prefer the higher dead space face masks to the Rendell-Baker type because of a better fit to the face, and in practice the dead space is less because of streaming of the fresh gas flow within the mask. A firm fit also enables distending pressure to be applied to spontaneously breathing patients, which prevents stridor, promotes gas exchange and prevents reduction in functional residual capacity.

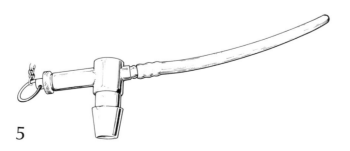

5

# 5

Plain Magill tubes with Cardiff connectors are used down to 2.5 mm inside diameter. The slightly greater wall thickness of the rubber tube makes it stiffer and thus easier to pass and less likely to kink in the oropharynx, and the Cardiff connector imparts a perfect curve for the tube in the mouth and pharynx.

# 6

The infant larynx lies higher in the neck (opposite the 4th cervical vertebra) and more anterior than in the adult and, as the epiglottis is relatively large, laryngoscopy is best performed with a small *straight-bladed* laryngoscope, the tip of which picks up the epiglottis.

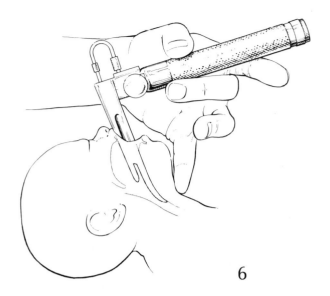

6

7

# 7

A small airway is put in the mouth alongside the tube to splint it and to prevent lateral movement. Perfect sizing, positioning and fixation of the endotracheal tube is central to paediatric anaesthesia and intensive care.

The oral tube is fixed to the face by two pieces of strapping, with secondary fixation to the forehead. The nasal fixation is similar, using a Tunstall connector, with primary strapping to the face and secondary fixation to the forehead, thus preventing accidental dislodgement of the tubes by pulling or twisting.

The correct size of tube is that which allows a small air leak between it and the mucosa of the cricoid at a peak inspiratory pressure of 25 cmH$_2$O. The cricoid ring is, of course, the narrowest part of the upper airway in a child and is easily damaged by too large an endotracheal tube, resulting in postoperative stridor or even subglottic stenosis (1 mm of mucosal oedema in the infant cricoid will reduce the airway by 60 per cent).

# General principles

The general principles of paediatric anaesthesia have not greatly changed recently. It is still taught that most neonates are better intubated awake (especially by anaesthetists in training) and that all babies weighing less than 5 kg should be intubated for anaesthesia, however minor the surgery.

Awake intubation is easily performed if the baby is held correctly (its shoulders should not be allowed to rise) and a straight-bladed laryngoscope is used (see *Illustration 6*). However, a pressure transducer placed over the anterior fontanelle during awake intubation shows a rise in intracranial pressure (ICP) which may be a problem if the patient is at risk from intraventricular haemorrhage or already has raised ICP.

## Inducing agents

Cyclopropane is still the finest agent for inhalational induction in paediatric anaesthesia, especially for the very sick small baby, but it requires that a premedication containing atropine is used. Because of its explosive properties this agent has unfortunately been removed from very many centres. In spite of the newer agents ketamine, methohexitone and etomidate, thiopentone in doses of 4–5 mg/kg is the preferred agent for intravenous induction and has become the standard by which all others are judged. Propofol (Diprivan) is a new non-barbiturate induction agent also suitable for children.

## Muscle relaxants

Sensitivity of the neuromuscular junction to non-depolarizing muscle relaxants exists during the first 2–3 weeks of life. This, together with individual variation, makes careful titration of dose with effect mandatory. D-tubocurarine (Jexin/Tubarine), for example, is diluted to 0.25, 0.5 or 1 mg/ml depending on the size of the child, and doses of 0.2 mg/kg are used for newborn babies, and 0.4 mg/kg for older children. The reported resistance to suxamethonium in this age group is caused by the dilution of a given dose in the larger extracellular fluid volume of the newborn. The independence of atracurium from hepatic and renal function possibly makes it the relaxant of choice for newborn babies, and it is frequently given by continuous infusion.

## Prevention of aspiration

Cricoid pressure to prevent aspiration of regurgitated gastric contents is as effective in babies as it is in adults if correctly applied and is used when indicated, for example in patients with pyloric stenosis or bowel obstruction.

## Ventilation

Intraoperative mechanical ventilation with T-piece occluding machines such as the Sheffield or Penlon 200 series with the Newton valve is very satisfactory for many cases. All mechanical ventilators must have a reliable alarm system. However, hand ventilation is essential during thoracic surgery in infants or in other situations of changing pulmonary compliance, or if there is tracheal compression. Controlled ventilation should be used for all newborn babies because the respiratory depressant effect of inhalational anaesthesia is so great at this stage, but older infants may be allowed to breathe spontaneously via a tube or a mask for periods up to one hour. Halothane or isoflurane is used. The reductive metabolism of halothane which may cause sensitization in postpubertal patients seems to occur very rarely in children[20]. Halothane may preserve blood flow to the liver better than other agents and is thus not contraindicated in patients with liver disease.

## Analgesic supplements

Analgesic supplements should never be given to newborn babies unless postoperative mechanical ventilation is planned, but older infants and children easily tolerate up to 10 µg/kg fentanyl and indeed this is an excellent anaesthetic. Narcotic supplements or local blocks are essential if the premedication has not included an analgesic.

## Fluid maintenance

Newborn babies do not need and should not be given clear fluids as maintenance during operation – the fluid given with drugs is adequate. Otherwise, inappropriate ADH secretion, shifts from the circulating blood volume to the third space and poor renal function will result in severe fluid overload. Blood losses approaching 10 per cent of the estimated blood volume are replaced by colloid in the form of plasma if the haemoglobin is above 15 g/dl, otherwise by whole blood. Older patients may be given intraoperative fluids at 6 ml/kg per hour as 4 per cent dextrose and 0.18 per cent saline.

## Caudal block

Sacral, lumbar and thoracic roots up to T10 may be blocked by caudal analgesia using 0.25 per cent plain bupivacaine. A dose of 0.5 ml/kg is sufficient to block sacral roots, but 1.25 ml/kg will be needed to block up to T10. This technique is widely used in paediatric anaesthesia, even in neonates. It is usually supplemented by light general anaesthesia, except in newborn babies, where the sedative effect of the absorbed bupivacaine is enough.

## Monitoring

All techniques of monitoring adult anaesthesia are entirely appropriate even for the neonate, but the precordial or oesophageal stethoscope is unsurpassed as a means of drawing the anaesthetist closer to his patient and of providing valuable respiratory and cardiovascular information[21]. A monaural earpiece also enables the anaesthetist to keep in touch with the conversation going on around him. This, together with electrocardiographic and automatic blood pressure monitoring (using the Dinamap for example) is recommended for most patients. Direct measurements of arterial and central venous pressures may be required for major cases.

Care must be taken with flushing devices and those of the Intraflo type are unsuitable for use in small babies, in whom a syringe pump at 0.5–1 ml/hour should be used. Temperature is measured by a nasopharyngeal probe. The normal difference between core and peripheral temperature is 2°C and peripheral cooling is a very sensitive guide in babies to cardiac output and the adequacy of cardiac filling. Transcutaneous $Po_2$ and $Pco_2$ electrodes are not frequently used in the operating theatre because at least 20 minutes are necessary before stability occurs and they may be affected in a non-linear way by anaesthetic gases. They may, however, give useful information about otherwise undetected swings in $Pao_2$, which can be significant, especially in premature babies at risk from retrolental fibroplasia before the retina is fully vascularized. Modern pulse oximetry has revolutionized the monitoring of oxygenation by non-invasive means and is now used routinely for all patients. Capnographs of the Hewlett Packard type which do not sample are very useful monitors as a continuous guide to the adequacy of ventilation, and in neurosurgery, as an early warning of air embolism. The paediatric cuvette can be further modified so that the increase in dead space is kept to an absolute minimum.

# Postoperative care

## Pain relief

Newborn babies may not need opiate analgesics unless they are having mechanical ventilation. Though they do feel pain, it is poorly localized and they settle if they are kept otherwise comfortable (e.g. by simple manoeuvres such as swaddling). Older babies weighing less than 6 kg may if necessary safely be given codeine phosphate 1 mg/kg intramuscularly. This is surprisingly effective in small children. However, only one dose should be given, as analgesics are poorly tolerated by newborn babies. They have poor liver function and an immature central nervous system so that the effects of even a single dose are profound and prolonged. For those over 8 kg, papaveretum 0.25 mg/kg intramuscularly is a suitable postoperative analgesic, to be administered 4-hourly as necessary. Babies being *fully* ventilated may be given morphine 0.2 mg/kg intramuscularly or intravenously at 4-hourly intervals. However, continuous infusion may be a safer and more effective way of administering opiates postoperatively, as it avoids the reduction in cardiac output occasionally seen with intramuscular and intravenous bolus injections of morphine or papaveretum. Morphine 0.5 mg/kg diluted in 50 ml of 5 per cent dextrose may be infused at a rate of 2 ml/hour. Such an infusion is unsuitable for non-ventilated patients below 6 kg body weight.

If the patient is having pancuronium it is important also to give a sedative (e.g. diazepam 0.2 mg/kg intramuscularly or intravenously) at regular intervals.

Analgesics and muscle relaxants should be withdrawn as soon as weaning from mechanical ventilation commences.

## Respiratory support

Postoperatively infants are extubated fully awake once spontaneous respiration is judged to be adequate. However, because of the low respiratory reserve at this age, respiratory failure may ensue. Acute respiratory failure is a clinical diagnosis based on a rising respiratory rate (above 60/min), pulse rate, cardiac output and oxygen dependency, and on an assessment of the work of breathing as shown by intercostal recession, tracheal tug, nasal flaring, restlessness and grunting. The inability to clear secretions or apnoeic attacks are further pointers. Blood gas levels may confirm the clinical impression and are measured to determine baseline values.

Distending pressure in the form of continuous positive airway pressure is indicated when an infant cannot maintain a $Pao_2$ of 50 mmHg (6·7 kPa) in 60 per cent oxygen. Mechanical ventilation is necessary if after an adequate trial of CPAP the $Pao_2$ remains above 60 mmHg (7·8 kPa) but the pH is less than 7.25 or if the $Pao_2$ is less than 50 mmHg (6·7 kPa) on 100 per cent oxygen.

Until recently intermittent positive pressure ventilation (IPPV) of infants, especially those with hyaline membrane disease, was accompanied by a very high morbidity and mortality. Gregory's discovery in 1971 of the advantages of CPAP was a milestone and, together with Reynolds' work on ventilator settings (especially with reference to the inspiratory:expiratory time ratio)[22], was the start of modern paediatric respiratory support.

Prolonged intubation requires nasal plain PVC tubes of the Portex type. All the complications of blockage, dislodgement and subglottic stenosis can be avoided by meticulous care. The tube must be of a size to allow ventilation, but also some airleak around it, or damage to the mucosa of the cricoid will result. Intubation may be continued if necessary for many weeks without resort to tracheostomy.

The art of ventilating small babies with modern infant ventilators such as the Bourn BP 200 consists of using the facilities of the machine to minimize the factors known to be associated with bronchopulmonary dysplasia (BPD). Infant lungs are particularly liable to be damaged by intubation and mechanical ventilation, with factors such as high inspired oxygen concentrations and high peak airway pressures being incriminated in the production of BPD. The lung architecture is progressively deranged with fibrosis and formation of cysts, which in turn demands higher oxygen and ventilator pressures to maintain adequate gas exchange. Unless the factors known to produce bronchopulmonary dysplasia are minimized, the condition will progress until ventilation becomes impossible. Machines must have the facility to allow high respiratory rates, square wave formation, variable I:E ratio, control of peak pressures and full humidification. They should also have an alarm system for disconnection and power failure, a facility for constant distending pressure and the ability to wean the patient from the ventilator by using intermittent mandatory ventilation

(IMV). This is a technique whereby the number of breaths from the ventilator is reduced gradually over a period of time, with the infant taking spontaneous breaths in between[23].

Constant distending pressure, whether used with IPPV (PEEP) or spontaneous breathing (CPAP), will improve the relation between functional residual capacity and closing volume in the lungs, and reduce R–L intrapulmonary shunting. By keeping the small airways distended it will also cause a fall in pulmonary resistance and in the work of breathing.

PEEP of up to 10 cmH$_2$O is used routinely after cardiopulmonary bypass and in other patients with increased pulmonary water. The distending pressure may save surfactant but, as PEEP is increased, pulmonary vascular resistance rises and there is an increased incidence of pneumothorax.

Formulae are of little help in setting up patients on ventilation because of the internal compliance of the machine and its tubing. However, 10 ml/kg tidal volume or 20–25 cmH$_2$O pressure are reasonable initial settings. Inspired oxygen concentration should be set at the level the child needed before mechanical ventilation was instituted.

Babies and children may be ventilated with simple sedation such as diazepam 0.2 mg/kg intravenously, morphine 0.2 mg/kg intravenously or chloral hydrate 30 mg/kg by nasogastric tube. However, it is increasingly necessary to use pancuronium to paralyse patients with severe pulmonary disease who need limitations of peak airway pressure and changes in the I:E ratio. There is

evidence that gas exchange may be improved in such paralysed patients so that they may need mechanical ventilation for a shorter period than those not paralysed.

Weaning takes place when cardiovascular stability has been achieved with a peak pressure of less than 30 cmH$_2$O, giving a Pa$CO_2$ of less than 45 mmHg (5·8 kPa) and a Pa$O_2$ over 100 mmHg (13 kPa) with an Fi$O_2$ less than 0.6. Distending pressure is used with IMV, which is the most convenient way of weaning from full ventilator support. IMV with the Bourn BP 200 ventilator is ideal, with continuous fresh gas flow and favourable I:E ratios during the reduction in mandatory breaths. The patient must be able to manage on 15–20 mandatory breaths before being ready to be weaned. The number of mandatory breaths is gradually reduced (the rate depending on the clinical progress of the infant) until the ventilator is delivering no breaths and the patient is on CPAP.

Patients are extubated when coping on 3 cmH$_2$O CPAP. Those with stiff lungs who are CPAP-dependent may continue on CPAP after extubation, using a nasal prong[24]. No patient is left to breathe through an endotracheal tube without distending pressure since without the physiological levels of CPAP the FRC will fall with increased resistance to gas flow, increased work of breathing and increased R–L intrapulmonary shunting.

Invasive and non-invasive blood gas analysis is essential for setting up and maintaining patients on mechanical ventilation, but plays very little part in monitoring them during the weaning process, when clinical observation of respiratory rate and effort is more important.

## References

1. Anonymous (1978) Paediatric anaesthesia. British Medical Journal, 2, 717

2. Smith, P. C., Smith, N. T. (1982) The special considerations of the premature infant. In: Some Aspects of Paediatric Anaesthesia, D. J. Steward (ed.), Monographs in Anesthesiology, 10, 273–329. London and Amsterdam: Excerpta Medica

3. Hislop, A., Reid, L. (1981) Growth and development of the respiratory system: anatomical development. In: Scientific Foundations of Paediatrics, J. A. Davis, J. Dobbing (eds.), 2nd edn., pp. 390–432. Baltimore: University Park Press

4. Haworth, S. G., Sumner, E. (1987) The respiratory system. In: Clinical Paediatric Anatomy, J. A. S. Dickson (ed.). Oxford: Blackwell (in press)

5. Dawes, G. S. (1968) Foetal and Neonatal Physiology: a comparative study of the dangers at birth. Chicago: Year Book Medical Publishers

6. Mott, J. C. (1980) Patent ductus arteriosus: experimental aspects. Archives of Disease in Childhood, 55, 99–105

7. Haworth, S. G., Hislop, A. A. (1981) Normal structural and functional adaptation to extrauterine life. Journal of Pediatrics, 98, 915–918

8. Sumner, E., Frank, J. D. (1981) Tolazoline in the treatment of congenital diaphragmatic hernias. Archives of Disease in Childhood, 56, 350–353

9. Hey, E. N. (1972) Thermal regulation in the newborn. British Journal of Hospital Medicine, 8, 51–64

10. Neuman, G. G., Hansen, D. D. (1980) The anaesthetic management of preterm infants undergoing ligation of patent ductus arteriosus. Canadian Anaesthetists Society Journal, 27, 248–253

11. Brown, T. C. K., Fisk, G. C. (1979) Anaesthesia for children: including aspects of intensive care. London and Oxford: Blackwell Scientific Publications

12. Chessells, J. M. (1979) Blood formation in infancy. Archives of Disease in Childhood, 54, 831–834

13. Kay, B. (1981) Intravenous fluid therapy. In: Paediatric Anaesthesia: Trends in Current Practice, G. J. Rees, T. C. Gray (eds.), pp. 169–188. London: Butterworths

14. Sumner, E., Facer, E. K. (1986) The paediatric patient. In: Preparation for Anaesthesia, A. J. Stevens (ed.), pp. 343–374. Tunbridge Wells: Pitman Medical

15. Leader (1979) Preventing endocarditis. British Medical Journal, 1, 290–291

16. Cohen, D., Keneally, J., Black, A., Gaffney, S., Johnson, A. (1980) Experience with day stay surgery. Journal of Pediatric Surgery, 15, 21–25

17. Pinkerton, P. (1981) Preventing psychotrauma in childhood anaesthesia. In: Paediatric Anaesthesia: Trends in Current Practice, G. J. Rees, T. C. Gray (eds.), pp. 1–18. London: Butterworths

18. Hatch, D. J., Sumner, E. (1981) Neonatal Anaesthesia. London: Arnold

19. Froese, A. B., Rose, D. K. (1982) A detailed analysis of T-piece systems. In: Some Aspects of Paediatric Anaesthesia, D. J. Steward (ed.), Monographs in anesthesiology, 10, 101–136. London and Amsterdam: Excerpta Medica

20. Steward, D. J. Matthews, U. F. (eds.) (1979) Manual of Pediatric Anaesthesia. London: Churchill Livingstone

21. Battersby, E. F. (1981) Monitoring during anesthesia for pediatric surgery. In: Monitoring During Anesthesia, G. R. Gerson (ed.), International Anesthesiology Clinics, 19, 95–122. Boston: Little Brown and Co.

22. Reynolds, E. O. (1974) Pressure waveform and ventilator settings for mechanical ventilation in severe hyaline membrane disease. In: Neonatal and Paediatric Ventilation, D. H. G. Kenskamp (ed.). International Anesthesiology Clinics, 12, 259–280. Boston: Little Brown and Co.

23. Goldsmith, J. P., Karotkin, E. H. (eds) (1981) Assisted ventilation of the neonate. Philadelphia: W. B. Saunders

24. Sumner, E. (1987) Artificial ventilation of children. In: Diagnosis and Management of Paediatric Respiratory Disease, R. Dinwiddie (ed.). London: Churchill Livingstone (in press)

Illustrations by Philip Wilson

# Choanal atresia

**John N. G. Evans**   MB, BS, DLO, FRCS
Consultant Ear, Nose and Throat Surgeon, The Hospital for Sick Children, Great Ormond Street and St. Thomas's Hospital, London, UK

## Preoperative

Choanal atresia occurs as a result of failure of canalization of the bucconasal membrane. Bilateral atresia causes total nasal obstruction and unless immediate treatment is initiated asphyxia will occur because the newborn will not breathe through the mouth. The diagnosis is confirmed when a catheter fails to pass from the nose into the nasopharynx.

### Investigation

## 1

After aspirating mucus from the nasal cavity, Gastrografin is instilled and a lateral supine radiograph will demonstrate the thickness of the atretic septum.

In 60 per cent of cases with a bilateral atresia another major congenital abnormality is present.

Unilateral atresia may also cause respiratory difficulty in the neonatal period, in which case immediate operation is advised. If nasal obstruction is not gross, surgical correction can be delayed until the age of 4–5 years.

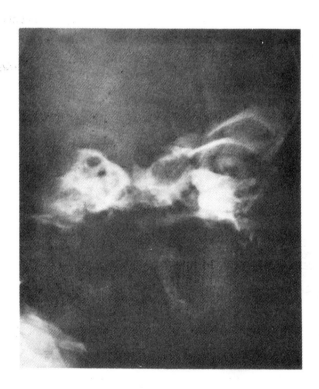

1

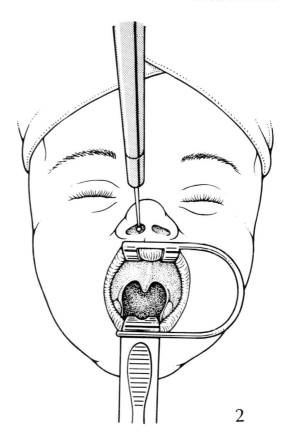

2

## Emergency treatment

An oral airway must be established and this is achieved by inserting a size 00 Guedel airway in the mouth and taping it to the mandibular region with adhesive strapping. Hydration is maintained by orogastric tube feeds. Blood is crossmatched for the procedure but is seldom necessary.

## Position of patient

## 2

A sandbag is placed behind the shoulders and a Boyle-Davis gag inserted. A 2.5 inch slotted tongue plate is used. The operator sits at the head of the patient. A headlight is used.

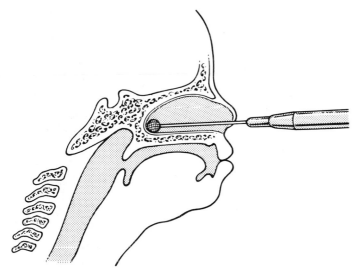

3

## The operation

## 3

The choanal septum is then perforated using a straight hand piece and electric drill. A 2 mm cutting burr effects the initial penetration of the septum. Great care must be taken to ensure that the drill is directed parallel with the floor of the nose. If this precaution is not observed the drill may penetrate the basi-sphenoid. The operator's forefinger is placed in the nasopharynx and as the burr penetrates the dorsal septum the burr may be felt with the pulp of the finger.

## 4

In order to avoid damage to the nostril margin the shaft of the burr is covered with 12 Fr Portex tubing. After the initial penetration of the choanal septum the hole is enlarged using a 5 mm diamond burr.

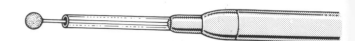

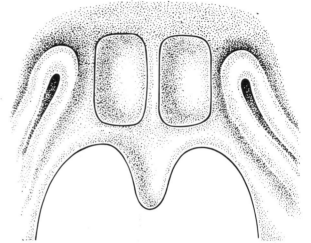

4

## 5–7

Illustration 5 shows a view of the choanal septa from behind. The choanal septum is drilled away superiorly, laterally and inferiorly. In addition at least 7 mm of the posterior edge of the nasal septum is removed.

5

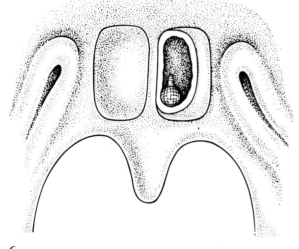

6

7

# 8

Having removed the choanal partition it is necessary to insert nasal tubes through the choanae to prevent subsequent stenosis. They are made from 12 Fr Portex tubing (nasogastric), a bridge of tubing being cut as shown. This holds the tubes apart and prevents damage to the columella.

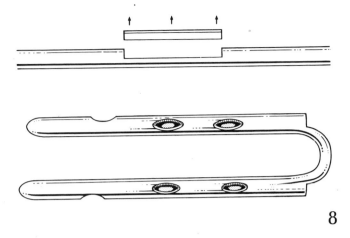

8

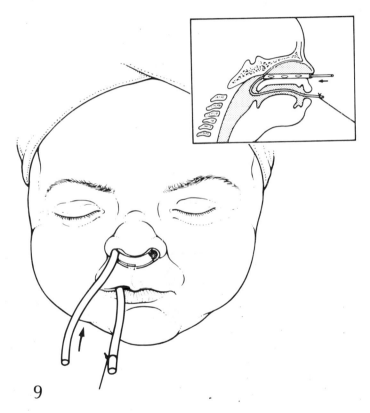

# 9

In order to prevent displacement of the nasal tubes a continuous nylon thread must be passed through the tubes and tied anteriorly.

9

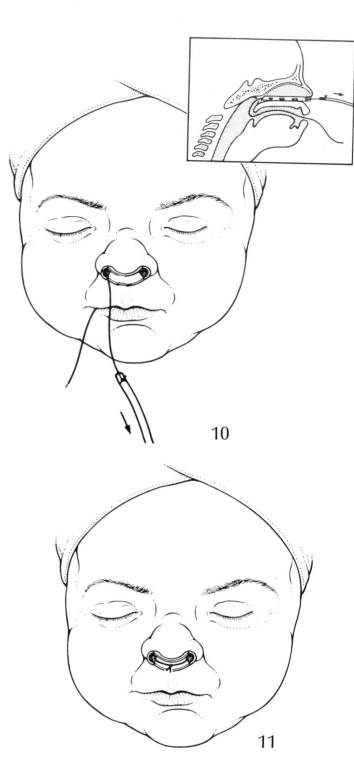

# 10 & 11

This is achieved by passing two fine catheters through the nasal tubes; the distal ends are delivered through the mouth and the nylon thread attached. The catheters are then withdrawn and the nylon thread tied in front.

Blockage of the tubes is prevented by the instillation of 0.5 ml of normal saline into each tube, followed by suction by means of a fine catheter long enough to pass through the tubes into the nasopharynx. The tubes are retained for 6 weeks.

10

11

# Harelip and cleft palate

**Ambrose Jolleys**  MD, FRCS
Paediatric Surgeon, Royal Manchester Children's Hospital and St Mary's Hospital, Manchester, UK

## Introduction

Cleft lip and palate is one of the more disabling congenital malformations. The degree of deformation varies considerably in different patients, but many have permanent physical stigmata, some have defective speech and impaired hearing. To obtain the best results a thorough knowledge of the normal and abnormal anatomies is needed.

The defects range from the most minor (notching in the lip, muscular defects in the lip or palate) to complete unilateral or bilateral clefts.

### BASIC ANATOMY

## 1

### Lip

To aid discussion of the operative procedures described here the features of the normal lip and nose are shown. In the repair the following points must be kept in mind.

1. Symmetrical Cupid's bow. Even in the most deformed unilateral clefts the mid-point and the peak of the Cupid's bow can be identified, although the latter is unduly high. In bilateral clefts they are not identifiable and have to be reconstructed.
2. The vermilion of the lip is everted.
3. The philtral ridges. The construction of the ridge on the cleft side is always difficult. Some elevation of the suture line results by incising the tissue at an angle and by the use of everting stitches. The knife is inserted so that the edges of the cleft are undercut.
4. Symmetrical nose.

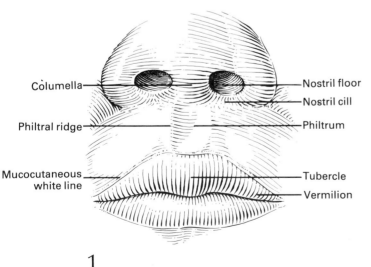

Columella — Nostril floor
— Nostril cill
Philtral ridge — — Philtrum
Mucocutaneous white line — — Tubercle
— Vermilion

1

# 2

## Nose

The alar cartilages are all important in maintaining the shape of the nostrils. They have medial and lateral crura, the former being adherent to one another.

## Classification

There have been many classifications. The Ritchie–Davis classification is still used.

Group I
   Prealveolar clefts (lip only)
      Unilateral or bilateral
      Complete or partial lip clefts
Group II
   Postalveolar clefts – palate only.
      Further classified according to length
Group III
   Complete alveolar
   Unilateral
   Bilateral (these were Group IV in Veau's classifiation).

Kernahan and Stark (1958) introduced a classification on an embryological basis. They pointed out that the fusion of the primary palate, consisting of the lip and alveolus, begins early in the third week of fetal life and that the fusion of the secondary palate occurred in the seventh and twelfth weeks. This is the bony and soft palate behind the incisive foramen.

Defects in the primary palate may occur: cleft lip with occasional extension into the alveolus.

Defects in the secondary palate correspond to post-alveolar clefts.

Defects in the primary palate are often followed by lack of fusion of the secondary palate, and result in complete clefts.

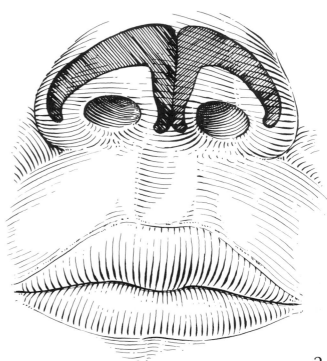

2

## DEFECTS OF THE PRIMARY PALATE

# 3 & 4

This will be a bilateral or unilateral harelip and will vary a good deal in extent. The alveolus is usually intact and does not show any deformity. The nostrils exhibit a moderate degree of distortion.

Less often there is a notch or cleft in the alveolus which is then distorted; the problem is discussed below. More deformity of the nostril will result.

In addition to the obvious cleft there will be deficiency in height at the cleft and an abnormal insertion of orbicularis oris to the bony maxilla near to the bony nares. Deformity of the nose includes deviation of the anterior nasal spine, the septum and columella, as well as lateral and posterior displacement of the alar base. The columella is short in bilateral cases.

When the alveolus is cleft unilaterally the end of the inner segment is rotated forward and laterally. In bilateral cases the premaxilla protrudes forwards and upwards.

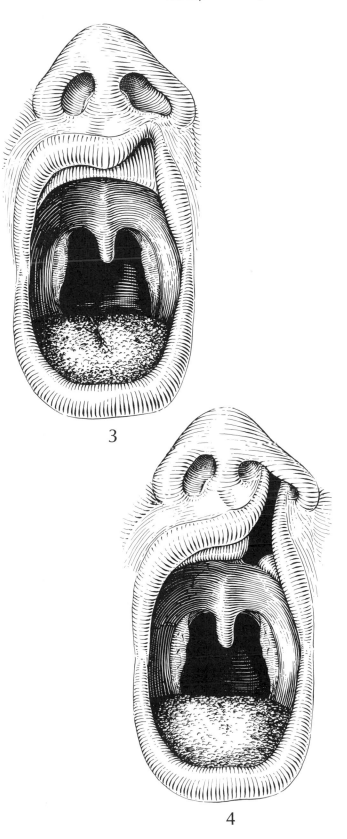

3

4

## DEFECT OF THE SECONDARY PALATE (POSTALVEOLAR CLEFT)

# 5 & 6

The lengths and widths of the clefts are variable. There is no deformity of the alveolar outline, although the size of the mandible is often deficient.

The width of the longer clefts is often maintained by the tongue which tends to be in the gap. In addition both the bone and the soft tissue of the palatal shelves are often deficient in the anteroposterior direction, and have an abnormal upward slope. The palatal muscles are abnormally inserted.

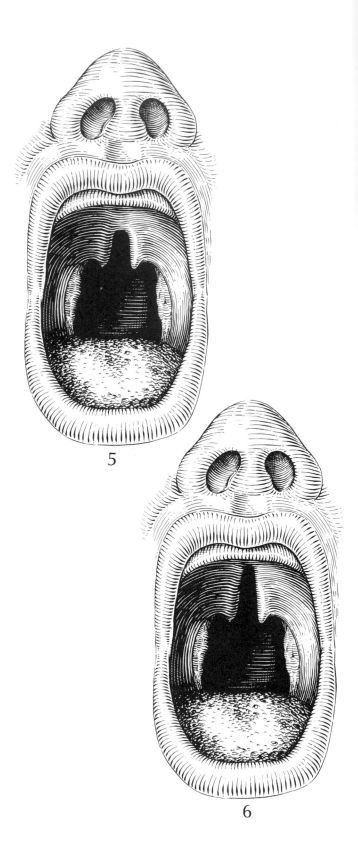

5

6

# 7

## COMBINED CLEFTS OF THE PRIMARY AND SECONDARY PALATES (COMPLETE CLEFTS)

The maximum degree of deformity is found in this group. Growth occurs in the face by sutural growth and by subperiosteal deposition. The main sutural activity is in the midline, and leads to displacement if the bony segments of the upper jaw are not attached to each other. In unilateral clefts the premaxilla is pushed forward, and tilts as it is attached on one side. It is also tilted forward and there is a step between it and the anterior end of the lesser segment. The anterior nasal spine is displaced away from the midline and there is a great difference in the width of the nostrils. The alar cartilage on the cleft side often assumes an S-shape.

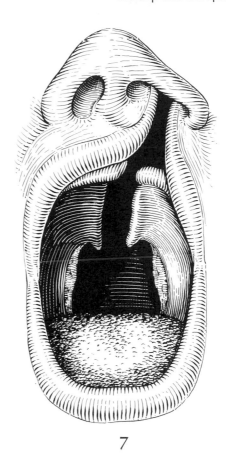

7

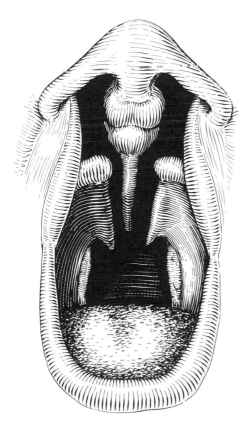

8

# 8

## DEFECT OF PRIMARY AND SECONDARY PALATES

Bilateral cleft of the lip and palate. Notice the forward displacement of the premaxilla and prolabium, with a short columella.

# Team management

A large team is necessary for the overall management of a child with a cleft deformity. As well as the surgeon an orthodontist should be involved, from an early stage and an ENT surgeon. Later a dental surgeon and a speech therapist will be involved and possibly a child psychiatrist and social worker. Supervision will be needed well into adolescence.

The parents should be interviewed at an early stage by the surgeon who can outline the plan of treatment and give some reassurance by doing so and by photographs illustrating the outcome of previous cases.

A consultation with the orthodontic surgeon within a few days of birth will determine if preoperative orthodontic treatment is necessary.

## OPERATIVE DISPOSITIONS

## 9

The infant is placed on an operating table fitted with a child's neurosurgical head rest, which allows a certain amount of mobility of the head. For operations on the palate extension of the head and neck is required.

Anaesthesia is given through an endotracheal tube passed through the mouth, and fixed to the midline, or just to one side of the midline. Distortion of the nostrils and lip must be carefully avoided. The eyelids are closed with Micropore tape.

The pharynx is packed with a moistened 2-inch gauze pack to prevent the aspiration of blood, and the assistant keeps the mouth and operative field clear with an angled sucker and dry and wet swabs.

In general, the surgeon sits or stands above the head, but does require to be mobile to view the repair from below and to insert some of the more difficult sutures.

The operative field, including the nostrils, should be cleaned with aqueous Hibitane solution.

Monitoring of the patient is achieved by a stethoscope strapped to the precordium, but the surgeon must accept some responsibility for ensuring that the airway and respiration are adequate.

Estimation of the blood loss must be made, and blood replaced if loss exceeds 5 per cent of the blood volume in a small baby; thus an intravenous drip must be set up in all cases.

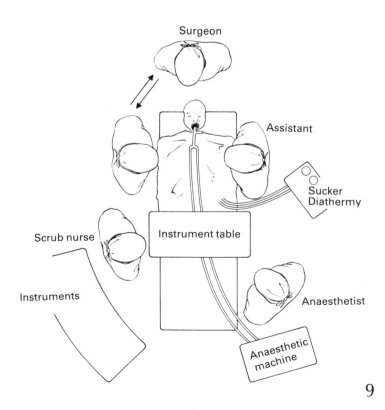

Surgeon

Assistant

Sucker
Diathermy

Instrument table

Scrub nurse

Instruments

Anaesthetist

Anaesthetic
machine

9

## INSTRUMENTS

# 10

### Kilner–Dott mouth gag

The Dott modification of this gag consists of a spiral spring attached to the main frame. It conveniently holds the ends of sutures.

The width of the mouth can also be adjusted by moving the prongs for the upper jaw.

# 11

### Dingman mouth gag

It is more bulky but allows the corners of the mouth to be retracted.

## SPECIAL INSTRUMENTS

Callipers, pen and ink are very useful for marking out incisions, and the naked eye itself is very accurate in judging symmetry. Deficiencies in lengths of less than 1 mm can be detected.

Skin hooks and small skin retractors are helpful.

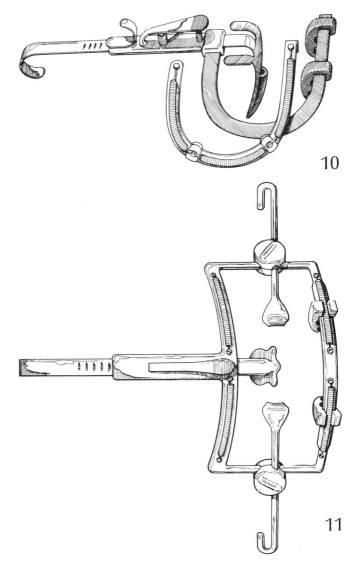

10

11

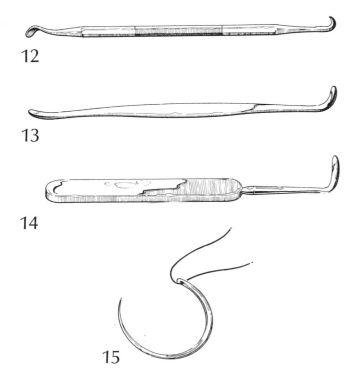

12

13

14

15

# 12–14

### McIndoe cleft palate raspatory and cleft palate elevators, angled and curved

These instruments are useful for lifting mucoperiosteal flaps, and generally separating soft tissue from the underlying bone.

# 15

### Denis Browne needle

This has a five-eighths circle and a cutting point, and although atraumatic sutures are now available it is useful in repairing the more awkward parts of the cleft palate. It comes in various sizes.

# Repair of harelip

## Introduction

All operations on cleft lips and palates must be done at the optimal time. Operations performed too early are unnecessarily difficult and the results are inferior. The baby's size and health must be good. In particular, infections in the area result in breakdowns, and preoperative swabs must be taken from the throat and nose. Haemolytic streptococci and other pathogenic organisms are contraindications to operation on the palate.

The possibility of infection from the child's relatives must be considered, and a preoperative period in hospital may reveal a developing problem.

Spoon feeding must be established before undertaking operation.

If a prosthesis has been worn it should be discarded for 2 days preoperatively.

The best time to operate on an uncomplicated harelip is at 5–6 months of age, but when it is part of a complete cleft, 3 months is a better age.

## Lip adhesion

To help preoperative orthodontic treatment it is sometimes necessary to do a temporary repair to bring into play the muscular forces in the lip to help close the gap. A simple repair only is indicated and a more formal operation is done after an interval.

Alternatively, in a bilateral complete cleft a bridge of skin across one nostril causes deviation of the premaxilla, and during orthodontics it may be necessary to divide it.

Certain general principles apply to all lip repairs. On the basis of the knowledge of the normal anatomy an attempt must be made to correct all the aspects of the deformity. The lines of the incisions must be carefully made with pen and ink, and the first cut is made, through the skin only, with a No. 15 blade. It is useful to hold the lip under tension with a skin hook or Allis forceps attached to the vermilion. The incision is completed with a larger triangular blade. It transfixes the full thickness of the lip and is held at an angle away from the cleft. When the undercut edges are brought together the skin will be elevated to produce a raised philtrum.

Initially the lower end of the incision is at the red margin, and flaps including the vermilion are turned down. They are finally trimmed and adjusted to each other. Each side of the lip must be undercut sufficiently to remove tension in the repair and to correct the shape of the nostril. On the lateral side the alar base is detached from the maxilla and the dissection taken along the lateral rim of the bony nares. Medially the dissection is taken to the nasal spine and beyond. The spine may be detached if it is displaced away from the midline. The incision is also taken backwards into the nostril to provide a shelf to form the nostril floor.

To diminish the bleeding it is useful to infiltrate the area with 1 per cent Xylocaine and 1:100 000 adrenaline, with a strict limitation on the total amount consistent with the baby's weight and to prevent puffiness of the tissues; 1.5 ml/kg bodyweight of solution must not be exceeded, and halothane anaesthesia avoided if adrenaline is used.

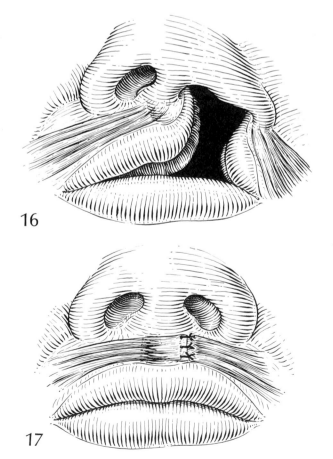

16

17

# 16 & 17

The components of the lip must be identified at the cut edge, by lifting the skin and mucosa from the orbicularis oris muscle, which tends to be bunched up and abnormally attached to the maxillary periosteum, particularly to the pyriform fossa at the base of the ala on the lateral side and at the base of the columella medially. The ends must be freed, fanned out, and sutured across the cleft.

# 18

## Simple repair

Only rarely is a simple repair undertaken, because the height of the lip on the cleft side is deficient. Quadrilateral or triangular flaps are usually fashioned.

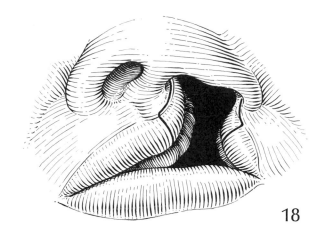

18

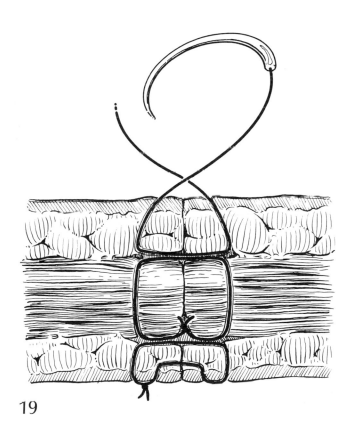

19

# 19

## Suturing

The layers of the lip are sutured separately. Fine mattress sutures of polyglycolic acid are used for the mucosa, and simple thicker ones for the muscle. Very fine Prolene is preferred for the skin.

## MILLARD'S REPAIR

This has the advantage of being a flexible plan and can be modified during the course of the operation. The Cupid's bow is preserved and the scars lie in good positions. Pouting of the lower lip is produced and it is the operation of choice for milder degrees of cleft. The good result usually persists because disproportionate growth of the parts rarely occurs. In the more severe cases the size of the lateral flap may be limited as the lateral vermilion would be reduced in width. Le Mesurier's quadrilateral flap is then to be preferred.

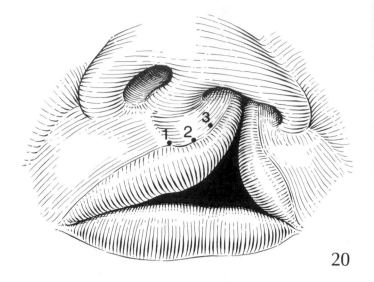

20

# 20–23

The point 2 in the midline and 1 at the top of the bow on the intact side are marked. Point 3 is chosen so that 2 lies midway between 1 and 3. An incision is carried upwards from 3 on the cleft side of the philtral groove and is then curved under the columella to point 5 just short of the normal philtral ridge. The extent will depend on the amount of rotation necessary to bring point 3 to the correct height. If necessary a back cut to x can be made.

The lateral advancement flap is made by incision 6–7, and length 6–7 must equal 3–5 or 3–5–X.

From 6 an incision is made laterally to complete the flap and may be carried round below the alar base to obtain more movement. Tissue may be removed from here to allow upward adjustment of the flap.

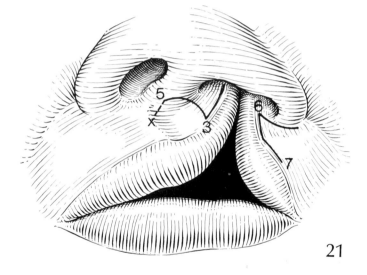

21

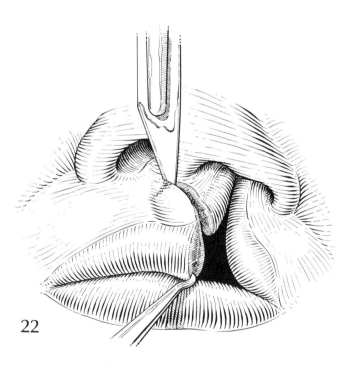

22

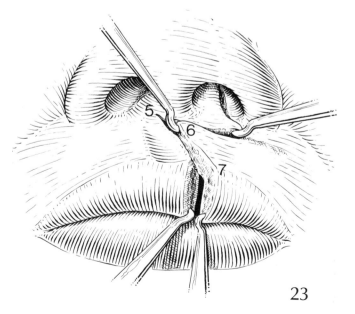

23

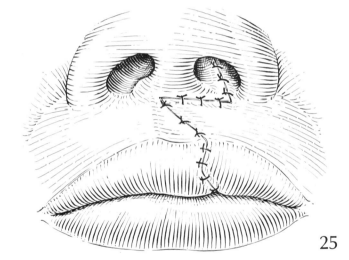

# 24 & 25

The medial flap has been rotated to produce a normal Cupid's bow. The lateral flap is pulled into position, after some undermining.

25

## MODIFIED LE MESURIER REPAIR

# 26

The normal side is measured and the repaired cleft side is made to correspond.

A point *a* is chosen in the normal nostril floor at the top of the philtral ridge. The distances from *a* to the base of the lateral alar crus and the insertion of the columella are measured and corresponding points *a'* and *a"* are marked on the cleft side. Point *p* is at the bottom of the normal philtral ridge, and *ap* is the height of the ridge.

On the medial side of the cleft *d* is marked on the mucocutaneous line where the vermilion border begins to narrow, and will preserve the apex of the Cupid's bow on that side. Lines *a"d* and *dc* are then drawn so that their total length equals the normal height of the lip *a"d + dc = ap*. The angle which *cd* makes with the medial vermilion edge must be slightly obtuse.

Points *b' c'* and *d'* are then marked on the lateral side of the cleft so that *a' b' = ad* and *c'd' = cd = b'c'*. The distance from *b'* to the vermilion edge must exceed *c'd'* by about 2 mm and *c'd'* must meet the edge of the lateral vermilion at slightly more than a right-angle.

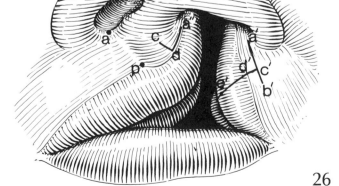

26

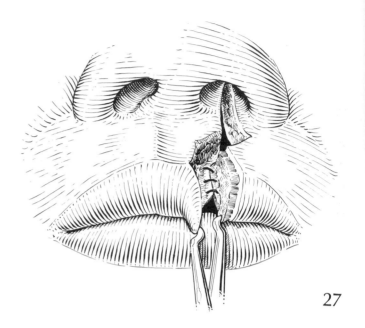

27

# 27 & 28

The balance of the Cupid's bow must be kept in mind so that the amount of vermilion on each side of the philtrum is equal.

Incisions are made into each buccal sulcus to mobilize the lip and the lateral alar crus from the periosteum. The midline of the nose is also mobilized by dividing the anterior nasal spine from the premaxilla.

The modified Le Mesurier's operation is the easier because the flaps can be accurately measured. However, once made they are difficult to adjust. The Millard operation depends more on the eye and freehand marking, but often gives a better result.

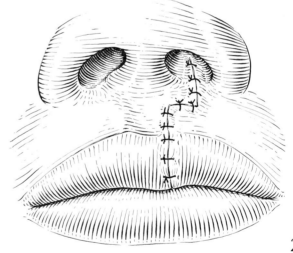

28

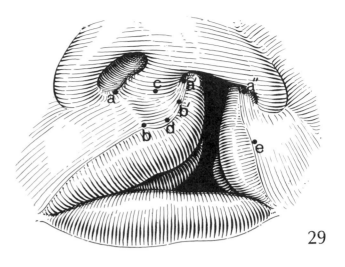

29

## TENNISON REPAIR

# 29–31

Instead of a quadrilateral flap, an inferiorly based triangular flap can be used as described by Tennison (1952).

*a* is a point on the floor of the uncleft side at the superior end of the philtral ridge;
*b* is the peak of the Cupid's bow on that side;
*c* and *d* are the midpoints of the columella and the Cupid's bow;
*a'* and *a''* are points on the cleft side corresponding to *a*, being measured from the columella and the alar base respectively;
*e* is the point at which the vermilion becomes narrower on the cleft side.

The following points are then drawn:

*b'* so that *bd* = *db'*,
Distance *x* = *ab* minus *a'b'*, i.e. the increase in height which is needed;
*b'f* is drawn perpendicular to *cd*;
*g* is the midpoint of line *fd*;
Arc, radius *x* is inscribed from *e*;
Arc, radius *a'b'* is inscribed from *a''*;
This gives point *b''*;
Now *y* is marked so that *ey* = *yb''* = *gb'*.

The columella and alar bases must be freed as described previously.

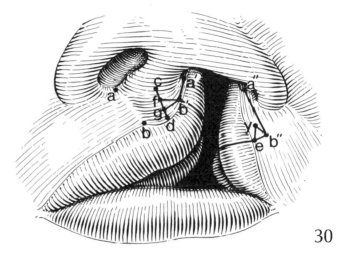

30

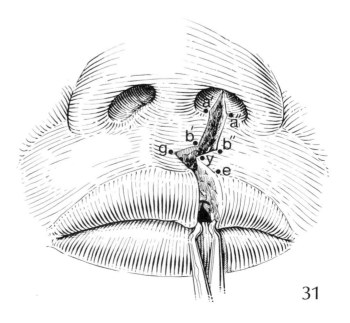

31

## REPAIR OF BILATERAL HARELIP

# 32 & 33

In bilateral harelips the muscle does not meet across the midline and makes attachments to bony points in the vicinity. The prolabium contains no muscle.

It is necessary to mobilize the muscle and bring it end-to-end in the midline, or in the case of a wide cleft to approximate the ends as far as possible, behind the skin of the prolabium.

The labial sulcus must be preserved to allow movement and development of the prolabium, which should provide the full vertical height of the middle of the lip. Skin flaps from the lateral segments must not be brought together in the midline below the prolabium. In fact the mucocutaneous ridge at its inferior border may be preserved, and the deficient prolabial vermilion is built up with vermilion flaps from the lateral segments. They can meet in the midline, or be overlapped to produce a central tubercle.

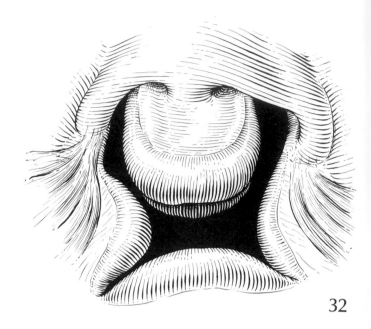

32

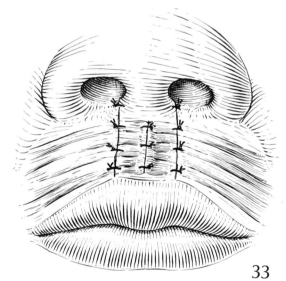

33

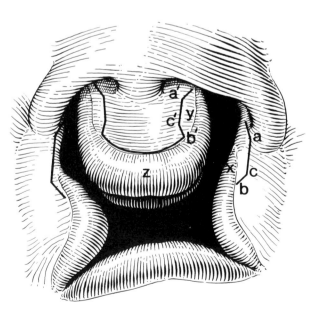

34

# 34

The line a' c' b' on the medial side should be close to the vermilion, and the remaining prolabial skin should be wider inferiorly. Point b is on the mucocutaneous border at the apex of the Cupid's bow. a c b is drawn to correspond to a' c' b' and c taken laterally will accentuate the tightness above the vermilion and the eversion of the latter.

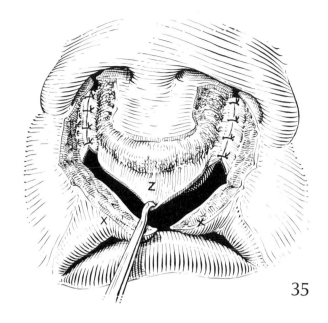

35

## 35

The mucosa is repaired posteriorly. Flap *X* retains as much bulk as possible to thicken the middle of the lip and produce a central tubercle. Skin is removed from it, leaving mucosa and muscle.

Excess skin in the floor of the nose is retained for a subsequent lengthening of the columella, and in fact the skin from flap *Y* may be banked in the nostril floor for this purpose (see Millard's operation below).

Normally $a'b'$ will be less than $ab$ and the prolabium will be stretched and advanced. However, if the lateral segment is too high a full thickness wedge can be removed immediately below the ala. The prolabium will generally enlarge postoperatively.

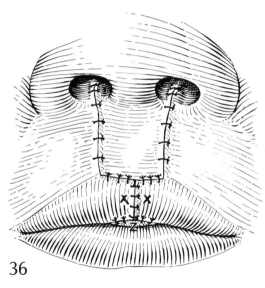

36

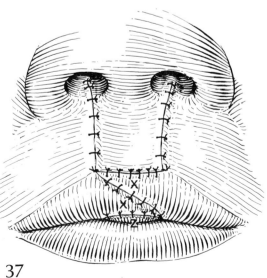

37

## 36 & 37

The mucosal *X* flaps are brought together in the midline, with the *Z* flap posterio-inferiorly. Sometimes (37) overlapping of the *X* flaps may be better.

## MILLARD REPAIR OF COMPLETE BILATERAL CLEFT LIPS WITH PROVISION FOR LATER COLUMELLA LENGTHENING

# 38

The philtrum is incised to provide a central skin flap which is wider below; a turned-down flap of vermilion and the lateral prolabial tissues are preserved. The incisions in the lateral segments are made so that in this case the white lines of the lateral mucocutaneous junctions are preserved to bring to the midline.

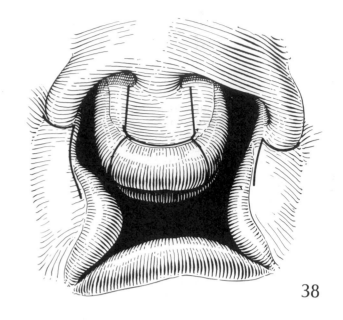

38

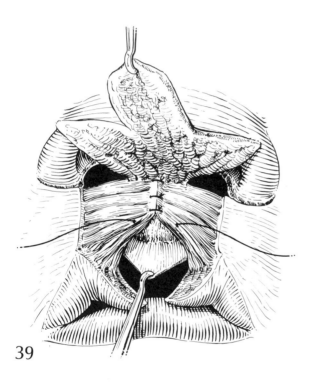

39

# 39

The lateral muscular segments are freed from the periosteum and then sewn together in the midline behind the prolabial skin. The alar base and cheek usually have to be mobilized.

# 40

Excess on the vermilion flaps is retained to build up the central tubercle. The forked flaps are turned laterally and sutured end on to the alar base flaps. Their raw surfaces are approximated to form a ridge in the nasal floor. The tissue is used for subsequent columella lengthening.

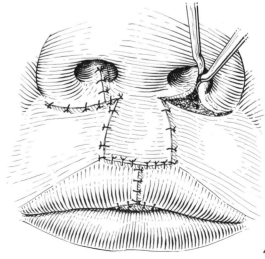

40

# Repair of harelip in complete clefts of lip and palate

## Preoperative orthodontic treatment

Preoperative orthodontic treatment is accepted as valuable for many cleft palates, particularly in complete clefts. The separate bony elements are both underdeveloped and badly positioned. Little can be done to stimulate growth, but the position can be altered by treatment given during the first few months of life when the elements are still mobile. It is necessary to control and mould growth, which is most vigorous during the very early months. Usually the outline of the upper alveolus can be adjusted to conform to the shape and size of the lower by the use of intraoral appliances and external pressure.

Considerable skill and careful attention is required for this work, which must be started within a few days of birth. Daily adjustment of the external forces is necessary and the intra-oral appliances will need remodelling at least once a month. The orthodontic surgeon can usually achieve considerable improvement in 3 months.

A number of advantages to the surgeon result. In general, the clefts, particularly at the front, are made narrower, the operations are easier, and repairs made under less tension. The soft tissues are in a more normal position, the amount of adjustment is less, and the operative results are better. The relationships of the bony bases in the anteroposterior direction are normalized and the results are more pleasing. The methods are most valuable in bilateral clefts, and the need to do staged operations has been removed. Less undermining of the lips is necessary. Lastly, because the bony segments of the maxilla have been brought into correct alignment with the lower alveolus they are more likely to remain in a good position after the operation and the repair should not deteriorate.

In the absence of expert orthodontic assistance the surgeon can produce some improvement by external strapping. Micropore tape is applied to the cheeks as a base for Elastoplast strapping, which is laid across the lip with its middle segment folded double and only the ends left sticky to apply to the Micropore. Cotton wool pads are used to concentrate pressure and to protect vulnerable areas. However, external pressure alone will only approximate the anterior ends, and if overdone may produce an unsatisfactory result. For instance, in a bilateral cleft the maxillary segments may be brought together behind the premaxilla.

Postalveolar clefts which involve the bony palate can also be helped by a preoperative appliance. The width of the cleft is related to the underdevelopment and increased angulation of the bony palatal shelves. Both these features are aggravated by the pressure and position of the tongue, which can be corrected by a thin plate worn in the mouth.

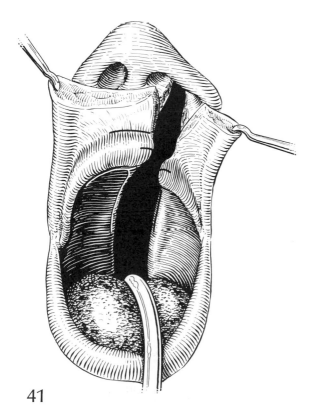

41

## CLOSURE OF ANTERIOR PART OF THE CLEFT IN COMPLETE UNILATERAL

# 41

The harelip in a complete cleft is usually repaired when the position of the bony segments has been improved by the preoperative orthodontics, at about the age of 3 months. The opportunity is also taken to repair the nostril floor, the alveolus, and the anterior part of the palate.

The incisions of the basic lip repair must be extended posteriorly into the nose so that flaps can be elevated on each side to form the nostril floor. The edges of the cleft are also incised, and a small flap, hinged posteriorly, is fashioned from the mucoperiosteum on the uncleft side.

The palatal flap is elevated. Incisions are continued on to the ends of the alveolus to provide flaps to bring across the alveolar gap. The greatest care must be taken not to injure the alveolar ends, which would result in restriction of growth and damage to tooth buds.

# 42

The repair is begun by suturing the nasal floor and nasal mucosa.

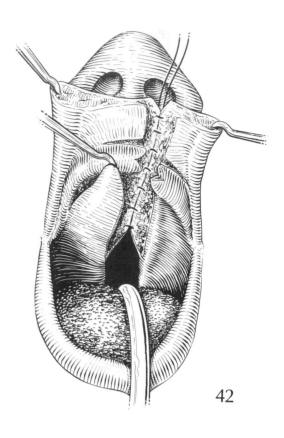

42

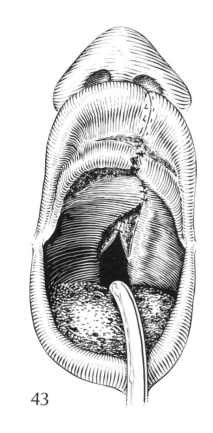

43

# 43

The palatal flap is brought across to the raw edge on the opposite side of the cleft and the alveolar ends are repaired with small flaps.

The lip is repaired last, in the usual manner.

## ANTERIOR PALATE REPAIR COMBINED WITH REPAIR OF BILATERAL CLEFT LIP

# 44–46

In bilateral complete clefts the anterior palate and the alveolar ends can be repaired at the same time, using flaps as described for unilateral clefts, as long as the alveolar gaps are not too large. Otherwise this part of the operation may be postponed or done in two stages. Preoperative orthodontic treatment should produce enough improvement in the position of the premaxilla to avoid the necessity to remove any septal bone from behind it.

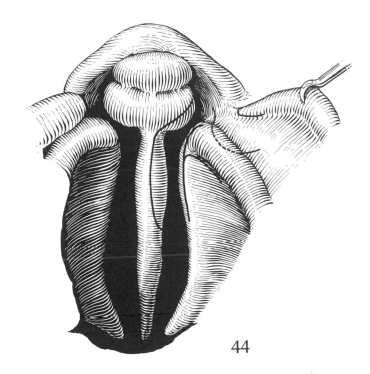

44

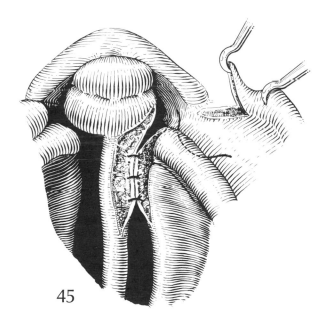

45

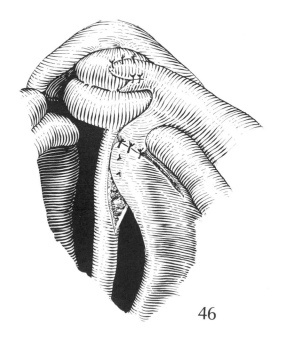

46

## FASHIONING THE NOSTRIL

# 47 & 48

The problem of fashioning the nostril is much increased in the wide complete clefts. Besides excising an ellipse of excess of skin from the inside of the nostril it is often helpful to separate the nasal skin from the underlying lateral crus. Blunt-ended scissors are used and can be taken round to the tip of the nose. Sometimes it is necessary to free the medial crus, but the blood supply from the nasal mucosa must be preserved.

The cartilage and skin can then slip over one another and will assume a better shape. The original lip incision, or a second one just inside the alar rim, can be used to gain access.

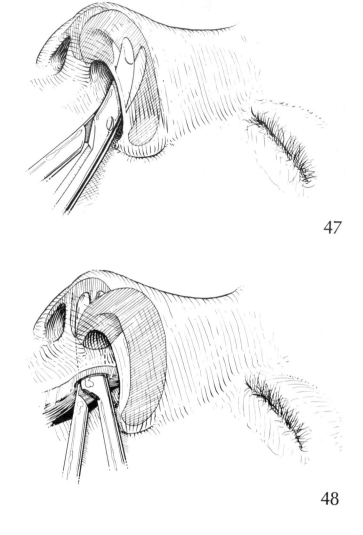

47

48

## PRIMARY BONE GRAFTING

After the position of the bony segments of the maxilla had been corrected by preoperative orthodontics, it was suggested that stabilization of the position could be achieved by bone grafts placed in the gap in the alveolus. It was hoped that deterioration in the shape, which often follows surgery, would not occur.

However, this hope has not been fulfilled and primary bone grafting has largely been abandoned.

Skoog and others showed that by swinging mucoperiosteal flaps across the alveolar gap, a pocket was left between the flaps, in which a bony strut would often develop, thus avoiding the transfer of a graft. However, as with bone grafts, such struts are probably disadvantageous.

# Repair of cleft palate

## Timing of operation

The correct time for operation is still not agreed. Modern anaesthesia and surgery have reduced the mortality to almost nil, and this hazard does not influence the timing. Operation is easier the older the child, and scarring is possibly reduced. It is generally considered that the palate should be repaired and functioning by the time the child begins to talk, which means that the operation ought to be done by 9 months of age. This ensures a palate which is longer, more mobile, and has a better muscular development.

In the belief that the earlier the operation is undertaken the greater the restriction in growth of the maxilla, some workers advise delay in closure of the hard palate. Schweckendiek and Hotz advise early closure of the soft palate and delay repair of the rest for 6–8 years in the case of complete clefts. This technique requires a good deal of close supervision and the use of intra-oral appliances.

However, there is no scientific evidence of benefit in this routine (Robertson and Jolleys). In the United Kingdom cleft palates are repaired at about the age of 1 year and preferably soon after 6 months of age.

## Preoperative care

The infant should be well and growing satisfactorily at the time of the operation. Checks must be made of the haemoglobin concentration and the bacteriology of the mouth, nose and throat. Pathogenic organisms, especially β-haemolytic streptococci and pyogenic staphylococci, increase the breakdown rate, and attempts must be made to eradicate them before surgery. Evidence of upper respiratory tract infections are contraindications to surgery.

Blood for transfusion should be available.

## General principles

Relieving incisions must always be made to allow the soft tissue of the palatal shelves to slide medially, so that the repair can be done without tension. With the angled cleft palate raspatories the mucoperiosteum is dissected as one layer from the bony shelves.

On the other hand, great care is necessary to avoid damage to the structures. Scarring must be kept to a minimum, and the blood supply preserved so as to avoid any damage which may limit the subsequent growth of the maxilla.

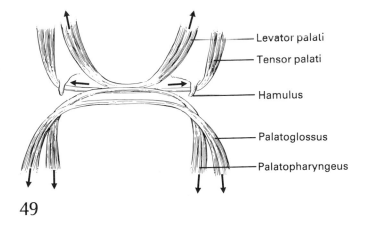

Levator palati

Tensor palati

Hamulus

Palatoglossus

Palatopharyngeus

49

## MUSCULAR SLINGS

# 49

The main purpose of the operation is to restore the correct functioning of the palatal muscles.

Two pairs of the muscles run downwards into the velum. The tensor palati runs around the hamulus so that its tendinous insertion runs almost horizontally.

The two levator palati muscles are very important for speech and are normally inserted into the middle of the velum, and lift it. A pair of palato-pharyngeus muscles and a pair of salpingo-pharyngeus muscles run upwards and are inserted into the palate from below.

## 50

When the soft palate is cleft the muscles on each side do not meet, and the series of U-shaped slings are disrupted. The muscles become inserted into the posterior edge of the bony palate.

When repairing the velum these muscles must be identified and detached from the bony edge so that they can be retroposed and brought together in the midline.

Removal of sutures from the mouth is always difficult in an infant. The use of polyglycolic acid material has been a benefit because it is quite persistent and causes little reaction in the oral cavity, but does not need to be removed.

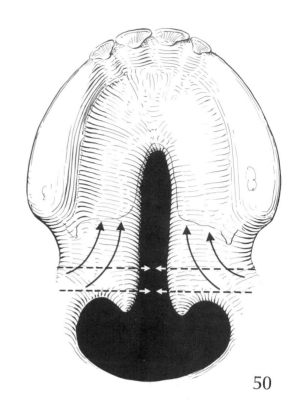

50

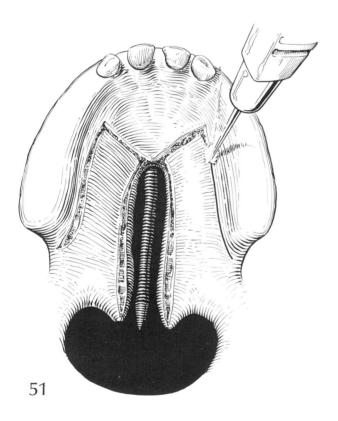

51

## WARDILL TWO-FLAP OPERATION

## 51

### Relieving incisions

The relieving incisions are made about 5 mm medial to the alveolus and pterygomandibular ligament to avoid both damage to the tooth buds and scarring which would interfere with mouth opening. Diathermy is useful. The incisions are taken down to the bone over the hard palate, and through the mucosa only in the posterior part. Here dissection is continued with blunt instruments into a bloodless space between the tensor palati and the medial pterygoid muscles. However, it must be limited to the necessary minimum to reduce postoperative scarring.

The incision at the edge of the cleft is made with a sickle-shaped knife and the edges must be opened up to expose the aponeurosis and muscles.

## Dissection

# 52

Provided that the incisions have gone through the periosteum there is no difficulty in elevating the mucoperiosteum with the angled elevators.

The hamulus is identified and the tendon of the tensor palati running around it. Division of the tendon and fracture of the hamulus are not necessary, but the tissue in this area must be carefully dissected.

Supplying the upper side of the flap which has been freed is the greater palatine artery emerging from the greater palatine foramen, anteromedial to the pterygoid hamulus. Tissue around it is freed to provide some mobility, but in addition the posterior bony wall of the foramen can be removed with small nibblers to allow posterior displacement of the flap and vessels (Limberg, 1927).

The nasal mucoperiosteum is separated from the upper side of the bony palate. After this mobilization posterior displacement of the soft palate is still restricted by the nasal mucosa, which is reinforced by fibrous periosteum. This can be divided, and small incisions made into the edges of mucosa. They should not be opposite each other, so that some inter-digitation is possible.

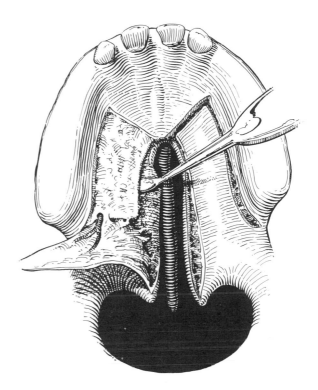

52

**Closure**

# 53 & 54

Suturing is begun anteriorly on the nasal side with 3/0 polyglycolic acid material inserted as horizontal mattress stitches. The repair is completed by suturing the oral side with vertical mattress stitches, which ensure that the muscles are well approximated. In general, a small atraumatic half-circle or a Denis Browne five-eighths needle is used. With limited access a Reverdin needle may be used.

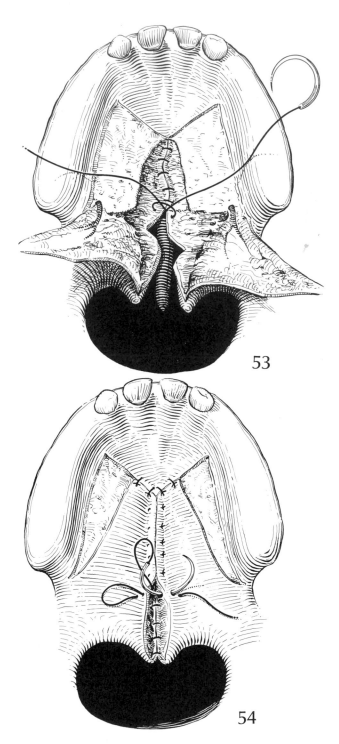

53

54

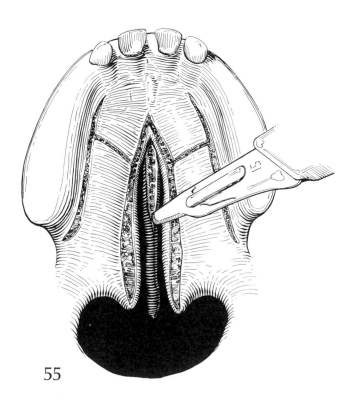

55

**Wardill four-flap operation**

# 55

When the cleft extends into the hard palate it is necessary to cut four flaps, because if the posteriorly hinged flaps are too long there is a risk of ischaemia of their anterior ends. The principle of retroposition remains the same. If the transverse incisions are made slightly asymmetrical the corners of the flaps do not all meet at the same point, with an advantage to healing.

# 56 & 57

In the postalveolar clefts the inferior edge of the vomer will be seen. An incision along this edge will allow flaps of nasal mucosa to be elevated on each side, and these are sutured to the nasal layers above the bony palate. Everting mattress sutures are generally applicable, and sutures are required between the nasal mucosa and the palatal flaps to obliterate the dead space.

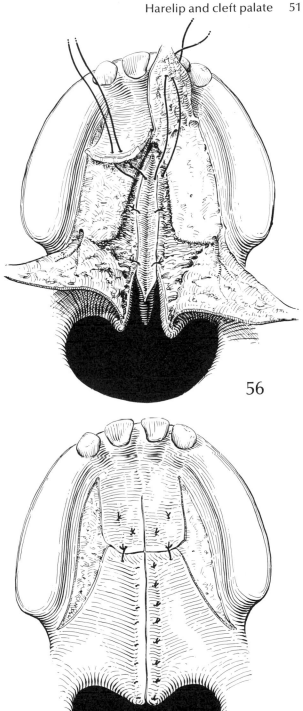

56

57

## POST-OPERATIVE CARE

The airways must be carefully cleared of blood and secretion at the end of the operation and the baby should at this point resume movement of the limbs and coughing. A semi-prone position with elevation of the chest over a pillow allows the tongue to fall forwards and secretions to run from the mouth.

It must be remembered that the operation will have reduced the airway, and close observation is necessary. Occasionally a severe problem can be overcome by inserting a stout stitch through the tongue, which can be pulled forward.

Splinting of the elbows prevents interference with the repair.

Feeding can be resumed on the first day with clear fluids. Next day the child will be remarkably well and will take milk. It has to be given by a spoon and then afterwards the milk is washed from the mouth by clear fluid drinks. Pyrexia occurs for a period of 48 hours. As the procedure is not undertaken in an aseptic field, broad-spectrum antibiotics are given for 4 days.

The raw areas resulting from the relieving incisions fill with granulation tissue very rapidly, and epithelialize over in about a week.

## SUBMUCOUS CLEFT PALATE

The submucous cleft is a rare form which may be missed. Especially during phonation or gagging, a median groove is seen on the underside of the velum where the muscles have failed to join, although the mucosa is intact. In addition there may be a notch or groove in the hard palate which can be felt, a missing posterior nasal spine, and a bifid uvula. The soft palate is short and with the disturbed muscular function there is frequently poor velopharyngeal closure, with a speech defect in about half the cases. Middle-ear damage may result.

Surgery is only indicated if hypernasality is present, and must be based on the principles already discussed. Detachment of the muscles from the posterior edge of the palatal shelves is followed by suturing in the midline, and the velum is retroposed.

Curiously, the functional result is more frequently unsatisfactory compared with repaired full-thickness clefts. This is possibly related to the fact that submucous defects are often diagnosed and treated in a later age group.

# Secondary procedures

### SECONDARY OPERATIONS ON THE LIP

Patients with clefts must be followed up throughout their growing period. Children with solitary lip problems are seen infrequently but cleft-palate patients are seen yearly, and joint consultations with dentist, orthodontic surgeon, and speech therapist are helpful.

Apart from programmes using delayed repair of the palate, orthodontic treatment is reserved for the second dentition. Routine dental care is pursued vigorously to conserve teeth, and includes the use of fluorides when indicated. Routine monitoring of the ears and hearing is needed.

Secondary adjustments are often necessary, and those involving the lip and nasal tip can be done before school age. Even major operations can be done, but if a poor outcome is the result of an underlying deformity of the maxilla, adjustment is delayed until 18 years of age and a full rhinoplasty is then performed.

Some of the basic general defects are discussed below.

### INCOMPLETE MUSCLE UNION

When for various reasons the muscle fibres have not been identified properly, or the continuity of the fibres has not been achieved, there is a bulging of the contracting muscle below the ala, or in bilateral cases the prolabium is immobile.

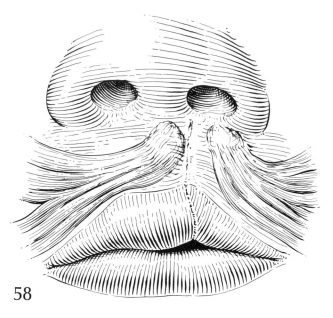

58

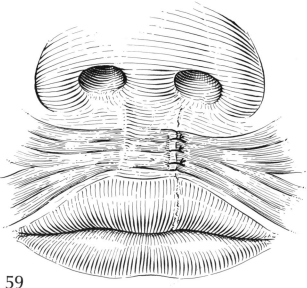

59

# 58 & 59

After division of the abnormal muscular attachments, the orbicularis oris is redirected and sutured end to end.

# 60 & 61

In bilateral cases the muscle is advanced into the prolabial segment where the fibres are very poorly developed. At the same time other adjustments are made to the skin and vermilion.

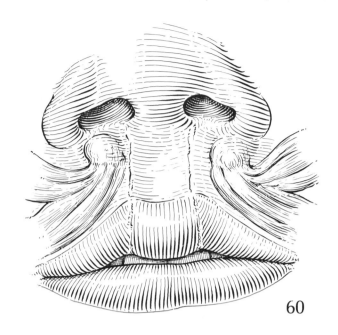

60

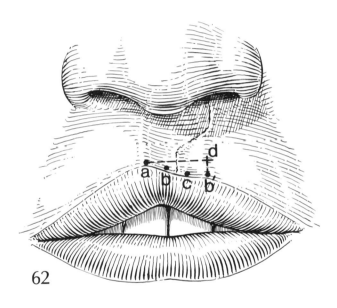

62

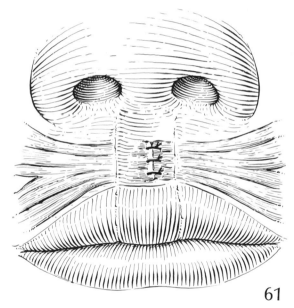

61

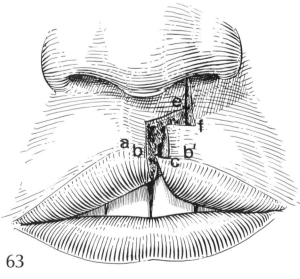

63

## DEFORMITIES AFTER ROTATION FLAP OPERATIONS

These are corrected by excision of the previous scar and modification of the flaps to correct the problem. Make *ab* = *cb'*.

# 62 & 63

Excessive length of the lip to the lateral side after Le Mesurier's operation is reduced by excision of tissue from the horizontal limb of the incision (*ef* is the reduction in height = *db'*).

# 64 & 65

Lack of height of the lip is remedied by re-doing the initial operation, making bigger flaps with more downward rotation.

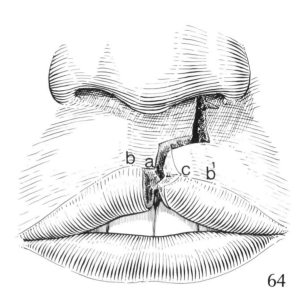

64

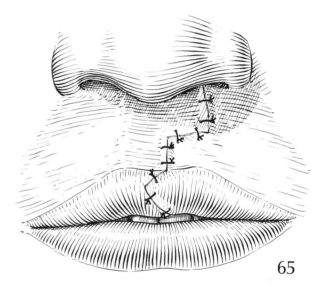

65

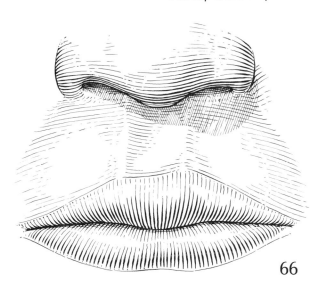

66

## MINOR MALALIGNMENT OF VERMILION

### V–Y Plasty to increase the thickness of the lip

# 66–69

By advancing tissue from the posterior aspect of the lip, an improvement in the shape can be achieved. It is necessary to take the incisions deeply and to undermine the tissue.

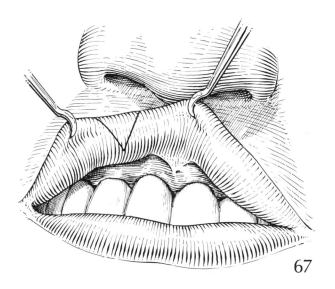

67

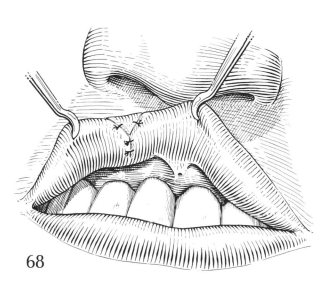

68

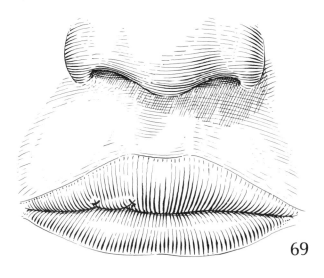

69

**Correction of irregularity at border of vermilion**

# 70 & 71

Corrections of vermilion irregularities are often quite simple. Excision and advancement will often suffice. Excess vermilion can be trimmed away with an elliptical incision. The amount of muscle to be excised has to be judged carefully.

Sometimes a notch at the margin can be treated by a Z-plasty.

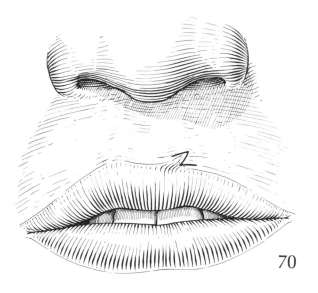

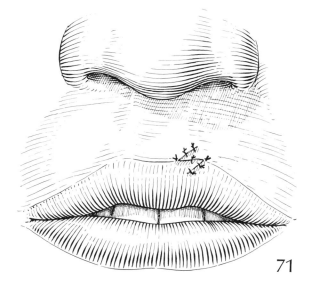

## CUPID'S BOW OPERATION

# 72–75

When making a Cupid's bow the skin marks must be drawn in an exaggerated fashion to make allowance for the contraction which will follow the operation. The skin is excised superficially and the dermis retained. The mucosa of the vermilion must be undermined quite deeply to include some muscle which is then advanced over the dermis, with a ridge at the vermilion border resulting. The vermilion can also be advanced towards the middle to produce a central papilla.

Such an operation may be required on one side only.

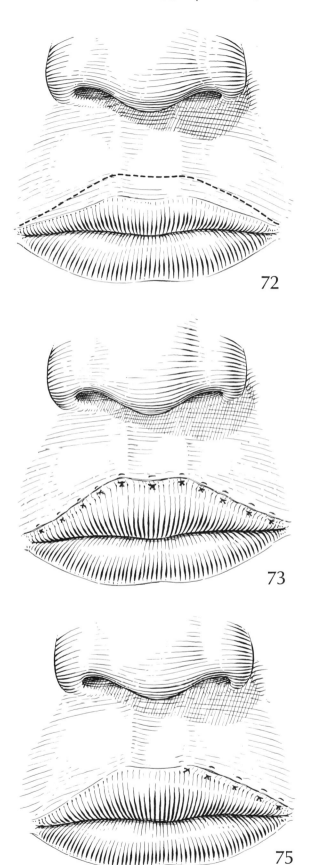

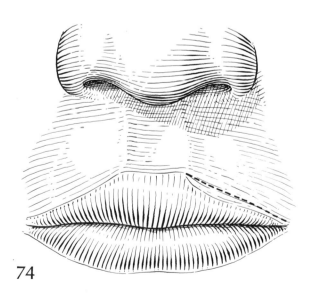

## ABBÉ FLAP FOR NARROW UPPER LIP

When the disparity in the width of the two lips is marked an Abbé flap is useful. The width and thickness of the upper lip is improved; the pouting lower lip is reduced.

# 76

A two-stage procedure is necessary, with nasal intubation for the anaesthetic. Most of the cases requiring the operation are bilateral clefts, but in any event the incision in the upper lip must be made in the midline to maintain symmetry; it is carried up to the base of the columella.

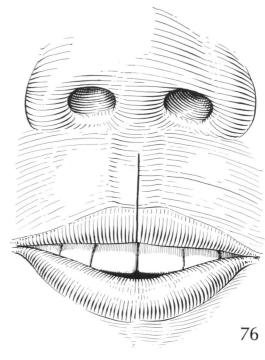

76

# 77 & 78

The tissues fall apart and the defect is assessed with a template. However, the size of the triangular flap taken from the lower lip must be a little smaller. It must also be cut symmetrically. The labial vessels are palpated in the proposed pedicle and preserved. The graft is then rotated through 180° and fixed in place with three layers of sutures. The latter must be inserted with small bites and tied loosely in order to preserve the blood supply.

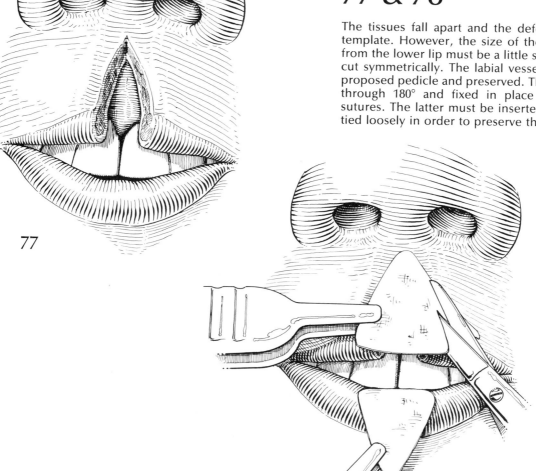

77

78

# 79–82

The cutaneous apex can be rounded off. The incision on the mucosal aspect is made wider and larger.

Some care must be taken to avoid a disruption of the repair as the patient recovers from the anaesthetic. Preoperative explanation and good nursing is necessary. A few strips of zinc oxide strapping suitably placed across the midline help, and may be removed with safety in an hour or so.

At a second operation, 9 or 10 days later, the pedicle is divided. The vermilion is adjusted. Further adjustment may sometimes be necessary after the healing is consolidated.

Feeding with fluids between the two operations is not a problem.

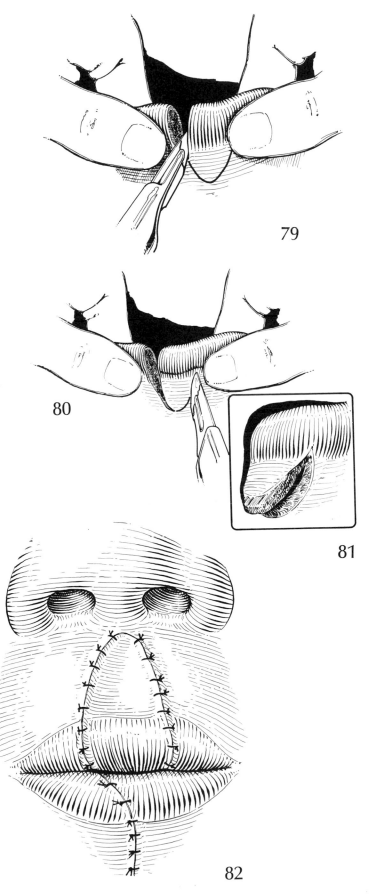

79

80

81

82

## DEFICIENT BUCCAL SULCUS

# 83–86

When the depth of the labio-gingival sulcus is insufficient, usually after a bilateral cleft, the fitting of a denture will be unsatisfactory and the lip is immobile. Prostheses may be necessary, not only to replace teeth but also to build up the lip to improve the profile. This problem may be avoided by rotational flaps at the time of primary surgery. Correction in later childhood is achieved by rotated mucosal flaps or by epithelial inlay. The latter is practical only in the second decade. The incision must be ample, but a fistula into the nasal floor must be avoided. A stent mould is then fashioned to fit the sulcus and a thick split-skin graft is prepared to cover it. After stitching the graft into place the mould is fixed either by sutures or by a bracket fixed to a cap splint.

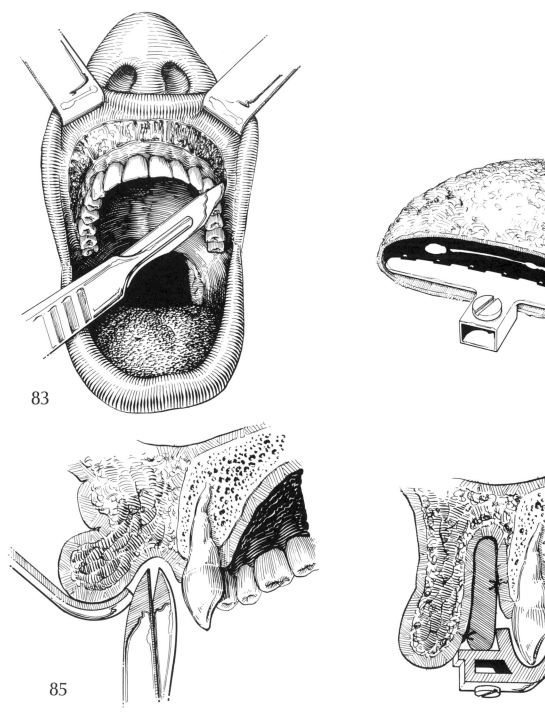

83

84

85

86

## SECONDARY OPERATIONS ON THE NOSE
## DEFORMITIES OF UNILATERAL CLEFT-LIP NOSE

# 87 & 88

It is accepted that in addition to mechanical distortion of the alar cartilages there is some inherent disturbance of growth in patients with cleft lips, because there has been failure of mesodermal invasion in the cleft area.

The medial alar crus on the cleft side is tilted and displaced posteriorly, resulting in a decreased projection of the dome. It is also displaced laterally so that the nasal tip shows bifidity, and the angle between the medial and lateral crura increases.

The alar base is displaced laterally and often downwards, resulting in a widened nasal floor and buckling of the alar cartilage.

Correction of these problems should be attempted at the time of the primary repair. Secondary procedures of a minor nature can be undertaken in early childhood. Major rhinoplasty procedures, if necessary, are probably best left until nasal growth has ceased at 16 years in females and a year or two later in boys. The nose is then fully developed and will not change. It may be necessary to undertake maxillary surgery beforehand. Maxillary expansion or secondary bone grafting is often useful, and other major reconstructions may be required and should only be done at this age.

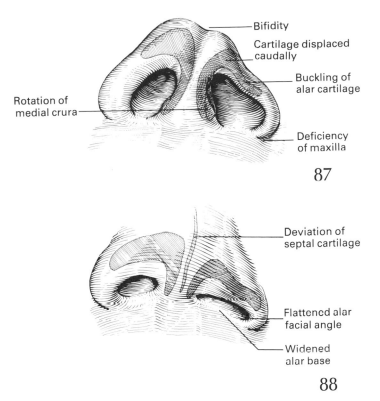

87

88

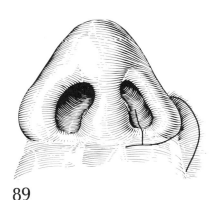

89

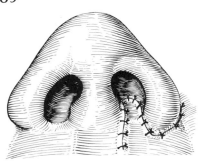

90

## MINOR CORRECTION OF ALAR BASE AND NOSTRIL FLOOR

The common deformity of a wide nostril floor accompanied by a recessed alar base can be corrected by the excision of an ellipse of tissue from the floor. The attachment of the lateral flap and lateral crus to the underlying bone must be freed completely. The lateral side can then be brought forward by suitably positioned subcutaneous sutures. At the same time minor adjustments can be made in the height of the alar base.

When a wide nasal floor is accompanied by an alar base which is too low, a flap can be swung into an incision inferior to the base.

# 89 & 90

Alternatively, a narrow nasal floor can be corrected by the insertion of a flap taken from below the alar base, as shown.

This is an example of a minor adjustment. In general the individual problems have to be analysed accurately and the appropriate operation undertaken. The cartilaginous framework may be adjusted by relocation and suture, by incision, by excision, and by graft augmentation. Z-plasties, excisions or rotation flaps may be needed for the skin.

The surgeon needs to be aware of the wide range of methods available.

# Deformities of the bilateral cleft-lip nose

The deformity is a bilateral form of the unilateral problem. However, because it is symmetrical, often more encouraging results can be obtained than in the unilateral case.

## 91

The medial crura are displaced posteriorly in the prolabium and the alar domes are separated and moved laterally, giving a bifid appearance to the nasal tip. It also seems flattened because the angle between the medial and lateral crura is increased, and the cartilage lateral to the dome is usually buckled inwards. The alar bases are displaced laterally and downwards, decreasing the alar-facial angles with a widened nasal floor. The columella is short.

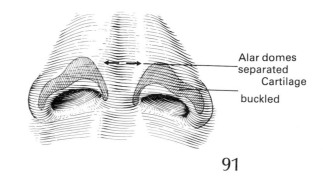

Alar domes separated
Cartilage buckled

91

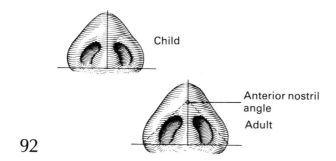

Infant

Child

Anterior nostril angle
Adult

92

## 92

It must be remembered that the nose is normally flatter and relatively broader the younger the patient (Piggott and Millard, 1971). An analysis of the defect and an appreciation of the normal nose proportions are necessary before undertaking secondary procedures, as correction of the underlying cartilages and manipulation of the skin by flaps or advancement may be necessary. Three basic procedures will be mentioned.

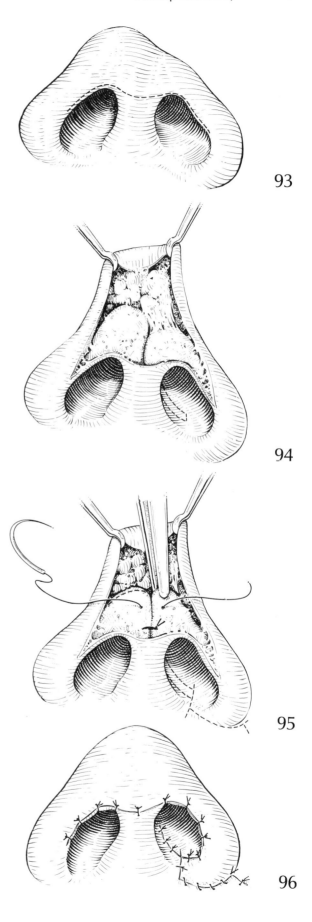

**FLYING WING OPERATION**

# 93–96

Deformities of the tip of the nose are amongst the most difficult to correct. This is an incision which makes a direct approach to the alar cartilages, and allows them to be adjusted relative to each other. Due regard must be paid to the blood supply to the cartilages and too much separation from the mucous membrane and from the skin must be avoided. In general, major operations of this nature ought to be delayed until the second decade. The primary incision is made just inside the edge of the nostril and across the underside of the columella.

The medial crus of the alar cartilage is freed from the opposite side until it can be advanced and fixed by suturing, to make the nasal tip symmetrical. Sometimes the building up may be augmented by the insertion of a cartilaginous graft. The lateral alar base is then adjusted. It generally needs to be elevated, advanced and medially rotated to make a matching nostril. Because the maxilla is hypoplastic on the cleft side, the rim of the pyriform fossa may be built up by the insertion of a bony or cartilaginous graft. Partial-thickness incisions into the alar cartilage will ensure that it bends smoothly, and other adjustments such as trimming the edge of the nostril may be done.

## COLUMELLA LENGTHENING BY A STELLATE FLAP

# 97–100

This is essentially a V–Y advancement with lateral wings attached which fall into the defect that results when incision X is made into the membranous septum. The upper ends of the incision can be extended around the inside of the alar rims to expose the cartilages, which are then mobilized, brought forward, and their domes approximated. The stellate flap is advanced and sewn into place.

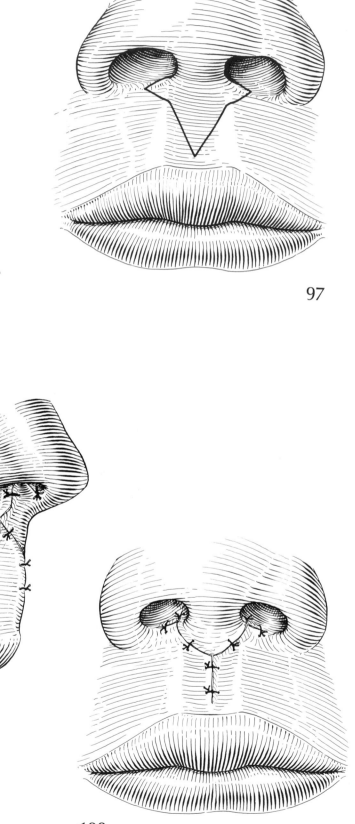

97

98

99

100

## COLUMELLA LENGTHENING BY MILLARD'S OPERATION USING FORKED FLAPS

# 101–103

Two flaps of skin are raised with their bases superiorly in continuity with the skin of the columella. The outer limbs of the incision again can be taken around the inside of the nostril rims. The medial crura are exposed and any tissue between them at the nasal tip is lifted, and they are advanced forward. The domes are brought together, thus the nasal tip is elevated and the skin flaps advanced.

However, it was realized that the fresh scars in the lip were often unsatisfactory so Millard (1971) introduced his two-stage operations for bilateral cleft lips. Then the forked flaps are saved at the original operation and banked in the floor of the nostril (see primary operation). Using this tissue the columella is lengthened in the pre-school period. The shape of the nostrils can be adjusted at the same time.

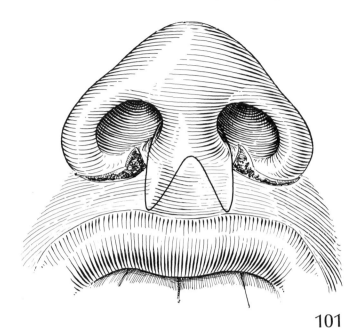

101

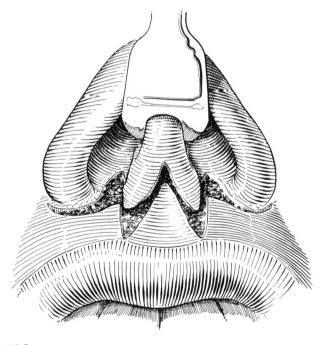

102

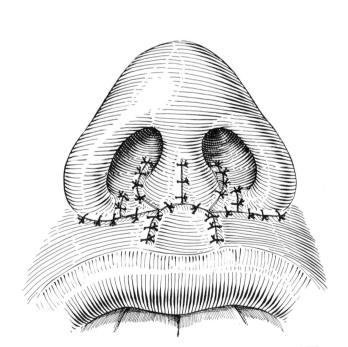

103

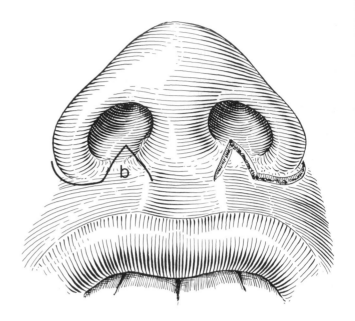

104

## ADJUSTMENT OF FLARING NOSTRILS

# 104 & 105

A flap *b* is raised from the nostril floor. A curved incision around the nostril base allows the base to be mobilized and rotated inwards. The resultant defect is filled by rotating the flap *b*.

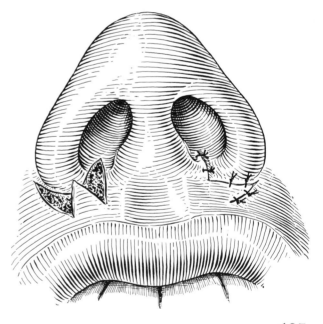

105

# Secondary operations on the palate

Palatal fistulas are usually closed, but only when the most active growth period has ceased, say after the age of 8 years. They rarely cause speech defects, but result in annoying leakages of food into the nose and interfere with the satisfactory seating of dentures. Closure can even be delayed until 18 years of age when it can be combined with rapid expansion of the maxilla and bone grafting.

Nasal speech results from velopharyngeal incompetence due to shortness of the palate, or from tightness or abnormal tethering of the muscles, and occasionally from paralysis. Speech abnormalities may be due to other factors, including poor lip function and tooth and alveolar deformity. The function of tongue and hearing must also be assessed.

## ASSESSMENT OF VELOPHARYNGEAL INCOMPETENCE

This begins with an aural assessment of speech, and more scientific assessments follow. Nasal airflow and pharyngeal pressure studies have been used, but the two investigations chiefly used are fluoroscopy and endoscopy. Examination of the velum from the mouth may be misleading because it does not reveal the point of contact, which is on the upper surface of the palate.

X-ray examination with still photographs is not very reliable and cine or videofluoroscopy in the lateral and sagittal planes, with or without augmentation with barium sulphate, are accepted as superior but require expensive equipment. X-rays can be combined with nasal endoscopy, and will generally confirm the degree of the velopharyngeal incompetence.

## NASENDOSCOPY

The Storz–Hopkins rigid 70 degree nasendoscope can be used in a high proportion of children over 8 years of age (Gilbert and Pigott, 1982). The patient, adjusted to a convenient height, sits facing the examiner and 4 per cent Xylocaine is used to provide local anaesthesia. A maximum of 1 ml is introduced by an intravenous catheter, to the tip of which is firmly attached a cotton wool bud with an external diameter of about 4 mm. Firstly the nose is cleared and the child given a sweet to suck. The catheter is introduced into the nasal vestibule and is allowed to rest there until the child is confident. It is then advanced about 1 cm and the Xylocaine introduced slowly. Progression continues until the catheter clears the posterior nares. Gagging usually occurs at this point and soon the catheter can be withdrawn, at the same time introducing the rest of the anaesthetic.

After clearing the nose the endoscope is passed slowly under direct vision after lifting the tip of the nose and taking care to run the instrument along the floor of the nose. Contact with the posterior pharyngeal wall must be avoided. All parts of the sphincter are watched during phonation.

## RE-OPERATION ON THE SOFT PALATE

In some cases it is clear that the muscular slings are defective because they have not been detached from the bony palate, or they have become re-attached. Then it is advisable to re-operate, paying particular attention to the proper alignment of the muscles, and to retropose the whole soft palate, using the Wardill type of posteriorly hinged flaps.

## ORTICOCHEA PHARYNGOPLASTY

# 106–110

Two lateral pharyngeal flaps are cut from the posterior pillars of the fauces so that they are superiorly based and contain palatopharyngeus muscle. They are reasonably long and wide, but the dissection is not taken too deep because of the adjacent internal carotid artery, and because the innervation from above must be preserved.

The transverse incision is made as high as possible and the superior edge is elevated. The lateral flaps are then sewn together end to end in the midline, taking care to include the muscular elements. Their medial edges are sewn to the superior edge of the horizontal incision, and their lateral edges are sewn together as far possible to produce a bulge of muscle, which is covered on its underside by the lateral margins of the mucosa.

This pharyngoplasty does not tether the velum as posterior flap operations do, and in fact may release any tightness in it. There are no problems with nasal discharge and it can be done after releasing posterior flap types of pharyngoplasties.

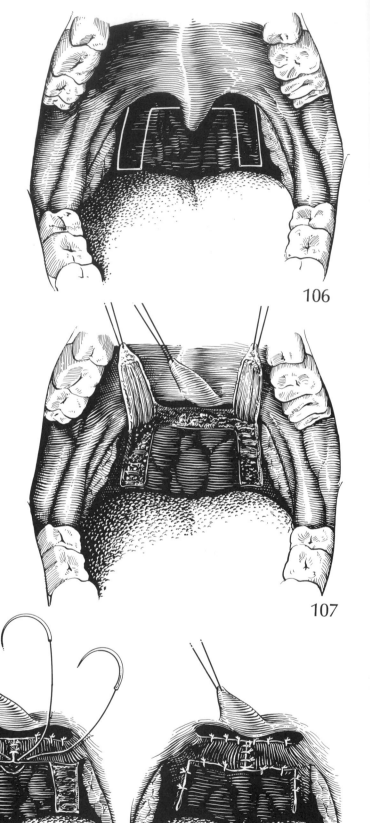

106

107

108                    109                    110

*Further reading*

## Anatomy and classification

Davis, J. S., Ritchie, H. P. (1922) Classification of congenital clefts of the lip and palate. Journal of the American Medical Association, 79, 1323–1327

Kernahan, D. A., Stark, R. B. (1958) A new classification for cleft lip and cleft palate. Plastic and Reconstructive Surgery, 22, 435–441

## Repair of the lip

Hamilton, R., Graham, W. P., Randall, P. (1971) The role of the lip adhesion procedure in cleft lip repair. Cleft Palate Journal, 8, 1–9

Le Mesurier, A. B. (1949) A method of cutting and suturing the lip in the treatment of complete unilateral clefts. Plastic and Reconstructive Surgery, 4, 1–12

Millard, D. R. (1964) Refinements in the rotation–advancement cleft lip technique. Plastic and Reconstructive Surgery, 33, 26–38

Millard, D. R. (1968) Extensions of the rotation–advancement principle for wide unilateral cleft lips. Plastic and Reconstructive Surgery, 42, 535–544

Millard, D. R. (1971) Closure of bilateral cleft lip and elongation of columella by two operations in infancy. Plastic and Reconstructive Surgery, 47, 324–331

Tennison, C. W. (1952) Repair of the unilateral cleft lip by the stencil method. Plastic and Reconstructive Surgery, 9, 115–120

Veau, V. (1938) Bec-de-Lièvre: formes cliniques, chirurgie. Paris: Masson et Cie

Wang, M. K. H. (1960) A modified Le Mesurier–Tennison technique in unilateral cleft lip repair. Plastic and Reconstructive Surgery, 26, 190–198

## Cleft palate

Braithwaite, F., Maurice, D. G. (1968) The importance of the levator palati muscle in cleft palate closure. British Journal of Plastic Surgery, 21, 60–62

Browne, D. (1935) An orthopaedic operation for cleft palate. British Medical Journal, 2, 1093–1095

Cronin, T. D. (1957) Surgery of the double cleft lip and protruding premaxilla. Plastic and Reconstructive Surgery, 19, 389–400

Cronin, T. D. (1957) Method of preventing raw area on the nasal surface of the soft palate in push-back surgery. Plastic and Reconstructive Surgery, 20, 474–484

Fara, M., Dvorak, J. (1970) Abnormal anatomy of the muscles of palatopharyngeal closure in cleft palates: anatomical and surgical considerations based on the autopsies of 18 unoperated cleft palates. Plastic and Reconstructive Surgery, 46, 488–497

Graber, T. B. (1964) Early Treatment of Cleft Lip and Palate. Berne and Stuttgart: Humber

Hotz, M. and Gnoinski, W. (1970) Comprehensive care of cleft lip and palate children at Zurich University. American Journal of Orthodontics, 70, 481–504

Jackson, I. T., McLennan, G., Scheker, L. R. (1983) Primary veloplasty or primary palatoplasty; some preliminary findings. Plastic and Reconstructive Surgery, 72, 153–157

Jolleys, A., Savage, J. P. (1963) Healing defects in cleft palate surgery – the role of infection. British Journal of Plastic Surgery, 16, 134–139

Limberg, A. (1927) Neue Wege in der radikalen Uranoplastik bei angeborenen Spaltendeformation. Zentralblat für Chirurgie, 20, 597–600

Robertson, N. R. E., Jolleys, A. (1974) The timing of hard palate repair. Scandinavian Journal of Plastic and Reconstructive Surgery, 8, 49–51

Slaughter, W. B., Pruzansky, S. (1954) The rationale for velar closure as a primary procedure in the repair of cleft palate defects. Plastic and Reconstructive Surgery, 13, 341–357

Schweckendiek, W. (1978) Primary veloplasty: long term results without maxillary deformity: a 25 year report. Cleft Palate Journal, 15, 268–274

Wardhill, W. E. M. (1937) The technique of operation for cleft palate. British Journal of Surgery, 25, 117–130

## Preoperative orthodontics and early bone grafting

Backdahl, M., Nordin, K. E. (1961) Replacement of the maxillary bone defect in cleft palate: a new procedure. Acta Chirurgica Scandinavica, 122, 131–137

Burston, W. R. (1958) The early orthodontic treatment of cleft palate conditions. Dental Practitioner, 9, (Nov) 41–56

Fish, J. (1972) Growth of the palatal shelves of post-alveolar cleft palate infants. British Dental Journal, 132, 492–501

Johanson, B., Friede, H. (1982) Discussion on 'The case for early bone grafting in cleft lip and cleft palate'. Plastic and Reconstructive Surgery, 70, 308–309

McNeil, C. K. (1956) Congenital oral deformities. British Dental Journal, 101, 191–198

Pruzansky, S. (1964) Presurgical orthopaedics and bone grafting for infants with cleft lip and palate – A dissent. Cleft Palate Journal, 1, 164–187

Robertson, N. R. E., Jolleys, A. (1983) An 11-year follow up of the effects of early bone grafting in infants born with complete clefts of the lip and palate. British Journal of Plastic Surgery, 36, 438–443

Rosenstein, S. W., Monroe, C. W., Kernahan, D. A., Jacobson, B. N., Griffith, B. H., Bauer, B. S. (1982) The case for early bone grafting in cleft lip and cleft palate. Plastic and Reconstructive Surgery, 70, 297–309

Skoog, T. (1967) The use of periosteum and Surgicel for bone formation in congenital clefts of the maxilla. Scandinavian Journal Plastic and Reconstructive Surgery, 1, 113–130

## Secondary operations on the lip and nose

Abbé, R. (1898) A new plastic operation for the relief of deformity due to double harelip. Medical Record of New York, 53, 477–478

Brown, J. B., McDowell, F. (1941) Secondary repair of cleft lips and their nasal deformities. Annals of Surgery, 114, 101–117

Converse, J. M. (1975) Correction of the drooping lateral portion of the cleft lip following the Le Mesurier repair. Plastic and Reconstructive Surgery, 55, 501–502

Converse, J. M., Hogan, V. M., Cupuis, C. C. (1970) Combined nose-lip repair in bilateral complete cleft lip deformities. Plastic and Reconstructive Surgery, 45, 109–118

Holdsworth, W. G. (1963) Later treatment of complete double cleft. British Journal of Plastic Surgery, 16, 127–133

Millard, D. R. (1958) Columella lengthening by a forked flap. Plastic and Reconstructive Surgery, 22, 454–457

Pigott, R. W., Millard, D. R. (1971) Cleft Lip and Palate. Boston: Little, Brown

## Secondary operation on the palate

Gilbert, T. S., Pigott, R. W. (1982) The feasibility of nasal pharyngoscopy using the 70 degrees Storz–Hopkins nasopharyngoscope. British Journal of Plastic Surgery, 35, 14–18

Glaser, E. R., Skolnick, M. L., McWilliams, B. J., Shprintzen, R. J. (1979) The dynamics of Passavant's ridge in subjects with and without velopharyngeal insufficiency: a multi-view videofluoroscopic study. Cleft Palate Journal, 16, 24–33

Jackson, I. T., Silverton, J. S. (1977) The sphincter pharyngoplasty as a secondary procedure in cleft palates. Plastic and Reconstructive Surgery, 59, 518–524

Lendrum, J., Dhar, B. K. (1984) The Orticochea dynamic pharyngoplasty. British Journal of Plastic Surgery, 37, 160–168

McWilliams, B. J., Glaser, E. R., Philips, B. J., Lawrence, C., Lavorato, A. S., Beery, Q. C. et al. (1981) A comparative study of four methods of evaluating velo-pharyngeal closure. Plastic and Reconstructive Surgery, 68, 1–10

Orticochea, M. (1968) Construction of a dynamic muscle sphincter in cleft palates. Plastic and Reconstructive Surgery, 41, 323–327

Orticochea, M. (1983) A review of 236 cleft palate patients treated with dynamic muscle sphincter. Plastic and Reconstructive Surgery, 71, 180–188

Riski, J. E., Serafin, D., Riefkohl, R., Georgiade, G. S., Georgiade, N. G. (1984) A rationale for modifying the insertion of the Orticochea pharyngoplasty. Plastic and Reconstructive Surgery, 73, 882–894

Skolnick, M. L. (1970) Videofluoroscopic examination of the velopharyngeal portal during phonation in lateral and base projections: a new technique for studying the mechanics of closure. Cleft Palate Journal, 7, 803–816

# Ranula

**R. J. Brereton**
Senior Lecturer in Paediatric Surgery, Institute of Child Health, University of London, London, UK

## Aetiology

A simple ranula (little frog) is a thin-walled cyst in the floor of the mouth, of uncertain aetiology, but said to arise either as a result of myxomatous degeneration of a mucous gland or from extravasation from a ductule of the sublingual or submandibular salivary gland. The latter aetiology would explain those cases in which there is a high concentration of amylase in the clear viscid liquid which gives the cyst a blue tinge when seen through the oral mucosa. The swelling arises on one side of the midline, but may reach enormous size, filling the whole of the mouth and causing respiratory problems, especially in the neonate.

The much rarer 'plunging ranula' may be of branchogenic origin and extends deeply, with communications to the structures of the neck and pharynx.

## Choice of treatment

Complete excision of a large cyst is a difficult and hazardous procedure. Marsupialization of the cyst into the floor of the mouth is by far the safest and simplest method of treatment.

## Preoperative

### Anaesthesia

For small lesions, general anaesthesia by means of an orotracheal tube may be possible, but for large lesions in young infants a nasotracheal tube and pharyngeal pack should be used.

### Position of patient and preparation

The patient is placed in the supine position. The mouth and lips are cleaned with 1 per cent cetrimide or aqueous povidone-iodine solution. A head towel to cover the anaesthetic tubing, hair and face (except for the mouth) is recommended, with additional towels over the neck and thorax.

## The operation

The mouth is held open with a gag; in small infants, a self-retaining retractor may be sufficient. A stitch or Allis forceps applied to the tongue helps to expose the lesion. The course of the distorted lingual vessels and submandibular ducts should be identified in order to avoid damage to these structures.

## 1

Three or four stay sutures of 3/0 silk may be inserted around the periphery of the proposed elliptical incision to help identify the mucosa of the floor of the mouth once the ranula has been punctured. The cyst is best uncapped by needle diathermy.

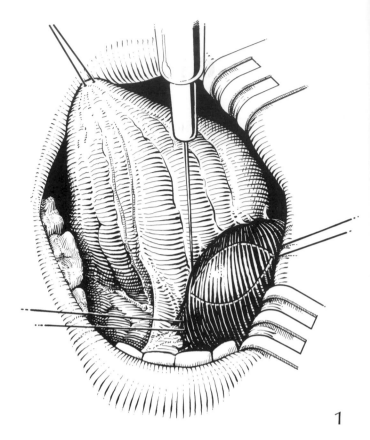

1

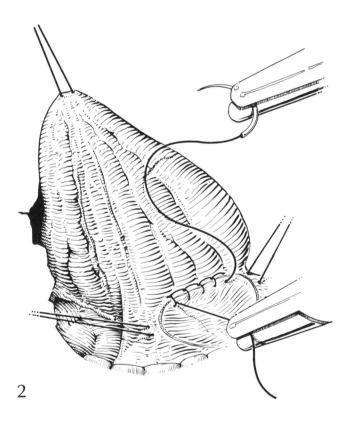

2

## 2

The edges of the cyst are sutured to the mucosa with a running locked stitch of 4/0 or 3/0 chromic catgut so that the postoperative oedema will tighten the stitch and prevent reactionary haemorrhage. In older children, infiltration of 0.5 per cent bupivacaine may be used to the same effect and also provides relief from pain.

## Postoperative treatment

No special care is required and oral feeds may be restarted after 3–4 hours.
 Recurrence is rare.

Illustrations by Kevin Marks

# Thyroglossal cyst and fistula

**R. J. Brereton**
Senior Lecturer in Paediatric Surgery, Institute of Child Health, University of London, London, UK

## Introduction

The thyroid gland develops mainly from the median bud of the pharynx and descends to its final position in the neck, leaving the thyroglossal duct, which extends caudally from the foramen caecum of the tongue to the pyramidal lobe of the gland, passing either anterior, through or posterior to the body of the hyoid bone. The duct normally disappears and the lateral lobes of the gland receive contributions from the fourth branchial cleft. Thyroid remnants may be found anywhere along the course of the thyroglossal duct[1,2].

Thyroglossal cysts most frequently arise just below the level of the hyoid bone and form the commonest anterior cervical swellings in children. Occasionally the duct deviates anterosuperiorly once it has passed the hyoid bone, giving rise to a thyroglossal cyst in the submental triangle, where it may be mistaken for a dermoid cyst. Although the latter may occur below the hyoid bone, they are more common in the submental triangle. They can be distinguished from thyroglossal cysts by their softer 'putty-like' consistency. Very occasionally, aberrant thyroid glandular tissue may be found along this track.

### Aims of surgery

The aim of surgery is to remove the entire duct, including the central part of the body of the hyoid bone, to the level of the foramen caecum[1,2]. Since side branches may arise from the duct within the muscles of the tongue, the intraglossal part of the duct should be removed with a surrounding cuff of muscle approximately 0.5 cm in diameter. Complete excision is essential in order to prevent recurrence and because of the risk of malignant degeneration[3]. All thyroglossal cysts, however small, should be excised once diagnosed since eventual inflammation and infection are common, making subsequent surgery more difficult and cosmetically less satisfactory.

## Preoperative

Preoperative isotope scanning or ultrasound examination to determine the precise location of the thyroid gland is recommended since, in thyroid hypoplasia, a small central area of aberrant ectopic thyroid tissue may be mistaken for a thyroglossal cyst and removal may be followed by hypothyroidism[4]. However, operation should not be deferred because of the lack of scanning facilities, as the incidence of such aberrant tissue is low (about 1 per cent of all thyroglossal abnormalities[5]) and the error should be easily recognized when the lesion is exposed.

Since occult staphylococcal infection is common, perioperative antibiotic cover is usually indicated. A penicillinase-resistant agent such as cloxacillin (Orbenin) or fusidic acid (Fucidin) is most appropriate.

### Anaesthesia

General anaesthesia using an orotracheal tube is recommended.

# The operation

## THYROGLOSSAL CYST

# 1

### The incision

The patient is placed supine with the head extended and the shoulders elevated on a small sandbag. A short transverse incision is made in a skin crease over the main prominence of the cyst. The length of the incision rarely needs to exceed 3 cm. Some authors recommend infiltration of the skin with adrenaline to prevent haemorrhage.

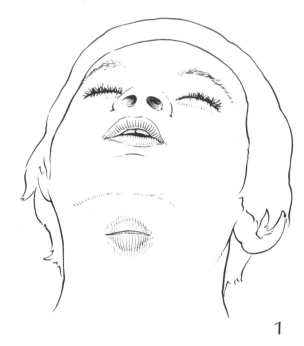

1

# 2

The subcutaneous fat, platysma and deep cervical fascia are incised in the line of the incision with a diathermy needle, and the cyst is freed from its superficial attachments by a combination of sharp and blunt dissection.

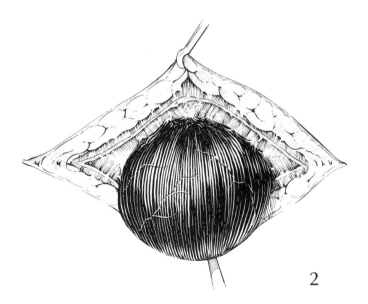

2

3

# 3

The tract is identified at its deep attachment to the cyst and traced between the sternohyoid muscles to the hyoid bone. Using a diathermy needle, the centrum of the hyoid bone is freed from the sternohyoid muscles below and the mylohyoid and geniohyoid muscles above. The thyrohyoid membrane is separated from the posterior aspect of the centrum using either artery forceps, a closed pair of scissors or a McDonald dissector. Bone cutting forceps or strong Mayo scissors are then used to divide the body of the hyoid 5 mm from the midline on each side. This manoeuvre is facilitated by grasping and steadying the bone with Kocher artery forceps.

## 4

A cylinder of geniohyoid and genioglossus muscles 0.5–1.0 cm wide (depending on the size of the patient) and including the duct is then excised up to the foramen caecum. This is best done with needle diathermy. It has been suggested that this part of the dissection is facilitated by asking the anaesthetist to use his or her finger to depress the foramen caecum into the wound, but this manoeuvre is seldom of practical value and potentially dangerous for the anaesthetist. Diathermy is used to secure meticulous haemostasis.

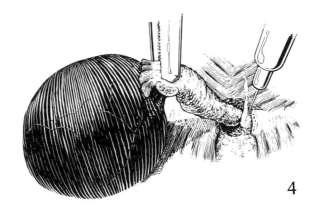

4

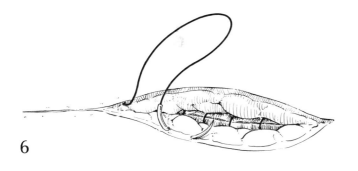

5

## Closure

## 5

The muscles are approximated in the midline using sutures of 3/0 polyglycolic acid or chromic catgut to aid haemostasis. It is not necessary to reconstitute the hyoid bone, the cut ends of which tend to be approximated by the sutures in the muscles.

## 6

The fascia and platysma are closed with a continuous suture of 3/0 or 4/0 polyglycolic acid or chromic catgut and the same suture is used in the subcutaneous layer to appose the skin edges. Alternatively, the skin edges may be approximated with self-adhesive wound tapes. Non-absorbable skin sutures or clips are not recommended, as their removal causes unnecessary anxiety and discomfort. Provided that good haemostasis has been secured, neither a drain nor a dressing is required.

6

## Postoperative care

It is important to ensure that the airway does not become obstructed by reactionary haemorrhage. Since infection is common and spreading cellulitis may cause airway compression, it is prudent to continue oral antibiotics for a further two or three days. The child is allowed home on the day following the procedure.

## Results

Local excision of the cyst is not recommended since more than 20 per cent of patients so treated later develop recurrences, which in some cases may not become evident for a decade or more. Removal of the central part of the hyoid bone reduces the recurrence rate to below 5 per cent, and if the cyst and duct are both excised, as recommended, recurrence is least likely[1, 2, 6].

### THYROGLOSSAL FISTULA

This usually results from rupture or incision of an inflamed thyroglossal cyst, but the orifice often appears quite low down on the neck. Recurrent discharge and inflammation are common symptoms.

The treatment is as for a thyroglossal cyst, all traces of the fistula being excised to the foramen caecum. The recurrence rate, however, is higher than for the uncomplicated cyst.

## 7

A small elliptical incision is made around the orifice of the fistula (sinus) in the neck.

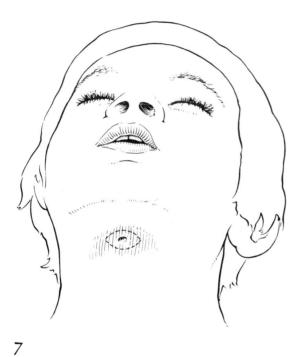

7

## 8

The ellipse of skin including the sinus and fistulous tract is traced through the subcutaneous tissues towards the hyoid bone.

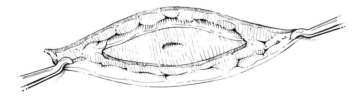

8

## 9

The centrum of the hyoid bone is resected *en bloc* with the fistulous tract.

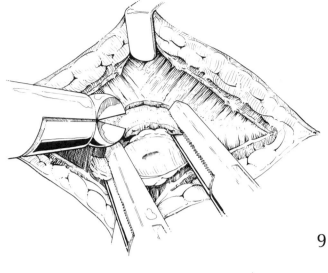

9

## 10

A core of geniohyoid and genioglossus muscles including the tract is excised up to the level of the foramen caecum.
Closure is as for a thyroglossal cyst. A drain may be necessary if perfect haemostasis cannot be guaranteed.

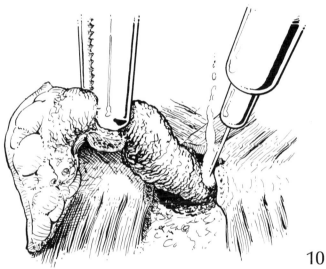

10

## References

1. Sistrunk, W. E. (1920) The surgical treatment of cysts of the thyroglossal tract. Annals of Surgery, 71, 121–123

2. Sistrunk, W. E. (1928) Techniques of removal of cysts and sinuses of the thyroglossal duct. Surgery, Gynecology and Obstetrics, 46, 109–112

3. Lui, A. H. F., Littler, E. R. (1970) Thyroid carcinoma originating in a thyroglossal cyst: report of a case. American Surgeon, 36, 546–548

4. Pulito, A. R., Shaw, A. (1973) Median ectopic thyroid gland. Journal of Pediatric Surgery, 8, 73–74

5. Gross, R. E. (1953) The Surgery of Infancy and Childhood, pp. 936–959. Philadelphia: W. B. Saunders

6. Brereton, R. J., Symonds, E. (1978) Thyroglossal cysts in children. British Journal of Surgery, 65, 507–508

# Branchial cyst and sinuses

**John F. R. Bentley**   FRCS, FRCS(Ed), FRCS(Glas)
Formerly Consultant Surgeon, Royal Hospital for Sick Children, Glasgow, UK

## Embryogenesis and anatomy

Five branchial arches form the neck and pharynx, the first giving rise to the mandible. Each arch has a core of cartilage, a muscle mass, a nerve, and an artery. Between the arches there are external depressions or clefts and internal depressions or pouches. The clefts are covered by squamous epithelium and the pouches are covered by columnar epithelium. The second arch grows quicker than those below and the consequent overhang produces the cervical sinus. The second arch ultimately droops caudally to fuse with the fifth, and the cervical sinus normally degenerates and disappears. Should degeneration of the cervical sinus be arrested, a branchial cyst or cervical branchial sinus results. The orifice of the sinus will be on the line of the anterior border of the sternomastoid muscle, and commonly just above the sternoclavicular joint. From the orifice a tract runs up along the anterior border of the sternomastoid to turn medially and pierce the deep fascia at the level of the upper border of the thyroid cartilage. It passes between the internal and external carotid arteries, below the posterior belly of the digastric muscle, to approach the tonsillar fossa, which represents the second branchial pouch. In so doing it is related closely to the facial, hypoglossal and glossopharyngeal nerves, and to the jugular and common facial veins.

Anomalous development can also involve the posterior end of the first branchial cleft, which is concerned with the external auditory meatus. A tiny blind accessory orifice can form on the crus helix of the pinna, or between the crus helix and the tragus. The tract of this preauricular sinus is surrounded by cartilage, and passes downwards and forwards for 5 mm or so. The lesion tends to occur in families.

A first arch cyst may arise in the submandibular region and may communicate with the external auditory meatus by a track in close proximity to the facial nerve. If infected, such a cyst is not uncommonly mistaken for a submandibular lymph gland abscess. Incision may be followed by a persistent submandibular sinus.

## Preoperative

### Indications for excision

There are no age limits for operation, but on general grounds elective excision is avoided in early infancy.

#### Branchial cyst

A branchial cyst is neither inherently harmful nor subject to sinister complications, but it persists and slowly increases in size. The obvious swelling draws more attention than the neat scar following excision, which also permits confirmation of the diagnosis.

#### Cervical branchial sinus

A cervical branchial sinus is not inherently harmful although it may be a minor source of annoyance (but seldom to the child) due to its occasionally exuding a spot of bland discharge. Infection is a rare complication and the effects can be mitigated with antibiotic treatment. As the clinical features are characteristic, the diagnosis is not in doubt. The lesion is almost imperceptible to a casual glance and often hidden by clothing. The scars following excision are more noticeable. On balance, excision may not be advantageous to the patient.

### Dangers and safeguards

#### Branchial cysts and cervical branchial sinuses

Operative damage to related anatomical structures and incomplete excision constitute the specific dangers. The safeguards are a knowledge of the anatomy, and meticulous haemostasis during dissection to ensure clear vision.

### Anaesthesia

Endotracheal inhalation general anaesthesia is preferred.

# The operations

### Excision of a branchial cyst

## Position of patient, skin cleansing and towelling

The patient is placed supine with a soft ring beneath the cranium and a sandbag beneath the shoulders so that the neck is extended. The foot of the table is lowered slightly to diminish venous blood pressure in the head and neck. The chin is turned away from the affected side. A diathermy plate is applied to a thigh. The skin is cleansed with 1 per cent povidine-iodine rather than chlorhexidine in 70 per cent of alcohol, as the former carries a much reduced risk of fire from the use of diathermy. Four towels are required. For a branchial cyst or cervical sinus, one towel is placed along each side of the neck, extending to cover the shoulder. The third towel is placed across the chest with the upper edge just below the clavicles. The fourth towel is first spread over the other so that its upper edge lies below the chin and it is clipped to the side towels at the level of the mastoid processes. The lower edge of this towel is then lifted upwards to raise the towel so as to cover the chin and face. For a preauricular sinus, the four towels are arranged to leave a 'window' exposing the pinna and tragus.

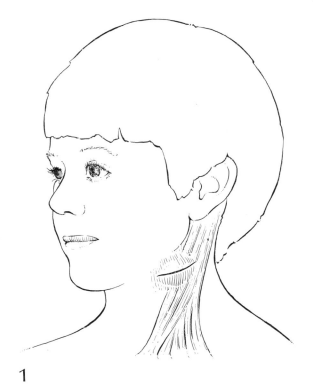

1

# 1

## Infiltration and incision

Infiltration of the overlying skin and the tissues adjacent to the cyst with dilute noradrenaline in isotonic saline (2 ml Levophed, 1:1000 in 500 ml isotonic saline) facilitates haemostasis and dissection. The volume injected is kept to a minimum consistent with effective infiltration. The needle tip is moved to a new position before each increment, the syringe plunger being withdrawn briefly before each injection to establish that no blood can be aspirated, thus avoiding undesirable intravascular dosage.

A collar incision is outlined overlying the cyst. This is done by applying a taut length of 2/0 ligature material firmly to the skin of the neck in the line of the proposed incision. When removed, a temporary indentation is apparent. Marking dye (Bonney's blue, brilliant green and crystal violet paint) is used to make cross lines for matching the closing sutures. (Scratch marks are avoided as they may form keloid.) The length of the incision will vary with the size of the cyst; it often extends from the centre of the ipsilateral thyroid cartilage to the centre of the belly of the adjacent sternomastoid muscle. A scalpel is used to incise the skin only, and subsequent dissection is with the diathermy needle.

# 2

## Exposure of the cyst

The incision is carried through the subcutaneous tissues and platysma to the deep cervical fascia. The flaps are then retracted upwards and downwards to expose the cyst. They are best held in place by a self-retaining retractor. The deep cervical fascia is divided at the anterior border of the sternomastoid muscle to allow the belly of the muscle to be retracted backwards, away from the cyst. Exposure is extended anteriorly by retraction of the sternohyoid muscle. Lifting and incising the overlying fascia exposes the superficial aspect of the cyst.

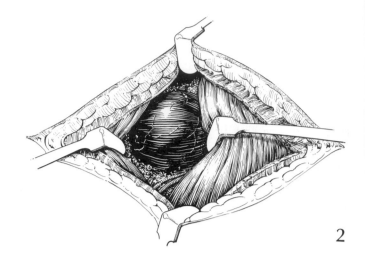

2

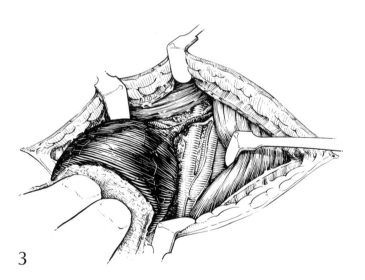

3

# 3

## Isolation and removal of the cyst

Rupture of the cyst is avoided, as the tense wall is easier to define. The adjacent structures are separated by gentle blunt dissection along the wall, special care being taken on the deep anterior aspect of the cyst where the jugular vein is an intimate relation. The pedicle of the cyst lies posterior to the jugular vein. When it is defined distinctly it is clamped and cut superficial to the clamp with a scalpel to allow the cyst to be removed. The pedicle is ligated with a 3/0 ligature applied deep to the clamp which is then removed. Haemostasis is secured before wound closure.

In dissection of the less common first cleft cyst, care must be taken to avoid damage to the adjacent facial nerve if there is a track leading up towards or into the external auditory meatus.

# 4

## Wound closure

The cervical fascia and platysma are closed with interrupted sutures of 4/0 polyglycolic acid. The skin is closed with interrupted sutures of 5/0 nylon which are removed on the fourth postoperative day. A plastic spray (OpSite) is applied as a wound dressing.

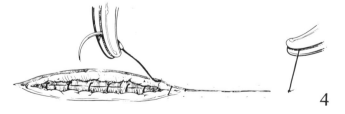

4

### Excision of a cervical branchial sinus

### Infiltration and incision

Haemostasis and dissection are made easier by preliminary infiltration of the skin in the line of the incision and the tissues around the sinus tract using dilute noradrenaline (Levophed, 2 ml 1:1000 in 500 ml isotonic saline). The volume of injection is only sufficient for effective infiltration. The needle tip is moved to a new position before each increment, and the plunger of the syringe is withdrawn to see that no blood is aspirated before the injection is made, so avoiding administration into blood vessels.

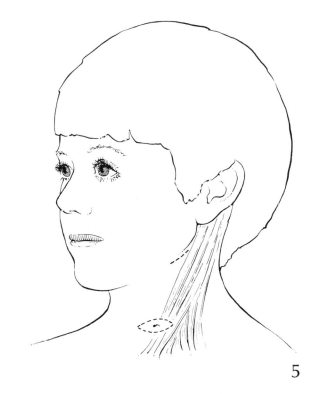

5

# 5 & 6

The use of a single low incision or two 'step-ladder' incisions is a matter of choice. If two incisions are used their combined length will equal that of the alternative single collar incision that may be made at the level of the sinus orifice. Such an incision is preferable, as the scar will often be hidden by clothing. In length it will equal the distance from the sinus orifice to the tonsillar fossa, and it will be centred on the orifice, which it surrounds elliptically. The incision may be outlined as indicated. The skin only is incised with a scalpel, and subsequent dissection is with the diathermy needle.

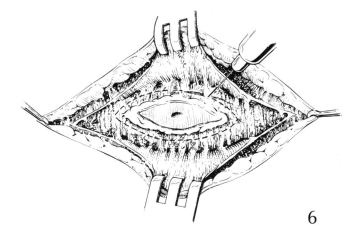

6

## Skin flaps

The platysma is divided to expose the deep cervical fascia and the upper flap is mobilized and retracted upwards to expose the superficial surface of the sternomastoid muscle.

# 7

## Dissection of the sinus tract

The deep cervical fascia is divided along the anterior border of the sternomastoid muscle to reveal the sinus tract. This is dissected free of the muscle with the help of gentle elevation of the mobilized orifice. The tract penetrates medially at the level of the upper border of the thyroid cartilage. The deep fascia is cleared from the carotid arteries and posterior belly of the digastric muscle at this level. The anaesthetist can then assist by placing a finger into the mouth to push the related tonsillar fossa laterally to facilitate the deeper dissection of the tract. When this is completed between the carotid vessels, a curved clamp is applied and the tract is ligated deep to the clamp with 3/0 chromic catgut. The sinus is then excised and the clamp removed. Haemostasis of the wound is then completed.

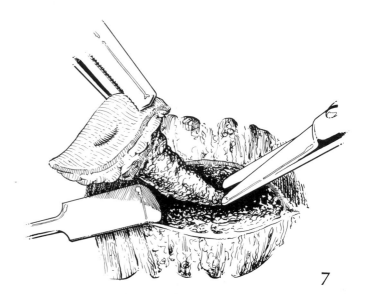

7

## Wound closure

The cervical fascia and platysma are closed with interrupted sutures of 4/0 polyglycolic acid. The skin is closed with interrupted sutures of 5/0 nylon which are removed on the fourth postoperative day. A plastic spray (OpSite) is applied as a wound dressing.

# External angular dermoid

**R. J. Brereton** FRCS
Senior Lecturer in Paediatric Surgery, Institute of Child Health, University of London, London, UK

This is one of the commonest sites for a dermoid cyst. In infancy and childhood there are few conditions that will cause diagnostic confusion. The cyst always lies in a shallow, saucer-like depression in the bone, but occasionally it is deeper, almost surrounded by bone. A tiny pit is invariably present in the base of the bony depression, through which the cyst receives its blood supply. Occasionally, the pit is larger and there may be a dumb-bell extension of the cyst which erodes the orbital plate of the frontal bone and lies in contact with the dura of the anterior cranial fossa.

The treatment is complete excision of the cyst.

## Preoperative investigation

A plain radiograph may be reassuring, but it is usually difficult to be certain of the size and depth of the defect in the frontal region.

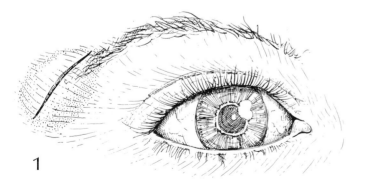

1

## The operation

### 1

In the majority of cases, the cyst can be totally excised through an incision 1.5 cm long and placed just above the hairline of the eyebrow on the affected side. The eyebrow should not be removed by shaving. Haemorrhage from the feeding vessels may be profuse, so facilities for electrocoagulation should be available.

## 2

The cyst is exposed by separating the fibres of the eyebrow muscle. A small margin of periosteum of the frontal bone, beyond the edges of the cyst, is cleared.

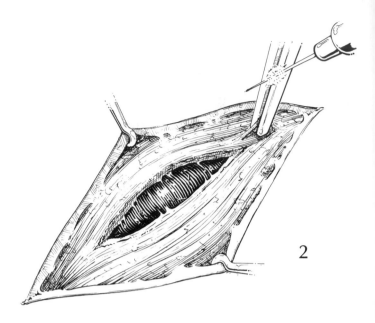

2

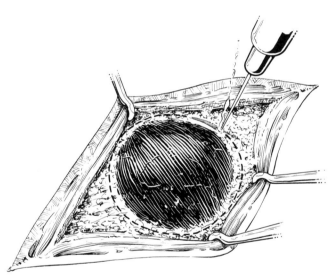

3

## 3 & 4

A fringe of periosteum 1 mm wide is incised around the cyst with needle diathermy. The periosteum is freed from the bone and used to hold the cyst. Instruments should not be applied directly to the cyst since this usually causes it to rupture, making removal more difficult. The periosteum is freed around the entire circumference of the cyst and then, using blunt or sharp dissection, the periosteum from the saucer-like depression in the frontal bone is elevated along with the cyst. Should the cyst rupture, simple excision of the remaining lining along with the periosteum from the frontal depression will suffice.

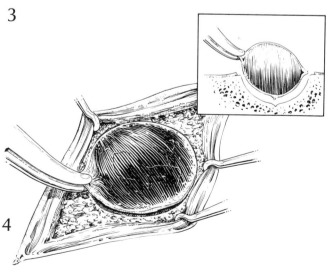

4

## 5

The feeding vessels passing through the pit of the bony depression are coagulated. Bleeding from the depression in the frontal bone which has been denuded of its periosteum is not a problem.

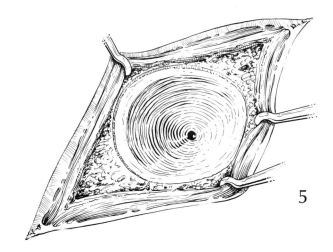

5

6

## 6

The wound is closed with a subcuticular suture to the skin.

In the rare event of an intracranial extension, an osteoplastic craniotomy will be required since the intracranial portion may be the larger of the two elements. It is not safe to attempt removal by simply nibbling away the orbital plate of the frontal bone.

# Sternomastoid (fibrous) torticollis

**Peter G. Jones**  MS, FRCS, FRACS, FACS, FAAP (Hon)
Surgeon, The Royal Children's Hospital, Melbourne, Victoria, Australia

## Clinical presentation

Fibrosis of the sternomastoid muscle may be recognized at one of three distinct phases:

1. In the infant aged 2–4 weeks, when it presents as a 'woody-hard tumour' located within the substance of the muscle. It occurs in 1 in 200 live births and is more common following breech delivery. In over 90 per cent of cases the tumour regresses spontaneously by 5–7 months of age, leaving no sequelae. In 1 per cent of cases torticollis develops.
2. In the toddler aged 6–24 months as a uniform, thickened and shortened sternomastoid muscle causing torticollis, restricting rotation of the head towards the affected side, and tilting to the opposite side.
3. In the older child in whom torticollis has only recently been recognized. There is a tight, narrow, 1–2 cm band within the shortened sternomastoid muscle, which also results in torticollis with restricted movement and more marked facial asymmetry (which may be more noticeable after correction, and hence should be pointed out to the parents before the operation).

## Indications for operation

'Established torticollis' rarely occurs before 8–9 months of age, and most children requiring operation present after the age of 2 years. A tight, fibrous and shortened sternomastoid muscle is present, with facial hemihypoplasia and diminution of the vertical (orbitomental) height. There will also be disuse atrophy of the ipsilateral trapezius muscle.

Other causes of torticollis (e.g. ocular, spastic or osseous) should be excluded.

# The operation

## Preparation

Apart from a photograph to demonstrate and record the effect on the growth of the face and an X-ray of the cervical spine to exclude hemivertebrae, the only preparation is the introduction of physiotherapy, which will be critical to the success of postoperative recovery.

## Anaesthesia

Endotracheal anaesthesia is employed to allow access to the neck and to permit a full range of rotation during operation in order to ensure that all secondary restricting structures in the adjacent fasciae have been divided. The tubing is carried over the forehead, where it is fixed in the midline with strapping.

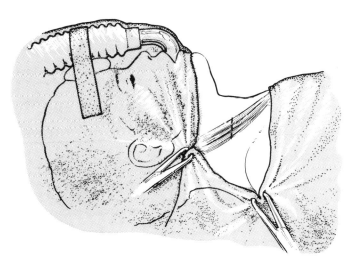

1

## Position

The patient is placed supine with the head slightly elevated and the neck slightly extended. This position is maintained by a small sandbag beneath the seventh cervical spinous process, and by a circular hollow sculpted in a block of sponge rubber to accommodate the occipital region of the head.

Slight rotation of the head away from the affected muscle is helpful in selecting the skin crease for the incision.

Loose or long hair is tied back in a 'pony tail', and short hair near the base of the mastoid process is plastered down with Vaseline or a dampened cake of soap. No shaving is necessary.

## Skin preparation

This should extend from the front of the shoulders across the upper sternum, up to the lower lip in the midline, and laterally to a point behind the anterior border of trapezius on both sides.

# 1

## Draping

One of the simplest methods is to use a full sheet extending downwards from the manubrium, and doubled small drapes passed beneath the head (held forward by the anaesthetist). The upper drape is then brought forward, its lower edge following the superior nuchal line, covering the ear, to meet the other half in the midline at a point just below the lower lip. The second small drape is then brought around each deltoid to be attached to the sheet covering the chest. The area is thus draped so that the neck can be put through a full range of cervical rotation during the operation without interfering with the sterility of the field.

## Level of division

The sternomastoid muscle may be divided at various levels:

1. at the upper end near the mastoid process;
2. at the lower end at the supraclavicular fossa;
3. at the upper *and* lower ends;
4. in the 'middle'.

Division of the muscle at the junction of the upper and middle thirds is recommended, as it is well below the course of the facial and accessory nerves. The ascending cutaneous nerves from the cervical plexus passing obliquely across the sternomastoid are easily identified and avoided.

## The incision

# 2 & 3

This is made in a convenient skin crease over the sternomastoid muscle. The actual site and direction of the incision is determined by the particular anatomy of the individual patient, and in all instances need not be more than 5 cm in length.

The incision is deepened through platysma, dividing the external jugular vein and also the anterior jugular vein when the line of the incision crosses them. The surface of the sternomastoid muscle is then cleared, and displayed by a pair of retractors.

The dissection is next carried around the deep aspect of the muscle, closely following the areolar planes which separate it from the carotid sheath and omohyoid muscle.

At the posterior border of the muscle, several branches of the cervical plexus emerge from the fascia colli to run upwards (auricular) and downwards (supraclavicular) on the superficial aspect of the muscle.

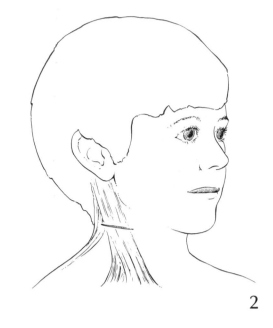

2

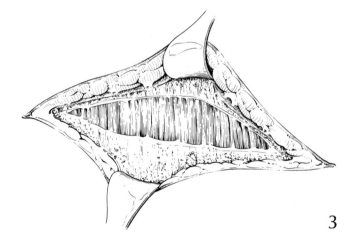

3

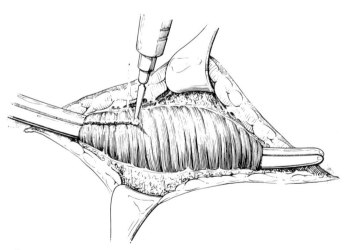

4

# 4

A curved artery forceps is then introduced in the plane between the internal jugular vein and the deep surface of the sternomastoid muscle.

# 5

The sternomastoid is then divided as follows:

1. the superficial fibres are divided using cutting diathermy applied to bundles of muscle fibres picked up between fine-toothed forceps;
2. the deepest fibres closest to the haemostat are divided with a scalpel, cutting outwards.

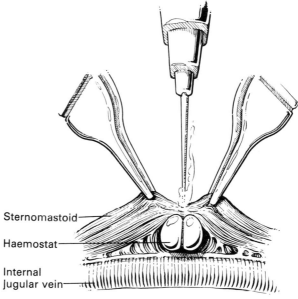

Sternomastoid

Haemostat

Internal
Jugular vein

5

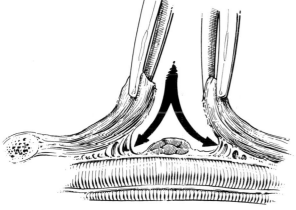

6

# 6

The ends of the transected muscle retract. Each end is picked up with toothed tissue forceps, and the deep surface of each segment completely freed from the carotid sheath. The lower end tends to have a posterior falciform ridge of fascia, which should be freed down behind its sternal and clavicular attachments.

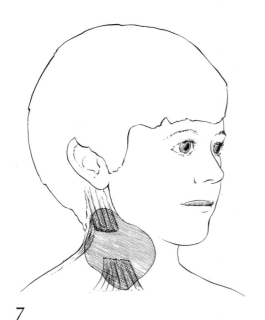

7

# 7

Any remaining contractures in adjacent soft tissue are then sought and divided, as far anteriorly as the midline, and posteriorly to the anterior border of trapezius (shaded area). In a minority of severe cases the carotid sheath itself may need to be divided down to the adventitia of the jugular vein. The omohyoid muscle, in contrast, is usually lax and elastic, and almost never requires division.

The head is then slowly rotated fully, to right and left, with an index finger in the wound to detect any remaining tight strands of fascia, which are divided as necessary.

Haemostasis is carefully checked, since a haematoma filling the gap in the muscle may vitiate the result.

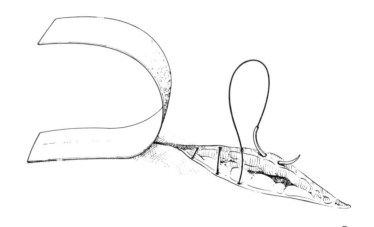

8

# 8, 9 & 10

The skin is closed with Dexon, 3/0 interrupted sutures in the platysma and subcutaneous tissues, and a 4/0 subcuticular to appose the edges of the incision.

A double dressing is applied: a Band-aid size piece of Dermahesive on the skin, covered by a wad of dressing held in place over the operation area with a loosely applied 3-inch crêpe bandage. This discourages venous oozing, and holds the head in a slightly overcorrected position.

On recovery from anaesthesia, the patient is nursed supine, without pillows, and with a large sandbag supporting the head on each side. This obviates the need for active use of the neck muscles while the head is kept still, in a neutral (anatomical) position, for forty-eight hours. Sedation, e.g. with chloral, may be required for patients less than 4 or 5 years of age.

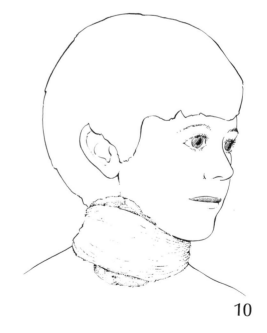

9

10

# Postoperative management

Two days later the outer dressing is removed, pillows are supplied progressively until the patient is sitting erect and able to walk without postural fainting. Normal bathing or showering can begin immediately.

A full range of physiotherapy is recommended immediately. Older children are taught before operation what will be required of them afterwards.

Lateral and anteroposterior flexion exercises are supervised for another 1 to 2 days in hospital, until patient, physiotherapist and parents are confident that exercises will be continued satisfactorily at home.

Retraining the neck-righting reflexes in front of a mirror is continued for three months, monitoring progress weekly for one month, and monthly thereafter.

# Complications

These are infrequent and seldom serious, except for intraoperative bleeding from injury to the jugular vein. With care this risk can be eliminated, remembering that occasionally a large, short vein draining the muscle opens directly into the jugular vein.

1. Bleeding can usually be controlled with finger-tip pressure while the muscle is divided, following which the bleeding can be readily controlled by a ligature, or rarely, a vascular suture such as 5/0 Ticron.
2. A haematoma can collect in the gap between the ends of the muscle, and may need evacuation if discretely localized.
3. Young children may not cooperate in physiotherapy, in which case an 'asymmetric' Zimmer collar maintaining overcorrection can be applied between exercises.
4. Recurrence of the torticollis can develop, even after careful complete division, but this should occur in less than 1 per cent of cases submitted to operation.
5. Cervical hypoaesthesia over an ill-defined area of 2 × 2 cm in the region of the submandibular triangle is occasionally found at a postoperative visit. This is usually a temporary neurapraxia following trauma to a nerve crossing the muscle. Very rarely the hypoaesthesia persists indefinitely but seldom bothers the patient.
6. Damage to the accessory nerve is a theoretical possibility, not yet encountered by the author in over a hundred operations.

Illustrations by Kevin Marks

# Protruding ears

**I. W. Broomhead**   MA, MB, MChir, FRCS
Consultant Plastic Surgeon, Guy's Hospital and The Hospital for Sick Children, Great Ormond Street, London, UK

## CLASSIFICATION

## 1–5

A normal ear is shown in Illustration 1, a protruding ear with a normal antihelix fold (*see Illustration 2*), a protruding ear with no antihelix fold (*see Illustration 3*), a 'rosebud' type of ear (*see Illustration 4*), a 'lop-ear' which has an excessive droop or overhang of the upper pole (*see Illustration 5*).

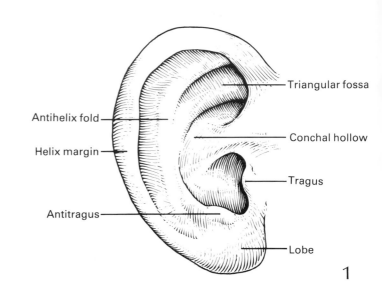

1

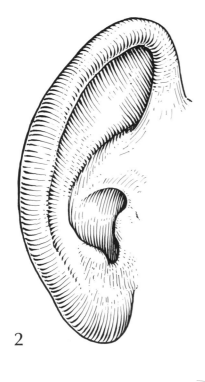

2

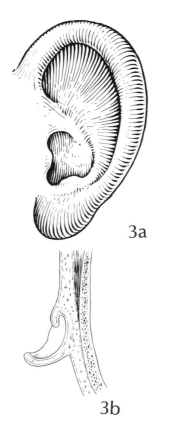

3a

3b

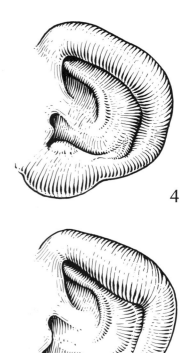

4

5

## Timing of operation

Although it is sometimes recommended that surgery is not carried out until the ear is fully grown, at about 7 years, many children will by this time have already suffered from teasing at school. On these grounds the operation is advisable at 3½ years of age and can be safely carried out at this time. Some flexibility is, of course necessary depending on the severity of the deformity.

No specific preoperative preparation is required except for a photograph, which is essential for complete records.

It is wise to cover the operation and postoperative period with antibiotics. Infection is rare, but the disasters which can follow a chondritis must be avoided.

# The operations

### CORRECTION OF EAR WITH EITHER NORMAL OR ABSENT ANTIHELIX FOLD[1]

Correction is achieved by excision of postauricular skin, and reshaping of the cartilage along the existing antihelix fold or, if the fold is absent, by cartilage excision.

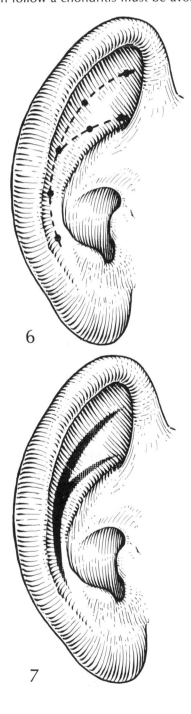

## 6

The skin is first marked along the prominence of the antihelix fold and triangular fossa with Bonney's blue. The cartilage is then tattooed at the points indicated by transfixing the ear with a straight cutting needle and then withdrawing the needle after applying Bonney's blue to its distal part.

## 7

The extent of cartilage to be excised (shaded area) depends on the severity of the protrusion.

## Skin excision

The width and direction of the skin excision in the postauricular region varies with each case, and depends on the severity of the deformity and the sites of maximum ear protrusion.

# 8

The helix margin is transfixed with a 3/0 silk stitch to assist in holding the ear forwards.

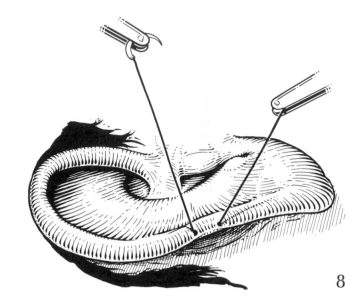

8

# 9

The ellipse is vertically placed if the protrusion is uniform and is marked on the back of the ear with Bonney's blue.

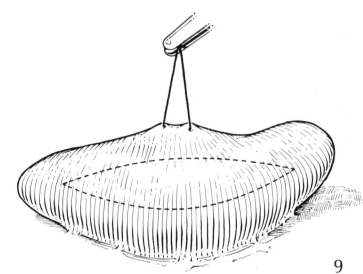

9

# 10

If the upper or lower poles of the ears show excessive protrusion, then the skin excision swings somewhat horizontally forwards at these sites.

10

## 11

The ellipse is usually placed ⅓ lateral and ⅔ medial to the blue tattooed dots, and is excised cleanly from the cartilage after incision by blunt stripping with sharp pointed scissors. The advantages achieved by removing the skin cleanly from the cartilage are (a) the majority of the bleeding points are on the medial aspect and can be controlled by diathermy coagulation, and (b) the blue tattooed dots on the cartilage can be seen clearly.

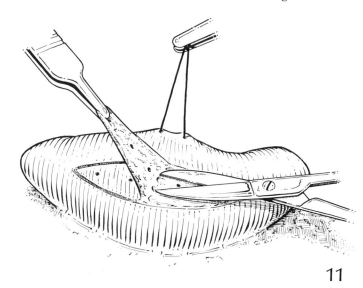

11

## 12

The cartilage is then incised along the line of the ink dots, taking care not to cut through the skin of the external aspect of the ear. Freeing of the cartilage from the external skin is carried out on the medial aspect of the incisions by blunt stripping with sharp pointed scissors, keeping the scissors parallel to the plane of dissection to avoid damaging the skin.

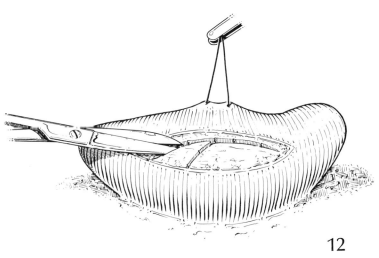

12

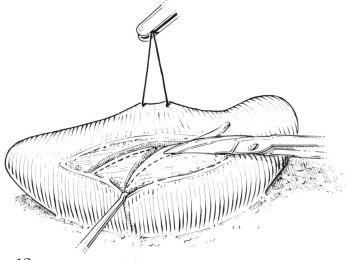

13

## 13

The excess cartilage to be excised is shown by the dotted lines.

The lower portion is first excised with curved scissors to produce a new and lower antihelix fold. The cartilage edge must be a perfect smooth curve or contour defects will result on the new fold.

# 14

To match the height of the new antihelix fold the cartilage excision is then carried out along the outer edge of the triangular fossa cartilage, after freeing this cartilage from the skin. The advantage of releasing the triangular fossa cartilage is that it can now be folded back by means of a single 3/0 plain catgut stitch to attach it to the edge of the conchal cartilage. This creates a new antihelix fold and also corrects the outward drooping of the upper pole of the ear. Great care is necessary in the accurate placing of this stitch. The tip of the triangular cartilage is transfixed with the stitch, the needle is then passed through the edge of the conchal cartilage at a slightly higher level (nearer the upper pole of the ear), so that the triangular cartilage buckles a little when the stitch is tied. This results in the triangular fossa being concave externally in its medial part and convex laterally where it forms the antihelix fold.

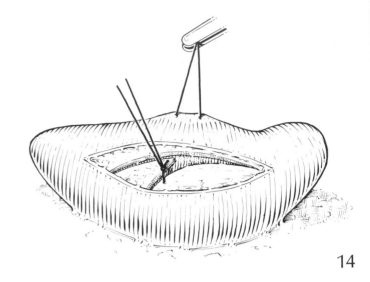

14

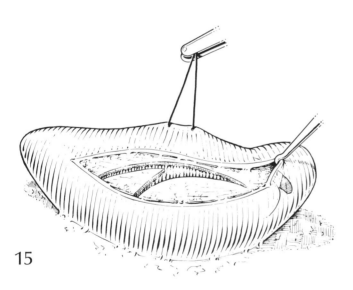

15

# 15

If the lobe of the ear shows excessive prominence prior to inserting the catgut stitch, the cartilage which extends into the ear lobe lateral to the original cartilage incision should be freed and excised. This removes the forward curve of the cartilage which produces the prominent lobe.

The skin is now closed with either 3/0 silk or Dexon. A subcuticular stitch can be used, but may give some difficulty in accurate placement when closing a curved suture line as it can give some longitudinal buckling of the ear. When using interrupted stitches it is wise to place firstly a central one and then one half-way above and one half-way below to assess the alignment of the ear and to make sure that the ear prominence has been uniformly corrected. Excessive skin excision in the centre, or inadequate skin excision at the upper and lower poles, can result in a deformity known as 'telephone ear'.

## CORRECTION OF PROTRUSION WITH NO ANTIHELIX FOLD[2]

# 16

The disadvantage of the previously described operation is that the new antihelix fold may be sharper than the normal soft curve of this part of the ear. This is particularly noticeable if the ear cartilage is thin.

To attempt to produce a smoother contour the cartilage can be weakened along the site of the absent antihelix fold.

The skin excision and markings are as described in the previous operation, but no tattooing is made along the lower edge of the triangular fossa.

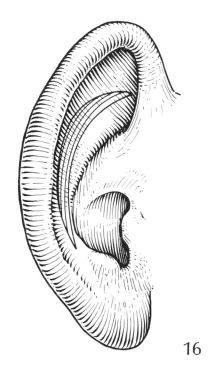

16

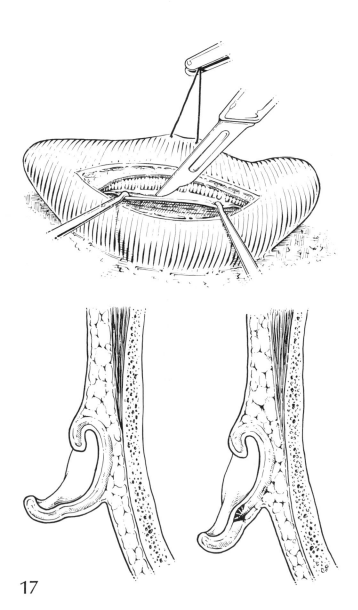

17

# 17

The cartilage is incised just lateral to the tattooed dots along the antihelix region. The cartilage is freed from the external skin on the medial side of the incision. Parallel longitudinal cuts are made on the outer aspect of this cartilage, thus allowing the cartilage to curve into a normal antihelix fold. In cases with only slight or moderate protrusion no cartilage is excised. If the protrusion is severe, 2–3 mm of cartilage should be excised from the medial edge of the cartilage incision, with fractionally more at the lower part.

Skin closure is as previously described.

## MUSTARDÉ'S PROCEDURE[3]

# 18

This operation achieves an antihelix fold by buckling the cartilage along the absent fold by using non-absorbable buried mattress sutures, such as 4/0 silk or 5/0 nylon. These stitches must be carefully sited to obtain a correct antihelix fold.

Skin excision and closure is as previously described.

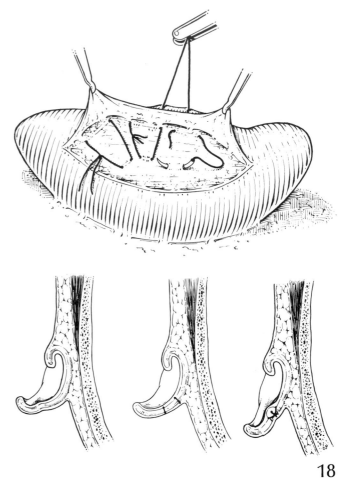

18

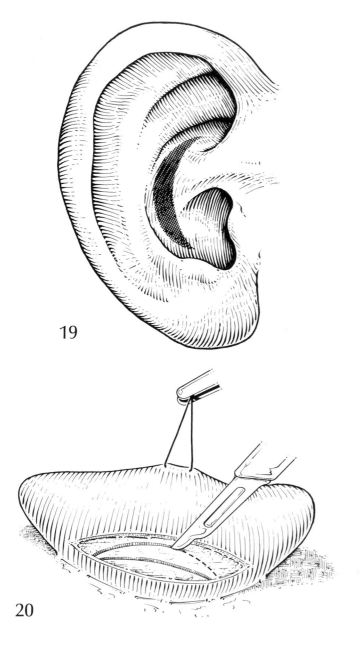

19

20

## CORRECTION OF PROTRUSION DUE TO EXCESSIVE CONCHAL CARTILAGE

# 19 & 20

This method is less frequently used, but is applicable to protruding ears with a normal antihelix fold but excessive depth of the conchal cartilage. The skin excision is as in the previous operations, but is placed a little closer to the root of the ear. An ellipse of conchal cartilage is excised in the deeper part of the conchal hollow, deep to the antihelix fold. The amount of cartilage removed depends on the severity of the protrusion and breaks the outward spring of the ear to allow it to sit closer to the head after skin suture.

Correction of 'rosebud' deformity is by the first operation described.

The main point to note is that the width of postauricular skin excised is greater than in the other types of protruding ear.

In the 'lop ear' deformities, again the first operative procedure is recommended, with a considerably greater amount of skin excision at the upper pole of the ear, with a marked horizontal component to correct the droop of the upper pole.

## Dressings

A meticulous technique is essential to give uniform pressure to the new cartilaginous shape, to avoid distortion, and to prevent haematoma formation. A retained haematoma not only increases the risk of infection but may lead to a 'cauliflower ear' as the haematoma becomes organized into scar tissue.

A single layer of 4 × 4 inch tulle gras is carefully moulded to the ear. Paraffin flavine wool is then packed into the contours of the ear to give uniform pressure, followed by a layer of dressing gauze, cotton wool and finally a 3-inch crêpe bandage, gently but firmly applied.

## Postoperative care

## 21

The dressing is removed on the seventh postoperative day and the stitches removed. The only indication for earlier removal is persistent bleeding or signs of suspected infection. Following removal of the stitches the ear is supported for 3–4 days by ¼-inch strips of zinc oxide strapping plaster, a thin wisp of cotton wool being placed in the postauricular sulcus.

A crêpe bandage or elastic head-band is worn at night for 3 weeks after removal of the stitches, to prevent the ear being accidentally bent forwards during sleep. Active sports should be avoided for about 4 weeks after the operation.

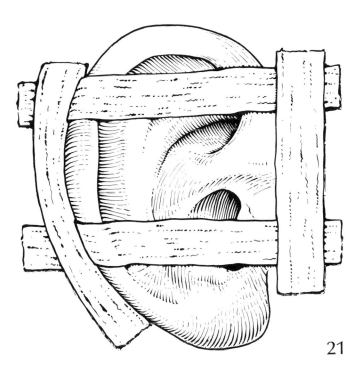

21

## Complications

### Haemorrhage

This is treated by firmer bandaging or a return to the operating theatre if it persists. Any haematoma should always be removed to prevent a 'cauliflower ear' deformity.

### Infection

This can have disastrous results if a chondritis leads to damage to the cartilage. Prophylactic antibiotics are advised and will normally be penicillin, as the haemolytic streptococcus is the organism most likely to cause severe cartilage destruction. If any fever develops in the postoperative period, the antibiotics should be changed, or commenced if not already being given.

### Telephone ear

This can be avoided by careful control of the skin excision. Secondary corrections may be necessary, either by further skin excision if the upper or lower poles of the ear remain too prominent, or even release of the central part and insertion of a full-thickness free skin graft if the central skin excision has been too radical.

Irregularities of the antihelix fold can be avoided by accurate and careful cartilage excision.

### Keloid scar

Fortunately this is rare. If present it is more commonly found and more severe in the upper part of the scar. Treatment is by injections of triamcinolone; or if surgery is necessary, excision of the keloid scar, application of a split skin graft, and postoperative X-ray therapy.

### References

1. McEvitt, W. F. (1947) Problem of the protruding ear. Plastic and Reconstructive Surgery, 2, 481–496

2. Tolhurst, D. E. (1972) The correction of prominent ears. British Journal of Plastic Surgery, 25, 261–265

3. Mustardé, J. C. (1964) The correction of prominent ears with buried mattress sutures. In: Modern Trends in Plastic Surgery, T. Gibson (ed.) pp. 233–236. London: Butterworths

Illustrations by Philip Wilson

# Tracheotomy

**John N. G. Evans**  MB, BS, DLO, FRCS
Consultant Ear, Nose and Throat Surgeon, The Hospital for Sick Children, Great Ormond Street, and St. Thomas's Hospital, London, UK

## Preoperative

A tracheotomy should be performed as an elective operation under general anaesthesia. In the paediatric age groups the child is usually intubated.

### INDICATIONS

1. Airway obstruction
   - (a) Congenital anomalies
     Laryngeal webs
     Subglottic stenosis
   - (b) Acute infection
     Epiglottitis
     Acute laryngotracheobronchitis
   - (c) Increasing laryngeal oedema with evidence of mucosal damage as a consequence of nasotracheal intubation
   - (d) Functional obstruction
     Recurrent laryngeal paralysis
     Cricoarytenoid fixation
   - (e) Tumours
     Haematoma; Lymphangioma
     Papillomata
   - (f) External trauma
     'Hanging' type injuries
   - (g) Extrinsic or intrinsic narrowing of the trachea.
2. Long-term respiratory support. After cardiac surgery or in cases of pulmonary pathology or thoracic dystrophy.
3. Clearance of secretions.
4. As a preliminary procedure to operations on the larynx, pharynx or temporomandibular joints.

## Anaesthesia

The operation is performed under general anaesthesia. In exceptional circumstances preliminary intubation of the trachea may be impossible, in which case a local anaesthetic using 1 per cent lignocaine with adrenaline 1:200 000 will be necessary.

# The operation

## 1

### Position of patient

The neck must be hyperextended. A sandbag, or rolled towel in the case of a neonate, is placed under the shoulders. The occiput is supported by a ring. The patient is tipped into the head-up position and a diathermy pad applied.

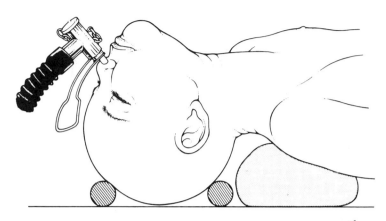

1

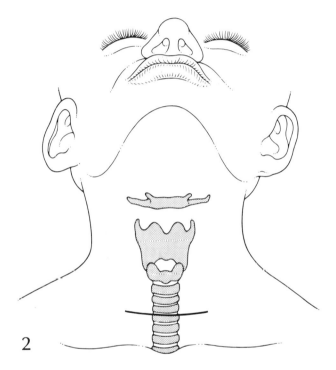

2

**TRACHEOTOMY**

## 2

### The incision

After carefully palpating the neck the hyoid bone and cricoid cartilages can be felt. The skin over the third tracheal ring is infiltrated using 1 per cent lignocaine with 1:200 000 adrenaline. This aids haemostasis. A transverse skin incision approximately 2 cm in length is made through the infiltrated area, cutting through fat and platysma.

## 3

The incision is deepened in a horizontal plane until the deep cervical fascia investing the sternohyoid and sternothyroid muscles is encountered. Branches of the anterior jugular vein will be seen during this dissection; these should be coagulated with diathermy and divided.

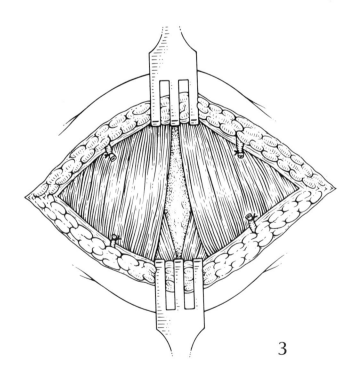

3

# 4

Having identified the strap muscles, a condensation of the investing layer of the deep cervical fascia will be seen running vertically between the sternohyoid and sternothyroid muscles. This interval is entered by blunt scissor dissection in a vertical direction and the strap muscles separated and retracted laterally.

## Exposure of the thyroid gland

Retraction of the strap muscles reveals the thyroid gland with the thyroid isthmus joining the two lobes of the gland. Above the isthmus the cricoid is seen, and even in a neonate it is easy to identify by feel.

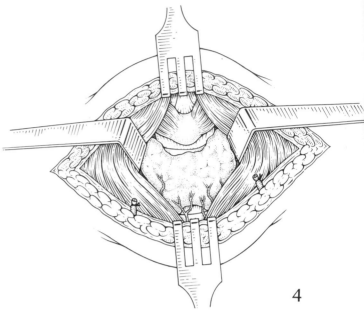

# 5

## Dissection of the thyroid isthmus

The size and relationship of the thyroid isthmus to the trachea is variable but in almost all cases the isthmus should be divided. A small incision is made through a condensation of the pre-tracheal fascia at the upper border of the isthmus, and the isthmus is then separated from the underlying trachea by blunt dissection. Branches of the inferior thyroid vein will be encountered at the lower border of the isthmus, and these should be diathermied.

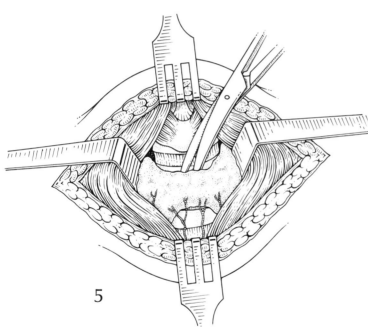

# 6

## Division of the thyroid isthmus

A haemostat is placed in each side of the isthmus which is then divided, the cut ends being secured by suture ligation.

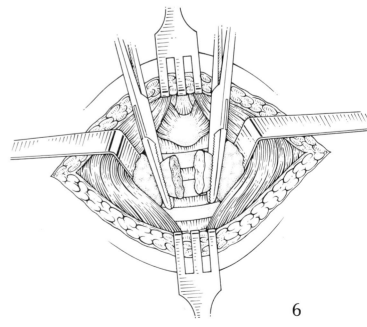

## Opening the trachea

Careful haemostasis is achieved and the tracheal rings counted: the first tracheal ring must *not* be included in the tracheotomy.

# 7

For a routine tracheotomy in children a vertical incision is made in the trachea through the second, third and fourth tracheal rings. If a subsequent reconstructive operation upon the larynx is planned, the incision in the trachea is made through the third, fourth and fifth tracheal rings. Care should be taken with a low tracheostome that the end of the tracheotomy tube is clear of the carina. A small sucker should be used to prevent blood entering the trachea.

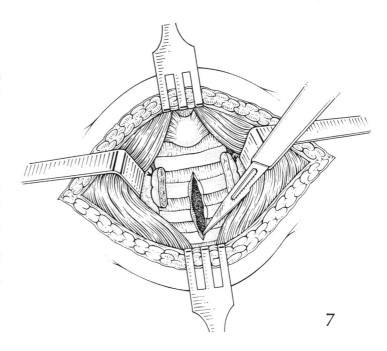

7

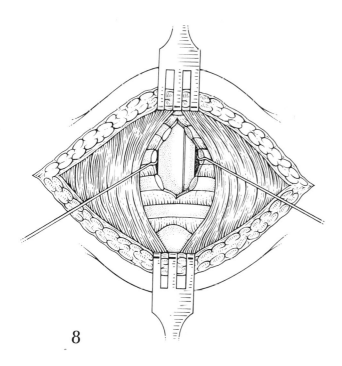

8

# 8

Fine skin hooks are now used to distract the cut edges of the trachea. The endotracheal tube will then be clearly seen.

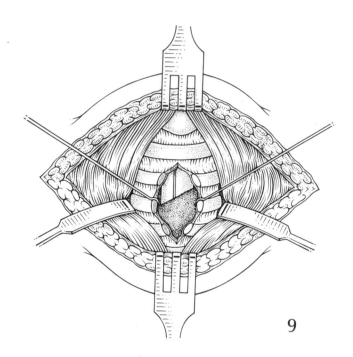

9

# 9 & 10

### Insertion of tracheotomy tube

The anaesthetist is asked to gently withdraw the endo-tracheal tube until its proximal end is just above the tracheostome. The tracheotomy tube is then inserted into the tracheal opening.

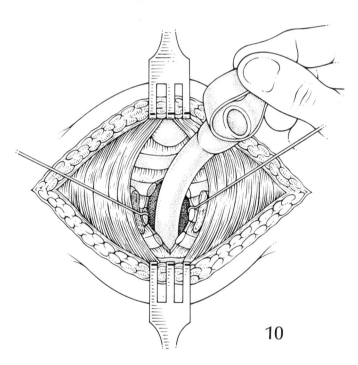

10

## Fixation of tracheotomy tube

When the tracheotomy tube is fully inserted it must be held by the assistant until it is properly secured. The skin edges are partly approximated with a suture on each side of the tube. It is essential to leave a gap around the tube to avoid postoperative surgical emphysema.

# 11

The sandbag is then removed from underneath the patient's shoulders and the tracheotomy tube is secured by tying the tapes with a reef knot with the *neck flexed*. It is extremely important to remember this neck flexion and to tie the tapes fairly tightly; failure to do this may result in the tube becoming dislodged. This must be avoided during the immediate postoperative period, as subsequent insertion of the tracheotomy tube can be difficult in the first few postoperative days. A non-adherent dressing is applied to the wound with a keyhole to accommodate the tracheotomy tube. This dressing should be changed when necessary and kept clean.

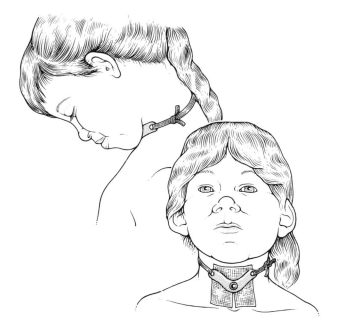

11

## Postoperative tracheotomy care

The following must be provided at the bedside:

(i) Tracheotomy tube of the same size as that in the patient;
(ii) Suction apparatus and sterile catheters with holes in the side;
(iii) A tracheal dilator;
(iv) A properly trained nurse!
(v) Humidification.

On return to the ward a chest X-ray should be arranged to check the length of the tracheotomy tube and its position with regard to its proximity to the carina, and to ensure that the right main bronchus has not been intubated. Suction is applied via the tracheotomy tube. This will be necessary half-hourly in the first few days after operation. Suction is facilitated by the instillation of 2 ml of sterile normal saline into the tracheotomy tube. A sterile catheter is inserted into the tracheal lumen gently but quickly, and suction is only applied as the catheter is withdrawn.

If the tracheotomy tube is properly positioned and functioning satisfactorily, respiration should be inaudible. If bubbling noises are heard, further suction is required.

Adequate humidification must be provided for a neonate in a head box; for a child in an oxygen tent, or for an older child using the thermostatically controlled humidifier connected to the tracheotomy tube. This will reduce the frequency of suction and the tenacity of secretions, and allow the tracheotomy tube to remain patent.

The tracheotomy tube is changed after the first week. If any difficulty is encountered during suction or if the breathing becomes noisy in spite of suction or if the child begins to phonate, then the tracheotomy must be changed immediately. This should be done with adequate help: the child's neck must be extended; good illumination is essential, and a headlight desirable. As the tracheotomy tube is withdrawn the tracheostome should be visible and a new tube is readily inserted under direct vision. If difficulty is encountered, a tracheal dilator must be inserted in the tracheal lumen, when subsequent intubation of the trachea should present no difficulty.

The commonest cause for difficulty in suction of the trachea is displacement of the tube in front of the trachea. This is always accompanied by audible respiration and by the child being able to phonate.

## COMPLICATIONS OF TRACHEOTOMY

### Operatively

1. Bleeding may be encountered from an abnormally high innominate artery. Careful controlled dissection of the structures in the lower part of the neck incision should avoid this.
2. Damage to the cervical pleura may cause a pneumothorax; dissection lateral to the trachea should be avoided.
3. Injury to the oesophagus should not occur if an elective tracheotomy is being performed.

### Postoperatively

1. *Blocking and displacement of the tracheotomy tube*   These complications are preventable by careful nursing and attention to detail when tying tracheotomy tube tapes.
2. *Postoperative pneumonia*   This risk is small if a sterile technique of tracheal toilet is used and effective humidification maintained. Adequate physiotherapy to encourage coughing is also desirable.
3. *Surgical emphysema*   If this occurs the wound should be opened fully. It is caused by suturing the wound too tightly around the tracheotomy tube.
4. *Haemorrhage*   Erosion of the anterior wall of the trachea may well occur if a metal tracheotomy tube of the incorrect curvature is used. The overlying innominate artery may also be damaged, in which event a frequently fatal haemorrhage will result.
5. *Stenosis*   This may occur at the tracheostome if cartilage is removed during the tracheotomy, or at the tip of the tube if suction is too vigorous or incorrectly applied.

# 12

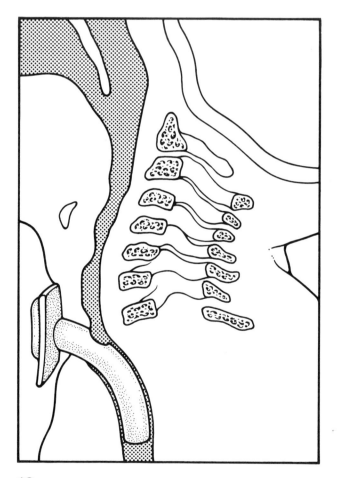

6. *Difficult decannulation*   In the absence of persisting pathology, decannulation may be facilitated by using a metal fenestrated tube which can be fitted with a blocker (Alder Hey pattern). Care must be taken to ensure that the fenestration of the tracheotomy tube is correctly positioned.
7. *Persistent tracheal fistula*   After prolonged tracheotomy, removal of the tube may result in a persistent fistula at the site of the tracheotomy. This is not serious. If it either fails to close or a persistent leak of mucus issues from it, the tract may be excised and a formal closure performed. In young children this may conveniently be done before they start school.

In an emergency, for example in the case of acute epiglottitis when sudden airway obstruction may occur and peroral endotracheal intubation may not be possible, a cricothyrotomy should be considered in preference to a crash tracheotomy which can be extremely difficult in the child whose trachea is soft and not always easy to identify.

# 13

## TECHNIQUE FOR CRICOTHYROTOMY

The child is held with its neck extended and the left hand is placed with the first finger over the cricoid cartilage and the second over the thyroid cartilage. A transverse stab incision is made through the cricothyroid membrane; the blade of the knife is then turned vertically, this will establish the airway and a tracheal dilator or any other tube of suitable size may be inserted to preserve the airway and to enable general anaesthesia to be undertaken safely. An elective tracheotomy is then performed.

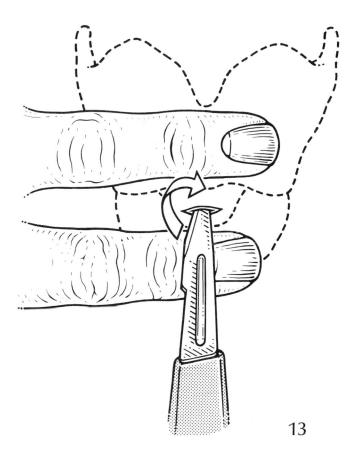

13

# Cystic hygromas

**E. M. Kiely**  FRCSI, FRCS
Consultant Paediatric Surgeon, The Hospital for Sick Children, Great Ormond Street, London, UK

## Introduction

Cystic hygromas may occur anywhere in the body but the most common sites are in the neck and axilla. Further discussion will be confined to the management of cervical lesions.

Excision of cystic hygromas is usually undertaken for cosmetic reasons. Untreated lesions are subject to repeated haemorrhage and infection, and may impinge on vital structures such as the airway or the eye. Rapid enlargement produced by haemorrhage or infection may on occasion necessitate urgent excision.

Surgery may be performed at any age. Most paediatric surgeons advocate early excision, although this is not usually necessary within the first few months of life. The scarring which results from recurrent inflammation may render excision more difficult.

Blood should be available at operation.

These lesions are often extensive and may envelop many vital structures in the neck. In order to preserve these, complete excision may not always be possible. Multilating surgery is unnecessary, however, because fragments of the lesion may be left *in situ*, provided that adequate postoperative drainage is employed.

## The operation

### Anaesthesia and position of patient

Surgery is performed under full intubated general anaesthesia. A roll is placed beneath the shoulders and the head is turned to the opposite side. Optical magnification is a considerable asset in precise dissection.

## 1

### The incision

A transverse cervical incision at least 2 cm below the angle of the mandible is made. The incision should extend to the limits of the lesion.

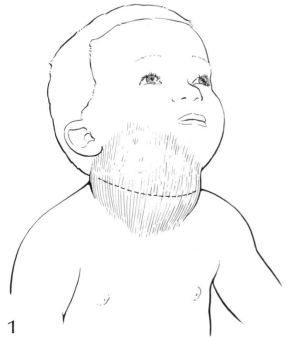

1

# 2–5

The platysma and deep cervical fascia are divided in the line of the incision and retracted with skin hooks or sutures. The skin flaps are dissected in turn, usually commencing with the inferior flap. The anterior and posterior limits of the hygroma are defined and subsequently the superior flap is freed. Blood vessels are diathermied prior to division if possible. The dissection is most easily accomplished with a knife.

Branches of the cervical plexus are sacrificed when encountered. The external jugular vein is also divided.

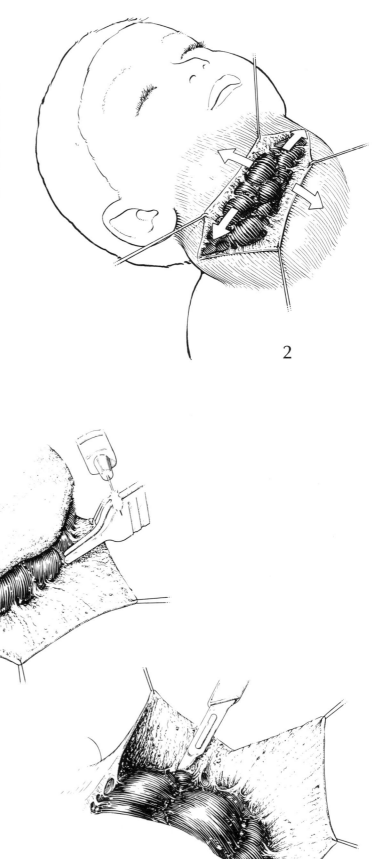

2

3

4

5

# 6 & 7

Dissection of the upper flap is undertaken with care to preserve the mandibular branch of the facial nerve. This usually does not enter the lesion and may be dissected free.

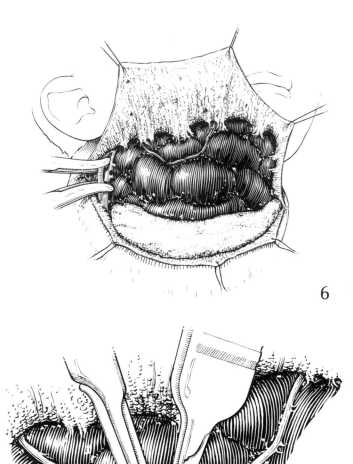

6

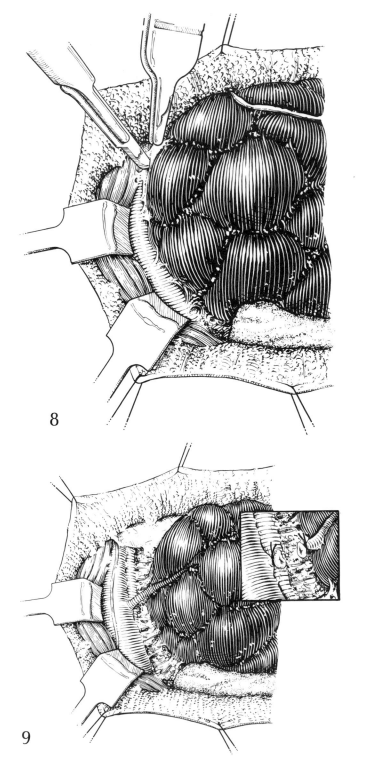

8

7

# 8 & 9

The deeper phase of the procedure involves the separation of the cystic hygroma from the major nerves and blood vessels of the neck. This is done by commencing inferiorly along the great vessels. The internal jugular vein is initially cut free from the hygroma, and this may involve division of the middle thyroid vein.

9

# 10

When the internal jugular vein has been completely mobilized, the common carotid artery and its bifurcation are encountered. Care is taken to preserve the hypoglossal nerve, but usually the facial artery is sacrificed.

The dissection advances anteriorly along the hypoglossal nerve, preserving this at all costs. Small fragments of hygroma may be left on the nerve but do not usually give rise to trouble. The lesion is then freed from the hyoid bone and its attached muscles; the submandibular gland is then encountered.

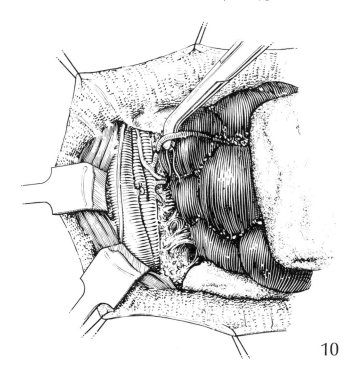

10

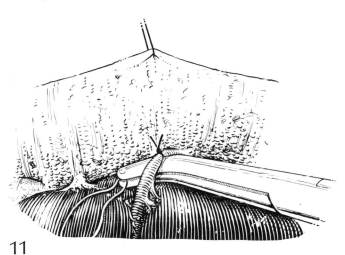

11

# 11

At this point the facial artery may again be encountered; the submandibular gland is usually excised *en bloc* with the specimen.

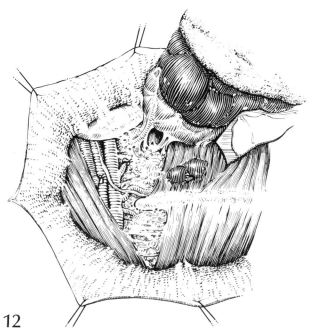

12

# 12

Involvement of the muscles of the tongue, as in this case, makes complete resection impossible. As much of the lesion as seems advisable is removed without excising an undue amount of the hyoglossus.

## 13

The wound is closed using continuous 5/0 or 6/0 polyglycolic acid sutures for the platysma, which is usually a more robust structure in its contracted state. The skin is closed with a subcuticular suture of the same material.

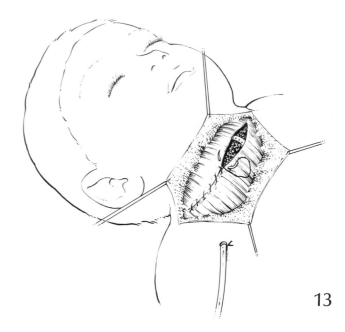

13

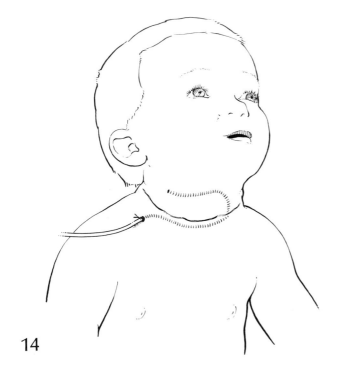

14

## 14

Drainage is mandatory in these cases. Suction drainage is very effective and particularly suitable in young infants.

## Postoperative care

Most infants may commence feeding within hours of surgery. Extensive dissection around the pharynx or floor of the mouth may temporarily impair swallowing. Patients are normally fit for discharge within 48 hours of surgery, but the drain should remain in place for at least seven days. The volume of drainage at that time will dictate the time for removal.

Illustrations by Kevin Marks

# Preauricular sinus

**R. J. Brereton**
Senior Lecturer in Paediatric Surgery, Institute of Child Health, University of London, London, UK

## HISTORY

This is a congenital sinus arising on the anterior aspect of the helix. The sinus passes through the skin anteriorly and inferiorly to end in a racemose group of preauricular cysts. They arise from imperfect fusion of the six tubercles which form the pinna. Symptoms are rare in early childhood. They usually present following an episode of infection. If untreated, recurrent infection results in a preauricular ulcer. The lesion may be unilateral or bilateral.

## PRINCIPLES

Complete excision is necessary to effect a cure.

# Preoperative preparation

Surgery should not be undertaken if there is active acute infection. This should be treated with antistaphylococcal antibiotics, since such organisms are almost invariably the cause of the suppuration. Oblique incisions to drain pus should be avoided as they are associated with unacceptable scarring and may result in an ulcer. In the chronically infected case, operation should be covered by appropriate antibiotics, commencing two or three days preoperatively and continuing for several days postoperatively.

## Anaesthesia

General anaesthesia by endotracheal tube is recommended, particularly for bilateral lesions. Infiltration with local anaesthetic may be used for co-operative older children.

## Position and towelling

Any hair immediately anterior to the pinna should be shaved. For bilateral cases standard head towelling is indicated, but when the lesion is unilateral a circumcision towel with a central aperture for the preauricular region suffices.

113

# The operation

The preauricular region should be infiltrated with 1:1000 adrenaline in saline solution or a local anaesthetic agent which also serves to reduce postoperative discomfort.

The injection of a coloured dye into the duct to outline the extent of the subcutaneous gland is generally unhelpful, and may even be misleading as the dye rarely outlines the full extent of the lesion. Rupture of the gland with escape of the dye may result in the excision of an unnecessarily large amount of normal tissue.

## 1

A purse-string suture of 5/0 nylon or 4/0 silk is inserted around the punctum and used for holding the skin flap to be raised.

An inverted L-shaped incision is made with the vertical limb running along the groove anterior to the pinna and the horizontal limb in the hairline.

The flap of skin so outlined is raised using fine needle-point diathermy which controls the haemorrhage. Damage to the preauricular nerve and vessels can be prevented by avoiding unnecessarily deep dissection immediately anterior to the pinna.

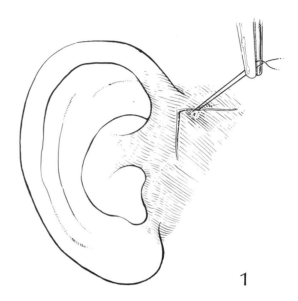

1

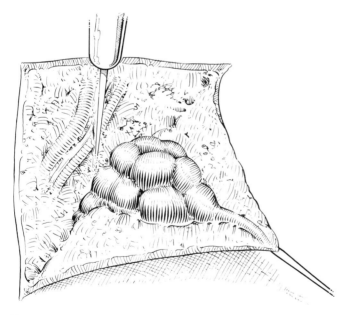

2

## 2

As dissection of the flap proceeds, the level of dissection is progressively deepened to avoid leaving any of the racemose gland. The gland is dissected anteriorly on the elevated flap.

## 3

Having dissected the gland completely from its facial attachments, it merely remains to detach the gland and its duct from the elevated skin flap. The flap is held vertically and the gland excised using a scalpel blade or the needle diathermy. Care should be taken not to buttonhole the flap.

The flap is repositioned using two or three subcutaneous sutures of 5/0 chromic catgut, and the skin edges approximated using small interrupted sutures of 6/0 polypropylene. The holding stitch is removed.

To prevent postoperative haematoma formation, the preauricular depression, crevices of the pinna and postauricular space should be lightly packed with proflavine wool and a pressure dressing of orthopaedic wool and crepe bandage applied. The dressing may be kept in place by a helmet made from Netelast.

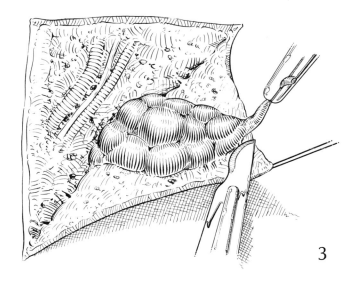

3

## POSTOPERATIVE TREATMENT

The pressure dressing is removed after 24 hours and the sutures after 5 days.

## RESULTS

Provided all the subcutaneous glandular tissue has been excised, a cure is assured, and the cosmetic result is excellent. In patients who have suffered recurrent infections the preauricular skin is usually very thin and scarred and the cosmetic result is less satisfactory.

## Further reading

Singer, R. (1966) A new technic for extirpation of preauricular cysts. American Journal of Surgery, 111, 291–295

# Oesophageal atresia and tracheo-oesophageal fistula

**Vanessa M. Wright** FRCS, FRACS
Consultant Paediatric Surgeon, Queen Elizabeth Hospital for Children, and University College Hospital, London, UK

## Clinical presentation

Prenatal inability to swallow may result in polyhydramnios and premature delivery. Postnatally the presence of frothy saliva requiring frequent suction to maintain an airway, accompanied by choking and cyanosis, is the commonest presentation of oesophageal atresia. To confirm the diagnosis a size 8 or 10 radio-opaque tube should be passed through the nose or mouth; in the presence of obstruction it cannot be advanced beyond about 10 cm.

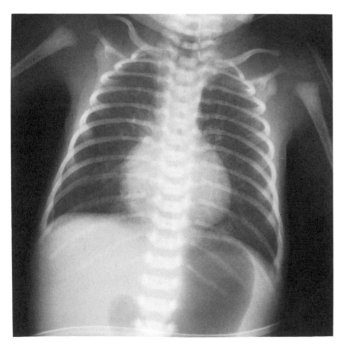

## Investigations

### 1

Plain X-ray of chest and abdomen will demonstrate the tube arrested in the upper mediastinum, and air in the intestine will confirm the presence of a tracheo-oesophageal fistula.

1

**2**

The absence of intestinal air suggests the diagnosis of a pure oesophageal atresia.

Contrast studies of the upper pouch in a case of oesophageal atresia with distal tracheo-oesophageal fistula are not indicated. However, evidence of aspiration on a very early chest X-ray raises the possibility of an upper pouch fistula, and in that instance a contrast study or intraoperative endoscopy examination is indicated. The absence of a distal tracheo-oesophageal fistula should also prompt a contrast study of the upper pouch to exclude an upper pouch fistula.

These specialized investigations should only be carried out in the institution where definitive surgery will be undertaken. The high incidence of major associated abnormalities in infants with oesophageal atresia necessitates very careful and repeated examinations. The initial X-rays may suggest cardiac, vertebral, rib, and other gastrointestinal anomalies such as duodenal atresia.

## Initial management

Immediate surgery in oesophageal atresia is rarely necessary; a period of 24–48 hours between diagnosis and operation allows a full assessment of the infant, and, if aspiration has occurred, resolution of the pulmonary changes can be expedited with appropriate physiotherapy and antibiotics, with or without assisted ventilation. Abdominal distension is rarely sufficiently severe to necessitate early division of the fistula. Before operation the upper pouch is continuously aspirated using a Replogle tube attached to low-pressure suction. Dextrose 10 per cent and saline 0.18 per cent intravenously maintains fluid and electrolyte balance and prevents hypoglycaemia. Vitamin K analogue should be administered routinely before operation.

## Choice of operation

In the vast majority of infants with oesophageal atresia and a distal tracheo-oesophageal fistula, division of the fistula and primary anastomosis of the oesophagus is possible. The possibility of this procedure is reduced if the infant is small (less than 1.8 kg), or if there are other major congenital abnormalities such as a Fallot's tetralogy with a right-sided aortic arch. This should be excluded preoperatively with echocardiography if such a diagnosis is suspected.

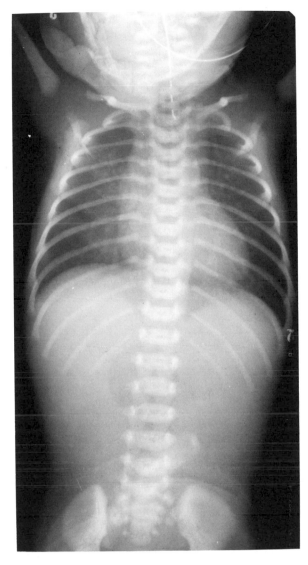

**2**

A short upper pouch as shown on the preliminary plain X-ray may also make a primary anastomosis difficult. However, the presence of a distal tracheo-oesophageal fistula requiring division dictates the necessity for right thoracotomy, and the possibility of obtaining a satisfactory primary anastomosis should not be ruled out until the anatomy has been inspected at the time of thoracotomy.

The absence of a lower pouch fistula is usually associated with a long gap between upper and lower oesophagus. This situation is usually managed by a preliminary feeding gastrostomy. If oesophageal replacement is the procedure of choice, a cervical oesophagostomy is necessary. The alternative is a delayed primary anastomosis after several weeks of gastrostomy feeding and upper pouch suction.

# The operations

## DIVISION AND PRIMARY ANASTOMOSIS

### Anaesthesia

Premedication is with atropine alone. The endotracheal tube requires careful positioning to permit adequate ventilation with minimal gas flow through the fistula. The majority of paediatric anaesthetists will control ventilation from an early stage following intubation. An intravenous infusion is sited in a limb other than the right upper limb.

The Replogle tube or a similar large-bore tube should be in position in the upper pouch. Careful attention is paid to maintaining body temperature, using a heating blanket, and to preventing heat loss by covering the infant with foil. Broad spectrum antibiotics should be administered either preoperatively or at the time of induction.

## 3

### The incision

The infant is positioned on his left side and stabilized with strapping or sandbags. The right arm is extended above the head and fixed. Care must be taken to ensure that the neck is flexed.

A curved incision is made around the lower border of the scapula, extending from the anterior axillary line to the paravertebral region posteriorly; division of the subcutaneous tissues and muscles is carried out with diathermy to minimize blood loss. Following division of the muscles the scapula is elevated and the rib spaces are counted by palpation.

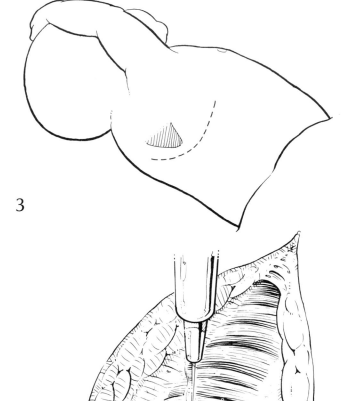

**3**

**4**

## 4

The thorax can be entered through the bed of the fifth rib, which is mobilized following incision of the overlying periosteum. An alternative and rather simpler approach is to divide the intercostal muscles of the fourth intercostal space. Whichever the approach, care is required to prevent incision of the pleura. Although the extrapleural approach is rather slower initially it confers substantial benefit and should always be used in the initial thoracotomy.

## 5

Having exposed the pleura through the intercostal space, stripping of the pleura from the chest wall is best carried out by the gentle insertion of a gauze swab into the extrapleural space. This is usually extremely well tolerated by both infant and anaesthetist. On withdrawing the swab an extensive area of dissection will have resulted; a rib spreader can then be inserted and the ribs gently separated. Further dissection of the pleura is achieved by using moist pledgets; a pair of pledgets used simultaneously is most satisfactory.

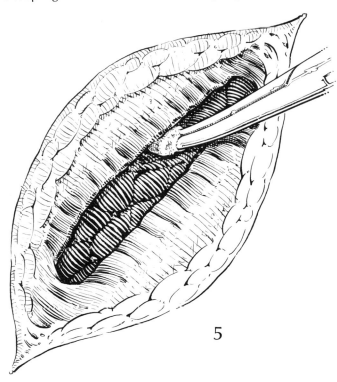

5

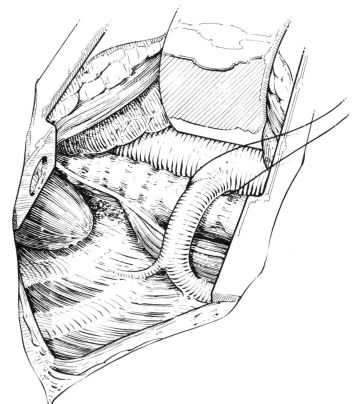

6

## 6

The azygos vein and the lower mediastinum should be exposed, enabling the lower pouch, upper pouch and fistula to be seen. Anterior dissection of the pleura should be sufficient to allow the ribs to be adequately spread. Very occasionally the size or position of the fistula may make it impossible for the anaesthetist to ventilate the lungs adequately. In that situation the more rapid transpleural approach to the fistula may be necessary. In order to expose the posterior mediastinum effectively, lung retraction is essential, but care must be taken to ensure that the retractor does not compress the mediastinum.

## Mobilization of lower oesophagus and division of fistula

The azygos vein is ligated and divided. The lower oesophagus may be obvious, distending with each inspiration as it lies in the lower posterior mediastinum. The close proximity of the vagus to the lower oesophagus helps identification.

## 7

Every attempt must be made during dissection to preserve the fibres of the vagus supplying the lower oesophagus. The lower oesophagus is dissected circumferentially just distal to the fistula and a tape is placed around it. Traction on this tape controls the fistula and enables the junction of the lower oesophagus and trachea to be recognized and dissected.

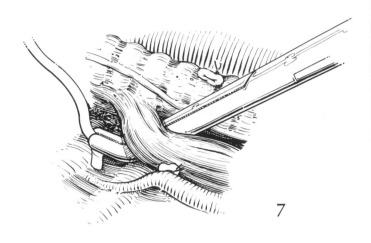

7

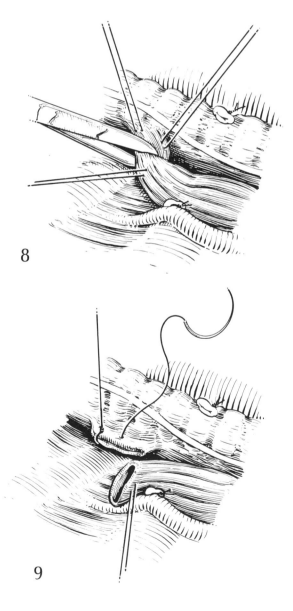

8

9

## 8 & 9

After carefully defining the junction between trachea and oesophagus, two 5/0 black silk sutures are placed in the trachea at the extremities of the fistula and the fistula is divided flush with the trachea. The trachea is closed with continuous or interrupted sutures. The air-tightness of the closure should be tested by filling the thoracic cavity with saline and watching for bubbles on ventilation. An alternative means of closing the fistula is to transfix it close to the trachea with a 5/0 suture.

A small tube is passed through the distal oesophagus into the stomach to ensure that an adequate lumen exists, and to enable air distending the stomach to be aspirated.

Dissection of the lower oesophagus needs care to preserve the vagal attachments and prevent damage to the adjacent thoracic duct and left pleura. A 5/0 stay suture allows traction on the lower oesophagus without excessive handling with forceps. It can be mobilized from surrounding structures down to the hiatus, but dissection should be the minimum required to achieve an anastomosis; some tension is acceptable.

## Identification of upper pouch

# 10

If the upper pouch is not immediately visible, pressure on the Replogle tube by the anaesthetist will usually advance it into the mediastinum. Dissection of the upper pouch should be minimal and only sufficient to allow an opening to be made in the distal end for an anastomosis to be performed. As with the lower oesophagus, branches of the vagus supplying the upper oesophagus should not be disturbed. Unnecessary dissection of the plane between oesophagus and trachea must be avoided. A stay suture can be placed in the muscular wall of the oesophagus to facilitate its exposure and minimize the need for forceps traction. When opening the upper oesophagus care should be taken to ensure that the opening is at the lowermost point; this is most reliably recognized by pushing the Replogle tube down and incising the oesophagus over the tip of the tube. The size of the opening in the upper oesophagus should correspond to the diameter of the lower oesophagus.

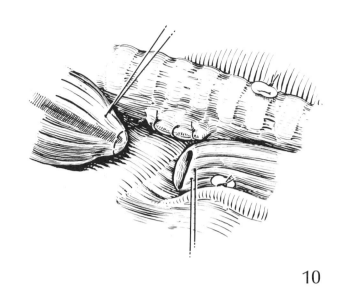

10

## Anastomosis

# 11

This is achieved using interrupted 5/0 sutures positioned along the posterior aspect of the anastomosis, particular care being taken to ensure that both mucosa and muscle are included in each stitch. An attempt is made to ensure that the knots are on the outside. It is rarely necessary to insert more than three or four sutures. Unless the two ends of the oesophagus are very close together the siting of these sutures before tying is essential.

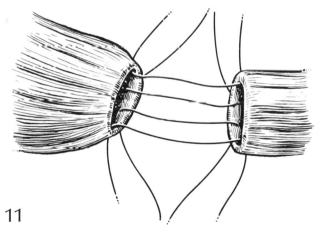

11

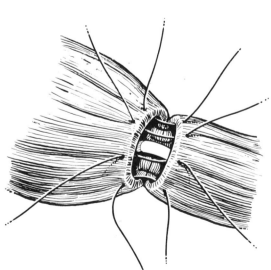

12

# 12

Following completion of the posterior layer of the anastomosis, a feeding tube should replace the Replogle tube and be advanced into the stomach. The anterior layer of the anastomosis is then completed over the tube. Once the anastomosis is complete, the intra-oesophageal tube may be withdrawn; if it is to be left *in situ* for feeding, its mobility should be checked to ensure that a suture has not inadvertently passed through it.

## Insertion of chest drain and closure of chest

# 13

A size 12 or 14 chest drain is inserted through a stab incision in a lower intercostal space in the midaxillary line. The drain should be adjacent to but not touching the anastomosis; a 3/0 chromic catgut suture through the periosteum of a rib to hold the chest drain away from the anastomosis is a sensible precaution. The lung is expanded following the placement of two pericostal 2/0 chromic catgut sutures. The muscles are closed with 3/0 Dexon, the subcutaneous layer with plain 4/0 catgut, and the skin with subcuticular 4/0 Dexon. The chest drain is securely anchored and connected to an underwater seal.

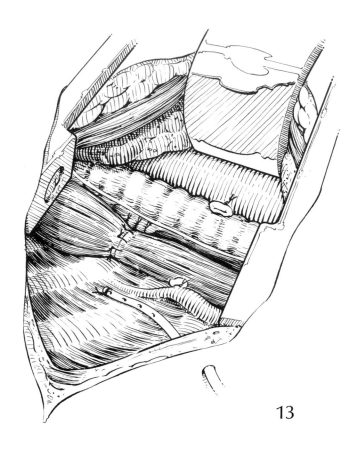

13

## POSTOPERATIVE MANAGEMENT

The infant is nursed in the neonatal intensive care unit. Intravenous fluids are administered and antibiotic prophylaxis is continued. Feeds via the transanastomotic nasogastric tube may be commenced on the second or third postoperative day. A contrast swallow is performed on the seventh postoperative day, and if no leak is identified the intercostal drain is removed. Oral feeding is now introduced. Regular chest physiotherapy, with nasopharyngeal suction as required, is carried out to avoid respiratory infection.

## COMPLICATIONS

### Mortality

This is directly related to the severity of associated congenital anomalies, especially cardiac malformations.

### Anastomotic leakage

Early leakage within 48 hours of the repair should be explored urgently with a view to secondary surgery.
Late leaks can be managed conservatively.

### Gastro-oesophageal reflux

Reflux should be treated conservatively, but if there is no response and the infant suffers repeated respiratory infections or apnoeic attacks, a surgical approach should be adopted.

### Tracheomalacia

This is a common occurrence and if severe should be treated by aortopexy (see chapter on 'Aortopexy' pp. 126–129).

### Recurrent tracheo-oesophageal fistula

Recurrent fistula should be suspected in the event of choking episodes associated with feeding, or recurrent bouts of pneumonia.

### Anastomotic strictures

Strictures usually respond to repeated dilatation, but gastro-oesophageal reflux as an aggravating factor should be excluded.

# ISOLATED TRACHEO-OESOPHAGEAL FISTULA

## Clinical presentation

The isolated or H-type tracheo-oesophageal fistula most commonly presents during the first few days of life, when the baby chokes on attempting to feed and/or has unexplained cyanotic episodes. The gaseous distension of the gastrointestinal tract may be sufficiently severe to mimic that of intestinal obstruction. The infant of a few weeks is likely to present with recurrent chest infections, particularly involving the right upper lobe.

## Investigations

# 14

The diagnosis of an H-type fistula is usually confirmed by careful contrast studies of the oesophagus, preferably using a technique which records the swallow on cine film.

Bronchoscopy with oesophagoscopy will confirm the presence of a fistula. If performed immediately prior to ligation of the fistula it may be possible to pass a fine tube such as a ureteric catheter through the fistula to aid subsequent identification.

Having accurately identified the position of the fistula a decision can be made on the most suitable approach. Some fistulae, including the recurrent ones associated with a previous oesophageal atresia repair, will be best approached through the thorax, but the majority of isolated tracheo-oesophageal fistulae can be divided through a cervical approach with adequate neck extension.

The thoracic approach to a tracheo-oesophageal fistula is similar to that previously described for oesophageal atresia with tracheo-oesophageal fistula.

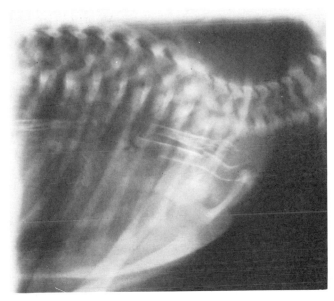

14

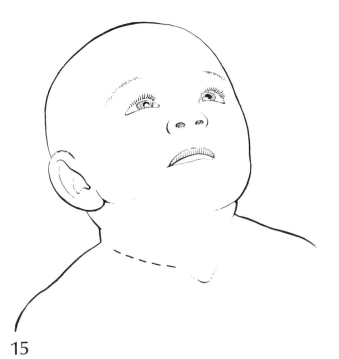

*The cervical operation*

# 15

### Position of patient

The child is placed on his back with the head turned to the left. Before extending the neck the site of the incision is drawn with a marker pen in a suitable skin crease 1 cm above the clavicle. Failure to mark the site of the incision before hyperextending the neck may result in a cosmetically unsatisfactory incision. A sandbag of appropriate size under the shoulder ensures adequate neck extension. An approach through the right side is usually preferred. A nasogastric tube of adequate size should be passed after induction of anaesthesia.

15

## 16

### Approach to fistula

Having incised the skin and subcutaneous tissues the sternomastoid is retracted posteriorly, dividing the sternal head if necessary to allow adequate exposure. The plane medial to the carotid sheath is identified, and dissection allows the sheath to be retracted posteriorly. The thyroid gland, trachea and oesophagus will lie medially. Palpation of the endotracheal and nasogastric tubes facilitates identification of these structures. The inferior thyroid artery and middle thyroid vein will be identified crossing the space between the retracted carotid sheath and the thyroid, and division may be necessary. The plane between trachea and oesophagus is gradually dissected, care being taken to identify and preserve the right recurrent laryngeal nerve.

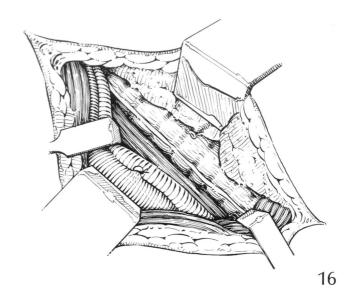

16

## 17, 18 & 19

### Dissection of the fistula

Identification of the fistula requires careful dissection and is usually rather higher than anticipated because of the hyperextension of the neck. Slings positioned around the oesophagus above and below the fistula will facilitate dissection, but extreme care is required to preserve the left recurrent laryngeal nerve, which will be difficult to visualize.

Having identified the fistula, a stay suture should be placed on the oesophageal side to mark its position, because following division of the fistula the oesophageal end may be difficult to identify. On the tracheal side a 5/0 black silk suture is placed at one limit of the fistula, and following division of the fistula the trachea is closed with a continuous or interrupted suture. The oesophageal end of the fistula is closed with one or two interrupted black silk sutures. A soft drain is placed down to the site of the oesophageal closure; the retracted tissues will assume a normal position. The wound is closed in layers with absorbable sutures and with a subcuticular suture for the skin.

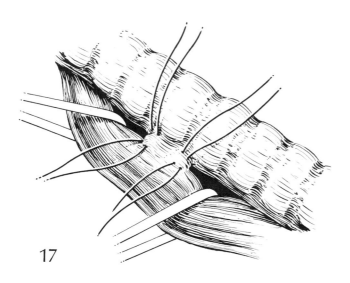

17

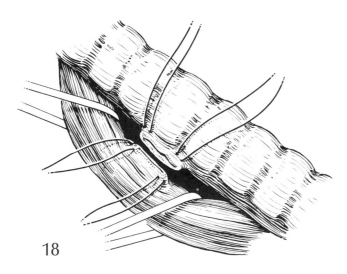

18

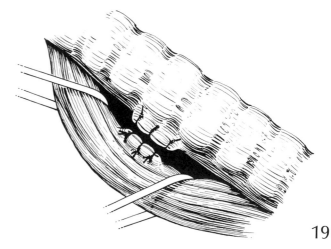

19

# Postoperative care

Extensive dissection of trachea and oesophagus is often required during this operation. Invariably this produces some tracheal oedema which may be minimal immediately postoperatively, but progress in severity for up to 48 hours. It is reasonable, particularly in the premature baby or one with pre-existing lung disease, to leave an endotracheal tube in position. It is unlikely that this can be removed in less than 5 days, and certainly no attempt should be made to extubate the baby during the first 48 hours.

Following extubation the movement of the vocal cords should be assessed. A significant proportion of these babies will require intubation for some considerable time and may have a tendency to stridor, particularly when crying or coughing for weeks or months afterwards. Feeds can be given through a nasogastric tube, or a gastrostomy may be preferred.

## Further reading

Holder, T. M. (1986) Esophageal atresia and tracheoesophageal fistula. In: Pediatric Esophageal Surgery, Ashcraft, K. W. and Holder, T. M. (eds.), pp. 29–52. Orlando, FL: Grune and Stratton

Koop, C. E., Schnaufer, L., Broennie, A. M. (1974) Esophageal atresia and tracheoesophageal fistula; supportive measures that affect survival. Pediatrics, 54, 558–564

Louhimo, I., Lindahl, H. (1983) Esophageal atresia: primary result of 500 consecutively treated patients. Journal of Pediatric Surgery, 18, 217–229

Myers, N. A. (1974) Oesophageal atresia; the epitome of modern surgery. Annals of the Royal College of Surgeons of England, 54, 277–287

Randolph, J. G., Altman, R. P., Anderson, K. D. (1977) Selective surgical management based upon clinical status in infants with esophageal atresia. Journal of Thoracic and Cardiovascular Surgery, 74, 335–342

Spitz, L., Kiely, E., Brereton, R. J. (1987) Esophageal atresia: five year experience with 148 cases. Journal of Pediatric Surgery, 22, 103–108

Waterston, D. J., Bonham-Carter, R. E., Aberdeen, E. (1963) Congenital tracheo-oesophageal fistula in association with oesophageal atresia. Lancet, 2, 55–57

Illustrations by Kevin Marks

# Aortopexy

**E. M. Kiely** FRCSI, FRCS
Consultant Paediatric Surgeon, The Hospital for Sick Children, Great Ormond St., London, UK

Severe, symptomatic tracheomalacia may be fatal if left untreated. The diagnosis is confirmed endoscopically when the trachea is seen to collapse during quiet respiration.

## 1

The slit-like endoscopic appearance of the trachea in tracheomalacia contrasts sharply with that of the normal trachea.

In infants who have had a tracheo-oesophageal fistula in the past the segment of collapse is usually above the entry site of the fistula. Almost complete obliteration of the trachea can sometimes be seen at endoscopy.

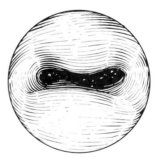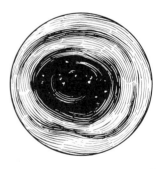

1

# The operation

# 2

### The incision

The infant is positioned supine with a small roll beneath the shoulders and the left arm abducted. The incision is made along the line of the 3rd rib and extends from just medial to the sternal border to the anterior axillary line. The incision runs well above the nipple.

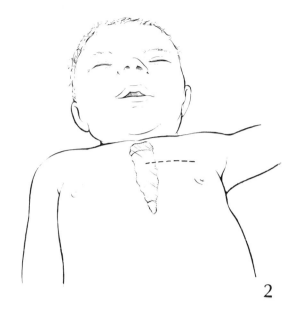

2

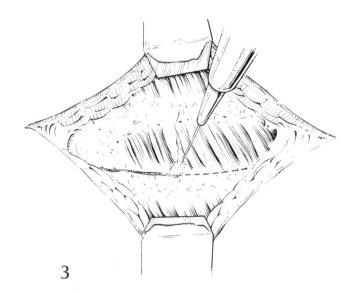

3

# 3

The pectoral muscles are divided in the line of the incision with diathermy medially, and are split laterally to expose the entire length of the third costal cartilage and the anterior half of the rib.

The perichondrium and periosteum are diathermied a few millimetres below the upper border of the rib and costal cartilage. The periosteum and perichondrium are then stripped with a periosteal elevator and the thorax entered through the bed of the 3rd rib.

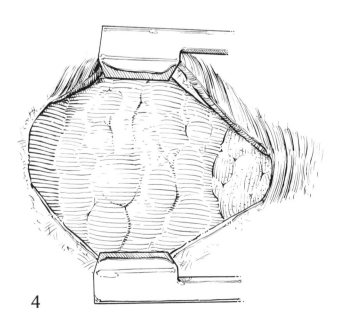

4

# 4

The thoracotomy is held open, aided by an infant-size Finochietto retractor. The left lung is then retracted laterally by means of a moist gauze and a malleable retractor.

# 5

The edge of the pleura is stripped from the left lobe of the thymus, taking care to preserve the phrenic nerve. The lobe is removed using sharp and blunt dissection with diathermy to the vessels.

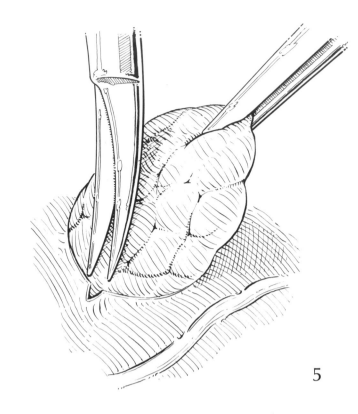

5

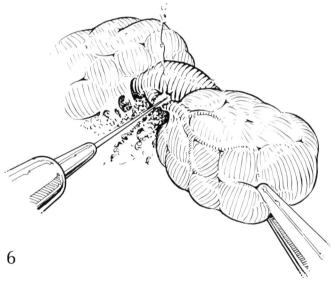

6

# 6

The left lobe of the thymus usually separates easily from the right lobe and the main venous drainage to the innominate vein is encountered. The vein is then coagulated and divided, and the lobe removed.

## 7

The pericardium is opened transversely just below its reflection on the arch of the aorta. Three sutures are inserted as shown. Each takes two or three bites of adventitia of the ascending aorta and perhaps pericardial reflection. Each suture in turn is then passed through the posterior aspect of the sternum and the sutures are left untied until all have been inserted. Polypropylene (4/0) is a suitable material.

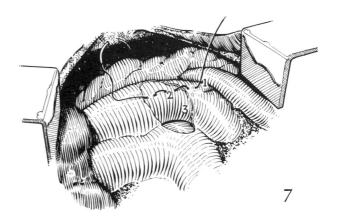

**7**

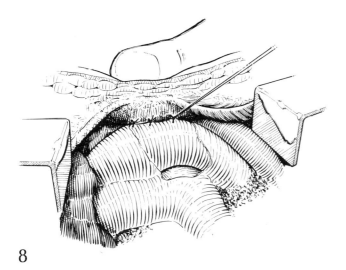

**8**

## 8

The assistant then depresses the sternum firmly posteriorly while the sutures are tied. The sternum is then released and the aorta is drawn anteriorly. This has the effect of pulling the anterior wall of the trachea away from the posterior wall, producing a wide open lumen of the trachea at the level of the aortopexy.

The wound is closed in layers, using continuous 4/0 or 5/0 polyglycolic acid sutures. The skin is closed with subcuticular sutures. A chest drain may be employed if necessary.

# Postoperative care

Oral feeding is commenced the same day, and discharge is possible within a few days.

### Further reading

Benjamin, B., Cohen, D., Glasson, M. (1976) Tracheomalacia in association with congenital tracheo-oesophageal fistula. Surgery 79, 504–508

Filler, R. M., Rossello, P. J., Lebowitz, R. L. (1976) Life-threatening anoxic spells caused by tracheal compression after repair of esophageal atresia: correction by surgery. Journal of Pediatric Surgery, 11, 739–748

Gross, R. E., Neuhauser, E. B. D. (1948) Compression of the trachea by an anomalous innominate artery: an operation for its relief. American Journal of Diseases in Childhood, 75, 570–574

Kiely, E. M., Spitz, L., Brereton, R. (1987) Management of tracheomalacia by aortopexy. Pediatric Surgery International, 2, 13–15

Spitz, L. (1986) Dacron patch aortopexy. Progress in Pediatric Surgery, 19, 117–119

# Oesophageal substitution

**John G. Raffensperger** MD
Children's Memorial Hospital, Northwestern University Medical School, Chicago, Illinois, USA

**Marleta Reynolds** MD
Children's Memorial Hospital, Northwestern University Medical School, Chicago, Illinois, USA

The indications for replacement of the entire oesophagus in children are becoming increasingly rare. Stretching of the proximal pouch, together with a circular myotomy, allows direct anastomosis in almost every infant with oesophageal atresia or atresia with fistula. Severe strictures of the oesophagus secondary to caustic ingestion are becoming less common, as a result of public education and early treatment with steroids, antibiotics and dilatation. The tremendous attention paid to gastroesophageal reflux and the development of effective operations to prevent reflux have decreased the incidence of oesophageal strictures secondary to oesophagitis.

The ideal oesophageal substitute should be sufficiently long to replace the entire thoracic oesophagus, be resistant to acid gastric juice, discourage reflux, and have some peristalsis. The right colon with an attached segment of terminal ileum, based on the middle colic artery, placed in the substernal position has been the most widely used oesophageal substitute since it was introduced almost 30 years ago[1-4].

An alternative approach is to place the transverse colon, based on the ascending branch of the left colic artery, in the posterior mediastinum[5,6]. This transplant provides an isoperistaltic conduit which is less bulky and less apt to become redundant than the right colon.

A reversed gastric tube, which receives its blood supply from the gastroepiploic vessels, may also be used to bypass the oesophagus[7,8]. This operation is preferred by many surgeons and is an excellent choice when a colon bypass has failed. In one series, however, there was a 63 per cent incidence of anastomotic leak and a 43 per cent incidence of anastomotic stricture with the gastric tube[9]. Lindahl et al. compared colon interposition with the gastric tube and found essentially no difference in function on long-term follow-up studies of 6 to 12 years.

Either conduit functioned satisfactorily; however, the gastric tube was easier to perform[10].

Our own preference is for an intestinal conduit consisting of a long segment of ileum with the ileocaecal valve and a portion of the ascending colon, based on the ileocolic artery. The ileum provides more peristalsis than a colonic segment and is nearly the same size as the proximal oesophagus. In addition, the ileocaecal valve prevents reflux of gastric contents into the upper conduit. We have now had the opportunity to follow-up 30 patients with a substernal colonic bypass from 7 to 25 years. Long-term function appears to be satisfactory. Follow-up cineradiographic studies in our patients demonstrate some motor activity; however, there is poor clearing of barium from the transplanted segment when the patient is in the recumbent position. Emptying is rapid when the patient is upright. Manometric studies have demonstrated peristalsis in the transplanted colon in response to the stimuli of swallowed water[11].

## PREOPERATIVE PREPARATION

The child with oesophageal atresia should be at least one year old before undergoing an oesophageal bypass. Normal nutrition is maintained via a gastrostomy tube, while saliva drains from a cervical oesophagostomy. Sham feeding is important until the definitive repair so that the swallowing habit is retained. A minimum of three days hospitalization should be allowed before the operation for mechanical and antibiotic intestinal preparation. An elemental diet, enemas and mild laxatives are given until the enemas are clear of solid faecal material. Erythromycin and neomycin are given in four divided doses during the 24 hours immediately before the operation.

# Terminal ileum/ascending colon

## TECHNIQUE

### 1

The child is placed supine on the operating table with a folded towel beneath his shoulders to hyperextend the head, which is turned to the right, away from the oesophagostomy. The entire neck, chest and abdomen are prepared and draped, and the gastrostomy tube is removed. One surgeon stands on the patient's left by the neck with his assistant opposite to isolate the oesophagus. The surgeon who is to mobilize the colon stands on the patient's right side. Each team works simultaneously, with one scrub nurse. A midline incision from the xiphoid to below the umbilicus is made, using the electrocautery for all layers except the skin. The cervical incision circumscribes the oesophagostomy and parallels the anterior border of the sternocleidomastoid muscle down to the upper border of the sternum.

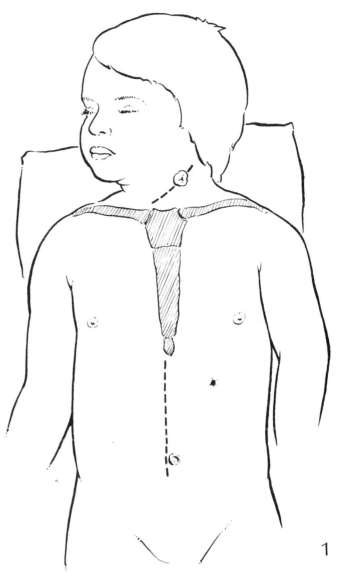

1

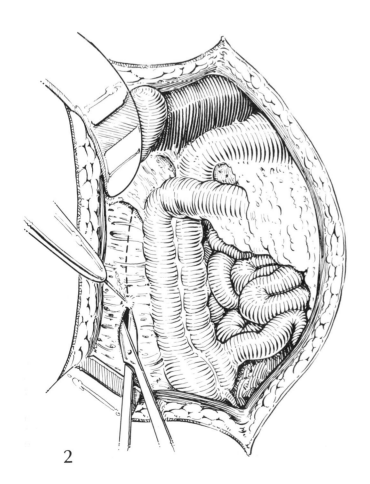

2

### 2

The terminal ileum, caecum, and ascending colon are mobilized by incising the lateral peritoneum with the electrocautery over the open blades of scissors. The areolar tissue behind the bowel is swept away with the scissors until the mesentery and bowel have been completely mobilized. Care is taken not to injure the mesenteric vessels and to identify the duodenum and ureter.

# 3

The middle, right and ileocolic arteries with accompanying veins are identified, and the marginal arteries inspected. The entire transplant, consisting of caecum, ascending and right colon, together with the terminal ileum, may be based on the middle colic artery. If possible, however, the ileocolic artery is chosen, because this allows a longer segment of ileum with less colon. The most likely segment of intestine is isolated with non-crushing vascular clamps. Bulldog clamps are placed across all vessels which will require ligation. Pulsations must then continue in the marginal vessels and the bowel must retain a normal colour. The blood supply is further evaluated by removing the appendix and observing blood flow from the appendiceal artery. If the segment does not appear to be perfectly satisfactory, another must be chosen. Great care must be taken to avoid damage to collateral and marginal vessels. Haematomas in the mesentery must be avoided absolutely. The leaves of the mesentery are separated and bloodless areas are divided with scissors.

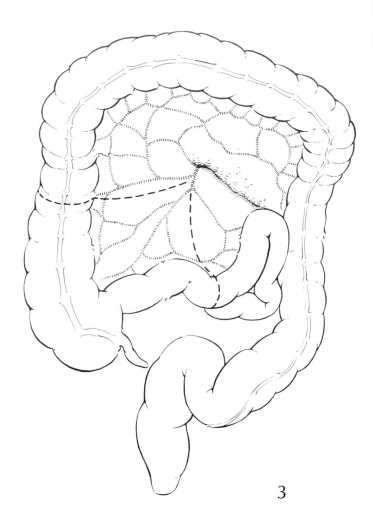

3

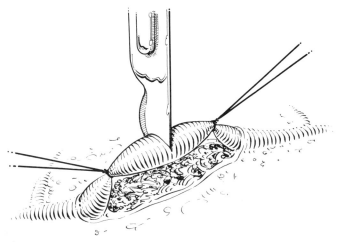

4

# 4

Each vessel is meticulously cleared of fat and lymph nodes, then ligated in continuity with 5/0 silk. Haemostats are not used to clamp mesenteric vessels for fear of damage to collateral blood supply. The ileum to be anastomosed to the oesophagus is divided between vascular clamps and sutured or, if desired, the bowel is stapled and divided.

## 5

Meanwhile, one surgeon has mobilized the cervical oesophagostomy from the skin and subcutaneous tissues by sharp dissection. It is essential to keep the operative field dry by coagulating the numerous small blood vessels with a needle-tipped electrosurgical unit. The oesophagus is closed with interrupted sutures, which are then used for traction to mobilize more oesophagus. The carotid sheath and sternocleidomastoid muscle are retracted laterally.

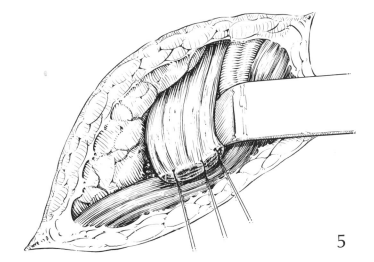

5

## 6

If the operation is being carried out for caustic stricture, the oesophagus will be intact. In this case it is encircled with a soft rubber drain and mobilized from the back wall of the trachea and the prevertebral fascia. The recurrent laryngeal nerve is avoided by keeping the plane of dissection immediately on the oesophagus as far down in the mediastinum as possible under direct vision.

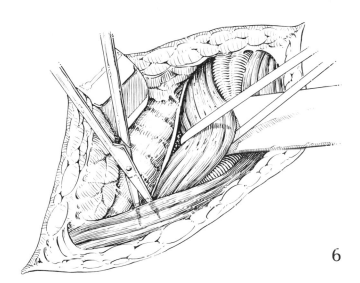

6

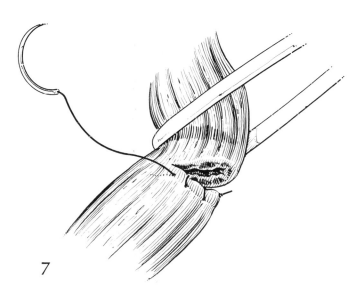

7

## 7

The oesophagus is divided for half its diameter and interrupted sutures are inserted to close the distal lumen. With these initial sutures held on traction, the remaining oesophagus is divided and sutured.

## 8

The upper, proximal oesophagus is now completely dissected for several centimetres.

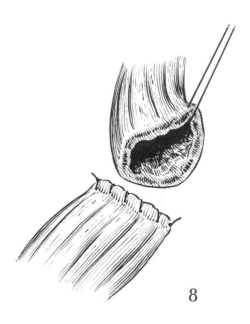

8

## 9

The upper border and posterior portion of the manubrium is exposed by dividing the cervical fascia and origin of the sternocleidomastoid muscle with the electrocautery. The sternoclavicular joint is also exposed. That part of the manubrium which curves backward is then removed with a rongeur, along with a segment of the joint. This is an essential part of the operation, because the curving sternum narrows the inlet to the anterior mediastinum. The posterior cut edge of bone is smoothed with a rasp, and bleeding is controlled with bone wax.

Failure to make a large opening into the upper, anterior mediastinum will result in venous obstruction in the transplanted bowel, necrosis, and leak at the anastomosis.

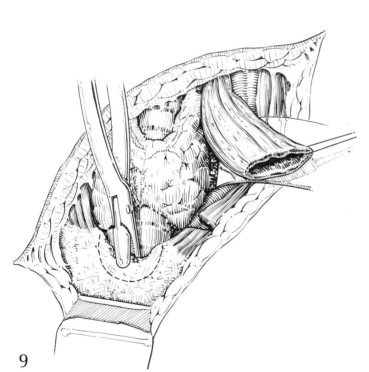

9

## 10

The substernal tunnel is then developed from the cervical incision between the back of the sternum and the thymus gland by blunt finger dissection. Meanwhile, the abdominal team has elevated the xiphoid and divided the attachments of the diaphragm to the undersurface of the lower sternum. The substernal tunnel must be large enough to accommodate two or three fingers.

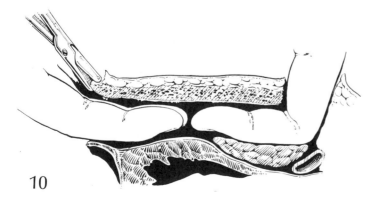

10

# 11

The stomach is mobilized and elevated with a soft rubber drain. Peritoneal folds at the root of the mesentery are divided so that the mesenteric vessels to the transplant are neither kinked nor under tension. The falciform ligament of the liver is divided. The transplant is drawn up behind the stomach, over the liver, and then up through the substernal tunnel. This step of the operation is performed with great care to ensure that there are no kinks or twists to obstruct the blood supply. Both surgeons must carefully evaluate the transplant to ensure that the blood supply is adequate and the tunnel is sufficiently large.

At this stage the abdominal team divides the colon in the abdomen at the point where it is to be anastomosed to the stomach. The distal colon is then brought back down from behind the stomach for anastomosis to the terminal ileum. This step is fraught with hazard! The dissection must proceed by dividing and ligating mesenteric vessels immediately on the wall of the bowel in order to prevent damage to the vessels supplying the transplant.

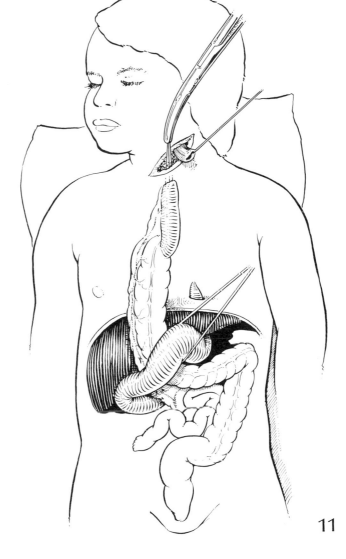

11

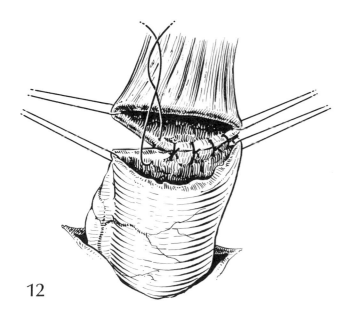

12

# 12

Excess ileum is resected in preparation for the anastomosis. There must be vigorous bleeding from the cut end of the bowel. 5/0 stay sutures are inserted to line up the seromuscular layer of the bowel with the muscular wall of the oesophagus. The anastomosis is made larger than either lumen by cutting the bowel and oesophagus at a 45° angle. Non-absorbable 5/0 sutures are then placed through the full thickness of oesophagus and bowel. Knots are placed on the inside on the back row, and on the outside in front. Neither the bowel nor oesophagus should be picked up with a tissue forceps or clamp. A drain is then placed into the anterior mediastinum and the wound is loosely closed.

## 13

Ideally, there should be sufficient length of ileum to reach from the oesophagus to the lower mediastinum. The anastomosis between caecum and stomach may then be made within 6–7 cm of the ileocaecal valve. Excess colon is resected and discarded so that there is no redundancy in the abdomen. The anastomosis to the stomach is carried out with an outer layer of non-absorbable interrupted sutures, and a full-thickness layer of continuous chromic catgut. A new gastrostomy is fashioned if necessary.

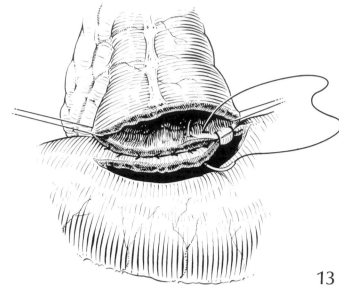

13

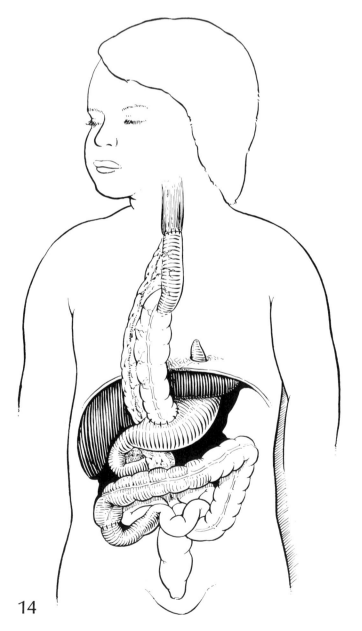

14

## 14

The operation is completed with an anastomosis between the terminal ileum and transverse colon. This illustration demonstrates the completed operation, with the blood supply to the transplant coursing behind the stomach and through the substernal tunnel.

### POSTOPERATIVE CARE

The gastrostomy tube is left on gravity drainage until there is evidence of peristalsis. It is then elevated and feedings are commenced. The cervical drain is removed after 48 hours. A barium swallow is obtained one week after the operation; if there is no leak at the anastomosis, feeding is commenced by mouth. We repeat the barium swallow six weeks and one year after the operation.

# Reverse gastric tube

### TECHNIQUE

Identical positioning and skin incisions are utilized in this technique of oesophageal replacement and are shown in illustration 1. Likewise, the mobilization of the cervical oesophagus and creation of the substernal tunnel follow the descriptions of illustrations 5–10.

## 15

The team working in the abdomen first inspects the gastric blood supply to ensure communication between the right and left gastroepiploic vessels, because the viability of the gastric tube will depend on this communication. The right gastroepiploic vessels are then divided approximately 2 cm proximal to the pylorus and the greater omentum is divided up to the splenic hilum.

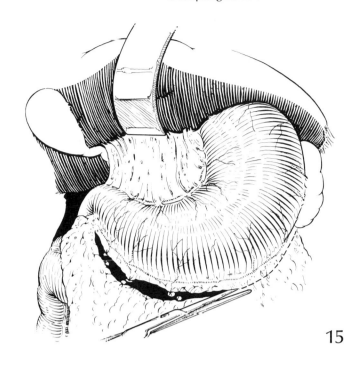

**15**

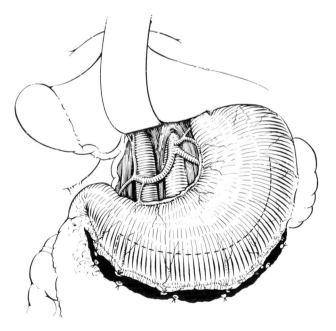

**16**

## 16

The gastric tube will be fashioned along the greater curvature of the stomach, incising both the anterior and posterior walls to conform to the size of an 18–24 Fr catheter.

# 17

The GIA stapler may be used for creating the gastric tube. Adequate length is assured by checking the length necessary to reach the neck. A two-layer closure of the stomach will provide haemostasis and a secure closure.

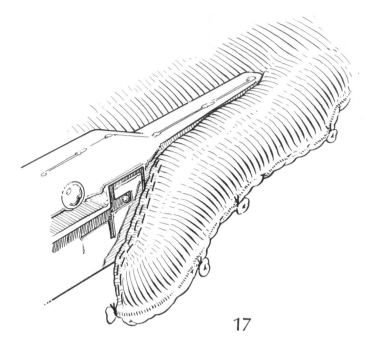

17

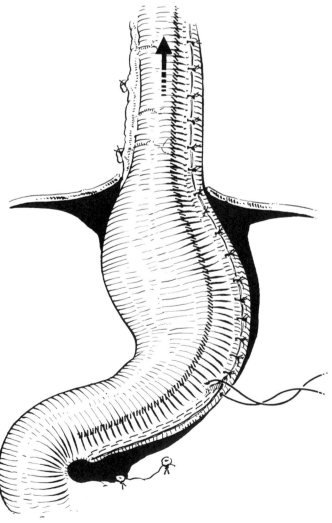

18

# 18

The gastric tube is then brought through the substernal tunnel, being careful to avoid any twist in the tube. After the two-layer cervical anastomosis is completed, the neck and mediastinum are drained and a gastrostomy created.

The postoperative management is the same as that described for the colon interposition.

# Resection and replacement of the lower one third of the oesophagus

Resection of the lower portion of the oesophagus is radical treatment for a benign stricture. Most often, strictures secondary to gastroesophageal reflux will respond to an antireflux operation and dilatation. On occasion, however, an oesophagus which has been damaged by previous caustic ingestion, as well as gastroesophageal reflux, will require resection.

## TECHNIQUE

## 19

The child is positioned with his left side partly elevated with towels. The left arm is allowed to fall across the upper chest, pulling the scapula upward. The operation is carried out through an incision at the ninth intercostal space, which is carried on across the upper abdomen almost to the midline. All layers except the skin are divided with a needle-tipped electrosurgical unit. The costal cartilage is divided so that the abdominal and thoracic incisions are continuous.

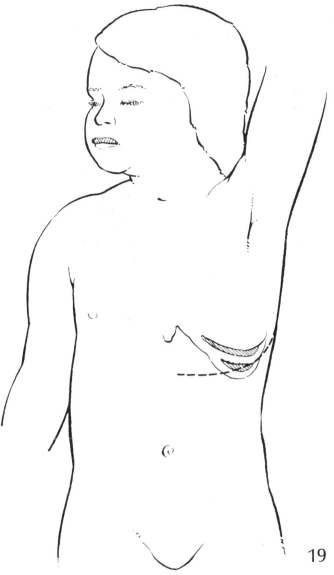

**19**

## 20

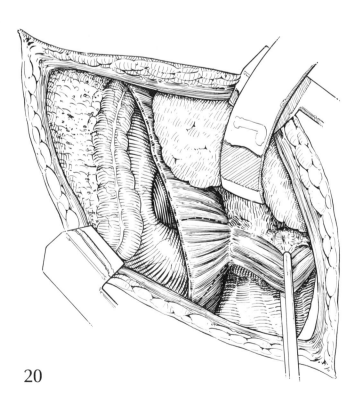

The chest is opened by gradually spreading a Finochietto retractor, while the diaphragm is separated at its periphery from the costal margin. The completed incision should expose the upper abdomen including the transverse colon, stomach, spleen, left lobe of the liver, and mesenteric vessels. In the thorax the lower lobe of the lung is elevated and the pulmonary ligament divided up to the inferior pulmonary veins. With the lung retracted, the pleura overlying the oesophagus is opened with scissors and the electrocautery from the oesophageal hiatus to the arch of the aorta.

Dissection around the oesophagus may be difficult due to perioesophageal fibrosis and reaction. Care must be taken to isolate, divide, and ligate oesophageal arteries which emerge directly from the aorta. When the oesophagus can be encircled with a soft rubber drain, it may be elevated and sharply dissected from the hiatus to above the stricture. Simultaneous endoscopy with a flexible oesophagoscope will locate the stricture precisely and will identify the extent of dissection required.

**20**

## 21

The oesophagogastric junction may be pulled up above the diaphragm through the hiatus and divided, or the stomach may be transected just below the hiatus from the abdominal side of the diaphragm. A paediatric GIA stapler will facilitate this step in the operation.

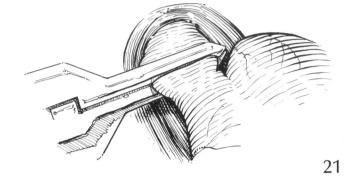

21

## 22

The oesophagus has been separated from the stomach and from the hiatus. It is held with traction sutures and dissected higher in the posterior mediastinum. It is absolutely essential to resect the oesophagus well above the stricture. If the anastomosis is not made in healthy tissue the patient is doomed to a recurrent stricture.

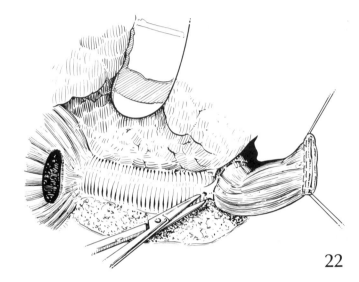

22

## 23

A segment of transverse colon based on the middle colic artery is selected for the transplant. The techniques described in illustrations 3 and 4 are utilized to identify and isolate the middle colic artery and to divide the mesenteric vessels.

23

# 24

The isoperistaltic segment of colon, with its blood supply, is then brought behind the stomach to emerge at the lesser curvature, and then through the oesophageal diaphragmatic hiatus. The anastomosis with the oesophagus and stomach are carried out as described in illustrations 12 and 13. The transverse colon is then anastomosed and a gastrostomy tube inserted. The wound is closed with a chest tube in place for pleural drainage.

A postoperative chest X-ray is taken to exclude significant pneumothorax.

## IMMEDIATE COMPLICATIONS

The most frequent complication of these three operations is leakage with subsequent stricture formation at the proximal anastomosis. Adequate drainage, together with gastrostomy feeding, will allow healing of small leaks. If there is reflux of gastric secretions and food, the gastrostomy tube must be kept on drainage, and total intravenous nutrition given until the anastomosis heals. Any strictures are then dilated with flexible mercury dilators.

24

## References

1. Longino, L. A., Woolley, M. M., Gross, R. E. (1959) Esophageal replacement in infants and children with use of a segment of colon. Journal of the American Medical Association, 171, 1187–1192

2. Dale, W. A., Sherman, C. D. (1955) Late reconstruction of congenital esophageal atresia by intrathoracic colon transplantation. Journal of Thoracic Surgery, 29, 344–356

3. Javid, H. (1954) Esophageal reconstruction using colon and terminal ileum. Surgery, 36, 132–135

4. Neville, W. E., Clowes, G. H. A. (1960) Colon replacement of the esophagus in children for congenital and acquired disease. Journal of Thoracic and Cardiovascular Surgery, 40, 507–516

5. Waterston, D. (1964) Colonic replacement of esophagus (intrathoracic). Surgical Clinics of North America, 44, 1441–1447

6. German, J. C., Waterston, D. J. (1976) Colon interposition for the replacement of the esophagus in children. Journal of Pediatric Surgery, 11, 227–234

7. Gavriliu, D. (1975) Aspects of esophageal surgery. Current Problems in Surgery, 12(10), 1–64

8. Anderson, K. D., Randolph, J. G. (1978) Gastric tube interposition: A satisfactory alternative to the colon for esophageal replacement in children. Annals of Thoracic Surgery, 25, 521–525

9. Ein, S. H., Shandling, B., Simpson, J. S., Stephens, C. A., Vizas, D. (1978) Fourteen years of gastric tubes. Journal of Pediatric Surgery, 13, 638–642

10. Lindahl, H., Louhimo, I., Virkola, K. (1983) Colon interposition or gastric tube? Follow-up study of colon–esophagus and gastric tube–esophagus patients. Journal of Pediatric Surgery, 18–1, 58–63

11. Benages, A., Moreno-Ossett, E., Paris, F. Ridocci, M. T., Blasco, E., Pastor, J. et al. (1981) Motor activity after colon replacement of esophagus. Manometric evaluation. Journal of Thoracic and Cardiovascular Surgery, 82, 335–340

Illustrations by Kevin Marks

# Gastric replacement of the oesophagus

**Lewis Spitz**   MB, ChB, PhD, FRCS(Eng), FRCS(Ed), FAAP(Hon)
Nuffield Professor of Paediatric Surgery, Institute of Child Health, University of London; Consultant Paediatric Surgeon, Hospital for Sick Children, Great Ormond Street, London, UK

## Introduction

An alternative means of replacing the oesophagus is by gastric transposition involving the whole stomach. This method has the advantage of involving only one anastomosis which is relatively well vascularized and is associated with a low leak rate.

The procedure may be performed either via a thoraco-abdominal approach, or trans-hiatally via the posterior mediastinum without having to resort to a thoracotomy. This latter method will be described in detail.

The importance of sham feeds before the definitive operation in simplifying the initiation of oral nutrition following the interposition should not be underestimated.

# The technique of mediastinal gastric transposition

The initial feeding gastrostomy should ideally have been sited on the anterior surface of the body of the stomach, well away from the greater curvature, in order to preserve the vascular arcades of the gastroepiploic vessels.

## INCISION

The stomach is exposed via an oblique left upper-abdominal, transverse muscle-cutting incision, encompassing the gastrostomy site. This incision may be extended into a thoracoabdominal incision, should the need arise. An alternative approach is via an upper-abdominal *midline* incision.

## PROCEDURE

The gastrostomy is carefully mobilized and the defect in the stomach closed in two layers with interrupted 4/0 polyglycolic acid sutures.

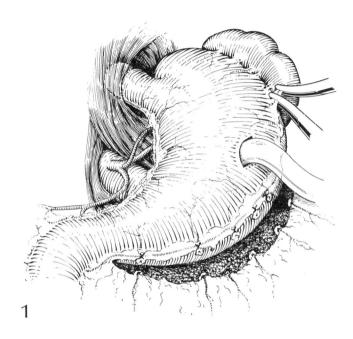

**1**

Adhesions between the stomach and the left lobe of the liver are lysed, taking care not to damage any of the major blood vessels.

The greater curvature of the stomach is mobilized by ligating and dividing the vessels in the gastrocolic omentum, and the short gastric vessels. The vessels should be ligated well away from the stomach wall in order to preserve the vascular arcades of the right gastroepiploic vessels. Meticulous care must be exercised to avoid damaging the spleen.

The lesser curvature of the stomach is freed by dividing lesser omentum from pylorus to the diaphragmatic hiatus. The right gastric artery is carefully identified and preserved, while the left gastric artery is ligated and divided close to the stomach. The lower oesophagus is exposed by dividing the phreno-oesophageal membrane, and the margins of the oesophageal hiatus in the diaphragm are defined.

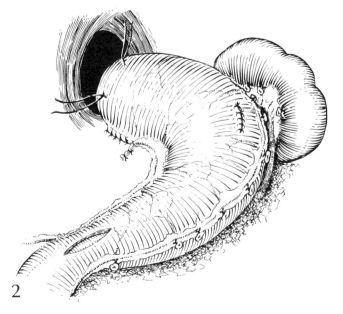

**2**

The inevitably short blind-ending lower oesophageal stump is dissected out of the posterior mediastinum by a combination of blunt and sharp dissection through the diaphragmatic hiatus. The vagal nerves may be divided during this part of the procedure. The body and fundus of the stomach are now free from all attachments and can be delivered into the wound.

The oesophagus is transected at the gastro-oesophageal junction and the defect closed in two layers with 4/0 polyglycolic acid sutures.

A pyloromyotomy (or pyloroplasty) is performed and a careful inspection made for mucosal perforation. The second part of the duodenum is Kocherized to obtain maximum mobility of the pylorus.

The highest part of the fundus of the stomach is identified and stay-sutures of different material are inserted to the left and the right of the area selected for the anastomosis. These sutures help to detect torsion of the stomach as it is pulled up through the posterior mediastinum into the neck. Attention is now turned to the neck, where the previously constructed cervical oesophagostomy (preferably performed on the left side) is mobilized via a 3–4 cm transverse incision, taking care not to damage the muscular coat of the oesophagus. The recurrent laryngeal nerve coursing upwards on the posterolateral surface of the trachea is identified and preserved.

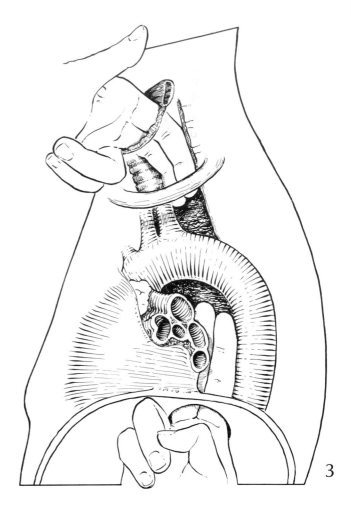

# 3

A plane of dissection between the membranous posterior surface of the trachea and the prevertebral fascia is established, and by blunt dissection immediately in the midline a tunnel is created into the superior mediastinum.

A similar tunnel is fashioned from below in the line of the normal oesophageal route, by means of blunt dissection through the oesophageal hiatus in the tissue posterior to the heart and anterior to the prevertebral fascia.

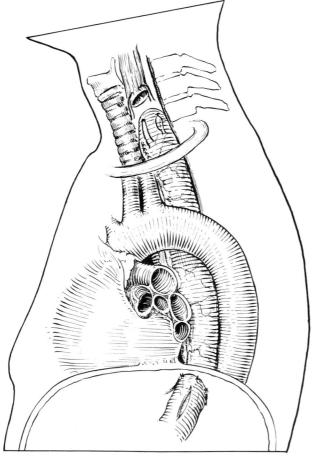

# 4

When continuity of the superior and inferior posterior mediastinal tunnels has been established, the space to be occupied by the stomach is developed into a 2–3 finger-breadth tunnel.

A long, blunt haemostat is passed into the posterior mediastinal tunnel from the cervical incision and the two stay-sutures on the fundus of the stomach grasped. The haemostat is gently withdrawn pulling the stomach up through the oesophageal hiatus and the posterior mediastinal tunnel into the cervical incision. Orientation of the fundus is checked by realigning the stay-sutures in their correct position.

# 5

The end of the oesophagus is anastomosed to the highest part of the stomach using a single- or two-layer technique with interrupted 4/0 polyglycolic acid sutures.

A large-calibre (No. 12 gauge) nasogastric tube is inserted into the stomach through the oesophagogastric anastomosis. This is left on free drainage and aspirated at regular intervals to prevent acute gastric dilatation in the early postoperative period.

A soft rubber drain is placed at the site of the anastomosis and the wound closed in layers.

The margins of the diaphragmatic hiatus are sutured to the antrum of the stomach with a few interrupted sutures (4/0 polyglycolic acid or braided polyamide (Nurolon)), so that the pylorus lies just below the diaphragm.

A polythene catheter is inserted via the oesophageal hiatus into the posterior mediastinum and placed in an underwater seal. This catheter will drain any blood or fluid which may accumulate in the mediastinum.

A fine-bore feeding jejunostomy has been found to be of considerable value in providing enteral nutrition in the first few weeks following the gastric transposition before full oral nutrition is established.

The abdominal incision is closed *en masse* or in layers.

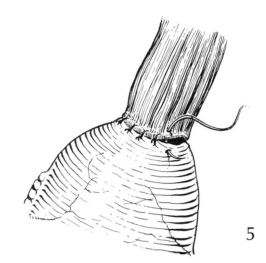

5

## Postoperative management

Careful monitoring of vital functions is essential in the early postoperative period. There has been a fairly extensive dissection in the tissues posterior to the trachea, and oedema may produce respiratory embarrassment. Elective nasotracheal intubation with assisted ventilation for a few days will simplify the postoperative course and reduce the incidence of respiratory problems.

The mediastinal drain may be removed 48 hours postoperatively. Jejunal feeds are instituted on the second or third postoperative day. The safest method of delivery of these feeds is by means of a slow continuous infusion rather than as a bolus which can provoke a 'dumping' effect. A contrast swallow is performed 7 to 10 days after surgery, and if no leak is identified at the anastomosis careful oral feeding may be commenced. The cervical drain is removed when the integrity of the anastomosis has been demonstrated.

*References*

1. Orringer, H. B., Sloan, H. (1978) Esophagectomy without thoracotomy. Journal of Thoracic Cardiovascular Surgery, 76, 643–654

2. Spitz, L. (1984) Gastric transposition via the mediastinal route for infants with long-gap esophageal atresia. Journal of Pediatric Surgery, 19, 149–154.

3. Spitz, L., Kiely, E., Sparnon, T. (1987) Gastric transposition for esophageal replacement in children. Annals of Surgery, 206, 69–73.

# Congenital diaphragmatic hernia and eventration

**Lewis Spitz**   MB, ChB, PhD, FRCS(Eng), FRCS(Ed), FAAP(Hon)
Nuffield Professor of Paediatric Surgery, Institute of Child Health, University of London; Consultant Paediatric Surgeon, Hospital for Sick Children, Great Ormond Street, London, UK

## DIAPHRAGMATIC HERNIA

### History

Ambroise Paré reported the first diaphragmatic hernia, which was of traumatic origin, in 1597. In 1848 Vincent Alexander Bochdalek published his description of the congenital diaphragmatic hernia that now bears his name. The defect as described by Bochdalek was a triangular slit between the lumbar portion of the diaphragm and the apex of the twelfth rib. He attributed the herniation to rupture of a previously intact membrane in the lumbo-costal triangle.

## 1a & b

### Types of hernia

The various areas in the diaphragm (excluding the oesophageal hiatus) through which hernias may occur are shown.

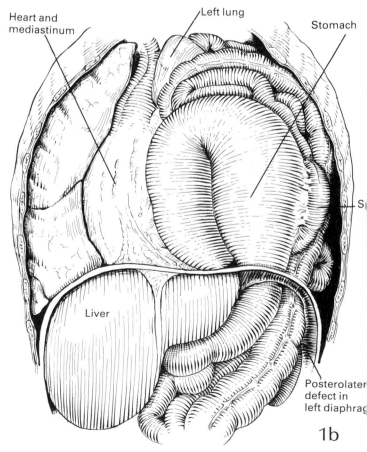

Parasternal (Morgagni) hernia

IVC

Oesophageal hiatus

Aorta

Agenesis of diaphragm (septum transversum defect)

Posterolateral (Bochdalek) hernia

1a

Heart and mediastinum

Left lung

Stomach

Liver

S

Posterolateral defect in left diaphragm

1b

## Diagnosis

Diaphragmatic hernia through the patent pleuro-peritoneal canal, generally referred to as the foramen of Bochdalek, usually presents as an acute emergency in the neonatal period. The classical diagnostic triad consists of respiratory distress, apparent dextrocardia and a flat 'scaphoid' abdomen. Breath sounds are diminished on the affected side and borborygmi may be auscultated in the chest. The presenting symptoms in cases manifesting at a later stage include recurrent respiratory infections, dyspnoea, especially after meals, and vomiting. The left side is affected in 85–90 per cent of cases. This has been attributed to the later closure of the left pleuroperitoneal canal during the eighth week of intrauterine development. Bilateral hernias are rare. Prenatal diagnosis of a diaphragmatic hernia can be established on antenatal ultrasound scan.

## 2

A chest radiograph, which should always include the abdomen, is usually diagnostic. The affected hemithorax is filled with gas-containing loops of intestine, the mediastinum is displaced to the opposite side, and there are relatively few intra-abdominal intestinal gas shadows.

The presence of a normal intestinal gas configuration with an apparently intact diaphragm is suspicious of congenital lobar emphysema or adenoid cystic malformation of the lung. Contrast studies of the gastrointestinal tract may be required to differentiate these two primary pulmonary conditions from a true diaphragmatic hernia.

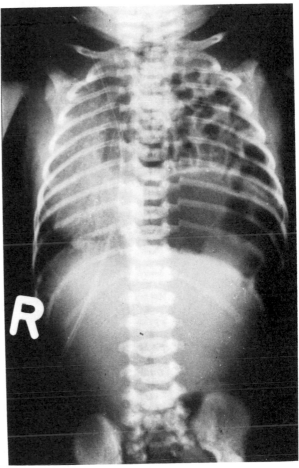

2

## Resuscitative measures

As soon as the diagnosis is suspected, a large calibre (No. 10 gauge) nasogastric tube should be introduced into the stomach and all swallowed contents evacuated. The infant is nursed in 100 per cent oxygen, and if this fails to improve the respiratory embarrassment, ventilatory assistance is administered via an endotracheal tube. Ventilation with a face mask is strictly contraindicated as this forces air into the stomach and intestines, further embarrassing the respiration. Sudden deterioration during resuscitation may be due to a tension pneumothorax. This is relieved by inserting a hypodermic needle (No. 21 gauge) into the affected pleural space. An intercostal drain with underwater seal can then be formally introduced in a relatively stable patient. Correction of acidosis should be attempted with extreme caution.

## Transportation

Where possible, transfer of the infant to a paediatric surgical centre should be carried out promptly while all resuscitative measures continue. This implies attendance by experienced medical and nursing personnel, ensuring as far as possible that the infant remains normothermic and adequately oxygenated and that the intestines remain decompressed.

Recently the previously accepted doctrine of emergency surgery for congenital diaphragmatic hernia has been challenged. The alternative approach is to stabilize the infant's cardio-respiratory status for a variable period (12–48 hours or longer) preoperatively before carrying out the surgical repair. This is achieved by elective mechanical ventilation and paralysis, correction of acid-base imbalance and hypoxia, and the judicious use of pulmonary vasodilators (tolazoline) and cardiocirculatory supportive agents (dopamine) (vide infra). The patient requires continuous close and meticulous monitoring including preductal radial artery pressure and blood gas analysis, central venous pressure and if possible pre- and postductal oxygen saturation with transcutaneous oximetry.

## Anaesthesia

This consists of standard neonatal anaesthesia with preoxygenation and awake endotracheal intubation (if this was not required during resuscitation) followed by hand ventilation with an Ayre's T-piece. Gentle ventilation, using inspiratory pressures of up to $25\,cmH_2O$ with $5\,cmH_2O$ end-respiratory pressure to maintain the functional residual capacity, is maintained throughout the operative period. Monitoring of electrocardiogram, core temperature (rectal probe), central venous and arterial pressures, blood gases and blood loss is carried out intraoperatively.

# The operation

### The incision

The abdominal approach is preferred for all left-sided congenital posterolateral diaphragmatic hernias. Correction of the associated intestinal malrotation and enlargement of the peritoneal cavity to accommodate the displaced viscera are more easily achieved through an abdominal incision.

A transthoracic approach may be used for the right-sided hernia where liver may be the only contents, or for recurrent hernias where adhesions prevent simple reduction of the herniated contents.

## 3

The abdominal approach is via a left upper abdominal transverse muscle-cutting (or alternatively a left oblique subcostal) incision placed 2 cm above the umbilical cord and extending from the midline to the tip of ninth costal cartilage.

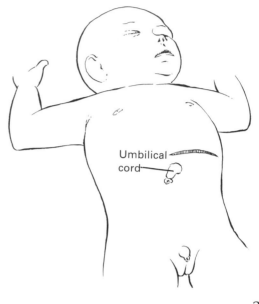

3

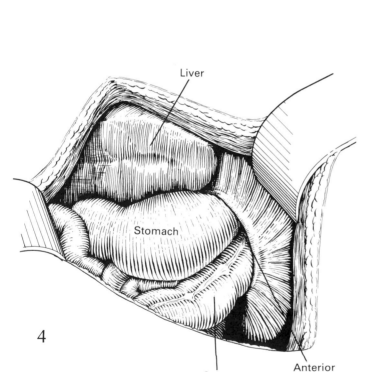

4

## 4

### Exposure of the diaphragmatic defect

The cranial part of the wound is retracted upwards to reveal the anterior well-muscularized diaphragm and the posteriorly located defect through which most of the abdominal viscera have herniated into the pleural cavity. The peritoneal cavity is relatively empty.

# 5

## Definition of the diaphragmatic defect

The herniated contents, which may include the entire small intestine together with a variable amount of the right colon, stomach, spleen and left lobe of liver, are gently withdrawn. The anterior rim of the defect is usually well defined and easily identifiable. The posterior rim is frequently adherent to the posterior abdominal wall in close proximity to the left adrenal and kidney. Occasionally the posterior rim is completely deficient but more commonly it gradually fades out laterally, where the margin of the defect merges with the chest wall.

Exposure of the margins of the defect may be facilitated by retracting the left lobe of the liver medially after dividing the left triangular ligament. A careful search is now made for a sac which is present in 10–15 per cent of cases. The sac may be extremely thin and closely applied to the pleura. The sac should be excised up to the margins of the diaphragmatic defect. A plastic drainage tube is inserted into the pleural cavity via the ninth intercostal space in the mid-axillary line. Some surgeons prefer not to drain the pleural space; others prophylactically insert catheters into both sides of the chest.

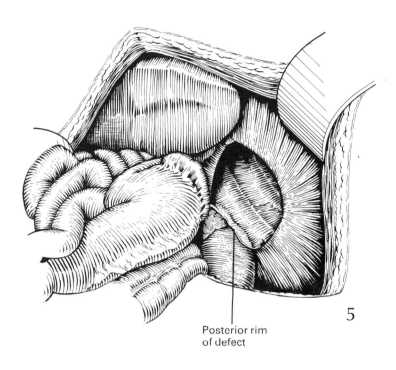

Posterior rim
of defect

5

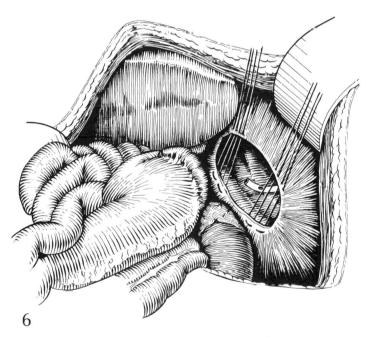

6

## Repair of the defect

The hernial orifice is closed in two layers by approximating the margins of the defect with interrupted non-absorbable suture material (2/0 or 3/0 silk or braided polyamine).

# 6

The first row consists of horizontal mattress sutures inserted 5 mm from the edge of the defect.

## 7

The second row approximates the everted rim.

Where the posterior rim is partially or totally absent the sutures should be placed around the adjacent rib to achieve a secure repair. Direct apposition of the hernial margins is occasionally difficult or would only be possible under tension. In these cases the defect is best closed with a prosthetic patch (Dacron, Teflon). Alternatively a flap of anterior abdominal wall may be rotated into the opening and sutured in position.

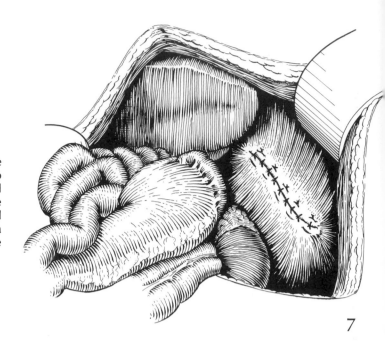

7

### Additional manoeuvres

The intestinal malrotation is corrected by dividing abnormal bands and splaying the root of the mesentery. The duodenal loop is straightened, and the small intestine placed in the right side of the abdomen with the caecum in the left upper quadrant. The peritoneal cavity is enlarged by forcibly stretching the muscles of the anterior abdominal wall.

### Closure of the abdomen

The abdominal incision is closed *en masse* or in layers with 3/0 polyglycolic acid sutures. A subcuticular 4/0 polyglycolic acid suture approximates the skin edges. In the very rare case closure of the abdominal wall cannot be achieved without profound tension which will further embarrass respiration. In these cases the establishment of a ventral hernia or accommodation of the intestine temporarily in a pouch fashioned with Silastic sheeting may be required.

The intercostal drain is connected to an underwater seal with 2–3 cmH$_2$O of negative pressure. We prefer to clamp the drainage tube, releasing it for a short period only every 6 hours. This manoeuvre allows gentle expansion of the ipsilateral lung while extreme to-and-fro shifting of the mediastinum is prevented. The intercostal drain is removed when full expansion of the lung has occurred or when a stable state has been achieved. No attempt at rapid re-expansion of the lung should be made.

## Postoperative care

All neonates presenting within 12 hours of birth are electively ventilated postoperatively. Monitoring consists of electrocardiogram, temperature, central venous pressure (via internal jugular vein catheter) and arterial pressure (via the right radial artery). Transcutaneous arterial $PO_2$ is measured in the upper part of the abdomen to give an early indication of ductal shunting of blood arising from increased pulmonary vascular resistance.

Fifteen per cent of infants are at risk of developing a transitional circulation (right-to-left shunting at ductal and atrial level) due to the pulmonary vascular resistance rising above systemic pressures. Such patients may respond dramatically to pulmonary vasodilators (e.g. tolazoline 1–2 mg/kg bodyweight per hour as an intravenous infusion). Dopamine (5–15 $\mu$g/kg per min) may be required in addition to improve the systemic circulation by its direct inotropic effect. Owing to the vasodilatory effects of both these drugs, large volumes of plasma expanders may be required. These requirements are best assessed by monitoring the central venous pressure.

Weaning of the infant from ventilatory assistance is accomplished slowly using intermittent mandatory ventilation once cardiopulmonary stability has been achieved. Prolonged ileus, particularly in the infant requiring ventilatory support, may indicate the need for parenteral nutrition for a variable period during the postoperative course.

## Results

The mortality rate is directly proportional to the degree of pulmonary hypoplasia. Infants presenting within 6–12 hours of birth usually have advanced pulmonary hypoplasia, whereas those infants in whom the diagnosis is not evident before 12–24 hours have little impairment of pulmonary development. The survival rate for infants presenting within 12 hours of birth is between 45–60 per cent, while few deaths should occur in infants older than 12 hours at the time of diagnosis. At the Hospital for Sick Children, London, 92 infants with diaphragmatic hernia were treated between 1979 and 1981. The overall survival rate was 74 per cent (68 infants). All the deaths, 24 cases, occurred in those infants presenting within 6 hours of birth (overall survival rate in this group 61 per cent, i.e. 37 of 61 patients).

# EVENTRATION OF THE DIAPHRAGM

This refers to an abnormally high position of one or both leaflets of the intact diaphragm as a result of paralysis, hypoplasia or atrophy of the muscle fibres. It is poorly tolerated by the young infant especially if bilateral. If there is a possibility that the damage to the phrenic nerve is reversible, the condition can be successfully managed with continuous positive airway pressure ventilation for a period of 4–6 weeks. Where the phrenic nerve injury is thought to be permanent or where there is a relapse following a trial of conservative management, surgery is recommended. The aim of surgery in eventration is to fix the paralysed diaphragm in the inspiratory position, thereby minimizing paradoxical movement and preventing shift of the mediastinum with respiration.

## The operation

### The incision

A thoracic or abdominal approach may be used. In bilateral eventration an upper abdominal transverse muscle-cutting incision is performed, while in unilateral cases, especially when the right hemidiaphragm is involved, a thoracic approach affords easier access and allows identification of the branches of the phrenic nerve. The lateral thoracotomy is via the unresected bed of the eighth rib.

Left phrenic nerve — Inferior vena cava — Right phrenic nerve — Pericardium — Oesophagus — Aorta

## 8

### Exposure of the diaphragm

The inferior pulmonary ligament is divided and the distribution of the branches of the phrenic nerve defined.

8

# 9–11

### Technique of plication

Four to six rows of 2/0 or 3/0 non-absorbable sutures (silk or braided polyamine) are inserted into the diaphragm from anterolateral to posteromedial. Each row comprises five to six pleats, avoiding the branches of the phrenic nerve. The suture should not pass through the full thickness of the diaphragm as underlying adjacent viscera may be traumatized. The sutures are left untied until all the rows are in position.

An intercostal drain with underwater seal may be inserted and removed when full expansion of the lung has been shown to have occurred. No special postoperative measures are necessary. Recovery is rapid and uneventful and complications rarely occur.

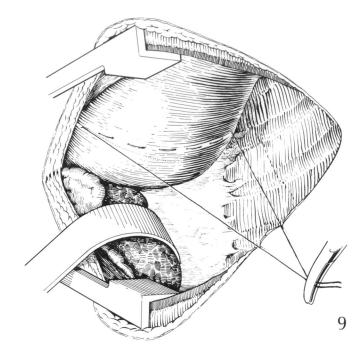

9

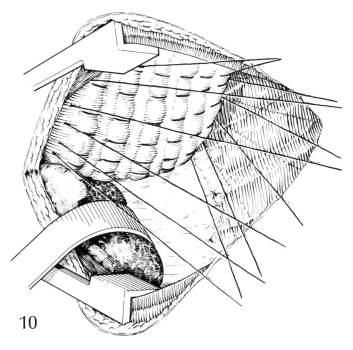

10

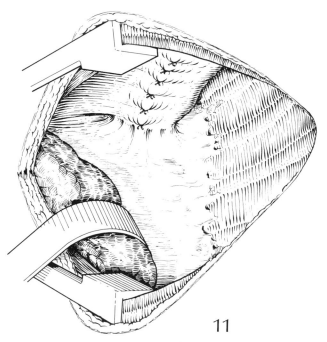

11

## Further reading

Bloss, R. S., Aranda, J. V., Beardmore, H. E. Congenital diaphragmatic hernia: pathophysiology and pharmacologic support. Surgery 1981; 89: 518–524

Carter, R. E. B., Waterston, D. J., Aberdeen, E. Hernia and eventration of the diaphragm in childhood. Lancet 1962; 1: 656–659

Haller, J. A., Pickard, L. R., Tepas, J. J., Rogers, M. C., Robotham, J. L., Shorter, N., Shermata, D. W. Management of diaphragmatic paralysis in infants with special emphasis on selection of patients for operative plication. Journal of Pediatric Surgery 1979; 14: 779–785

Miyasaka, K., Sankawa, H., Nakajo, T., Akiyama, H. Congenital diaphragmatic hernia: is emergency radical surgery really necessary? Japanese Journal of Pediatric Surgery, 1984, 16, 1417–1422

Sakai, H., Tamura, M., Hosokawa, Y., Bryan, A. C., Barker, G. A., Bohn, D. J. Effect of surgical repair on respiratory mechanics in congenital diaphragmatic hernia. Journal of Pediatrics, 1987, 111, 432–438

Schwartz, M. Z., Filler, R. M. Plication of the diaphragm for symptomatic phrenic nerve paralysis. Journal of Pediatric Surgery 1978; 13: 259–263

Sumner, E., Frank, J. D. Tolazoline in the treatment of congenital diaphragmatic hernias. Archives of Diseases in Childhood 1981; 56: 350–353

Illustrations by Kevin Marks

# Lung surgery in infants and children

**T. R. Karl**  MD
Kaiser Permanante Medical Center, San Francisco, California, USA

**J. Stark**  MD, FRCS
Consultant Cardiothoracic Surgeon, Cardiothoracic Unit, The Hospital for Sick Children, Great Ormond Street, London, UK

## INTRODUCTION

Lung surgery in infants and children is peformed far less frequently than in adult patients. The conditions requiring early surgery in childhood are obstructive lobar emphysema, lung cysts (both congenital and acquired), sequestration, tumours and infections of the lung and pleura.

Many principles of surgical approach and technique are similar to those used in adult patients. In this chapter we shall confine our remarks to those aspects that are different or even unique in infants and children.

# Thoracotomy

A thoracotomy in infants and young children differs from that commonly performed in adults. The configuration and elasticity of the chest wall make a transverse lateral incision ideal for most operations. The posterior and upward curving part of the adult incision should be avoided, even when a posterior exposure is desired. Good exposure can be obtained through the fourth or fifth intercostal space without transecting or removing a rib.

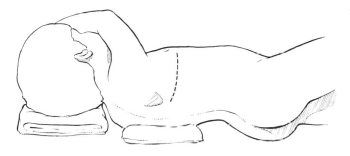

**1**

## 1

### Position of patient and incision

The patient is placed in the full lateral position with the arm over the head. Sandbags are placed to support the chest anteriorly and posteriorly. It is advantageous if the patient lies slightly obliquely across the table with the shoulders closest to the surgeon. In this position the ribs will lie more perpendicular to the operator.

The skin is painted with antiseptic solution and drapes applied. The nipple, spine, scapular tip and costal arch should all be in the operative field as they serve as landmarks, and the inferior exposure facilitates placement of chest drains.

The skin incision is made well below the nipple to avoid damage to breast tissue. This is particularly important in young infants in whom the dimensions are short. It is a straight incision starting usually 2–3 cm posterior to the nipple and staying below the inferior tip of the scapula. The skin is incised with a scalpel; subsequent layers with a diathermy needle.

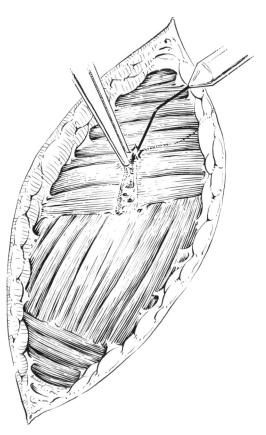

**2**

## 2

The pectoralis major and serratus anterior muscles are incised in older children and part of the latissimus dorsi may also be divided. Bleeding points are controlled with diathermy current. The scapula is lifted upward with a retractor, and the ribs are counted to determine the correct interspace. The highest rib palpable is usually the second. Most operations (excluding those on the diaphragm) can be done easily through the fifth interspace.

# 3

Diathermy is used to divide the intercostal muscles for a few centimetres along the upper border of the rib, avoiding the neurovascular bundle. The intercostal muscles are spread with a fine artery forceps to facilitate the incision.

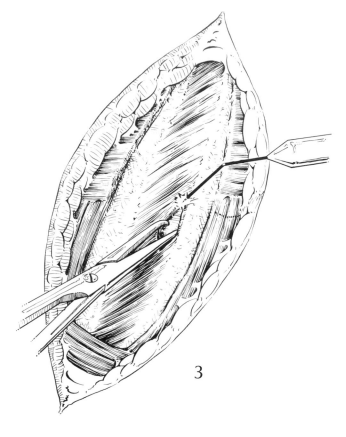

3

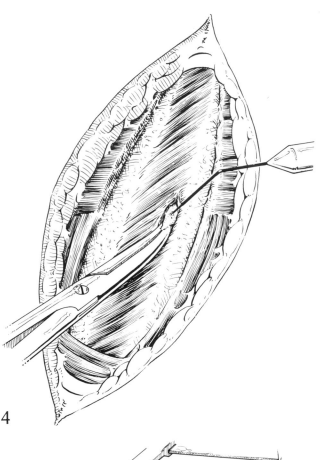

4

# 4

The anaesthetist deflates the lungs, the pleura is punctured with artery forceps, a small swab (peanut) is placed beneath the intercostal muscles and the diathermy tip is pressed against it, resulting in a quick and bloodless thoracotomy.

# 5

Towels are placed over the wound edges and a Finochietto retractor is inserted and partially opened. Exposure is increased by extending the intercostal incision anteriorly and posteriorly beyond the limits of the skin incision. If necessary, the subcutaneous tissue can also be undercut from inside the chest. A completed opening is shown.

When the operation is completed the chest drain is inserted. A short skin incision is made 3–4 cm below the thoracotomy incision at the midaxillary line. A suture is placed to fix the drain and can also be used to close the tract left after its removal. An artery forceps is passed through the chest wall one to two interspaces below the thoracotomy and the drain pulled through. If a lung resection has been performed two drains are placed, one anteriorly and apically and the second posteriorly to drain both blood and air.

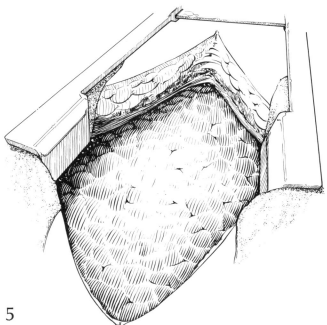

5

## 6

Non-absorbable sutures (0 Ethibond for infants, 1 or 2 Ethibond for older children) are used to encircle the ribs, taking care to avoid the intercostal bundles. Two or three sutures are used. The needle holes are checked for bleeding on both sides of the chest wall. The sutures are then tied while the assistant crosses the adjacent ones. At this point, chest drains should be connected to underwater seals and the lung fully inflated by the anaesthetist.

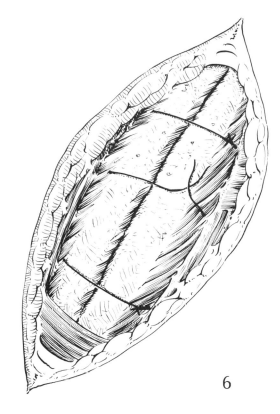

6

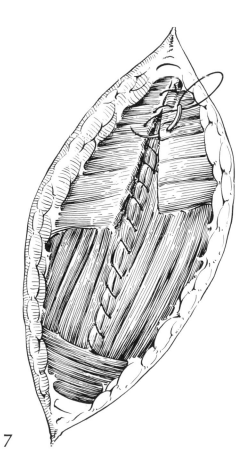

7

## 7

The divided muscles are closed in anatomical layers with continuous Dexon sutures. Careful muscle closure provides a superior cosmetic and functional result. The subcutaneous tissue is sutured with running Dexon, and intracuticular Dexon closes the skin.

A lateral thoracotomy is well tolerated in infants and children. After 24 hours the dressings are removed and the incision can be exposed. If there is no air leak the drains are usually removed on the first postoperative day. If an air leak is present the drains are left in place for a further 24 hours after the leak has stopped. Wound infections are unusual and dehiscence rare.

# Lobectomy

A lobectomy is usually performed for obstructive lobar emphysema, extensive cystic malformation, or occasionally for tumour or a very large acquired cyst. Pneumonectomy is only very rarely indicated. The severe physiological consequences of pneumonectomy in children (kyphoscoliosis, or tracheal obstruction by rotated great arteries)[1] make a conservative approach desirable. Most surgeons will try to preserve at least a portion of the lung if possible, rather than opt for pneumonectomy.

## Technique

A left upper lobectomy is described, as this is most commonly performed for obstructive lobar emphysema. The principles apply to the other lobes as well as to pneumonectomy. The key to any resection is good visualization and adequate dissection of the pulmonary veins and arteries.

The chest is opened through the fifth interspace. Any adhesions between the lung and chest wall are diathermied and sharply divided. Once freed, the left upper lobe is delivered into the operative field and gentle traction is applied in an inferior and posterior direction. The thin pleura overlying the hilar vessels is opened with scissors. Bleeding is controlled with low diathermy current applied to a fine forceps.

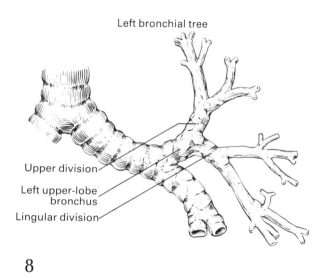

Left bronchial tree

Upper division

Left upper-lobe bronchus

Lingular division

8

# 8, 9 & 10

Normal anatomy of the bronchus, pulmonary artery and pulmonary vein bronchus is shown. The pulmonary artery exits beneath the aortic arch and crosses the left upper-lobe bronchus. The segmental pulmonary artery branches to the left upper lobe (usually three in number) are encircled with fine silk ties. When these branches are divided and ligated, the upper-lobe bronchus becomes visible. The superior pulmonary vein usually has three segmental branches which are encircled, ligated and divided. The main trunk of the superior pulmonary vein is also ligated. Prior to division it is essential to confirm the presence of a lower-lobe pulmonary vein. A vascular clamp is placed across the left upper-lobe bronchus and free inflation and deflation of the left lower lobe is confirmed. The upper-lobe bronchus is then divided and a swab taken for bacteriological examination.

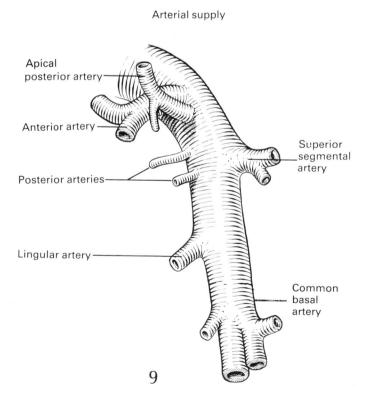

Arterial supply

Apical posterior artery

Anterior artery

Posterior arteries

Lingular artery

Superior segmental artery

Common basal artery

9

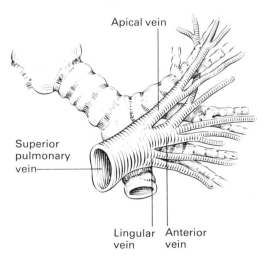

Venous drainage of left upper lobe

Apical vein

Superior pulmonary vein

Lingular vein

Anterior vein

10

# 11 & 12

The bronchial stump is closed with a running fine polypropylene suture. Usually a continuous mattress and then over-and-over stitch are used. In infants with obstructive lobar emphysema the bronchus is usually soft and of small calibre. In such cases suture ligation is adequate and safe. The bronchial closure is tested for leakage by filling the chest with water and inflating the left lower lobe to a pressure of about 40 cm. The inferior pulmonary ligament is divided up to the inferior pulmonary veins to free the lower lobe. The chest is closed with anterior and posterior drains as described above.

If a pneumonectomy is performed some authors have suggested filling the empty chest with a prosthetic material such as Silastic foam. This may be particularly important after right pneumonectomy in infants as the heart may rotate to the right and posteriorly, and subsequent shift of the great arteries can cause severe obstruction of the trachea by the transversely lying aortic arch.[1]

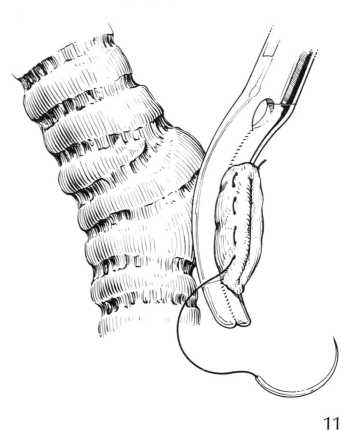

11

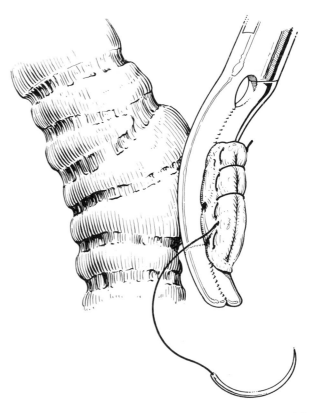

12

# Obstructive lobar emphysema

This condition is characterized by hyperinflation of a lobe or lobes, causing mediastinal shift and compression of the remaining lung tissue. The left upper lobe is the one most commonly involved. Air trapping in the lobe is usually due to the deficiency of bronchial cartilages.

Progressive tension and mediastinal shift can cause acute distress and circulatory collapse in newborns and small infants. The majority of cases present within the first 6 months of life, and many will be admitted in respiratory distress in the newborn period.[2–4]

13

# 13

Diagnosis is made from the clinical presentation and chest X-ray. The unilateral hyperlucent chest can be distinguished from tension pneumothorax and lung cyst by the presence of fine vascular markings in the cystic lobe seen under the bright light. The collapsed lobe is seen as a small triangular shadow just above the diaphragm or near the apex, depending on whether the upper or lower lobe is involved.

Ventilation and perfusion scans, although not usually necessary for diagnosis, may show obstructed and delayed ventilation in the affected lobe. In older children with mild symptoms bronchoscopy may be indicated to exclude the presence of a foreign body. As associated congenital heart lesions are frequently present they should be ruled out by echocardiography and/or catheterization studies.

## Indications

Urgent operation is required when respiratory distress is present. Removal of the diseased lobe is effective. In the rare case involving several lobes a more extensive resection may have to be considered. Extrinsic lesions compressing the bronchus should be relieved, but the lobectomy may still be necessary. In children with mild symptoms the extrinsic obstruction only is relieved. If the child improves no further, operation (lobectomy) is necessary.

## Preparation of patient

Newborns should receive vitamin K preoperatively. Precautions against heat loss in the theatre are essential. The anaesthetic should not be given until everything is ready for rapid thoracotomy, as positive-pressure ventilation may acutely increase the mediastinal shift, resulting in cardiovascular collapse. Lobectomy is performed following the principles described above.

Operative mortality for lobectomy for congenital lobar emphysema was 18 per cent in our early series.[3] The presence of congenital heart defects in 36 per cent of these patients undoubtedly had an unfavourable effect on survival. At late follow-up most patients are clinically well, with only minor or no abnormalities detectable on pulmonary function testing.[5] Failure to improve after lobectomy may imply residual areas of cartilagenous defect in other bronchi or a diffuse form of the disease.

# Lung sequestration

Pulmonary sequestration is a non-functioning portion of a lung that has developed independently of surrounding normal parenchyma, usually in the posterior basal region of the lower lobe. The sequestered tissue receives its blood supply from the systemic circulation, usually from the thoracic or abdominal aorta. The venous drainage may be normal to the left atrium or abnormally into a systemic vein, the right atrium, or portal vein. The sequestered lung does not have a normal bronchus, although in some cases there is a poorly formed communication with the tracheo-bronchial tree. Communication with the oesophagus is also occasionally seen. The term 'extralo-bar' is used to describe a sequestration having its own investment of visceral pleura completely separating it from the remaining normal lung. The 'intralobar' form is the most common type, presenting as recurrent infections in one lobe, accompanied by a dense mass on chest X-ray. The extralobar sequestration may be an incidental finding on chest X-ray (triangular perihilar mass in the lower lung field), or at thoracotomy for associated diaphragmatic hernia. Congenital heart disease, and chest-wall, vertebral and foregut anomalies may also be associated with extralobar sequestration.

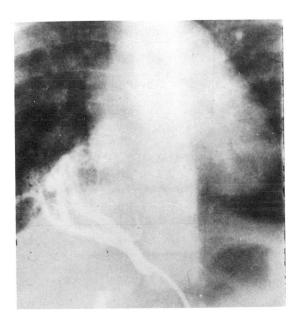

14

## 14

Diagnosis is based on presentation and chest X-ray findings. Ventilation perfusion radionuclide scans are helpful. Patients with non-ventilated segments should have aortography to demonstrate the exact nature of systemic arterial blood supply. This is of great practical importance to the surgeon, as avulsion or transection of an unsuspected artery in the inferior pulmonary ligament, chest wall, or diaphragm may lead to fatal haemorrhage. This is particularly so if dense adhesions are present following previous infection or empyema.

Pulmonary venous drainage from the sequestrated segment and from the rest of the lung should be assessed by cardiac catheterization and pulmonary angiography. It is important to distinguish the sequestration from the 'scimitar' syndrome.[6] The main feature of the scimitar syndrome is drainage of the entire right lung into the inferior vena cava, or the right atrium/inferior vena caval junction. In addition, the right lung may be hypoplastic, with hypoplasia of the pulmonary artery and bronchial anomalies. Major collateral arteries originating in the thoracic or abdominal aorta supply part of the lung.

### Treatment

Recurrent localized infection may cause empyema. Rupture of and haemorrhage into sequestrations have been reported, and operation is therefore recommended even for asymptomatic patients. The sequestrated segment can sometimes be removed. In many patients a lobectomy is the safer operation, particularly when infection and inflammation have been present. For extralobar sequestration excision of the sequestrum is easily performed.

Respiratory infections should be treated as thoroughly as possible preoperatively. Thoracotomy is covered by administration of antibiotics one hour preoperatively, and this is continued for three doses postoperatively.

# 15

It is of utmost importance to know the number and exact position of the anomalous vessels to the sequestrated lobe. These are dissected and divided between ligatures immediately after opening the chest.

Adhesions to the chest wall may be quite vascular. The phrenic nerve may have a course lateral to the abnormal lobe and can thus be injured during dissection. When the arterial blood supply is controlled, venous drainage from the sequestered lobe should be carefully visualized, doubly ligated, and divided.

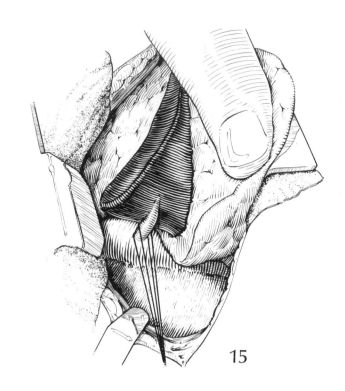

15

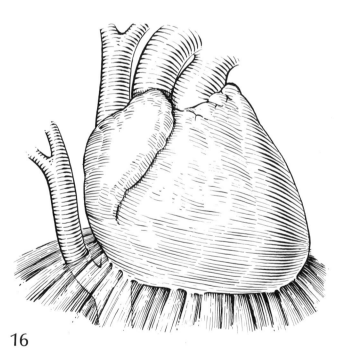

16

# 16

Care must be taken not to overlook the rare situation in which the sequestered segment and normal lung drain into a single venous channel running to the right atrium or inferior vena cava (scimitar syndrome). In this situation we recommend ligation of the arterial supply to the sequestered lobe instead of removal of the lobe[6].

Alternatively, occlusion of collateral arteries can be accomplished by insertion of coils or balloons at catheterization. Ligation or even partial occlusion of the common pulmonary venous channel may result in haemorrhagic infarction of the entire lung, requiring emergency pneumonectomy, as we have encountered in one of our infants[6].

Extralobar sequestration normally does not present a technical problem. The vascular pedicle is divided between two ties or transfixing ligatures. The sequestered segment is then removed with diathermy and all residual bleeding points checked. The chest is closed as described previously, with one intercostal drain connected to an underwater seal.

Sequestration is a localized disease and resection should be curative. In the absence of associated anomalies the operative mortality is low and the long-term outlook good.[7,8]

# Lung cysts

## 17

*Congenital lung cysts.* These usually occur within a lower lobe and may be multilocular. They are lined with a mucus-secreting epithelium, and have a fibrous capsule. Symptoms of tension and compression may result from air-trapping within a cyst which communicates with the bronchus. In older children recurrent infections are common. Chest X-ray shows a hyperlucent space surrounded by lung parenchyma. Mediastinal shift may be evident. Air/fluid levels within a cyst are also common. Symptomatic cysts require surgical treatment. We recommend surgery even for asymptomatic cysts, because of the possibility of secondary infection leading to abscess or empyema.

Preoperative decompression of a cyst is indicated only for life-threatening cardiovascular problems resulting from air-trapping and tension. Multilocular cysts usually require lobectomy, although large, solitary cysts can occasionally be enucleated.

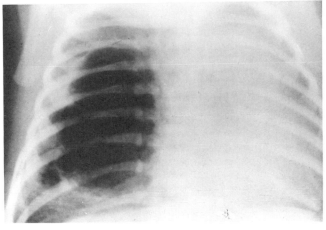

17

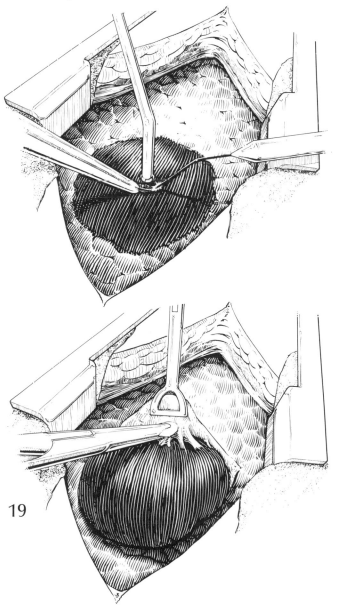

## 18, 19 & 20

The operative technique aims to open the lung tissue above the cyst and then dissect in the plane between the wall of the cyst and the lung. If the removal of the cyst proves difficult it can be opened widely and the inner surface diathermied. The opening of any small bronchus into the cyst must be carefully oversewn. Results of surgery for congenital cysts are good, with low operative mortality and good long-term pulmonary function.

*Acquired lung cysts.* These include pneumatoceles and echinococcal cysts (hydatids). Pneumatoceles are air-filled cysts which develop during staphylococcal pneumonia, generally in infants. Spontaneous resolution is the rule if the staphylococcal pneumonia can be controlled with antibiotic therapy. An observation period of a few months is therefore indicated in such patients. Decortication is very rarely necessary.

19

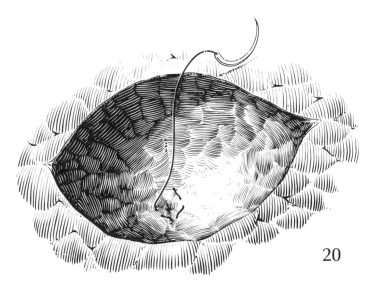

20

## 21

Conversely, echinococcal cysts always require surgery, as rupture may cause dissemination or anaphylaxis. In children coming from an endemic area, a large, round, sharply defined opacity in the lung fields on chest X-ray is highly suggestive of hydatid disease. The cysts may be multiple. Symptoms will arise from compression of a bronchus or other mediastinal structure as the cyst enlarges. Serological tests to confirm the diagnosis are useful when positive but they are not 100 per cent sensitive.

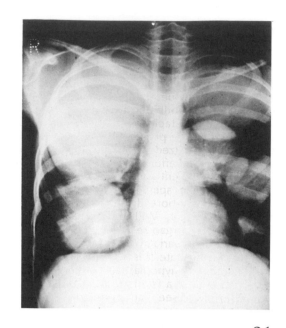

21

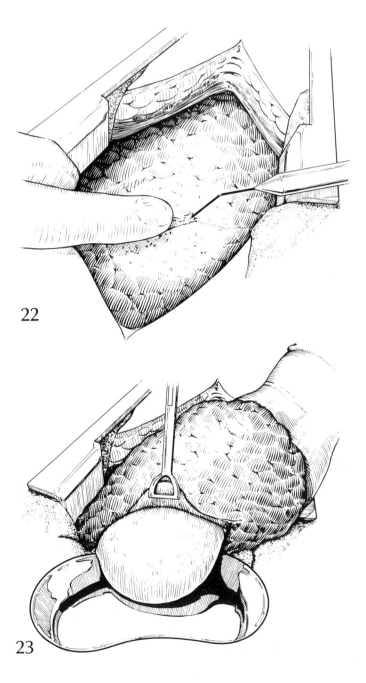

22

## 22 & 23

The cysts can usually be enucleated. With the healthy lung draped away, a diathermy needle is used to open the pseudocapsule of compressed lung infesting the cyst. The cyst is then enucleated without opening the true capsule.

Remaining air leaks are closed with fine sutures, and the cavity space obliterated with a running stitch. Enucleation of these cysts is curative from the pulmonary point of view; however, it should be remembered that the echinococcal larvae enter the body through the gastro-intestinal tract and reach the lung by way of the liver. Careful preoperative investigation for liver and other abdominal cysts is mandatory and chemotherapy may be indicated.

23

# Empyema

*(See also chapter on Empyema thoracis).*

Empyema continues to be a childhood problem despite the widespread use of antibiotics.The pleural suppuration is usually secondary to staphylococcal and Gram-negative pneumonia. In the acute phase a thoracic empyema may produce severe generalized symptoms along with radiographic signs of a pleural effusion, which may be loculated. At this stage the treatment consists of adequate drainage with a chest tube and specific antibiotic therapy. It is important to use large-bore drains to evacuate the pus rapidly and completely. With time, an inadequately treated empyema will organize into a thick, fibrous peel, covering visceral and parictal pleurae and trapping the lung in a collapsed state.This can lead to permanent consolidation and even hypoplasia of the underlying lung.

We allow a period of a few months' observation in an otherwise well child to see if any spontaneous resolution occurs. If not, a thoracotomy and decortication is performed. The potential for blood loss during decortication is significant, and an adequate amount of blood should be cross-matched. Through a lateral thoracotomy the thick lung is freed to allow improved expansion. Procedures used in adult empyema, such as rib resection and open drainage, are rarely necessary in children.

# Lung tumours

Childhood lung tumours are rare and the majority are metastatic from primary lesions elsewhere, notably Wilms' tumour and osteosarcoma. When the primary tumour has been controlled, excision of isolated or even multiple lung metastases may be indicated as adjunct therapy, with or without radiation and chemotherapy depending on the number and location of nodules. Wedge excision using the TA-55 stapler is ideal for peripheral lesions, whereas lobectomy may be necessary for central nodules. Results will vary considerably according to the histology and extent of the disease.

Of the primary childhood lung tumours, bronchial adenomas are most common. These may be silent for some time, or produce cough, haemoptysis and wheezing. Bronchoscopy is useful to assess the location and extent of the tumour. If only a lobar or distal bronchus is involved, lobectomy is the procedure of choice. About 5 per cent of bronchial adenomas in childhood are malignant. High cure rates following resection have been reported[9].

# Pneumothorax

Pneumothorax can be caused by trauma, including traumatic birth, by rupture of a cyst, or during chest aspiration for effusion or empyema. It may occur repeatedly in patients with cystic fibrosis. The diagnosis is made from clinical signs and confirmed by chest X-ray. It is very important not to mistake obstructive emphysema for pneumothorax. Aspiration or insertion of needles or catheters into the emphysematous lobe may result in acute tension pneumothorax with severe haemodynamic consequences.

Tension pneumothorax must be directly relieved by insertion of a chest drain. In an emergency, placement of a plastic cannula (Medicut, Angiocut) may be sufficient, but a drain is preferable. After insertion the drain is connected to an underwater seal.

Repeated pneumothoraces, which usually occur with cystic fibrosis, should be treated aggressively by chest drainage. If the lung does not expand fully following insertion of chest drains, some authors recommend early thoracotomy, with abrasion of parietal and visceral pleura. Sclerosing agents have been injected through the drain, with less predictable results.

## References

1. Szarnicki, R., Maurseth, K., de Leval, M., Stark, J. (1978) Tracheal compression by the aortic arch following right pneumonectomy in infancy. Annals of Thoracic Surgery, 25, 231–235

2. Hendren, W. H., McKee, D. M. (1966) Lobar emphysema of infancy. Journal of Paediatric Surgery, 1, 24–39

3. Lincoln, J. C. R., Stark, J., Subramanian, S., Aberdeen, E., Bonham-Carter, R. E., Berry, C. L. et al. (1971) Congenital lobar emphysema. Annals of Surgery, 173, 55–62

4. Haller, J. A., Golloday, E. S., Pickard, L. R., Tepas, J. J., Shorter, N. A., Sherineta, D. W. (1979) Surgical management of lung bud anomalies: lobar emphysema, bronchogenic cyst, cystic adenomatoid malformation and intra-lobar pulmonary sequestration. Annals of Thoracic Surgery, 28, 33–43

5. Demuth, G. I., Sioan, H. (1966) Congenital lobar emphysema: Long term effects and sequelae in treated cases. Surgery, 59, 601–607

6. Alivizatos, P., Cheatle, T., de Leval, M., Stark, J. (1985) Pulmonary sequestration complicated by anomalies of pulmonary venous return. Journal of Paediatric Surgery, 20, 76–79

7. Burtain, W. L., Woolley, M. W., Mahour, G. H. Issacs, H., Payne, V. (1977) Pulmonary sequestration in children: a 25-year experience. Surgery, 81, 413–420

8. Canty, T. G. (1981) Extralobar pulmonary sequestration: unusual presentation and systemic vascular communication in association with a right-sided diaphragmatic hernia. Journal of Thoracic and Cardiovascular Surgery, 81, 96–99

9. Wellons, H. A., Eggleston, P., Golden, G. T., Allen, S. (1976) Bronchial adenoma in childhood. American Journal of Diseases of Children, 130, 301–304

Illustrations by Kevin Marks

# Management of empyema thoracis

**P. Upadhyaya**  MS, FRCS(Eng), FAMS
Professor of Paediatric Surgery, King Faisal University, Dammam 31451, Saudi Arabia

## Introduction

Empyema is essentially an abscess – a localized accumulation of purulent exudate in the pleural cavity secondary to inflammation of the underlying lung, usually pneumonia but sometimes lung abscess or bronchiectasis. Direct contamination of the pleural cavity by external trauma or following thoracic or gastro-oesophageal surgery can cause empyema, but serious pleural sepsis in the presence of a normally expanding healthy lung is very rare in children.

The incidence and clinical picture of empyema have greatly altered with the advent of antibiotics. Streptococcal and pneumococcal empyema are now infrequent. Most empyemas in children are due to penicillin-resistant *Staphylococcus aureus*. Other organisms are seen in neonatal empyema and cases of inadequately treated pulmonary sepsis. Empyema is sometimes tuberculous, and may rarely be caused by fungi.

Staphylococcal pneumonia in infants may be a primary infection or superimposed on viral infections like measles, chickenpox, or influenza. An extensive interstitial inflammatory reaction manifests as multifocal pneumonia. Suppuration and necrosis produce multiple small abscesses. Peripheral abscesses may break through the visceral pleura causing empyema or pyopneumothorax. Central abscesses produce pneumatoceles by eroding through the walls of adjacent bronchioles.

Pneumatoceles are air-filled cavities in the lung parenchyma with no epithelial lining. They often resolve under antibiotic therapy but are potentially dangerous. They can attain an enormous size, displacing the mediastinum or lung parenchyma and producing respiratory distress. They may become infected or rupture into the pleura causing a bronchopleural fistula.

# 1a-d

Depending on the duration of symptoms, pleural sepsis can be divided into four stages: early stages of exudative pleurisy; stage of established empyema; late-organizing empyema; and chronic empyema.

# 1a

Early stage of exudative pleurisy – duration of symptoms 2–3 weeks. The inflammatory fluid is thin and can be easily *aspirated,* allowing full expansion of the lung.

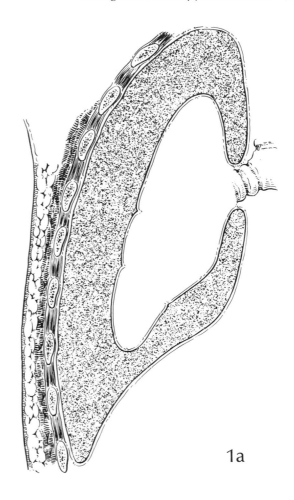

1a

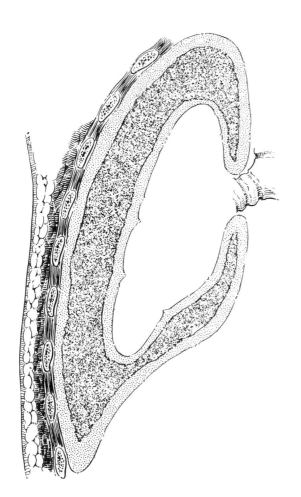

1b

# 1b

Stage of established empyema (fibrinopurulent stage) – duration of symptoms 3–6 weeks. The accumulated fluid is thick and purulent, the pleural walls thicken with inflammatory oedema and fibrin deposition. *Intercostal tube drainage* will be needed for several days to remove the fibrinopurulent exudate.

# 1c

Late-organizing empyema (fibropurulent stage) – duration of symptoms 6–9 weeks. The pleural cavity contains tenacious purulent exudate and slough which tends to block free drainage of pus. Intercostal tube drainage, therefore, will not be adequate. These cases need *open drainage* or *surgical debridement followed by water-seal tube drainage* to allow expansion of the lung. Once the infection is controlled, pleural thickening will resolve in the course of time.

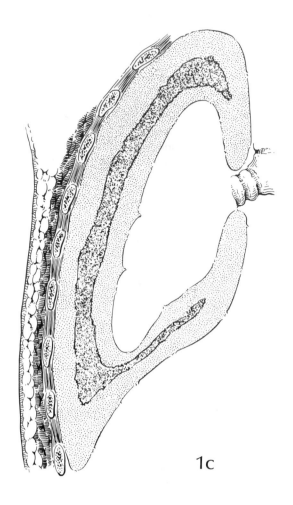

1c

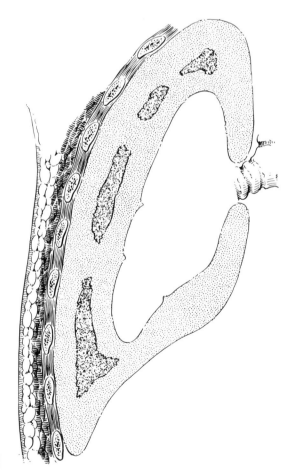

1d

# 1d

Chronic empyema – duration of symptoms 9–12 weeks. Long-standing pleural infection, improperly drained and inadequately treated with antibiotics, leads to the chronic phase. The lung becomes encased in thick fibrous tissue which invades the visceral and parietal pleura as a result of the ingrowth of new capillaries and fibroblasts. Not only is the thickened pleura resistant to antibiotics, but also it does not allow expansion of the lung, until the latter is freed by *decortication*. Children with chronic empyema are frequently anaemic and debilitated. Other signs include scoliosis and chest-wall deformity.

# 2

# Clinical presentation

Empyema usually presents as a delayed recovery or clinical deterioration following pneumonia. There are clinical and radiological signs of accumulation of fluid. X-ray of the chest often shows bilateral disease, more severe on one side, with opacification of a hemithorax due to accumulated pus with or without pyopneumothorax. The lung parenchyma may show one or more pneumatoceles. If antibiotics had been given for pneumonia, the empyema may have an indolent course and the aspirated fluid may be sterile. Sterile pus in the presence of antibiotics does not indicate a cured or controlled empyema. Frequent X-ray examinations of the chest are required during the course of the disease.

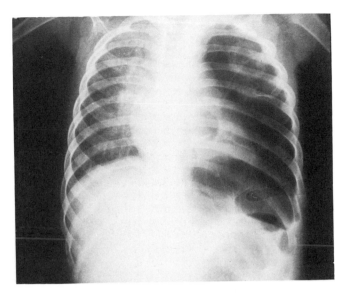

2

## ENCAPSULATED EMPYEMA

Encapsulated empyema usually develops secondary to a lung abscess. If the localization is incomplete, a multilocular empyema may develop.

Localized empyema may be posterior, interlobar, parietal, apical, basal or paramediastinal. Initially the symptoms are minimal and the condition may remain undetected for some time. Classically, encapsulated empyema produces a sharp oval outline adjacent to the lateral chest wall, the diaphragm or the cardiac shadow. If there is a communication with the air passages or if air has been introduced during aspiration, an air–fluid level will be evident. The radiological picture may lead to an erroneous diagnosis of collapse or consolidation of a lobe of the lung, a lung abscess or a cyst of the lung. A spherical, well-circumscribed empyema may be confused with a hydatid cyst or a mediastinal tumour. Interlobar empyema must be carefully differentiated from a collapsed middle lobe. Posteroanterior and lateral X-rays of the chest are required. In some cases CT scanning of the thorax and thoracic ultrasonography are necessary to resolve the diagnosis.

## ACUTE COMPLICATIONS

1. Pyopneumothorax.
2. Pneumothorax, pneumomediastinum and subcutaneous emphysema.
3. Bronchopleural fistula.
4. Suppuration of the lung.
5. Lung abscess.
6. Septicaemia.

## LATE SEQUELAE

1. Chronic empyema.
2. Residual bronchial fistula.
3. Postinflammatory lung cyst.

# Diagnosis

The diagnosis of empyema is suggested by the history and physical findings and confirmed by radiology and thoracocentesis. Posteroanterior and lateral X-rays are the cornerstone of diagnosis, but it may be difficult to interpret the findings because of coexisting parenchymal lesions of the lung. Injection of a small quantity of Lipiodol helps to outline the cavity. Computerized tomography (CT) scans of the thorax, and thoracic ultrasonography are useful to diagnose and localize empyema and the underlying lung disease with greater clarity and accuracy.

Diagnostic thoracocentesis should follow. The pleural cavity is tapped with a long, wide-bore needle and the aspirated pus submitted for (1) Gram staining; (2) bacterial aerobic and anaerobic cultures; (3) culture for fungi and tuberculosis; (4) cell count and protein content.

In approximately half of the cases the culture is sterile because of prior antibiotic therapy. It is also desirable to carry out sputum culture because the organisms present are often responsible for both the pneumonia and the empyema. If aspirated pus has a protein content greater than 2.5 g/dl and white cell count greater than 500/μl the diagnosis of empyema is confirmed, even if the culture is sterile.

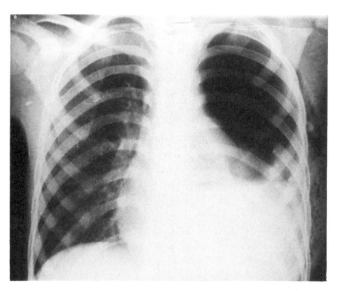

3

# 3

## PYOPNEUMOTHORAX

Rupture of a lung abscess or a staphylococcal pneumatocele may produce pyopneumothorax, causing sudden onset of pain, dyspnoea and, less frequently, cyanosis. X-rays of the chest will show an air–fluid level.

## EMPYEMA WITH BRONCHOPLEURAL FISTULA

The lateral X-ray will reveal an air–fluid level traversing the entire pleural cavity, unlike the case with lung abscess. If there is significant coexistent thickening of the pleura, differentiation from a lung abscess may be impossible.

## ANAEROBIC EMPYEMA

Anaerobic empyema is more common than is generally appreciated. It may coexist with aerobic infections. It is caused by (1) direct extension of a suppurative process within the lung; (2) haematogenous spread; or (3) contamination of the pleural cavity by external trauma. The pus is frequently putrid or foul smelling. *Bacteroides fragilis*, a commonly isolated anaerobic bacteria, is resistant to antibiotics and requires metronidazole therapy together with early and aggressive surgical drainage.

## CHRONIC EMPYEMA

Chronic empyema is usually the result of a neglected or inadequately treated acute empyema. Unwarranted reliance on pleural aspiration, inadequate intercostal drainage, or withdrawal of the drainage tube before the empyema cavity is collapsed are some of the common causes of chronicity. If the empyema cavity is not obliterated after 6–9 weeks of intercostal drainage, it is very likely to become chronic.

# Treatment

Treatment must first deal with the underlying lung infection, and secondly allow full expansion of lung as promptly as possible. These objectives are achieved by:

1. prompt and adequate drainage of pus;
2. prolonged administration of antibiotics as indicated by culture and sensitivity reports;
3. clearing the pleural infection and ensuring collapse of the empyema cavity by tube drainage, debridement or decortication;
4. simultaneous expansion of the lung by physiotherapy;
5. if necessary, surgical treatment of the underlying lung pathology such as lung abscess and bronchiectasis by drainage, lobectomy or pneumonectomy;
6. general improvement in health by adequate nutrition.

# Pleural aspiration

Aspiration of the pleural cavity may be either diagnostic, as mentioned above, or therapeutic. In parapneumonic empyema, large quantities of thin, seropurulent fluid producing respiratory embarrassment can be completely removed, and 5 megaunits of penicillin in 5 ml saline instilled in the pleural cavity.

## PROCEDURE

Pleural aspiration can be performed at the bedside, using aseptic precautions. It is preferable, however, to perform it in a minor operation room so that intercostal drainage can be undertaken if the aspiration fails to remove the thick, tenacious pus. Local infiltration anaesthesia is adequate, but in apprehensive children this should be supplemented with a mild sedative. The site for aspiration should be selected according to the radiological findings. The upper limit of the fluid level is seen as a crescent-shaped radio-opaque margin.

For a diffuse collection of pus the patient is placed in a semi-reclining position, slightly on the unaffected side, so that the posterior aspect of the chest wall is accessible. The sixth intercostal space in the posterior or midaxillary line is selected for aspiration. Multilocular or encapsulated empyemas may require several attempts at different sites.

After raising an intradermal weal with 2% lignocaine, the anaesthetic is infiltrated in the muscles and in the vicinity of the pleura. A wide-bore aspiration needle with a stilette is passed. By proper localization and careful technique, the risk of rupturing the lung or producing pyop-neumothorax can be avoided. The aspiration needle is connected to a three-way stopcock and the accumulated fluid aspirated. A specimen of the pus is sent for bacteriological examination and the total quantity withdrawn measured. Before removing the aspiration needle, penicillin solution (5 megaunits in 5 ml) is instilled into the pleural cavity. Antibiotic therapy is based on the culture and sensitivity report.

At the end of the aspiration an X-ray of the chest is taken to ensure that no fluid remains and the lung has expanded fully. If the fluid reaccumulates and becomes thicker, intercostal drainage with a water-seal will be required.

# The operations

### INTERCOSTAL DRAINAGE

Intercostal drainage under negative pressure is the most commonly practised primary procedure in the management of empyema. Its purpose is to remove air and pus as promptly as possible, obtaining early expansion of the lung and promoting adhesions between the visceral and parietal pleura.

## Site of drainage

In diffuse empyema the fifth or sixth intercostal space in the posterior or midaxillary line is selected as the site of drainage. The general principle is to achieve intercostal drainage one space above the lowest limit of the empyema cavity, as indicated by posteroanterior and lateral X-rays. This avoids the possibility of the drainage tube becoming blocked as the diaphragm rises with the collapse of the cavity. In cases of pyopneumothorax two tubes are needed, the second tube being inserted in the second or third intercostal space in the midclavicular line. Multilocular or encapsulated cavities may require multiple tube drainage.

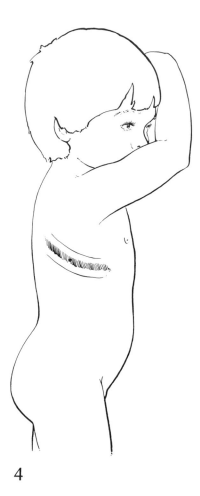

4

# 4

## Position of the patient

The patient is placed on his back or slightly tilted to the unaffected side in a half-reclining position. The child with a bronchopleural fistula should be kept sitting up with the trunk leaning forwards, to avoid spillage of infected material into the bronchial passages.

## Anaesthesia

Local infiltration anaesthesia under mild sedation is usually adequate.

## The incision

A small incision is made in the skin over the intercostal space selected for drainage, using a No. 15 blade. The intercostal muscles are divided midway between the borders of the adjacent ribs and an opening made, small enough to hold the drainage tube tightly.

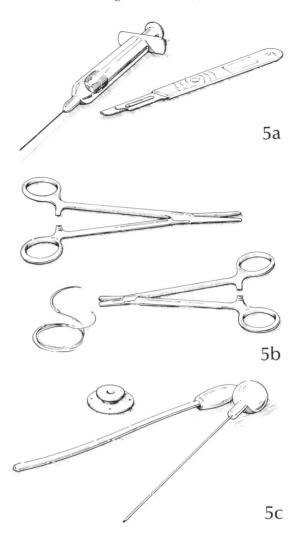

5a

5b

5c

# 5a-c

## The instruments

The instruments used are shown in the accompanying figure. These include a syringe for local anaesthesia, an artery clamp, a needle holder, skin sutures and an intercostal drainage tube with a metal introducer and guard.

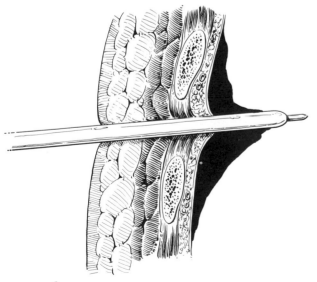

6

# 6

## Introduction of intercostal catheter

Disposable intercostal catheters (Argyle or Vygon type) of suitable sizes, with a radio-opaque line for easy detection on X-rays, and with length markings, are available. These have a pointed metal introducer, and a collar for securing the tube after insertion into the empyema cavity. The metal introducer facilitates introduction of the catheter with minimal risk of injury to the underlying lung. Alternatively, a Malecot catheter stretched over a metal introducer can be inserted into the pleural cavity after dividing the intercostal muscles.

The effectiveness of drainage depends on the choice of a tube of correct calibre, consistency and length.

# 7

## Withdrawing the introducer and securing the catheter to the chest wall

Using a blunt dissection forceps the catheter is held at the site of entry, while the introducer is gradually withdrawn. To prevent entry of air, the catheter is blocked with an artery clamp before withdrawing the introducer completely. The drainage catheter is secured firmly to the chest wall with the help of the plastic collar. If a Malecot catheter is used, it is secured to the skin with silk sutures.

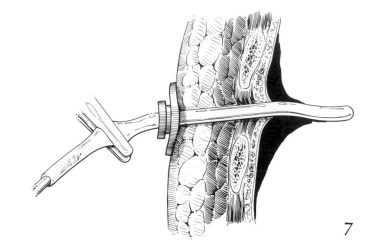

# 8

## Connecting the catheter to the drainage bottle

The drainage catheter is now connected to a graduated underwater seal drainage bottle and the artery clamp removed. Glass connections to the tubing and the drainage bottle are checked and firmly secured with adhesive tape to prevent entry of air into the drainage system. The skin incision and site of drainage are painted with povidone-iodine and a firm dressing applied; the drainage catheter is further anchored to the dressing with adhesive tape. The outlet of the drainage bottle is attached to a low negative pressure of 15–20 mmHg (20–30 cmH$_2$O).

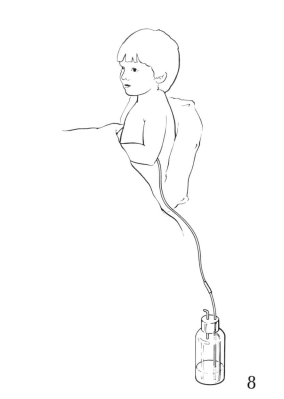

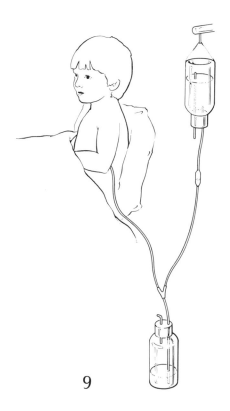

# 9

## Cyclical irrigation

The drainage is sometimes slow, and to achieve a more rapid resolution, the technique of cyclical irrigation is recommended. The pleural space is irrigated with fluid containing antibiotics or an antiseptic such as noxythiolin or povidone-iodine. The cavity is filled for 3 hours; this is followed by drainage for 1 hour, in repeated 4-hour cycles.

# Postoperative care

The child should be nursed in a semi-sitting position. The tubing connecting the drainage catheter to the collecting bottle must be free from kinks and dependent loops and must be checked periodically for any blockage by slough or thick pus. The site of entry of the drainage tube should be dressed daily. In debilitated children on prolonged intercostal drainage, infection may cause widening of the entry wound. Inadequate support of the tube allowing pressure on the wound edges is another cause of widening. In such cases atmospheric air may be sucked into the drainage system and give a false impression of bronchopleural fistula.

If the catheter does become blocked or loose at the point of entry, it will need replacement by one of larger diameter. Alternatively, another catheter may be introduced through a fresh site. Intensive physiotherapy and postural drainage are important to ensure early lung expansion. Anaemia should be corrected by blood transfusion as required, and a high-protein diet given to compensate for loss of protein in the pus.

The drainage bottle should be changed every day and progress monitored by serial chest X-rays. The intercostal tube is removed only when pyrexia subsides, drainage of pus ceases, any air leak from a bronchopleural fistula resolves, and no residual empyema cavity remains.

## THORACOTOMY AND SURGICAL DEBRIDEMENT

In late organizing empyema, intercostal drainage is inadequate. The pus is too thick and the tube frequently becomes blocked by slough. If pyrexia and loculated pus continue in spite of adequate intercostal drainage, there is a clear indication for open surgical treatment. If the operation is delayed, the condition will progress to chronic empyema and the more extensive procedure of decortication will be required.

The site of incision is selected with the guidance of chest X-rays and by a diagnostic pleural tap. Injection of a small amount of water-soluble radio-opaque contrast medium accurately outlines the base of the cavity. Systemic antibiotics are administered as indicated by culture and sensitivity tests.

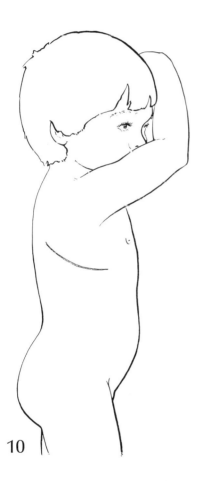

10

# 10

### The incision

A posterolateral incision is preferred. The patient is turned onto the unaffected side with a small sandbag under the lower chest. The ipsilateral arm is drawn forwards over the head. The skin incision is made over the fifth or sixth intercostal space, starting at the lateral border of the erector spinae muscle, and does not usually need to extend anteriorly beyond the nipple line.

Part of the latissimus dorsi may need to be divided, while the serratus anterior muscle can usually be retracted anteriorly.

# 11

### Entering the pleural cavity

The periosteum along the upper border of the sixth rib is incised with electrocautery and is separated from the deep surface of the rib. The pleural cavity is entered through the posterior periosteum and a self-retaining rib retractor inserted. Rib resection is rarely necessary.

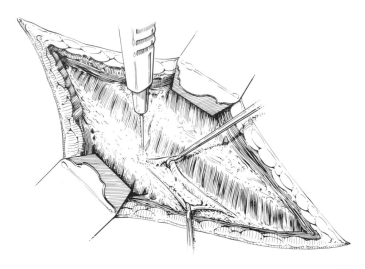

11

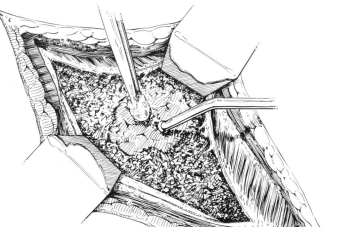

12

### Debridement

# 12 & 13

Debridement of the pleural cavity is carried out through the incision. Gauze pledgets on sponge-holding forceps, and finger dissection are used to break loculi, and the purulent material is removed by suction.

An intercostal tube is placed at the bottom of the cavity, usually in the seventh or eighth space in the midaxillary line, secured with a bootlace stitch, and connected to an underwater seal drainage bottle. The thoracotomy wound is closed in layers.

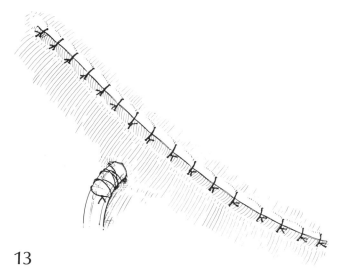

13

## THORACOTOMY AND DECORTICATION

### Indications

Most cases of empyema will respond to the above methods. However, 8–10 per cent progress to chronic empyema. Decortication should be undertaken if conventional treatment by antibiotics and intercostal drainage fails, as manifested by persistent pyrexia, loculated pus, continued debility, and respiratory distress. The empyema will have become a thick-walled sac lined by unyielding fibrous tissue which does not allow the lung to expand. Often the underlying lung will have suppurated and there may be an associated bronchopleural fistula. In these cases decortication will have to be combined with debridement of necrotic lung or removal of the affected lobe.

### Preoperative measures

1. Chest X-rays, occasionally bronchography and bronchoscopy to delineate the underlying lung pathology.
2. Culture of pus and sensitivity of organisms.
3. Appropriate antibiotic therapy.
4. Cross-match of blood, as haemorrhage can be copious.

### Anaesthesia

General anaesthesia by endotracheal intubation.

### The incision

The patient is turned onto the unaffected side unless there is a bronchopleural fistula, in which case the semi-sitting position is preferred. A wide thoracotomy incision is made in the fifth or sixth intercostal space, as described for surgical debridement.

### Opening the chest

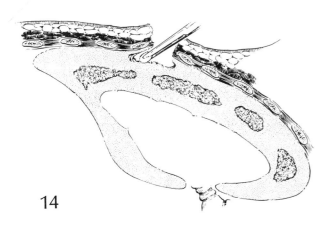

14

## 14

After separating the periosteum along the upper border of the fifth or sixth rib, an incision is made in the periosteal bed and the extrapleural endothoracic plane is entered. Thereafter, blunt dissection with the fingers or gauze pledgets mounted on artery clamps creates sufficient room to insert a rib retractor.

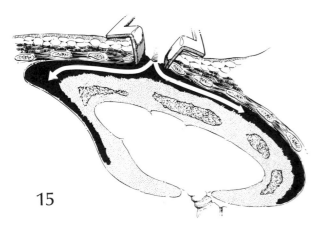

15

## 15

Blunt dissection in the extrapleural plane is continued until the thick-walled pleural membrane is separated from the parietes up to the apex of the lung above and the costophrenic sulcus below. The membrane is often quite pliable and separates easily. However, being soft it ruptures easily and may be removed in numerous large fragments. No attempt is made to dissect the membrane from the mediastinum as this may endanger underlying structures such as the phrenic and vagus nerves, the great vessels, and the pericardium.

## 16

After removing the parietal pleural membrane, the visceral membrane is removed from the surface of the lung as a separate step, leaving the mediastinal membrane *in situ*. The visceral membrane is carefully incised over the lung, until the shiny visceral pleura is seen.

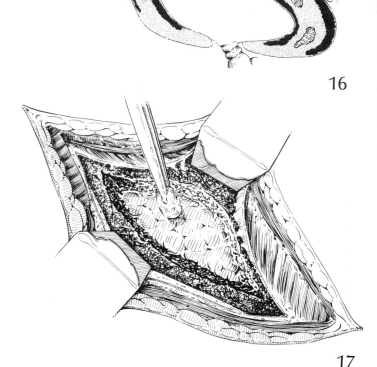

16

## 17

By a combination of sharp and blunt dissection the membrane is gently stripped off the visceral pleura over the entire peripheral surface of the lung. Fibrous tissue remnants and interlobar adhesions are carefully removed until the lobes of the lung are seen to be expanding freely with positive-pressure ventilation.

Necrotic pulmonary tissue, if present, is sharply debrided to healthy lung parenchyma, which is then closed with an absorbable running locked suture. Lobectomy is performed if the entire lobe has been destroyed.

17

18

## 18

At the end of the dissection, minor air leaks are often seen over the expanding surface of the lung. Because of these, and the oozing of blood from the raw surface, it is necessary to leave two tubes in the pleural cavity to drain both the base and the apex of the lung. The drainage tubes are led out through separate stab incisions one space below the thoracotomy incision, and connected to separate underwater seal drainage bottles, to which continuous negative pressure of 20 mmHg is applied.

### Closure of the wound

The thoracotomy wound is closed in layers, using interrupted non-absorbable sutures to close the periosteal gap, and continuous catgut for muscles and subcutaneous tissue. The drainage tubes are firmly secured to the chest wall with silk Roman bootlace sutures.

# Postoperative care

1. Closed underwater seal drainage using a negative pressure (15–20 mmHg) is maintained until the lung is fully expanded.
2. Antibiotics are continued until all chest drainage has ceased.
3. Serial X-rays of the chest are taken to monitor re-expansion of lung and to adjust the site of the tube.
4. Breathing exercises, physiotherapy and postural drainage are carried out regularly to encourage expansion of the lung.

The drainage tube is removed when there is complete obliteration of the cavity as shown by a contrast study. Residual pleural thickening will disappear in the course of time and should not be a cause for anxiety.

## Further reading

Adebonojo, S. A., Grillo, I. A., Osinowo, O., Adebo, O. A. (1982) Suppurative diseases of the lung and pleura: a continuing challenge in developing countries. Annals of Thoracic Surgery, 33, 40–47

Benfield, G. F. (1981) Recent trends in empyema thoracis. British Journal of Diseases of the Chest, 75, 358–366

Clagett, O. T. (1973) Changing aspects of the etiology and treatment of pleural empyema. Surgical Clinics of North America, 53, 863–866

Collis, J. L., Clarke, D. B., Smith, R. A. (eds.) (1976) d'Abreu's Practice of Cardiothoracic Surgery. London: Edward Arnold

Editorial (1982) Thoracic empyema. Lancet, 1, 722–723

Fraedrich, G., Hofmann, D., Effenhauser, P., Jauder, R. (1982) Instillation of fibrinolytic enzymes in the treatment of pleural empyema. Thoracic and Cardiovascular Surgery, 30, 36–38

Jain, S. K., Mishra, R. M., Gupta, R. K., Rehman, H., Mishra, J. K. (1981) A study of different methods of treatment in childhood empyema thoracis. Indian Pediatrics, 18, 237–240

Kosloske, A. M., Cushing, A. H., Shuck, J. M. (1980) Early decortication for anaerobic empyema in children. Journal of Pediatric Surgery, 15, 422–426

Poradowska, W., Reszke, S., Kubicz, S. (1972) Surgical Lung Diseases in Childhood. Warsaw: Polish Medical Publishers

Rahman, H., Mishra, J. K., Srivastava, A. K., Agarwal, V. K., Kumar, P. (1981) Treatment of empyema thoracis with intercostal tube drainage. Indian Journal of Pediatrics, 48, 105–107

Rosenfeldt, F. L., McGibney, D., Braimbridge, M. V., Watson, D. A. (1981) Comparison between irrigation and conventional treatment for empyema and pneumonectomy space infection. Thorax, 36, 272–277

Rowe, L. D., Keane, W. M., Jafek, B. W., Atkins, J. P. Jr. (1979) Transbronchial drainage of pulmonary abscesses with the flexible fibreoptic bronchoscope. Laryngoscope, 89, 122–128

Samson, P. C. (1971) Empyema thoracis: essentials of present-day management. Annals of Thoracic Surgery, 11, 210–221

Sokal, M. M., Nagaraj, A., Fisher, B. J., Vijayan, S. (1982) Neonatal empyema caused by group B beta hemolytic streptococcus. Chest, 81, 390–391

Stiles, Q. R., Lindesmith, G. G., Tucker, B. L., Meyer, B. W., Jones, J. G. (1970) Pleural empyema in children. Annals of Thoracic Surgery, 10, 37–44

Villalba, M., Lucas, C. E., Ledgerwood, A. M., Asfaw, I. (1979) The etiology of post-traumatic empyema and the role of decortication. Journal of Trauma, 19, 414–421

Illustrations by Kevin Marks

# Mediastinal masses

**D. K. C. Cooper**  MA, MD, PhD, FRCS
Cardiothoracic Surgeon, Oklahoma Transplantation Institute, Baptist Medical Center, Oklahoma City, Oklahoma, USA;
formerly Associate Professor of Cardiothoracic Surgery, University of Cape Town Medical School, Cape Town, South Africa

**Marc de Leval**  MD
Consultant Cardiothoracic Surgeon, Hospital for Sick Children, Great Ormond Street, London, UK

# Preoperative

### Investigation

A mediastinal mass may be symptomless and may be recognized only on a chest radiography taken as part of a routine examination. Symptoms and physical signs are usually the result of pressure on other organs or structures within the limited confines of the thoracic cavity. The mass acts as a space-occupying lesion, leading to expiratory stridor, a harsh, brassy cough, dyspnoea or tachypnoea (pressure on the trachea, bronchus or lung), dysphagia and/or vomiting (pressure on the oesophagus), venous engorgement (pressure on the major veins) or neurological sequelae (pressure on thoracic nerve roots, spinal cord or sympathetic chain – Horner's syndrome). Thoracic neurofibromas may be associated with the neurofibromatosis of von Recklinghausen's disease, and, like neuroblastomas and ganglioneuromas, may present as dumb-bell tumours with associated scoliosis. Rarely, malignant tumours erode through the chest wall.

Occasionally tumours present with systemic rather than local symptoms and signs (e.g. lymphomas, thymomas, catecholamine-secreting neurogenic tumours). Symptoms from distant metastases may be the presenting feature of malignant tumours.

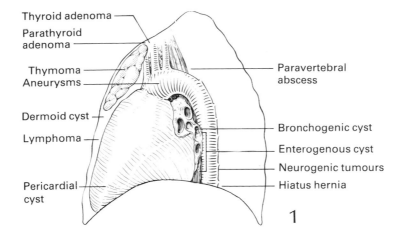

Mediastinal masses may be solid or cystic, tumours (malignant or benign), or developmental anomalies, abscesses, haemangiomas or hernias; the site of the lesion frequently suggests its nature. It should always be remembered that in developing countries, tuberculous lymph nodes are the commonest cause of such a mass. In the vast majority of cases, such lymph nodes do not require surgical intervention for either investigation or treatment.

Anteroposterior and lateral chest X-rays reveal the site of the mass in most cases, but occasionally in infants and young children the mass may be 'hidden' in the normal mediastinal shadow and cannot be distinguished in either view. In such cases, which may present as increasing stridor of unknown cause, radiographs taken in the lateral plane during the infusion of barium into the oesophagus may confirm the presence of a space-occupying lesion by displacement of the oesophagus posteriorly and of the trachea anteriorly. This has proved a valuable investigation in our experience. A barium meal may also exclude diaphragmatic hernias, the management of which is discussed elsewhere (see chapter on 'Congenital diaphragmatic hernia', pp. 146–153). To exclude a Morgagni or right diaphragmatic hernia conclusively, a barium meal and follow-through is necessary. Special radiological studies may be required if the lesion is suspected of arising from the heart or great vessels, or extending to and compressing the spinal cord (dumb-bell tumour). Involvement of such structures necessitates consultation with surgeons experienced in cardiovascular and neurological surgery. Special radiographs of the vertebral column and myelograms should be obtained whenever there is any suspicion that a mediastinal tumour extends through a spinal foramen. Laminectomy for the removal of such dumb-bell extensions should precede thoracotomy whenever spinal compression threatens.

Radiographs of the lower cervical and upper thoracic spine may be helpful in suggesting the nature of the mass, as duplication cysts (whether bronchogenic or enterogenous) are not infrequently associated with vertebral body abnormalities, particularly hemivertebrae, in these regions.

Bronchoscopy and oesophagoscopy may provide further information, particularly when infiltration of the wall of the trachea, bronchus or oesophagus by a malignant tumour is suspected. Mediastinoscopy is difficult and not without hazard in children, and probably plays no part in the investigation; it is particularly contraindicated where tracheal compression is already a problem. Although it is important to differentiate anterior mediastinal masses such as lymphomas and leukaemias, which may be treated successfully by cytotoxic therapy, from those which require surgical excision, such pathology can usually be differentiated by excision biopsy of other involved and more accessible lymph nodes or by examination of the blood. Percutaneous needle biopsy may provide valuable diagnostic information in anterior mediastinal masses, especially when a lymphoma is suspected on clinical grounds and when no other accessible lymph node appears to be affected.

As mentioned above, estimation of the absolute and differential white blood count may indicate the presence of an abscess, lymphoma or leukaemia-associated lymphadenopathy. Bone marrow examination may clarify the diagnosis in these important cases.

If the symptoms – sweating, tachycardia, failure to thrive, hypertension – suggest a catecholamine-secreting neurogenic tumour, the diagnosis can be confirmed by measuring either urinary vanillylmandelic acid (VMA) excretion or, preferably, urinary concentrations of noradrenaline and metadrenaline.

Ultrasound studies using a special sector cardiac probe scanner (rather than a linear array scanner) may differentiate cystic from solid masses, particularly in the anterior mediastinum or pericardium. They are much less helpful in demonstrating posterior masses, as the presence of intervening air in the lungs between scanner and lesion severely degrades the image obtained.

Computerized axial tomography (CAT) may again be helpful in determining the exact anatomical site of the lesion, and ascertaining whether it is solid or cystic and whether there is infiltration of surrounding organs. It is particularly helpful in investigating posterior mediastinal tumours in demonstrating whether there is intervertebral foramen involvement and whether the vertebral body itself has been invaded. CAT scanning allows views in the transaxial plane and may provide further information when used with intravenous contrast enhancement to show up vascular structures. (In the future, nuclear magnetic resonance imaging will provide even clearer information.)

## Indications

Except where a lymphoma or leukaemia-associated lymphadenopathy has been shown to be present, the chest should be explored and the mass removed (unless there are serious contraindications on general grounds). The nature of such lesions is frequently uncertain and the possibility of a malignant tumour can rarely be absolutely excluded. Growth of the mass, whether rapid or slow, will lead to increasing compression of the mediastinal structures.

## Special equipment

Facilities for blood replacement are essential. A rib or sternal spreader, such as a Finochietto self-retaining retractor, is essential. If a midline sternotomy approach is to be used, a bone-cutting saw or shears will be required.

## Preoperative preparation

Time spent preoperatively in preparing the child, particularly an infant, may diminish the risk of operation and lead to rapid postoperative recovery. If the mass has been compressing the trachea or bronchus, atelectasis or respiratory infection may have occurred, particularly in infants. Improvement may be obtained by physiotherapy, the administration of an antibiotic, and nursing in a humidified oxygen tent, head box or incubator, but thoracotomy should not be delayed unduly.

When a catecholamine-secreting neurogenic tumour is known to be present, operation should be deferred if at all possible until the systemic effects have been maximally controlled by courses of alpha (e.g. phenoxybenzamine) and beta (e.g. propranolol) blocking agents. Such medication should be given for at least 48 hours, and preferably for 5 days, before the operation. The advice of an expert in this field should be sought.

In children, enlargement of the thymus or thymic tumours may rarely be associated with myasthenia gravis, and this condition should be stabilized medically as much as possible before operation.

If there is respiratory distress, arterial blood gases should be measured and any acidosis corrected. Rarely, mechanical ventilation of the patient may be required. Similarly, acid-base imbalance or fluid depletion resulting from vomiting should be corrected. The haemoglobin should be checked in all cases and severe anaemia treated.

There is no sound scientific evidence that prophylactic antibiotics are beneficial. If at operation the mass should prove to be an abscess or other infective lesions, then a postoperative course of a specific antibiotic should be administered.

## Anaesthesia

If the child's condition is particularly poor, it may be wise to give no premedication. In all other cases, premedication should be carried out with atropine, together with a suitable sedative (preferably one which does not lead to severe respiratory depression) in older children. If the patient's condition is poor, it is preferable to set up both central venous and arterial pressure monitoring lines before induction of anaesthesia. These cannulae may also be used for the withdrawal of blood for gas and acid-base estimations, if indicated, and are essential when the risk of excessive blood loss is considered to be high or when the mass is known to be a hormone-secreting tumour. A separate venous cannula for infusion of blood and/or clear fluids should also be inserted.

Induction of anaesthesia should be gaseous in small children and intravenous in older children. Great care must be taken during the induction phase, particularly in stridulous patients. An uncuffed endotracheal tube, passed through the mouth, is essential in all cases; a cuffed tube should never be used in children. Once the airway has been secured, a muscle relaxant should be given in all cases except when myasthenia is present.

Insertion of an oesophageal stethoscope is valuable in providing auditory confirmation of adequate ventilation and for monitoring heart sounds.

## Choice of approach and applied anatomy

If the mass is known to be in the anterior mediastinum or anteriorly placed in the superior mediastinum, a midline sternotomy gives excellent access, although a lateral thoracotomy can be used. Masses elsewhere in the mediastinum should be approached through a left or right lateral thoracotomy. The choice of side will naturally be indicated in most cases by the situation of the mass, but occasionally the mass is centrally placed. Access to the midline is more difficult in the superior and middle mediastinum from the left side because of the presence of the arch and descending aorta. When choosing the side of approach it should also be remembered that, once the chest is opened, the lung on that side should be partially collapsed to allow the surgeon access to the lesion; hence, if complete atelectasis of one lung is already present, thoracotomy should be performed on that side whenever feasible.

## 2

The major structures on the right side of the superior mediastinum are: thymus, superior vena cava, phrenic nerve, trachea, vagus nerve, oesophagus, sympathetic chain. Those in the middle and posterior mediastina are: the heart in the pericardial cavity, phrenic nerve, pulmonary vessels and bronchi, oesophagus with over-lying vagus nerve, thoracic duct, sympathetic chain.

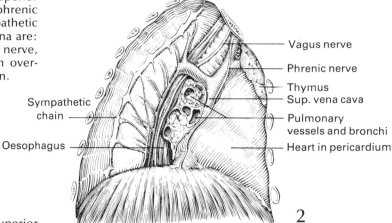

Vagus nerve
Phrenic nerve
Thymus
Sup. vena cava
Pulmonary vessels and bronchi
Heart in pericardium
Sympathetic chain
Oesophagus

2

## 3

The major structures on the left side of the superior mediastinum are: thymus, carotid and subclavian arteries arising from the aortic arch, phrenic and vagus nerves, oesophagus, thoracic duct, sympathetic chain. Those in the middle and posterior mediastina are: the heart in the pericardial cavity, phrenic nerve, pulmonary vessels and bronchi, vagus nerve with its recurrent laryngeal branch, descending aorta, sympathetic chain.

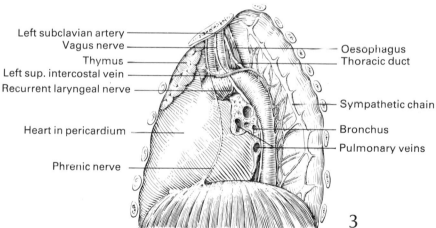

Left subclavian artery
Vagus nerve
Thymus
Left sup. intercostal vein
Recurrent laryngeal nerve
Heart in pericardium
Phrenic nerve
Oesophagus
Thoracic duct
Sympathetic chain
Bronchus
Pulmonary veins

3

## Position of patient for right or left thoracotomy

For a right thoracotomy, the child is placed in a lateral position lying on the left side, with the right arm drawn well forwards and upwards against the side of the face so as to draw the scapula out of the line of the incision.

Similarly, the left arm is drawn upwards when a left thoracotomy is intended. The child should be firmly maintained in this position by sandbags or chest and arm supports, together with adhesive strapping as necessary.

After skin preparation with povidone-iodine or other effective agent, towels should be draped to expose the area of the incision. Other towels are arranged, with the help of the anaesthetist, over a screen in such a way as to allow the anaesthetist to observe the face of the patient and have access to the endotracheal tube throughout the operation. If heart rate and blood pressure are not being continuously monitored, it is essential that the anaesthetist should be in a position to monitor pulse rate and upper limb blood pressure himself.

## Position of patient for midline sternotomy

The child should be supine, with the table 'broken' under the thorax to hyperextend the thoracic spine 30° from the horizontal. A foam-rubber pillow or sandbag placed under the back just below the shoulders, with the head piece of the table slightly lowered, has a similar effect in 'presenting' the sternum to the surgeon. The entire table should be tilted so that the patient's head is slightly higher than the feet, partly to prevent venous engorgement of the head and neck, and partly to improve access for the surgeon.

# The operations

## REMOVAL OF A MEDIASTINAL MASS BY LATERAL THORACOTOMY (LEFT OR RIGHT)

## 4

### The incision

A horizontal incision is made beginning 2.5–7.5 cm (1–3 inches) below the nipple, and continued to a point just posterior and inferior to the inferior angle of the scapula. In children there is no need to extend the incision upwards behind the scapula. If the mass arises in the superior mediastinum, the chest should be entered through the fourth intercostal space; if elsewhere, the fifth intercostal space is chosen. Occasionally, for masses in the costophrenic recess, a lower space is preferred. This is particularly necessary for some neurogenic tumours which may extend below the diaphragm. A thoracoabdominal approach may rarely be necessary, the initial thoracotomy incision in the seventh intercostal space being extended anteriorly if required. The intercostal muscles may be divided by cutting diathermy along almost the entire length of the rib, but a subperiosteal approach is likely to cause less bleeding. It is unnecessary to remove a rib to gain adequate exposure.

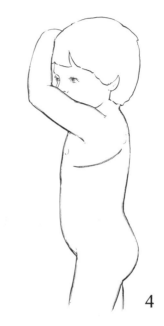

4

## 5

### Exposure

The pleura is opened and the ribs are widely separated by a self-retaining retractor. Depending on its site of origin, the mass of the tumour, cyst or abscess may lie in the *superior mediastinum* pushing the lung downwards, *anterior* to the lung, pushing it backwards, or *posterior*, pushing it forwards. The lung is retracted to gain maximum exposure of the mass. (Throughout the operation, both surgeon and anaesthetist should take care to ensure that airway obstruction does not occur as a result of traction on the trachea. Similarly, kinking of the major head vessels must be avoided.) Should further exposure be required, particularly for large anterior mediastinal masses, the sternum may be divided transversely. The internal mammary vessels on one or both sides will then require division between ligatures.

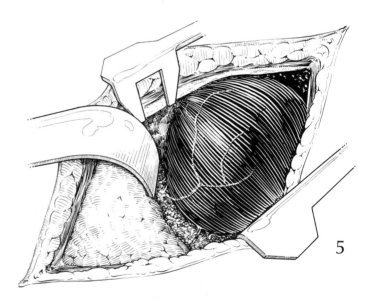

5

### Aspiration of cyst

Unless there is any suspicion of hydatid disease, where the mass is cystic and large enough either to make mobilization and removal difficult or even impossible, or to be causing serious respiratory embarrassment, reduction by aspiration may be beneficial. (In hydatid disease, the characteristic white ectocyst can clearly be seen at operation, and aspiration is absolutely contraindicated for fear of contamination of the pleural cavity.) A purse-string suture is placed in the wall of the cyst, its contents are aspirated through a large needle inserted within the purse-string, and the suture is tied down after removal of the needle. Contamination of the pleural cavity should be avoided whenever possible, as the fluid may be extremely acid or may contain malignant cells or bacteria.

Enterogenous cysts are not uncommonly lined by gastric mucosa and the pH of the fluid contents of the cyst may be very low; this can be tested easily in the theatre with litmus paper.

## Mobilization

The mediastinal pleura is incised around the margin of the mass (except where a malignant tumour has invaded the pleura, in which case the pleura over the mass should be widely excised with the mass).

### Mobilization of a cyst

In many cystic lesions (e.g. enterogenous cysts) the mucosal lining of the cyst can easily be peeled away from the attached structures by firm 'wiping' with a wet swab, leaving the non-epithelial portions of the wall.

Enterogenous cysts may communicate with the oesophagus or gastrointestinal tract, or penetrate the diaphragm and end blindly in the abdomen. Such communications should therefore be sought and closed by ligation or suture if present. With other types of cyst it may be necessary to dissect out the cyst completely.

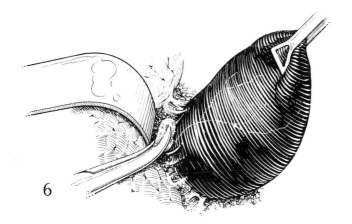

6

## 6

### Mobilization of a solid mass

The mass is dissected out of the space in which it lies, taking care to avoid unnecessary harm to underlying structures. This dissection may be digital or by scissors or swabs, and may be facilitated by retracting the mass, either by swab pressure or by tissue forceps, away from the neighbouring structure, so that the connective tissue between it and these structures can be put under sufficient tension for safe division. Handling of catecholamine-secreting tumours may result in sudden episodes of hypertension which can be minimized by preoperative autonomic blockade and the use of relatively deep anaesthesia. Sodium nitroprusside by continuous intravenous infusion is valuable in controlling such episodes if they occur during the operation.

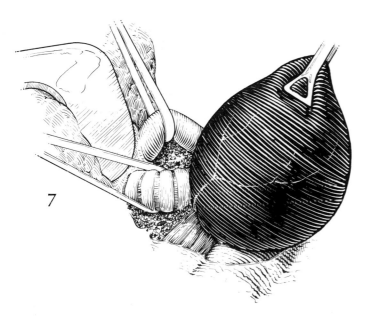

7

## 7

### Exposure of deeply placed masses

Exposure of masses arising deep in the mediastinum can be facilitated by retraction of nearby structures. The arch or descending aorta can be retracted considerably with a suitable retractor, although great care must be taken not to avulse any of the intercostal arteries arising from it. The major pulmonary vessels and bronchi can be retracted by rubber slings or tapes placed around them. Identification of the trachea can frequently be facilitated by palpation of the indwelling endotracheal tube. Similarly, in difficult cases, the oesophagus can be recognized by palpation through its wall of a stomach tube passed specially for this purpose. If the pleura of the opposite chest is inadvertently opened during this dissection, it should be repaired if possible, the anaesthetist cooperating to prevent collapse of the opposite lung. (This feature should be checked at the end of the operation by a chest radiograph, and an intercostal tube inserted if a significant pneumothorax persists.)

# 8

## Removal of mass

In most cases, whether the mass is cystic or solid, it is fed by a pedicle containing one or more arteries and veins; in many solid tumours, multiple vascular pedicles may be present. Such pedicles, except when of minimal size, should be divided between ligatures. The mass can then be removed. Ligation of the major vascular pedicle of a catecholamine-secreting tumour may be accompanied by a sudden fall in blood pressure despite the administration of preoperative autonomic blocking agents. Intravenous fluids and inotropic drugs should be readily available and administered immediately if necessary.

Where removal of a malignant mass is considered to be incomplete, the application of radio-opaque tantalum clips to the residual mass and surrounding tissues will allow more accurate localization of subsequent radiotherapy, should this be indicated.

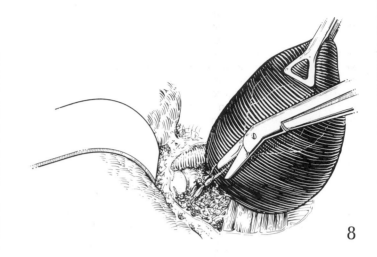

8

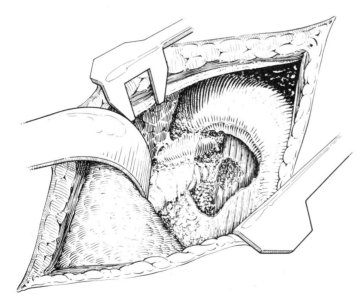

9

# 9

## Final inspection and closure

The bed from which the mass has been removed is carefully inspected for bleeding points and damage to underlying structures. Such damage should be repaired whenever possible. Covering of the area by pleura is unnecessary. Particularly when dissection has taken place in the posterior mediastinum, a careful search should be made for leakage of lymph from the thoracic duct or other major lymphatic channel. Suture-ligation should be employed to stop such leakage. The lung is fully reexpanded by the anaesthetist before final closure.

# 10

## Intercostal tube drainage

A single intercostal tube of adequate size is inserted through a stab wound which should be situated antero-laterally to avoid the possibility of the child lying on the tube postoperatively. The tube is retained in place by a skin stitch tied around it. A further mattress suture should be placed through the stab wound for subsequent tying down when the tube is removed. The tube is attached to underwater-seal syphon drainage. If dissection of the mass has resulted in an air leak from the lung, two intercostal tubes should be inserted, one to lie posteroinferiorly in the chest and the other anterosuperiorly. The two tubes should ideally be connected to separate bottles. Suction is rarely necessary and can be dangerous in small children and infants; it should be avoided except in exceptional circumstances. It is unnecessary to place sutures around adjacent ribs, as the chest can be adequately closed by repairing the intercostal muscles and periosteum. The muscle and fascial layers of the chest wall should be repaired individually. A subcuticular polyglyco-lic acid absorbable suture (Dexon) can be used to re-appose the skin edges if there is no sign of infection, or the skin may be closed with continuous or interrupted non-absorbable sutures.

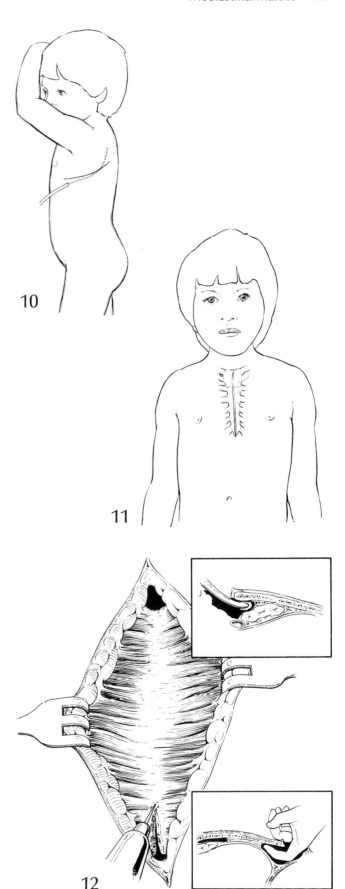

10

11

## MEDIAN STERNOTOMY AND THYMECTOMY FOR REMOVAL OF AN ANTERIOR MEDIASTINAL MASS ARISING IN THE THYMUS (THYMECTOMY FOR MYASTHENIA GRAVIS)

# 11 & 12

## The incision

A skin incision is made in the midline extending from just below the suprasternal notch to a point just below the tip of the xiphoid process. Dissection is carried out in the suprasternal notch and the tissues are mobilized off the posterior aspect of the manubrium. The xiphoid is divided with heavy scissors or diathermy and a finger passed up behind the body of the sternum freeing pericardial attachments to allow the heart to drop backwards.

12

# 13

## Division of sternum

The sternum is then split longitudinally in the midline with a rotating or other bone saw or shears. The anaesthetist should temporarily decrease or discontinue ventilation while this is being done to diminish the risk of opening one or both pleural cavities. Periosteal bleeding points are cauterized and bone wax is applied sparingly over the cut surface of the bone. A self-retaining retractor is inserted, and the bone edges are gently retracted for only a short distance at this stage, as wide retraction before any substernal tissues have been divided may lead to compression of the heart or tearing of one or both pleura.

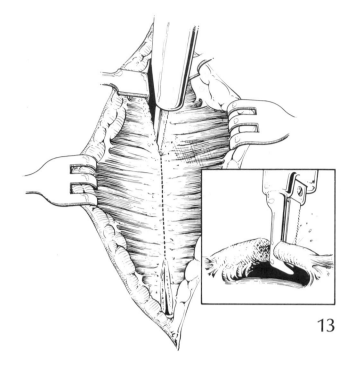

13

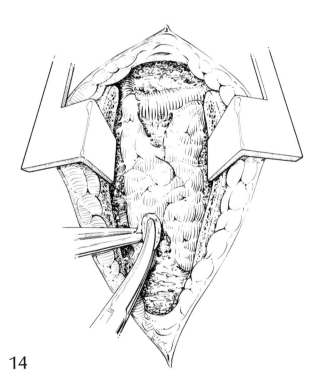

14

# 14

## Mobilization of thymus

Inspection will reveal whether the anterior mediastinal mass originates from the thymus, whose H-shaped outline can be identified within the mediastinal fat and connective tissue. (If the mass originates from another structure, e.g. the pericardium or a lymph node, dissection should proceed along the lines described in the approach by thoracotomy.) The thymus is now dissected off the pericardium and pleura using a combination of blunt and sharp dissection. The pleural cavities are less likely to be opened if blunt dissection (with small gauze pledgets held in haemostats) is used in the relevant areas. Care must be taken not to damage the phrenic nerves lying on the pericardium when dissection proceeds far laterally. The self-retaining retractor can be opened further as dissection continues.

# 15

## Removal of thymus

Small arteries frequently enter the gland laterally and at the upper pole; it is wise to ligate these pedicles before final division. Where thymectomy is being performed for myasthenia gravis, it is essential to remove all thymic tissue. The upper poles may extend into the root of the neck, and considerable care and extensive mobilization are necessary to ensure that thymic tissue is not overlooked at these sites. The major thymic vein is single and usually found in the midline, passing superiorly to the left innominate vein. This relatively large vein should be carefully mobilized and doubly ligated before division. However, it is frequently very short, making double ligation difficult; if so, or if torn, a fine vascular suture should be placed around the entry point of the vein where it joins the left innominate vein. If other thymic veins are found to be present, these should be dealt with similarly.

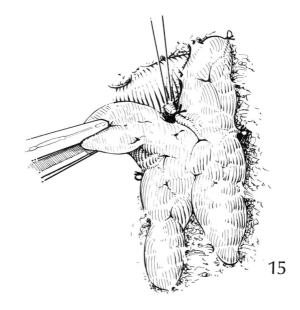

15

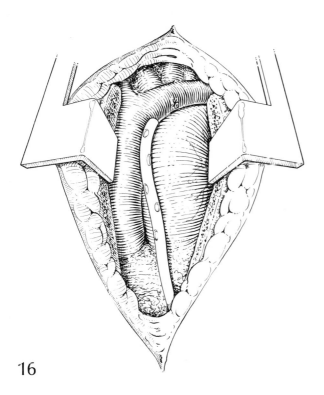

16

# 16

## Final inspection

Any small bleeding points should be identified and dealt with by cautery or ligation. The pleura should be inspected for small holes. If it is found to have been perforated, it is wise to open the pleura widely. It is generally not necessary to insert an intercostal drainage tube, as air from the pleural space will escape through a retrosternal drain.

# 17 & 18

## Closure

Even if the pleura remains intact, it is mandatory to insert into the retrosternal space one or two continuous vacuum suction drainage catheters of the Redivac variety, through separate stab wounds inferolateral to the xiphoid process. Six wire or heavy thread sutures should be placed through or around the sternum, and ligated, thus apposing the two parts of this bone. The deep fascia and periosteum should be closed as a single layer with a continuous suture of an absorbable material. Subcutaneous and subcuticular continuous Dexon sutures, or interrupted or continuous non-absorbable skin sutures complete the closure. (It is wise to take a chest radiography immediately after operation to exclude a pneumothorax which may have been missed at operation.)

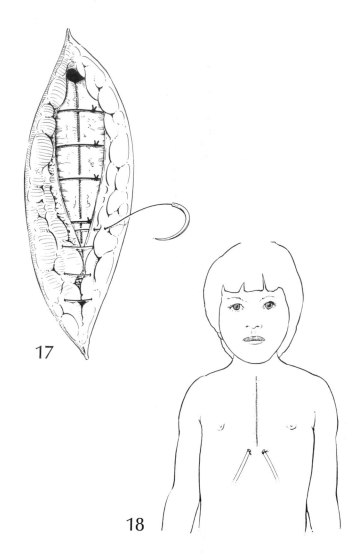

17

18

# Postoperative care and complications

## Management of the airway

At the end of the operation, the majority of infants and children will breathe adequately and can be extubated without difficulty. The child can be allowed to breathe spontaneously in either a humidified oxygen tent, head box or incubator. In infants and small children, it is frequently beneficial to replace the orotracheal tube with one introduced nasally and to connect it to a continuous positive airway pressure circuit with or without intermittent mandatory ventilation (IMV). A nasotracheal tube is preferred to an oral tube when it is likely to be *in situ* for more than a few hours, as it causes less irritation to the upper airways and is less likely to become displaced. An uncuffed tube is obligatory, as it is much less likely to cause tracheal damage. It is also essential that the indwelling endotracheal tube should not be tight within the trachea: it should be small enough to allow a slight leak of air around it when the ventilator inspiratory pressure is 15 cmH$_2$0. These features are particularly important in children under the age of 10 years.

Intermittent positive pressure ventilation (IPPV) or IMV with continuous positive airway pressure (CPAP) may be required postoperatively if respiratory efforts or cough are inadequate, secretions are profuse, or if there has been severe airway compression. Elective postoperative IPPV is desirable in all myasthenic patients. CPAP is helpful in maintaining airway patency and preventing alveolar collapse, particularly in small patients. Blood gases and acid-base balance should be estimated at intervals in any child being nursed on a ventilator, the frequency of the estimations depending on the clinical condition of the patient. The rate of IMV should be steadily reduced to zero, but CPAP should be maintained. Unless there is persisting collapse of lung tissue, prolonged IMV for more than a few hours is rarely necessary. In young children and infants, an interval on CPAP is frequently beneficial after a period of mechanical positive pressure ventilation as a preliminary to the return to unsupported respiration.

The endotracheal tube should be removed once it is clear that the child is breathing spontaneously without difficulty, and it is not essential for the aspiration of secretions which it is considered the child will be unable to cough up.

Skilful and frequent physiotherapy is an important factor in keeping the airway clear and preventing atelectasis. In patients with an endotracheal tube, this must be firmly secured to avoid any possibility of dislodgement or kinking. Meticulous nursing attention is necessary to maintain its patency, especially when thick mucus secretions are present.

## Intercostal drainage

The intercostal tube should be removed when there is clinical and radiological evidence that the lung has been completely re-expanded for 24 hours, and when all significant bleeding has stopped. A serous discharge down the tube is common and, unless excessive, is not a contraindication to removal of the tube. A chest radiograph should be taken after its removal to confirm that the lung remains fully expanded. The suture closing the drain site may be removed after 5 days.

If fluid collects in the pleural cavity subsequently, it should be aspirated, and possibly analysed to ascertain its nature. If it is blood, re-exploration may be necessary; if it is clear fluid, a thoracic duct or other major lymphatic injury should be considered. Such an injury can usually be managed successfully by the reinsertion of an intercostal drain, but if chyle continues to accumulate, operative exploration may be necessary.

Following midline sternotomy, the Redivac drains can be removed when all significant bleeding has ceased. A firm dressing should then be applied.

## Antibiotics

Although there are exceptions, in general antibiotics should only be prescribed when there are definite signs of infection (e.g. of sputum or wound), and when organisms have been cultured and antibiotic sensitivities determined.

## Management of the wound

A light dressing is used to cover the main wound and left in place for 7 days. It should not be removed to inspect the wound unless there are definite features suggesting infection.

## Analgesia and sedation

Adequate analgesia should be provided for all children for 24 hours, and sedation continued in all those on a ventilator. Intravenous morphine 0.1–0.15 mg/kg body weight is valuable in both situations, but the child must be observed carefully for signs of respiratory depression, although this is extremely unlikely with these dosages. Alternatively, morphine 0.2 mg/kg body weight may be given intramuscularly.

## Intravenous fluids

Intravenous fluid administration should be continued until there are clinical signs of bowel function. This will generally occur within 6 to 8 hours after operation, at which time the child may begin taking fluids orally. When intravenous fluids are required, a general guide is to use 4 ml/kg body weight in children weighing less than 10 kg, and 3 ml/kg in children of greater weight. A suitable dextrose and electrolyte solution should be administered.

## Special problems

After operation for myasthenia gravis, IPPV is usually electively continued for 12–24 hours until the patient's condition appears stable. With the discontinuation of ventilation, and during the subsequent postoperative period, neostigmine or pyridostigmine is administered, the dose being based on the patient's clinical condition, and on the results of the tensilon test and tests of basic ventilatory function (e.g. vital capacity). The management of such patients can be very difficult and should only be undertaken by those with experience in this field.

Similarly, in patients in whom a catecholamine-secreting tumour (which are extremely rare in children) has been resected, alpha- and beta-blockade medication can be discontinued immediately, but increased intravenous fluids and inotropic support of blood pressure may be necessary. If excision of the tumour is considered to have been incomplete, the behaviour of the patient should be carefully observed, as treatment with alpha- and beta-blockers may have to be restarted.

Where the mediastinal mass was found to be a malignant tumour, postoperative irradiation and/or chemotherapy may be indicated, particularly if removal of the tumour is thought to have been incomplete.

Illustrations by Kevin Marks

# Surgical treatment of chest-wall deformities in children

**J. Stark** MD, FRCS
Consultant Cardiothoracic Surgeon, Cardiothoracic Unit, The Hospital for Sick Children, Great Ormond Street, London, UK

**T. R. Karl** MD
Kaiser Permanante Medical Center, San Francisco, California, USA

# PECTUS EXCAVATUM

Pectus excavatum is the most common of the chest-wall deformities. Its incidence is 7.9 per 1000 births, with a male preponderance[1]. The deformity is due to unbalanced growth of the costochondral region. This results in sharp posterior curvature of the sternal body. The lower costal cartilages are bent dorsally and form a depression with sharply angled lateral borders. Sometimes the sternum is rotated towards one side and the deformity becomes asymmetrical. Pectus excavatum is usually present at birth and may be progressive.

## Indications for operation

Ravitch[2], Wada[3,4] and others reported patients with respiratory symptoms, arrhythmias and decreased exercise tolerance. Although such symptoms can occur we have not seen them in any of our patients. It is our view that psychological and social problems usually dominate the picture. It is, therefore, important to discuss the deformity extensively with the parents and in the case of an older child he or she should be closely involved in the discussion. If the deformity is severe we expect the psychological impact to become important, especially during puberty. We recommend operation for severe deformities, but stress the cosmetic nature of such an operation. When the deformity is moderate to mild we are more conservative. We usually recommend exercises to develop and strengthen the pectoral muscles and to improve the posture. This often improves the overall appearance. If the patient or the parents are still concerned we consider surgery even for moderate deformities.

# The operations

Many operations have been recommended. We have experience with the sternal turnover[3,5] and with the Ravitch[2] operation. We use flucloxacillin and gentamicin as antibiotic cover. The first dose is given with premedication, and antibiotics are continued for 48 hours. Standard endotracheal anaesthesia is used. Satisfactory venous access for drugs and transfusion is required. The skin is prepared with povidone-iodine, and Steridrapes are used.

## STERNAL TURNOVER

The operation was first described by Nissen in 1944.[5] Subsequently it has been used extensively by Wada.[3,4] We have used it for symmetrical deformities during the past 8 years with excellent results.

## 1

A submammary transverse incision gives a good exposure and is cosmetically superior to the midline incision. A scalpel is used for the skin, and all subsequent layers are cut with a diathermy needle.

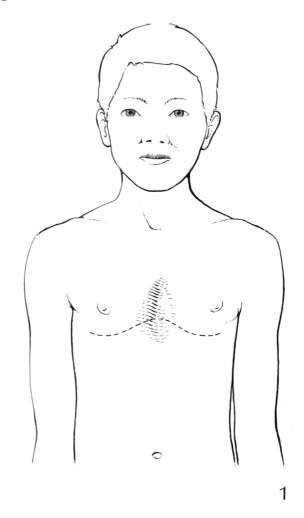

1

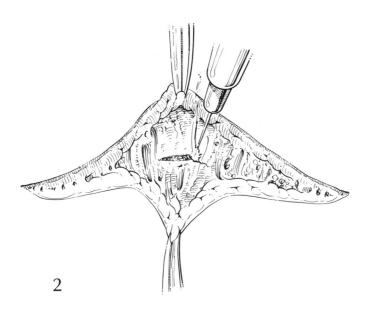

2

## 2

The skin flaps are developed superiorly to the manubrium and inferiorly to the xiphoid process and lower costal margins. Great care must be taken to avoid injury to the skin flaps. Towels are then sutured to the subcutaneous tissue. Throughout the procedure the tissues are kept moist with warm saline. Flucloxacillin and gentamicin can be added to the saline.

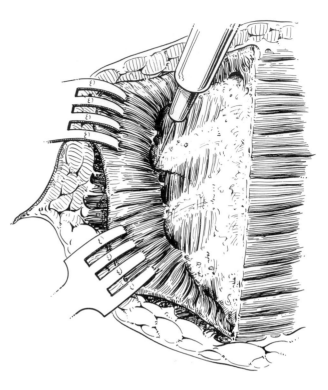

3

# 3 & 4

### Muscle mobilization

The midline incision is then carried down to the
periosteum of the sternum and the pectoralis major
muscles are dissected laterally to expose the costochondral junctions. Inferiorly the xiphoid process is freed and
detached, retaining the insertions of the rectus abdominis
muscles. It is advisable to detach the xiphoid with
periosteum; reattachment at the end of the operation is
then facilitated.

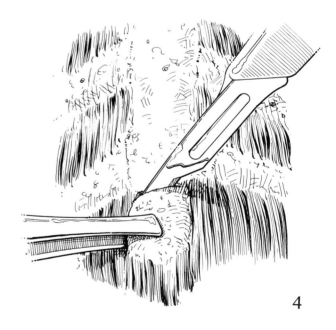

4

## Mobilization of sternum

The lower end of the sternum is grasped with Kocher forceps and elevated. The mediastinum is dissected bluntly with a finger and wet swabs. Care is taken to displace both pleural sacs laterally to avoid injury, but this is only rarely achieved. If pleural spaces are opened they should be drained. The perichondrium is then cut with a diathermy needle and the cartilage is divided with a scalpel.

# 5

The incision is made at the lateral border of the deformity. Intercostal vessels are identified, doubly ligated, and divided.

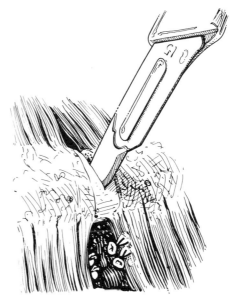

5

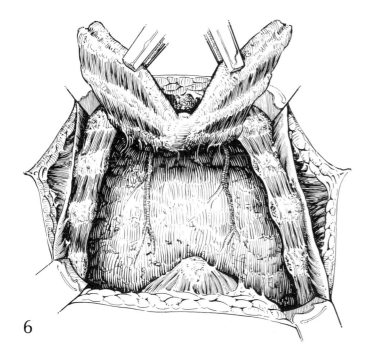

6

# 6 & 7

When all cartilages (except the first and second) have been divided on both sides, the sternum is elevated, the internal mammary vessels are ligated and the sternum is transected at the junction with the manubrium. Then the sternum with all adjacent cartilages is removed.

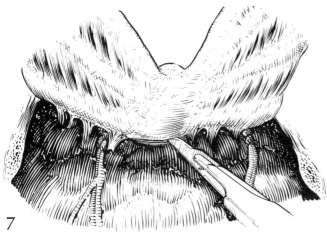

7

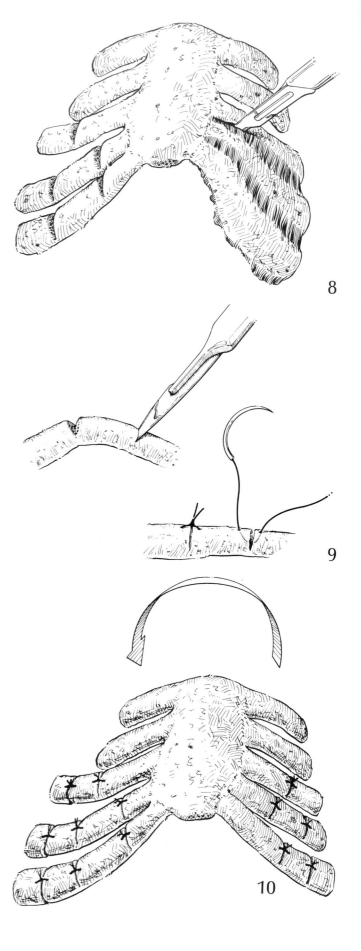

# 8, 9 & 10

## Remodelling of plastron

The sternum with the adjacent cartilages is placed on a board and all the attached soft tissues, including intercostal muscles, are excised. Wedge resection and resuture of some of the cartilages will remodel the sternal plastron. The sternum is then turned upside down. Shortening of some of the cartilages may be required. All pieces of resected cartilage are kept in a bowl of saline to which gentamicin and flucloxacillin have been added. They may be required to lengthen the shorter side of the plastron. If the sternal depression was deep, corrective wedge osteotomy of the sternum may also be required.

Whilst the plastron is being prepared the assistant carefully controls all bleeding points, and if the pleural spaces were opened chest drains are inserted. The lateral ends of the costal cartilages may be broken and turned upwards to further remodel the thoracic cage. The whole plastron is repeatedly bathed in warm saline with antibiotics.

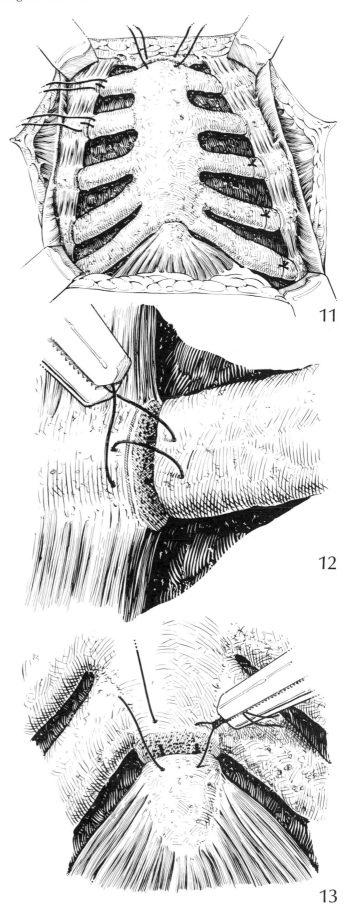

11

12

13

# 11, 12 & 13

### Reinsertion of plastron

The plastron is turned upside down and placed into the defect. The sternum is then sutured with two wires to the manubrium. The length of the cartilages is then considered. Additional resections on one side with insertion of the resection pieces on the other side is occasionally necessary. Cartilages are sutured with mattress or figure-of-eight sutures of non-absorbable material (Ethibond 2/0 or 3/0 depending on the size of the patient). The xiphoid process is then reattached to the lower end of the sternum with wire sutures.

# 14 & 15

## Closure

Pleural spaces, if opened, are drained with Argyle drains. The pectoralis muscles are reattached in the midline, using 2/0 Dexon. The rectus muscles are also sutured together and superiorly attached to the pectoralis muscles. Several single stitches are placed to achieve symmetrical reattachment of the skin flaps. Redivac drains are placed under the skin flaps. A running suture of 3/0 or 4/0 Dexon is used for subcutaneous tissue, and the skin is closed with intracuticular Dexon.

## Postoperative care

Adequate sedation and pain relief is recommended for the first 24–48 hours. We prefer a morphine drip (0.5 mg morphine/kg body weight in 50 ml of 5 per cent dextrose, given at 2 ml/hour). Chest drains are usually removed the following morning, and the Redivacs after 24–48 hours. After the chest drains are removed the child is allowed out of bed and usually discharged 1 week postoperatively. The child is allowed to return to school after 4 weeks but contact sports should be avoided for a period of 3 months.

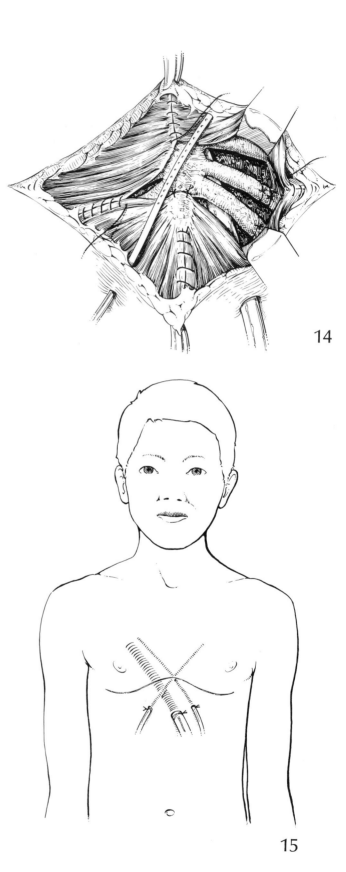

14

15

## THE RAVITCH PROCEDURE

The Ravitch[2] repair can be performed through the same type incision as the sternal turnover. Skin flaps are raised and the muscles reflected in a similar fashion. The sternum is mobilized posteriorly, using the finger and moist swabs technique.

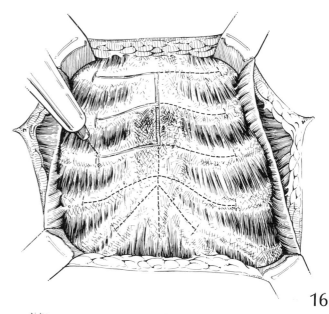

**16**

# 16–19

## Freeing the perichondrium

The perichondrium is incised longitudinally from the sternum to the lateral extent of the deformity, using the diathermy needle. A 'T' incision is made at either end. A fine periosteal elevator is used to free the perichondrium from the cartilage. The edges of the perichondrium are grasped with several arterial forceps and the dissection continued. This technique causes less bleeding than a trans-perichondrial resection. The bone can also regenerate from the residual perichondrium, resulting in better chest-wall stability. The dissection is completed with the right-angled periosteal elevator.

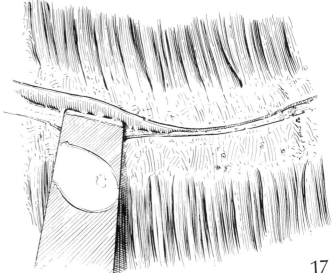

**17**

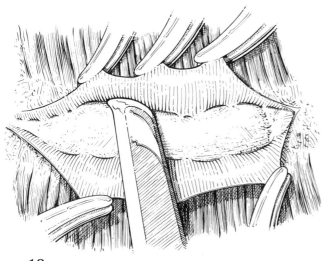

**18**

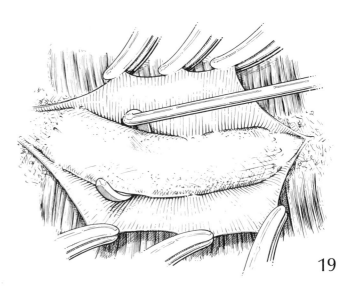

**19**

# 20 & 21

The cartilage is then transected close to the costochondral junction. The end is elevated with Kocher clamps and disarticulated at the chondrosternal junction. The extent of resection depends on the type of deformity; usually three to five cartilages are resected bilaterally.

When the cartilages have been resected the intercostal vessels are identified, doubly ligated and divided. The lowest non-deformed cartilage (usually the second or third) is then transected 1 cm lateral to its sternal articulation. The transection is made oblique to facilitate stabilization of the sternum after elevation. The incision runs from the anteromedial to posterolateral aspect. This step allows the sternum to move anteriorly, hinged in the interspace above the lowest normal cartilage, thus relieving the deformity.

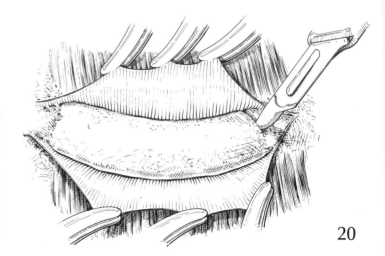

20

### Posterior osteotomy

The oesteotomy can be made anteriorly or posteriorly, but the latter will give the best result. Osteotomy is performed with a Gigli saw which is passed behind the sternum. Only one cortex is broken (greenstick fracture).

# 22

### Stabilizing the sternum

Various techniques to stabilize the sternum have been described. We prefer to use a stainless steel bar. It is passed under the lower part of the sternum and attached to the ribs or cartilage on both sides. The bar is removed 6–12 months later.

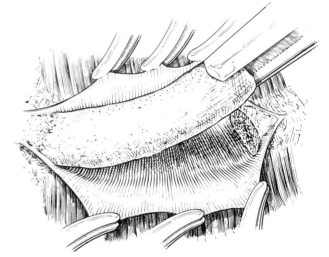

21

### Closure

Closure and postoperative care do not differ from that in the sternal turnover operations already described.

### Results

The current operative mortality should approach zero. One can expect over 60 per cent excellent and 20 per cent good cosmetic results (Ravitch[1]). The best results are obtained in younger children with symmetrical central deformities. Long-term follow-up suggests that there is continued growth of the inverted or mobilized sternum and continued improvement of the chest contour with age. Recurrence of the pectus deformity is rare after either procedure, but may be treated by a secondary operation if indicated.

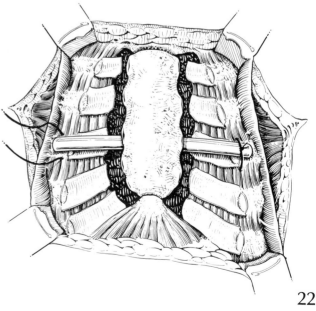

22

# PECTUS CARINATUM

The carinatum deformity is about one-tenth as common as the excavatum type. It is probably caused by overgrowth of the costal cartilages, with forward displacement and secondary deformity of the sternum. There is a considerable variability in degree of asymmetry and rotation. Synostosis or complete non-segmentation of the sternum is typical but not clearly aetiologically related. As with pectus excavatum this deformity presents a cosmetic problem with associated psychological and social complications. Lester performed the first corrective operation for this condition in 1953, employing cartilage and partial sternal resection.[6] Ravitch[7] has stressed that the pathology is in the costal cartilages and his repair, described in 1960, recommends resection of the costal cartilages and preservation of the sternum. We have followed Ravitch's principles.

## The operation

Indications for operation are similar to those described for pectus excavatum.

The transverse inframammary incision is used. This is performed as in the pectus excavatum repair, including raising of skin and pectoralis flaps and detachment of rectus muscles from the sternum and costal arches. The upper margin of muscle reflection usually need not be above the third cartilage.

The perichondrium is incised with a diathermy needle and freed from the cartilage, using the technique described under the Ravitch operation (see *Illustration 16*). All deformed cartilages are then resected with strong shears or a scalpel. In older children the resection may extend into the bony rib for 1–2 cm if necessary. Interrupted 2/0 Ethibond mattress sutures are used to plicate the perichondrial beds to eliminate the carinatum defect. It is usually not necessary to divide the intercostal neurovascular bundles.

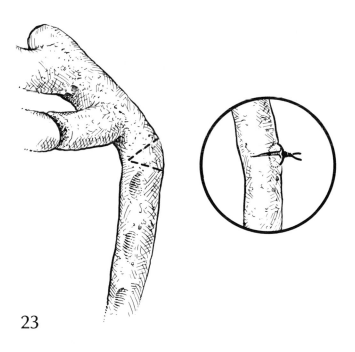

23

## 23

If an osteotomy is required, it is performed as illustrated.

Closure is identical to that in the pectus excavatum repair. One or two Redivac drains are left under the skin flap for 24–48 hours.

## Results

Mortality should approach zero for this operation. The cosmetic results are very satisfactory and recurrence is rare. Growth and development of the anterior chest is normal following the operation.

# STERNAL CLEFT

Failure of fusion of the primitive sternal bars results in a cleft which may be partial or complete. Simple cleft sternum usually involves the manubrium and variable parts of the body but may extend to or through the xiphoid. The cleft can be 'V'-shaped, or broad and 'U'-shaped. True ectopia cordis is associated with variable degrees of cleft. Major intracardiac and other developmental abnormalities are commonly present. Cantrell's pentalogy is a complex anomaly involving lower sternal, midline abdominal, intracardiac and other severe defects[8]. The simple sternal cleft is most amenable to surgical repair and is considered here.

## Indications for operation

Despite the alarming appearance of the sternal cleft, with the beating heart visible through its attenuated skin covering, patients are usually asymptomatic. The heart and great vessels are, however, vulnerable to injury. Operative correction is best undertaken in the first few months of life, as it is both safer and easier at this time. Later on the infant's cardiopulmonary system will accommodate to the size of the thorax, making closure a physiological compromise. Furthermore, the chest wall becomes increasingly firm with age. Preoperative investigation (cross-sectional echocardiography and/or cardiac catheterization and angiocardiography) should exclude any associated intracardiac defects. Endotracheal anaesthesia is used.

## The operation

### The incision

A standard midline incision from the level of the clavicular heads to the xiphoid is used. The proximity of pericardium and heart to the skin should be kept in mind.

# 24

Skin flaps are developed with sharp dissection laterally to expose the entire sternum. The dissection is carried out in the plane just superficial to the sternum and pectoralis muscles. The sternal edges are mobilized from underlying mediastinal structures with blunt dissection.

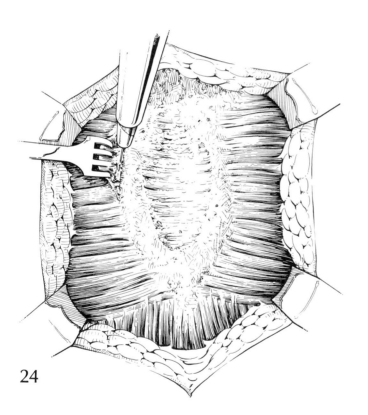

24

## Approximation of sternum

# 25

Ethibond sutures (2/0 and 0) are passed through the manubrium and around the sternum at each interspace. With a 'U'-shaped defect a wedge of distal sternum and xiphoid may be resected to facilitate closure. The sternal bars can be notched to straighten them and improve alignment, although in small infants this is usually unnecessary. Patients beyond early infancy may require multiple chondrotomies to attain safe closure. These can be made subperichondrially in an oblique manner to retain sternal stability. The suture holes are checked for bleeding anteriorly and posteriorly. Sutures are then crossed and a trial apposition of the sternum is made while blood pressure and ventilation are observed for any signs of a thoracic compression. If satisfactory, the sutures are tied.

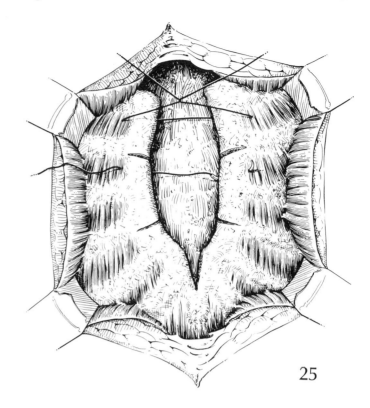

25

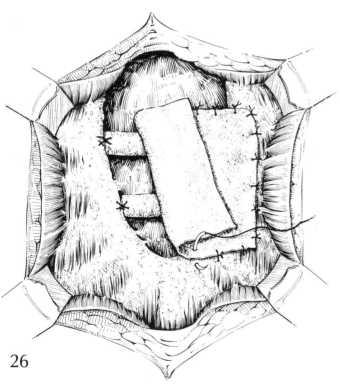

26

# 26

Patients who do not tolerate apposition of the sternal bars can be treated palliatively with a Marlex or Silastic mesh to bridge the sternal defect, and thus to improve protection of the underlying heart and great vessels. These may be strengthened by rib grafts placed under the mesh.

## Closure

The fascia and subcutaneous tissues are closed with continuous Dexon sutures, and the skin with fine nylon interrupted mattress sutures. Redivac drains may be placed under the skin flaps. As the skin in this area is often quite attenuated, great care should be taken to avoid injuring it with forceps during the closure.

# Results

With current techniques of neonatal anaesthesia, surgery and postoperative care, a good result can be expected. The long-term outlook is related to the severity of any coexisting defect.

# POLAND'S SYNDROME

This curious syndrome was reported in 1841 by Poland.[9] Features include deficiency or absence of the pectoralis major and minor, serratus and external oblique muscles. Syndactyly and agenesis of the middle phalanges are also common. Varying numbers of ribs may be malformed, hypoplastic, or completely absent. In the latter case the deficit begins near the sternal edge. The defect extends from some distance laterally, where the ribs may fuse. The defect is commonly unilateral, and the ipsilateral breast may be hypoplastic or absent.

## Indications

The muscular deficit, while disfiguring, is not a severe physiological handicap. It is, therefore, the rib anomalies that are brought to the attention of the surgeon. An extensive deficit requires operative correction in order to protect the underlying heart, lung and mediastinum. In addition, the missing segment results in a flail chest with paradoxical movement during breathing, and resulting ventilatory compromise. Repair of the deficit should be undertaken in early childhood as the ribs bordering the deformity may bow with time, thus increasing the problem.

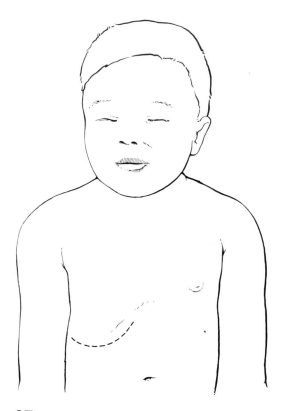

27

# The operation

# 27

## The incision

The patient is placed supine and the entire anterior and lateral chest is painted with antiseptic solution. The incision is made inferior and parallel to the border of the defect. The incision should be kept over the bony portion of the chest wall and not over the defect.

# 28

The area of the breast should be avoided in order to facilitate future mammoplasty in girls. Skin flaps are developed to expose the entire defect.

## Harvesting ribs

An adequate length of rib is harvested from the contralateral chest. The rib is exposed through an incision directly over it, after retracting and splitting the interposed muscle. An adequate length of rib is scored with a diathermy needle and then a periosteal elevator is used to expose the bony portion. This is excised with rib shears. The rib is split longitudinally with an oscillating saw to provide two grafts. If three grafts are required, a second donor rib is used. The donor incision is closed in layers with continuous Dexon.

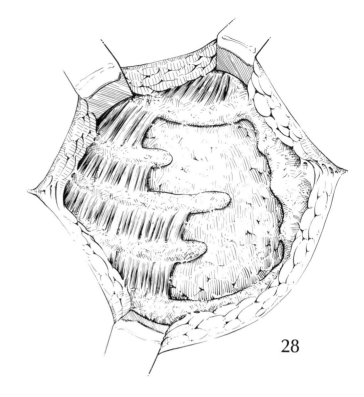

28

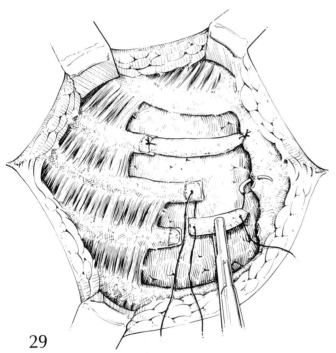

29

# 29

## Placing the grafts

The rib end to be placed medially is sharpened with a scalpel and pressed into a recess in the lateral sternum which has been created with a Kelly clamp. This is secured with 2/0 Ethibond sutures or fine wire placed through the rib and sternum. Lateral ends are secured subperichondrially or subperiosteally to the recipient rib ends using the same suture material. The convex surfaces of the ribs should be placed facing exteriorly.

# 30

## Stabilizing the grafts

A sheet of Marlex or Silastic mesh is cut to the shape of the deformity and sutured to the edges of the defect and to the rib grafts themselves, using 2/0 Ethibond sutures. This serves to stabilize the chest wall and to prevent rotation of the rib grafts, providing a better cosmetic and functional result.

## Closure

Any fascia present, and subcutaneous tissues, are closed with continuous 3/0 Dexon sutures. A subcuticular suture completes the operation.

# Postoperative care

No specific problems are anticipated.

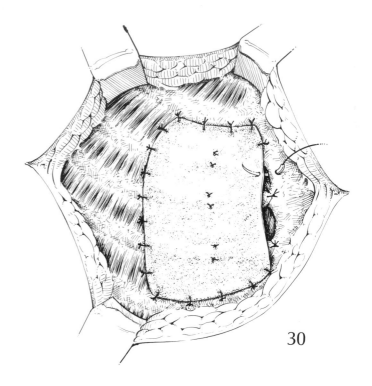

30

# Results

This syndrome is rare and a large series is not available for review. Results in individual cases have, however, been gratifying, in terms of both chest-wall stability and cosmetic appearance. Subsequent implantation mammoplasty has been performed with good results in some female patients.

## References

1. Clark, J. B., Grenville-Mathers, R. (1962) Pectus excavatum. British Journal of Diseases of the Chest, 56, 202–205

2. Ravitch, M. M. (1977) Pectus excavatum. In: Congenital Deformities of the Chest Wall and their Operative Correction, pp. 78–205. Philadelphia: W. B. Saunders

3. Wada, J. (1981) Surgical correction of the funnel chest 'sterno-turnover'. Western Journal of Surgery, Obstetrics and Gynaecology, 69, 358–361

4. Wada, J., Ikeda, K., Ishida, T., Haegawa, T. (1970) Results of 271 funnel chest operations. Annals of Thoracic Surgery, 10, 526–532

5. Nissen, R. (1944) Osteoplastic procedure for correction of funnel chest. American Journal of Surgery, 64, 169–174

6. Lester, C. W. (1953) Pigeon breast (pectus carinatum) and other protrusion deformities of the chest of developmental origin. Annals of Surgery, 137, 482–489

7. Ravitch, M. M. (1960) The operative correction of pectus carinatum (pigeon breast). Annals of Surgery, 151, 705–714

8. Cantrell, J. R., Haller, J. A., Ravitch, M. M. (1958) A syndrome of congenital defects involving the abdominal wall, sternum, diaphragm, pericardium and heart. Surgery, Gynecology and Obstetrics 107, 602–614

9. Poland, A. (1841) Deficiency of the pectoral muscles. Guy's Hospital Reports, VI, 191–193

Illustrations by Gillian Oliver

# Inguinal hernia and hydrocele

**J. D. Atwell**  FRCS
Paediatric Surgeon, The Wessex Centre for Paediatric Surgery, The General Hospital, Southampton, Hampshire, UK

## Introduction

The majority of inguinal hernias in infants and children are indirect. The M.F sex ratio is 10:1. Right-sided hernias are commonest (60 per cent), left 25 per cent and bilateral 15 per cent on presentation. In males the most usual content is bowel, but in females the ovary and Fallopian tube are often found, especially in the infant under 2 years of age. In older children omentum may be a content.

The diagnosis depends on an accurate history from the mother of an intermittent swelling in the groin especially noticeable on crying. Confirmation of the diagnosis depends on seeing or reducing the swelling, the *silken* feel of the cord as it is rolled under the index finger and checking the position of the ipsilateral testis.

## Preoperative

### Indications

There is no place for the conservative management of an inguinal hernia in either infancy or childhood, as the incidence of incarceration is highest within the first 3 months of life and is even higher in premature infants. Incarceration may result in strangulation of the intestine in the male or of the ovary and Fallopian tube in the female; testicular atrophy may be a late sequelae of incarceration.

In patients with a unilateral inguinal hernia there is an increased risk of developing a hernia on the contralateral side (right inguinal hernia – 33 per cent; left inguinal hernia – 66 per cent). Despite the increased risk of developing a contralateral hernia, routine exploration of both sides is not recommended[2].

### Anaesthesia

General anaesthesia is required and the operation is suitable at all ages for day care,[3] thus avoiding many of the upsets caused by an in-patient admission with separation of the child from the family.

### Principles of the operation

Inguinal herniotomy is the treatment of choice as the hernia is due to congenital persistence of the processus vaginalis. In the female infant with a sliding hernia of the ovary and Fallopian tube and in inguinal hernia associated with spina bifida and exstrophy of the bladder, secondary factors are of aetiological significance and a repair of the hernia may be required.

### Management of the incarcerated inguinal hernia

Incarceration of an inguinal hernia results from a loop of bowel being trapped in the hernial sac by the external ring. The resultant swelling is painful and tender to touch and there is intestinal obstruction with abdominal pain and vomiting.

Treatment is by early reduction of the hernia. The infant is sedated and the limbs are elevated to allow gravity to assist with manipulative taxis. The aim is to reduce the sac by *gentle* pressure on the fundus with the right hand, whilst the thumb and the first and second fingers manipulate the contents of the hernia at the external ring back into the peritoneal cavity.

Successful reduction of the hernia should be followed by operative inguinal herniotomy after an interval of 48 hours. This delay allows the oedematous thickening and friability of the sac to settle.

# The operations

Minor differences of technique are used depending upon the age and sex of the patient and therefore the operations are considered under four sub-headings:

1. Inguinal herniotomy in the male infant or child under 2 years of age.
2. Inguinal herniotomy in the male child over 2 years of age.
3. Inguinal herniotomy in the female infant or child.
4. Surgical treatment of a hydrocele.

### Inguinal herniotomy in the male infant or child under two years

## 1

### The incision

A skin-crease incision in the fold of the skin above the external inguinal ring gives adequate access. An oblique incision should be avoided.

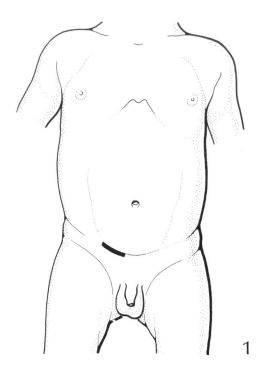

## 2

### Exposure of the spermatic cord and the external inguinal ring

Haemostats are placed on the subcutaneous tissue and lifted thus allowing the subcutaneous tissues to be cut with dissecting scissors. Blunt dissection in this manner along the line of the spermatic cord is used until the cord is seen emerging from the external ring. This may be difficult in the small infant as the incision is sited above the external ring but the cord is easily recognized by its glistening appearance.

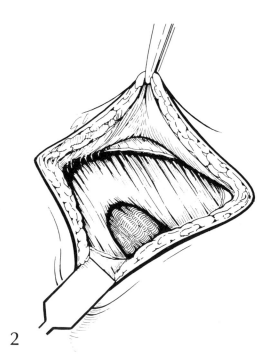

## 3

### Mobilization of the spermatic cord

Once identified the cord may be mobilized to allow later dissection of the cord structure. Isolation of the cord is often easier if a haemostat is passed behind the cord and then clipped to the edge of the operation towels.

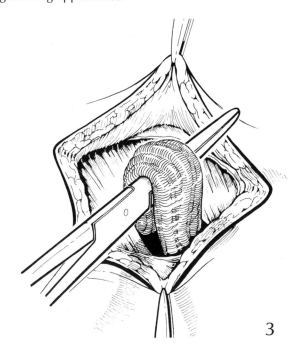

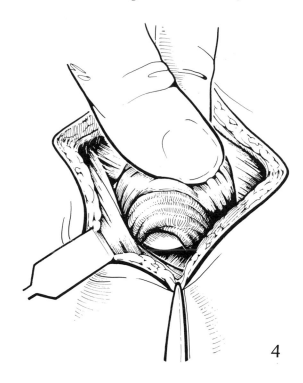

## Isolation and separation of the sac

### 4

In many infants the cremaster derived from the internal oblique is a well-defined layer of hypertrophied muscle fibres and can be separated along the length of the cord by blunt dissection with fine dissecting forceps. This procedure is easier if the cord is held on the stretch between the thumb and first finger.

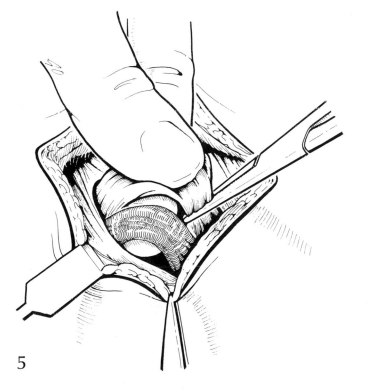

### 5

The hernial sac is then visible and may be either thin-walled (as in a complete inguinal hernia) or moderately thick-walled and with a fundus (as in an incomplete inguinal hernia). The vessels and the vas deferens are then gently dissected off the hernial sac and a haemostat can be placed on the fundus of the sac. Gentle traction on the fundus of the sac together with blunt dissection with a gauze swab or pledget frees the vessels and vas deferens, to expose the internal inguinal ring demonstrating the extraperitoneal fat at the neck of the sac which is now visible distal to the external ring (due to the short, straight course of the inguinal canal in the infant).

Difficulty may be experienced at this stage with the complete thin-walled sac. If so the sac may be opened and separated from the vessels and vas deferens by blunt dissection.

## 6

### Exploration of the hernial sac

The fundus of the sac is opened and the contents inspected and reduced.

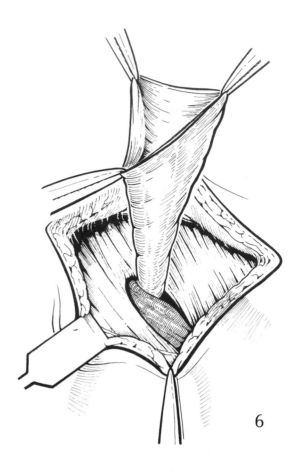

6

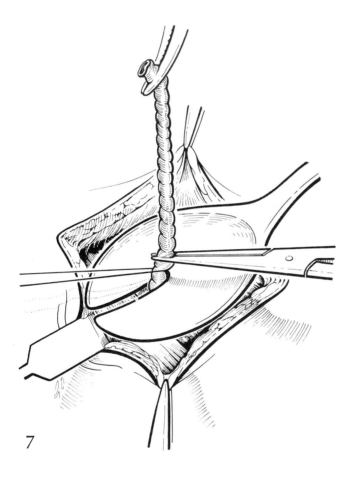

7

## 7

### Transfixation of the hernial sac

The sac is then twisted to ensure reduction of the contents and the neck of the sac is transfixed with a 3/0 polyglycolic acid or braided polypropylene suture. The sac is divided and the internal ring then retracts into the inguinal canal.

The Denis Browne 'hernia spoon' illustrated is invaluable in keeping other structures away during the transfixation of the sac.

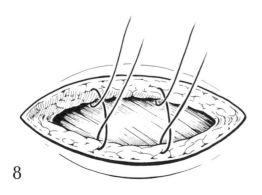

8

## 8

### Closure of the superficial fascia

The subcutaneous tissues are closed with one or two interrupted polyglycolic acid or chromic catgut sutures.

## Closure of the skin

## 9

The skin is closed with a continuous subcuticular stitch of 5/0 white Vicryl; each end of the suture is cut flush with the skin, the end then retracts into the subcutaneous tissues. Steristrips (½ inch) or an OpSite dressing is applied to hold the edges of the wound together.

At the end of every inguinal herniotomy the position of the ipsilateral testis must be checked carefully to avoid producing an iatrogenic undescended testis.

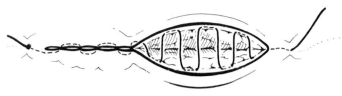

9

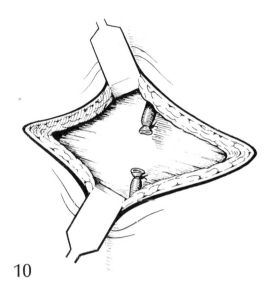

10

### Inguinal herniotomy in the male child over 2 years of age

The operative technique described above for infants has been modified for use in the older male child although the principles of the operation are unchanged.

## 10

### The incision

Due to the obliquity of the inguinal canal in the older child, the incision is made in a skin crease centred over the superficial epigastric vein which is often easily seen. The vein is then either diathermled or divided between ligatures.

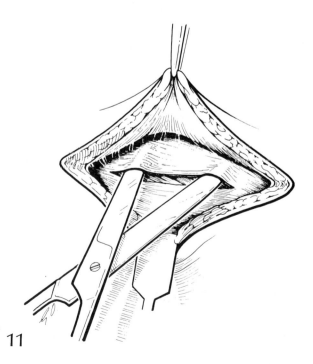

11

## 11

### Exposure of the external oblique aponeurosis

The superficial fascia (both layers) is then incised to expose the aponeurosis of the external oblique and the inguinal ligament is identified. (In infants and young children the deeper membranous layer of the superficial fascia is a well-defined layer and may be mistaken for the external oblique aponeurosis.)

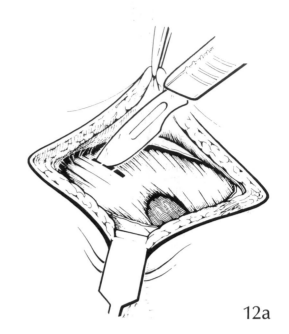

12a

# 12a & b

### Opening of the inguinal canal

A small incision is made in the external oblique aponeurosis along the line of its fibres and a haemostat is placed on the free cut edge. Care is taken to preserve the integrity of the external inguinal ring. The cord is thus exposed covered with the cremaster, *but before isolation of this the inguinal ligament should be identified from within the canal.*

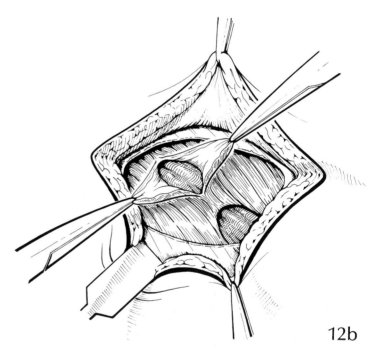

12b

# 13a, b & c

### Identification and isolation of the hernial sac

The cremaster muscle is split longitudinally in the line of the muscle fibres. The thin, flimsy internal spermatic fascia is divided between fine artery forceps to expose the underlying hernial sac and cord structures. The vas deferens lies medially and the testicular vessels laterally, with the sac between them. Isolation, transfixation and excision of the sac proceeds in the same manner as shown in *Figure 7*.

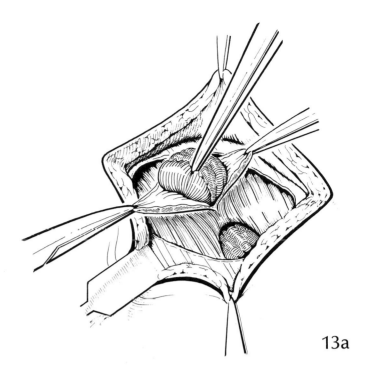

13a

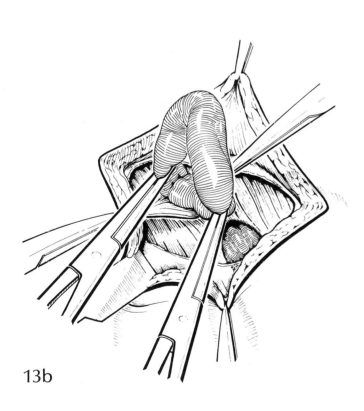

13b

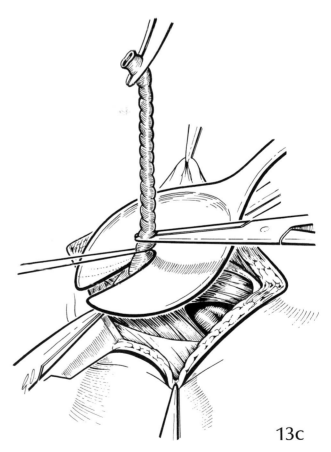

13c

# 14a & b

### Closure

The external oblique is closed with two interrupted absorbable sutures. Closure of the subcutaneous tissues and skin is similar to that described in *Figure 9*.

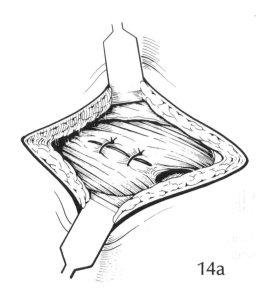

14a

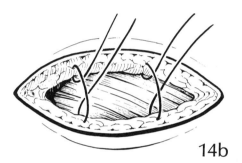

14b

### Inguinal herniotomy in the female infant and child

Minor modifications of technique are required in this group of patients.

Due to the rare association of inguinal hernia with the testicular feminization syndrome, nuclear sexing may be carried out either preoperatively or at operation by examination of a buccal smear or peripheral blood film for sex chromatin[4,5].

### Exposure and isolation of the hernial sac

The hernial sac is identified together with the round ligament in a manner similar to that described for the male infant and child, except in infants and children under 2 years of age when it becomes necessary to identify both limbs of the external inguinal ring, and place haemostats upon them.

### Isolation, reduction of contents and transfixation of the hernial sac

In female infants the hernia sac often contains the ovary which may be reduced after opening the sac. At the neck of the sac the Fallopian tube may be seen at the junction of the free and fixed portion within the broad ligament. Care must be taken to avoid this structure when transfixing the neck of the sac. No attempt should be made to dissect these structures from the sac wall in a sliding hernia.

### Closure of the canal

In the sliding hernias complete excision of the sac is not possible. In such patients the canal may be closed by suturing the edges of the external ring. Previous identification of these edges assists in this manoeuvre. Non-absorbable sutures are used (3/0 braided polypropylene).

## Surgical treatment of a hydrocele

### Indications

Hydroceles in infancy and childhood are due to the persistence of a communication between the peritoneum and the tunica vaginalis thus allowing fluid from the peritoneal cavity to collect in the tunica vaginalis. Secondary hydroceles are rare in infancy and childhood, and the idiopathic hydrocele is not seen in this age range. Therefore hydroceles in infancy and childhood are considered a variant of an inguinal hernia and the treatment, with minor exceptions, is similar.

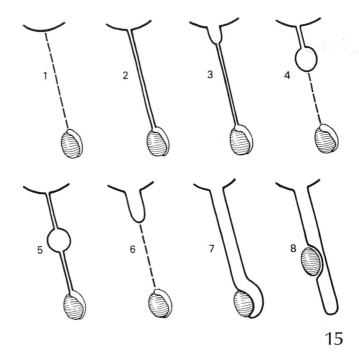

# 15

Variants of the clinical and operative findings of a persisting communication between the tunica vaginalis and the peritoneum are shown.

Many hydroceles of a communicating type disappear spontaneously in the first year of life, due to obliteration of the tract; thus operation should be delayed until over 1 year of age unless an associated 'clinical' hernia is found.

Operation is carried out under general anaesthesia and the operation is suitable for a day case admission.

15

### Contraindications

A hydrocele in an infant or child should *never* be aspirated, nor should sclerosing fluids be injected as a form of treatment. (Aspiration may occasionally be indicated to examine the testis.)

### The incision

This is as for infants and children for an inguinal herniotomy.

### Isolation of the communication

Excision of the hydrocele sac is not necessary, but identification of the communication is essential. The communication is then divided, dissected to the internal ring, and transfixed and excised. The fluid remaining in the hydrocele may be allowed to absorb spontaneously, but to avoid parental anxiety the hydrocele may be aspirated or emptied by a stab incision through the sac which can be pushed upwards from the scrotum into the wound.

### Closure

Similar to that for inguinal hernias.

# Complications and results

The results of surgery are excellent and complications are usually avoidable.

### Haematoma

Some swelling of the scrotum and along the cord may follow inguinal herniotomy in infants. It can usually be avoided by meticulous technique, gentle dissection and careful haemostasis.

### Infection

Despite the young infant being wet and in nappies wound infection is rare.

### Iatrogenic undescended testis

This may follow inguinal herniotomy at any age but especially in young infants. It can be avoided by careful checking of the position of the testis during and at the end of the operation.

### Recurrence

This is rare (0.1 per cent) and is a result of the treatment of complicated hernias or to technical problems.

### Damage to cord structures

These should be avoidable by careful technique.

### Bladder complications

Rarely the bladder may be damaged at the time of transfixation of the hernial sac.

### Fever

A transient rise in temperature in the first postoperative 24 hours is almost invariable.

## References

1. Sloman, J. G., Myliuf, R. E. (1963) Testicular infarction in infancy: its association with irreducible inguinal hernia. In: Stephens, F. D. Congenital Malformations of the Rectum, Anus and Genito-urinary Tracts, p. 321–324. Edinburgh and London: Livingstone

2. De Boer, A., Potts, W. J. (1963) Inguinal hernias in children. Archives of Surgery, 86, 1072–1074

3. Atwell, J. D., Burn, J. M. B., Dewar, A. K., Freeman, N. V. (1973) Paediatric day-case surgery. Lancet, 2, 895–897

4. Atwell, J. D. (1962) Inguinal hernia in female infants and children. British Journal of Surgery, 50, 294–297

5. Atwell, J. D. (1962) Inguinal herniae and the testicular feminization syndrome in infancy and childhood. British Journal of Surgery, 49, 367–371

Illustrations by Gillian Oliver

# Umbilical, supra-umbilical and epigastric hernias

**J. D. Atwell** MD, ChB, FRCS
Consultant Paediatric Surgeon, Wessex Regional Centre for Paediatric Surgery, The General Hospital, Southampton, UK

# UMBILICAL HERNIA

## Introduction

The defect in the anterior abdominal wall found in infants with an umbilical hernia is due to failure of the extra-abdominal coelom to close completely at the site of the umbilical vessels. This results in a small defect through the umbilical scar, with a relatively narrow neck through which the peritoneal sac protrudes.

Umbilical hernia is commoner in premature than in full-term infants (84 per cent of cases occurring in infants weighing 1000–1500 g, and only 20.5 per cent in infants weighing 2000–2500 g)[1]. The umbilicus is one of the commonest sites for a hernia in infancy.

The swelling seen when the infant cries or strains often causes considerable anxiety to parents. Incarceration, strangulation and rupture of this thin-walled sac have been described but are exceptionally rare events and should not be cited as an indication for surgical treatment.

Fortunately, the majority of umbilical herniae decrease in size and then close spontaneously, usually between the ages of 1–7 years[2].

## Preoperative

### Indications

The size of the defect at the umbilicus is the main factor determining the time of operation. Defects less than 1.5 cm in diameter usually close by school age but with larger defects closure may be delayed beyond this and operative closure is then indicated.

### Anaesthesia

The operation is carried out under general anaesthesia and is suitable for day care admission.[3]

## The operation

# 1

### The incision

A curved transverse incision is made immediately above or below the umbilicus. Traction with tissue forceps on the hernia ensures symmetry of the incision.

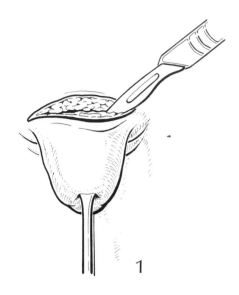

# 2 & 3

### Exposure of hernial sac

The hernial sac is exposed just distal to the neck, leaving the fundus of the sac adherent to the overlying skin. When this is completed, the scissors are passed behind the sac, which is still held on traction.

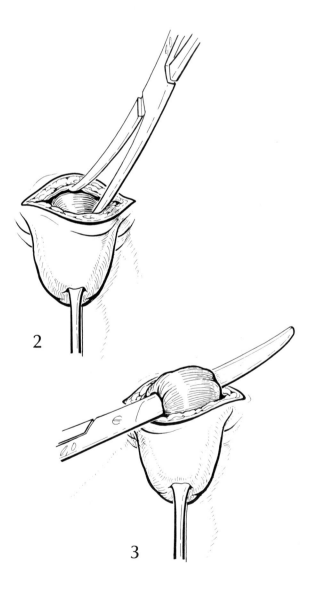

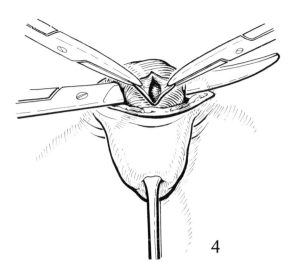

4

# 4 & 5

## Opening the sac

The superior aspect of the sac is then opened and any contents inspected and reduced.

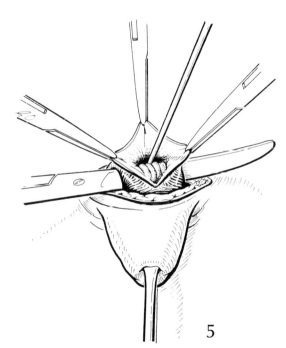

5

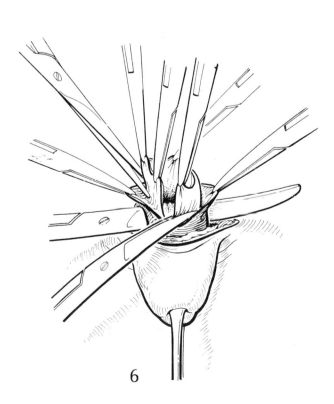

6

# 6

## Mobilization of hernial sac

The peritoneal sac is then separated from the fascial covering of the hernia.

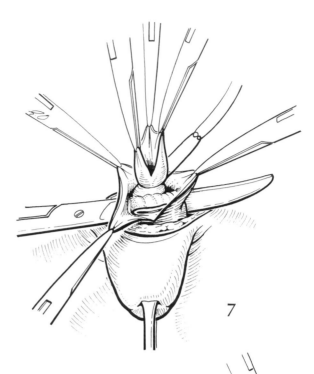

7

# 7 & 8

### Transfixation of hernial sac

Once mobilized, the peritoneum can be closed with
single or multiple absorbable sutures and the excess
fascial covering is excised to expose the free margin of the
defect.

8

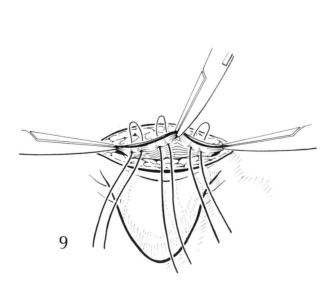

9

# 9

### Repair of hernia

The defect is repaired with interrupted non-absorbable
sutures. The lateral sutures are placed initially and traction
is then applied, thus making it easier to insert the two or
three intermediate sutures. If the defect is large,
overlapping of the edges allows a Mayo type of repair.

## 10

### Invagination of hernial sac

After invagination of the skin overlying the fundus of the sac, the remaining peritoneal sac may be dissected free, although this is not essential and the remnant of the sac may quite safely be left behind.

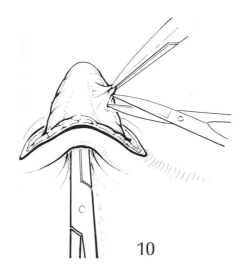

## 11

### Suturing the umbilical scar to anterior abdominal wall

A single 3/0 absorbable suture is then inserted and tied to suture the dermis of the umbilicus to the line of the repair.

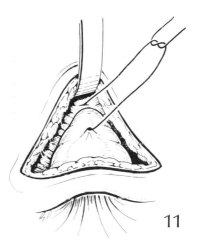

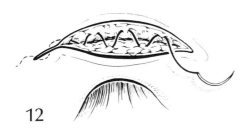

## 12

### Skin closure

The skin incision is closed with either subcuticular Vicryl or interrupted silk sutures. A pressure dressing is applied to obliterate any dead space under the incision. This may be removed after 24–48 hours.

## Postoperative care

A pressure dressing is applied for 48 hours to reduce the chance of a haematoma developing and possible secondary infection.

For pain relief during the first 24–48 hours, paracetamol (60 mg/kg body weight) is all that is required.

# SUPRA-UMBILICAL AND EPIGASTRIC HERNIAS

## Preoperative

### Indications

Supra-umbilical and epigastric hernias can be considered together, as the pathology is similar and in both, the defect is in the linea alba. A supra-umbilical hernia is sometimes difficult to distinguish from an umbilical hernia, as the defect may be almost contiguous with the umbilical cicatrix. A supra-umbilical hernia always has a hernial sac and thus differs from many epigastric herniae which contain only a pad of extraperitoneal fat. Surgery is always indicated, as there is no natural history of spontaneous cure.

### Anaesthesia

General anaesthesia is required and the procedure may be carried out on a day care basis[2].

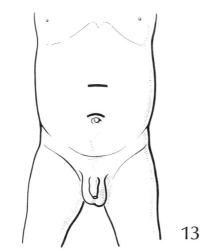

13

## The operation

## 13

### The incision

A small transverse incision is made over the defect. In children with epigastric hernia, because of the small size of the defect, it is advisable to mark the exact site with a skin pencil before anaesthesia, as on the operating table small defects can be extremely difficult to localize accurately.

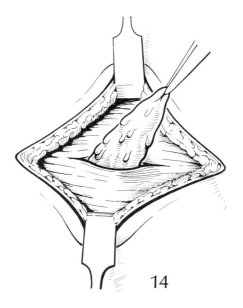

14

## 14

### Isolation of 'hernial' sac

The pad of extraperitoneal fat coming through the defect in the linea alba is isolated and, if small and without a hernial sac, may be excised or returned to the abdominal cavity.

## 15

### Transfixation of hernial sac

If there is a hernial sac, this is now opened and the contents inspected and reduced. The sac is then transfixed and excised.

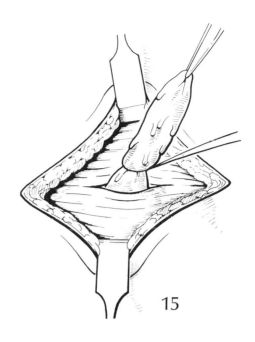

15

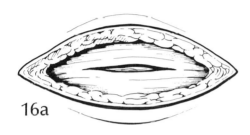

16a

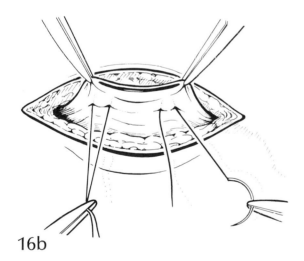

16b

## 16a–c

### Repair of defect

The defect in the linea alba is defined and repaired with overlapping interrupted linen sutures (Mayo repair). In small defects, a repair with two mattress sutures is all that is required.

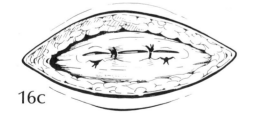

16c

# 17

### Skin closure

An absorbable 5/0 Vicryl subcuticular suture is used to close the wound.

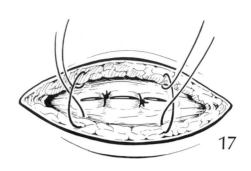

17

# Complications

1. Potentially, the umbilicus is an unclean area and this, together with the loose tissue planes and predisposition to haematoma formation beneath the wound, increases the risk of infection.
2. Haematoma formation and thus the risk of secondary infection can be avoided by applying a pressure dressing for 24–48 hours postoperatively.
3. Infection following the use of non-absorbable linen sutures for the repair may result in extrusion of the sutures.
4. Recurrence of the hernia is rare and usually due to faulty technique.

## References

1. Evans, A. G. (1941) The comparative incidence of umbilical hernias in coloured and white infants. Journal of the American Medical Association, 33, 158–160

2. Walker, S. H. (1967) The natural history of umbilical hernia. Clinical Pediatrics, 6, 29

3. Atwell, J. D., Burn, J. M. B., Dewar, A. K., Freeman, N. V. (1973) Paediatric day-case surgery. Lancet, 2, 895–897

Illustrations by Gillian Oliver

# Femoral hernia

**J. D. Atwell**  MB, ChB, FRCS
Consultant Paediatric Surgeon, Wessex Regional Centre for Paediatric Surgery, The General Hospital, Southampton, UK

Of all the hernias in childhood, femoral hernia is the rarest. However, the diagnosis should always be borne in mind when examining any swelling in the inguinal region, especially in young girls.

# Preoperative

### Indications

It is a rare event to diagnose a femoral hernia in an infant or child. If found, it is usually in a girl between 5 and 10 years of age and there is often a family history of the condition. Conservative treatment is contraindicated because the high incidence of strangulation in later life and the uselessness of wearing a truss. The risk of strangulation is due to the rigid margins of the femoral ring at the entrance to the femoral canal. A Richter's hernia is particularly dangerous in patients with a femoral hernia.

### Anaesthesia

General anaesthesia is required and the operation is suitable for day care unless complicated by the presence of strangulation. I have never seen a strangulated femoral hernia in infancy or childhood.

### Choice of operation

There are three approaches to the repair of a femoral hernia. The 'low' operation (Langenbeck), the 'high' operation (Lotheissen) and the abdominal extraperitoneal operation (McEvedy). In childhood, because of the rarity of strangulation, the 'low' operation is satisfactory and only this is described here. If there is clinical evidence of strangulation of the bowel, the McEvedy approach is the treatment of choice although the Lotheissen operation is very adequate.

### Principles of operation

The femoral hernial sac must be isolated and excised after reduction of the content, which is usually omentum. In addition, a repair is required to obliterate the femoral canal, preferably at the level of the femoral ring. This may be done by suturing the medial end of the inguinal ligament either to the pectineus fascia or to Sir Astley Cooper's ligament. The latter procedure is the treatment of choice although it is more difficult to perform.

# The operation

## The incision

### 1

A skin-crease incision is made over the swelling in the inguinal region. This extends from medial and just below the pubic tubercle to a point just lateral to the pulsation of the femoral artery.

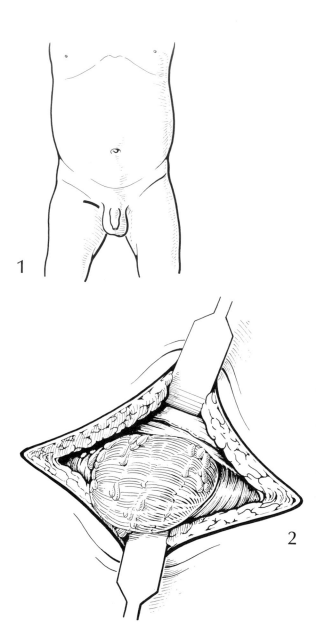

### 2

The wound is deepened to expose the bulge of the hernia covered with the cribriform fascia. The sac may overlie the femoral vein and pass superiorly to cover the inguinal ligament.

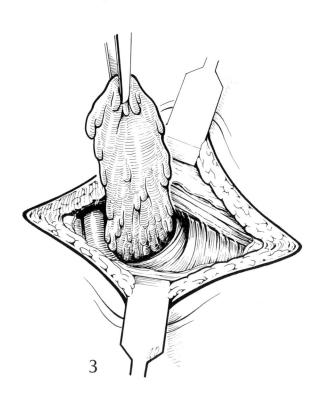

## Exposure and mobilization of sac

### 3

The cribriform fascia and condensed fatty tissue covering the sac are incised and separated to expose the sac. This is eased by applying traction to the fundus of the hernial sac.

The neck of the sac is traced upwards to the femoral canal and the boundaries of the femoral ring are identified, i.e. the inguinal ligament anteriorly, the lacunar ligament medially, the pectineus with its fascia and the pubic ramus posteriorly covered by Cooper's ligament, and the femoral vein laterally.

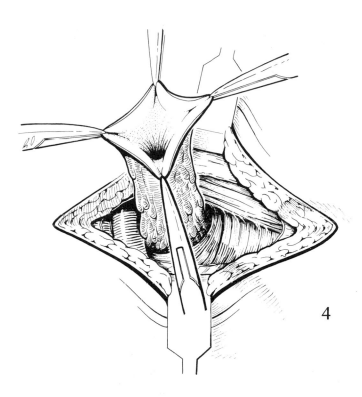

4

## Excision of sac

# 4 & 5

The peritoneal sac is often small with a relatively large condensation of extraperitoneal fat around it. The contents have often reduced spontaneously by this stage of the operation.

The sac is opened to confirm that it is empty, and then transfixed at its highest point and cut off. The stump should then retract or be pushed upwards well above the entrance of the femoral canal.

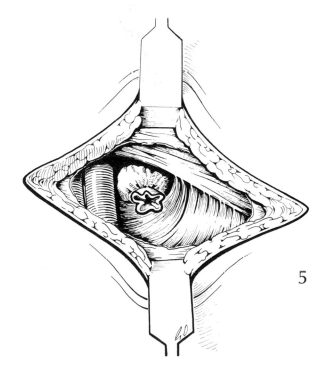

5

## Repair

# 6 & 7

A small retractor is used to lift the inguinal ligament superiorly to expose the pectineus fascia and Cooper's ligament. Two or three non-absorbable sutures are then placed between the inguinal ligament and Cooper's ligament, care being taken to avoid damaging the femoral vein lying laterally. These sutures should all be inserted before being tied individually with care to avoid compressing the femoral vein.

The subcutaneous tissue is closed with two or three interrupted absorbable sutures.

### Skin closure

The skin edges are approximated with a continuous subcuticular Vicryl suture (4/0 or 5/0) and 12.5 mm Steri-Strips. In young patients in nappies an OpSite dressing (Smith and Nephew) provides excellent protection of the wound.

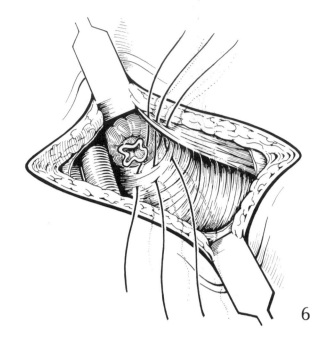

6

# Postoperative care

Steri-Strips or an OpSite dressing to protect the wound closed with subcuticular Vicryl is all that is necessary. The dressing should be left on until the 5th postoperative day.

Relief of pain may be required in the first 24 hours. Paracetamol is a suitable analgesic.

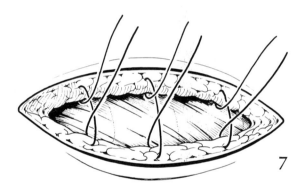

7

# Complications

1. Injury to the femoral or external iliac vein can be avoided by careful lateral retraction of the vein at the time of inserting the sutures between the inguinal and Cooper's ligament.
2. Constriction of the femoral vein may follow excessive narrowing of the femoral canal by the sutures between the inguinal and Cooper's ligament.
3. A protrusion of the bladder may be included in the extraperitoneal fat around the sac and may be caught by the transfixation suture, resulting in a urinary fistula.
4. Congenital inguinal and femoral hernia may be found in the same patient on rare occasions.
5. Wound infection may occur secondary to haematoma formation; this may be avoided by careful haemostasis and ligation of the superficial veins in relation to the saphenous opening.

Illustrated by Gillian Oliver

# Exomphalos/omphalocele

**J. A. S. Dickson**   MB, ChB, FRCS, FRCS(Ed),
Consultant Paediatric Surgeon, Children's Hospital, Sheffield, UK

Exomphalos or omphalocele is a useful term to cover the major congenital abdominal-wall defects at the umbilicus.

## EMBRYOLOGY

Two processes affect the umbilicus during development:

1. Mesoderm migrates medially to form the abdominal wall muscles, eventually replacing the amniotic sac.

2. During this development the early rapid growth of the midgut leads to herniation into the amniotic sac in the cord, followed by its later return, rotation, and adherence to the posterior abdominal wall as the coelom expands. The whole process should be complete by the 12th week of intrauterine life.

## Hernia into the cord

### 1

Simple persistence of the physiological hernia is the commonest of the defects, 'hernia into the cord'. Adherence of gut or a Meckel's diverticulum within the sac provides an obvious explanation of some of the cases. Others appear to be due to delayed closure of the defect in the linea alba, the umbilical ring. The size of lesion is dictated by the amount of herniated gut. The abdominal cavity is of normal capacity and only adhesions within the sac may prevent simple reduction; thus the size of the visible sac does not usually affect surgical management.

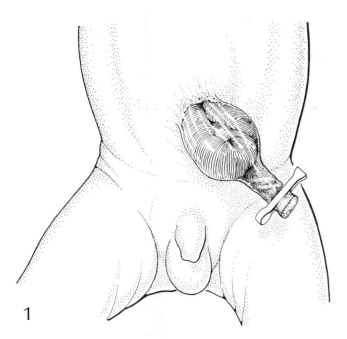

1

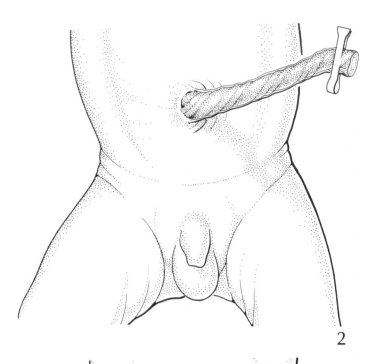

**2**

## CONSERVATIVE TREATMENT

# 2, 3, 4

Occasionally it is appropriate to empty the sac by twisting it and maintaining the reduction with strapping on the abdominal wall, although any adhesions within the sac will prevent this.

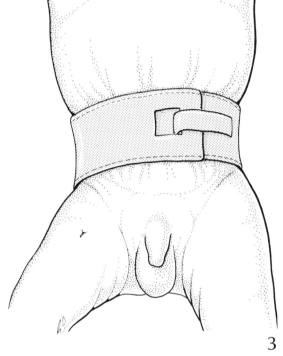

**3**

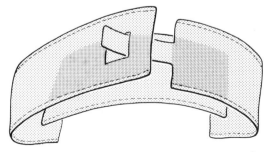

**4**

## OPERATIVE TREATMENT

Rarely, an abnormal tongue of liver will also be found in the sac, and here it is generally better to repair the defect under general anaesthesia. The sac is excised, the abdominal-wall defect repaired and the skin closed with an attempt to produce an 'umbilicus'. It is usually desirable to inspect the gut for abnormalities and check on the rotation and fixation, but if problems with abdominal wall closure are expected minimal handling may occasionally be preferable to avoid increasing gut distension.

# Omphalocele

## 5

Failure of migration of the mesoderm leaves a defect with a wide base, a deficient anterior abdominal wall, and a sac containing liver. This is frequently associated with other anomalies. If the mesodermal defect extends cranially there are sternal, diaphragmatic and pericardial defects with thoraco-abdominal ectopia cordis and congenital heart lesions, including a diverticulum of the left ventricle – 'the pentad of Cantrell'. Caudal extension is associated with varying degrees of extroversion of the bladder up to vesicointestinal fissure. The rectus abdominis muscles are always intact around the circumference of the base of the defect.

The abdominal-wall defect varies in extent from minor, less than 5 cm at the base, to very extensive with an entirely extra-abdominal liver. In the case of a minor defect with a base diameter of less than 5 cm simple excision of the sac and repair of the abdominal wall, as for a hernia into the cord, is satisfactory. However, in large defects the abdominal-wall deficiency renders closure difficult.

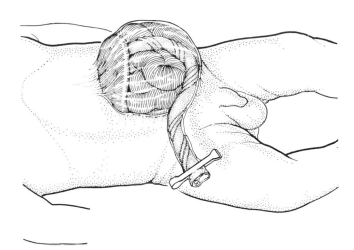

5

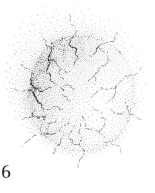

6

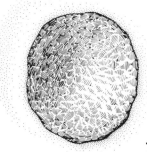

7

## CONSERVATIVE TREATMENT

## 6 & 7

If the sac is painted with alcoholic mercurochrome it will form a firm, dry membrane which remains uninfected and is gradually replaced by ingrowing epithelium. Other therapeutic agents, povidone iodine, flavine dyes, and multi-antibiotic sprays, have also been used on the membrane to prevent infection in the sac. Mercurochrome, as the first application, produces the best tanning effect on the sac, but repeated applications of mercury compounds may lead to potentially toxic levels of mercury absorption. Iodine-containing compounds similarly lead to iodine absorption, with possible effects on thyroid function. This conservative treatment is particularly suitable for small or premature infants and for those with severe congenital heart disease.

### Advantages

Operation is avoided at the time of the greatest risk.

### Disadvantages

Healing takes about 3 months, and a late repair of a large ventral hernia will still be required.

## OPERATIVE TREATMENT

The techniques available to assist closure are:

1. Skin only, with or without retaining the amniotic sac. The skin can virtually always be mobilized adequately for closure. An intact sac requires more extensive mobilization of the skin, and does not permit inspection of the gut for abnormalities or the diaphragm for anterior defects, but does reduce the risks of adhesion of the gut to the skin flaps, and also protects the gut if the skin closure fails.

2. If the sac is excised some stretching of the abdominal wall, which will facilitate final closure, is possible, and the defect can be repaired with either a biological implant, e.g. lyophylized human dura or bovine pericardium, or a prosthetic implant; reinforced silicon rubber has been recommended, but an implant which can be incorporated into the tissues, e.g. Marlex mesh or Gore-tex, is to be preferred.

3. The use of a deliberately fashioned reinforced silicon rubber pouch which can gradually be reduced to give a delayed primary muscle closure has been largely replaced because of the complications of early separation of the membrane, infection, and perforation of the gut.

Most methods leave a ventral hernia for later repair. Except in the massive forms with most of the liver outside the abdomen, the hernia tends to reduce with growth, and repair can be safely deferred for several years. It should be performed before the child goes to school.

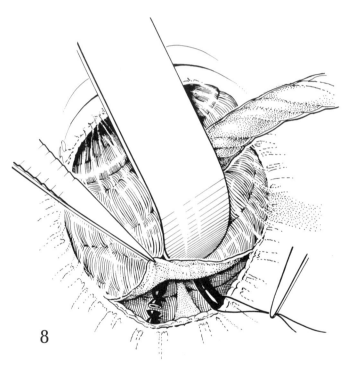

8

## Technique

The sac is excised, with ligation of the umbilical vein and arteries, closure of the umbilical defect in layers, and reconstruction of the umbilical cicatrix.

## 8

The junction of the sac and skin is incised and the umbilical arteries underrun and ligated. *They are brittle and will be cut by artery forceps.*

## 9

The urachus may also require ligation. The much larger umbilical vein lies in the left side of the sac and passes to the cleft in the liver suspended from the abdominal wall by the falciform ligament.

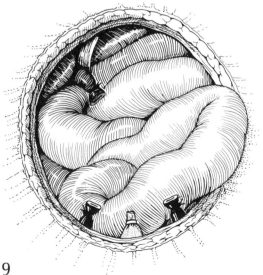

9

## 10

Sharp dissection separating skin from deep layers is now undertaken.

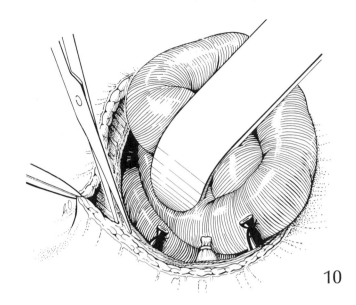

## 11

The peritoneum and linea alba is repaired with 3/0 Vicryl, Dexon or PDS sutures.

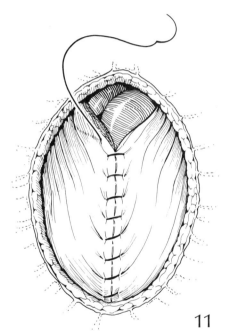

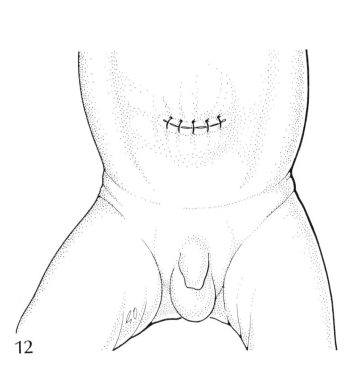

## 12

The umbilicus is then reconstructed.

## Major defects in fit babies

Skin cover can be achieved by undermining the abdominal skin widely and suturing it over the sac.

# 13 & 14

Dissection of skin from the sac and abdominal wall muscles may be undertaken. The sac may be excised as in illustrations 8–12, or left intact.

### Disadvantages

Tight closure may lead to early breathing difficulties and, later, suture-line separation. A late ventral hernia repair will be required.

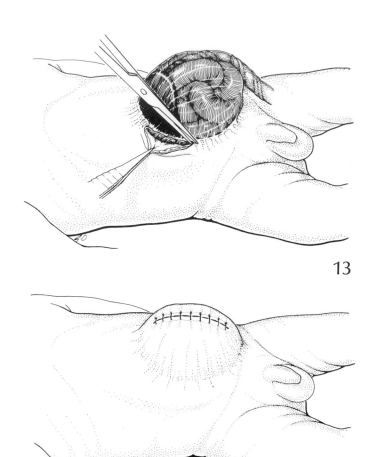

13

14

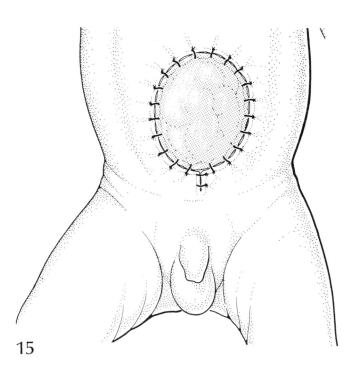

15

## Use of a prosthesis

# 15

The abdominal wall defect may be repaired with reinforced silicon rubber (0.007 inch thickness), but lyophyllized dura, Goretex, or Marlex mesh, which are incorporated into the tissues, are better. The skin should be closed as near to the midline as possible.

## BECKWITH–WIEDEMANN SYNDROME

Exomphalos is one of the features of the Beckwith–Wiedemann syndrome, which also includes macroglossia, organomegaly and hypoglycaemia. The importance of recognizing this syndrome lies in the special need to treat the severe hypoglycaemia, which can cause mental retardation.

# Gastroschisis

# 16

The term gastroschisis is restricted to the condition in which a variable length of a thickened abnormal gut protrudes through a short, transverse, slit-like defect to one side of the umbilical cord (in over 90 per cent this defect is right-sided). There is no sac. The most plausible explanation for this is an antenatal rupture of the amniotic sac, right-sided because of the obliteration of the right umbilical vein.

The natural tendency of the defect to close may result in strangulation of the extruded intestine and lead to atresias. Growth of tissues, including epithelium, can separate the defect from the umbilical cord. The thickened abnormal state of the gut is due to exposure to amniotic fluid, while the protruding gut maintains the abdominal-wall defect.

The technical problems in treatment are:

1. The gut is grossly thickened and shortened.
2. The abdominal cavity is deficient.
3. There may be ischaemia or atresias in the gut.
4. The gut is contaminated and potentially infected.
5. Recovery of gut motility is delayed.
6. The babies are frequently small or premature.

Anomalies in other systems are relatively uncommon: an incidence similar to that seen with 'hernia into the cord'.

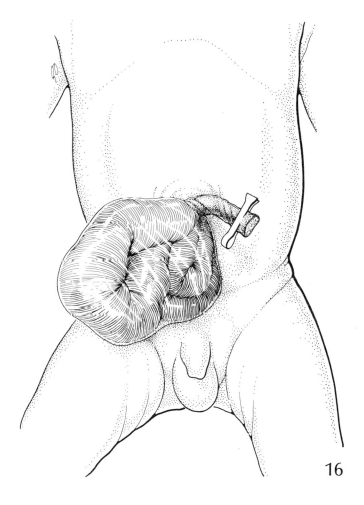

16

## OPERATIVE TREATMENT

# 17, 18 & 19

The abdominal-wall defect must be enlarged either longitudinally or transversely. The abdominal wall can then be stretched with fingers to enlarge the available space, and contents expressed from the gut to reduce its bulk. Milk small bowel content to the stomach where it can be sucked out, and large bowel content towards the anus where it can be expressed. Use saline rectal irrigation in preference to undue force.

Stripping of the covering pellicle off the gut is not advised.

Primary closure, when this does not obstruct breathing, is best. If breathing problems appear inevitable the use of a reinforced pouch of silicon rubber is helpful (*see* Use of a prosthesis, p. 234).

### Problems

1. Hypothermia is common both before and during operation.
2. Infection may occur under the membrane.
3. A long delay of 2 or 3 weeks before gut function returns is usual, and intravenous feeding is advised from the time of operation.

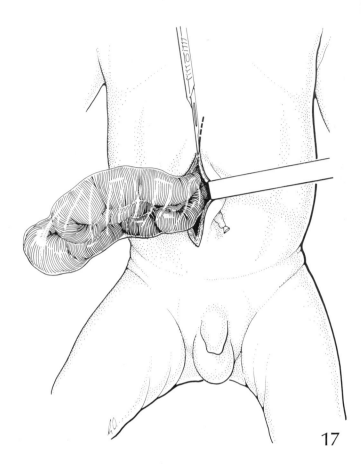

17

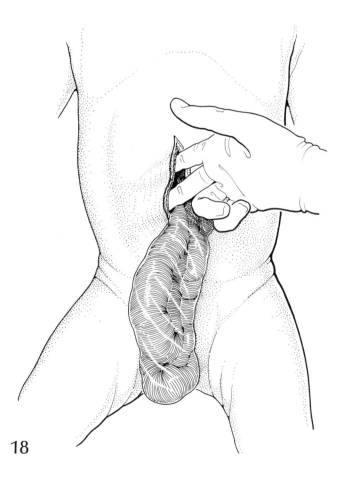

18

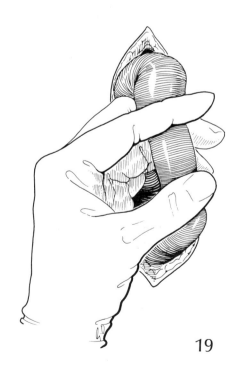

19

### Use of a prosthesis

## 20

A reinforced silicon rubber membrane 0.007 inches thick (Silastic, Silon) can be sutured over the sac to the layers of the abdominal wall. This artificial pouch is progressively reduced in size over the next 10–14 days, followed by a formal closure. The skin–membrane suture line should be sprayed with povidone iodine aerosol to keep it dry and non-infected.

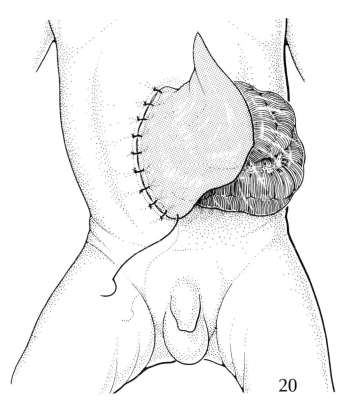

20

## 21

The membrane should pass deep to the peritoneum, permitting two rows of silk sutures, one to muscle and one to skin. If membrane with a mesh 'skirt' is available, the skirt should be sewn to the muscle layer.

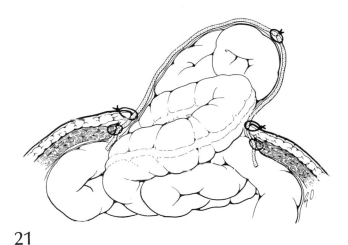

21

## 22

Progressive tucks are taken in the sac. A 'sewing-machine' stitch, which is easily inserted and removed, is useful.

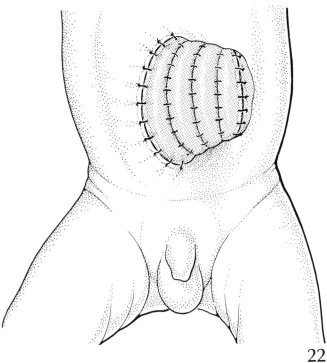

22

## 23 & 24

After about 2 weeks full closure should be possible. Deep tension sutures are shown.

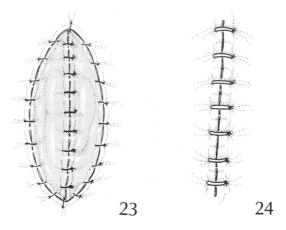

**23**      **24**

### Problems

1. Sepsis at the sac to abdominal wall suture line is common.
2. The membrane may break away from the suture line.
3. There are risks of damage to the underlying gut.

There are still difficulties with delayed return of peristalsis, and persisting obstruction due to the retention of inspissated meconium, which can be relieved by a Gastrografin enema. Intravenous feeding is usually required. Late onset of necrotizing enterocolitis has been seen in association with obstruction.

## Results

The survival rate is directly related to the severity of associated abnormalities. There should be no technical surgical problems with the hernia into the cord and minor omphalocele groups. In omphalocele major the survival rate in many series is just over 60 per cent. It is in the gastroschisis group that there has been the most dramatic improvement in results, with 80–90 per cent survival in recent series, compared with the previously nearly uniformly fatal outcome.

## 25 & 26

Transverse extension and closure is possible if preferred.

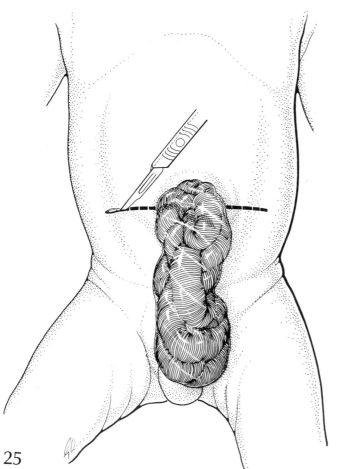

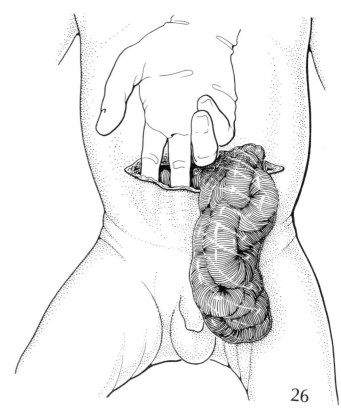

**25**

**26**

## Further reading

Aaronson, I. A., Eckstein, H. B. (1977) The role of the silastic prosthesis in the management of gastroschisis. Archives of Surgery, 112, 297–302

Amoury, R. A., Ashcraft, K. W., Holder, T. M. (1977) Gastroschisis complicated by intestinal atresia. Surgery, 82, 373–381

de Vries, P. A. (1980) The pathogenesis of gastroschisis and omphalocele. Journal of Pediatric Surgery, 15, 245–251

Duhamel, B. (1963) Embryology of exomphalos and allied malformations. Archives of Disease in Childhood, 38, 142–147

Eckstein, H. B. (1963) Exomphalos. A review of 100 cases. British Journal of Surgery, 50, 405–410

Ein, S. H., Rubin, S. Z. (1980) Gastroschisis: primary closure or Silon pouch. Journal of Pediatric Surgery, 15, 549–552

Glick, P. L., Harrison, M. R., Adzick, N. S., Filly, R. A., deLorimier, A. A., Callen, P. W. (1985) The missing link in the pathogenesis of gastroschisis.

Gough, D. C. S., Auldist, A. W. (1979) Giant exomphalos – conservative or operative treatment? Archives of Disease in Childhood, 54, 441–444

Grob, M. (1963) Conservative treatment of exomphalos. Archives of Disease in Childhood, 38, 148–150

Grosfeld, J. L., Dawes, L., Weber, T. R. (1981) Congenital abdominal wall defects: current management and survival. Surgical Clinics of North America, 61, 1037–1049

Irving Irene, M. (1971) The "E.M.G." syndrome (Exomphalos, Macroglossia, Gigantism): a study of eleven cases. In: Progress in Pediatric Surgery, Rickham, P. P., Hecker, W. C. L., Prevot, J. (eds.) pp. 1–61, Baltimore: University Park Press

Knight, P. J., Buckner, D., Vassy, L. E. (1981) Omphalocele: treatment options. Surgery, 89(3), 332–336

Luck, S. R., Sherman, J. O., Raffensperger, J. G., Goldstein, I. R. (1985) Gastroschisis in 106 consecutive newborn infants. Surgery, 98, 677–683

Mollitt, D. L., Ballantine, T. V. N., Grosfeld, J. L., Quinter, P. (1978) A critical assessment of fluid requirements in gastroschisis. Journal of Pediatric Surgery, 13, 217–219

Moore, T. C. (1977) Gastroschisis and omphalocele: clinical differences. Surgery, 82, 561–568

Moore, T. C., Nur, K. (1986) An international survey of gastroschisis and omphalocele (490). Pediatric Surgery, 1, 46–50

Pokorny, W. J., Harberg, F. J., McGill, C. W. (1981) Gastroschisis complicated by intestinal atresia. Journal of Pediatric Surgery, 16, 261–263

Rubin, S. Z., Ein, S. H. (1976) Experience with 55 Silon pouches. Journal of Pediatric Surgery, 11, 803–807

Schuster, S. R. (1967) A new method for the staged repair of large omphaloceles. Surgery, Gynecology and Obstetrics, 125, 837–850

Schwaitzberg, S. D., Pokorny, W. J., McGill, C. W., Harberg, F. J. (1982) Gastroschisis and omphalocele. American Journal of Surgery, 144, 650–654

Shaw, A. (1975) The myth of gastroschisis. Journal of Pediatric Surgery, 10, 235–244

Towne, B. H., Peters, G., Chang, J. H. T. (1980) The problem of "giant" omphalocele. Journal of Pediatric Surgery, 15, 543–548

Illustrations by Kevin Marks

# Nissen fundoplication

**L. Spitz**  MB, ChB, PhD, FRCS(Ed), FRCS(Eng), FAAP(Hon)
Nuffield Professor of Paediatric Surgery, Institute of Child Health, University of London; Consultant Paediatric Surgeon, Hospital for Sick Children, Great Ormond Street, London, UK

## INTRODUCTION

Gastro-oesophageal reflux is commonly encountered during the first year of life, but due to maturation of the lower oesophageal sphincter mechanism, spontaneous resolution occurs in 90–95 per cent of cases. The reflux may be precipitated by associated pathology such as oesophageal atresia, malrotation, or anterior abdominal wall defects, and is frequently present in children with disorders of the central nervous system, e.g. cerebral palsy.

## PATHOLOGICAL ANATOMY

Reflux may or may not be accompanied by an associated hiatus hernia. Two types of hiatus hernia are recognized:

# 1

Sliding hiatus hernia characterized by ascent of the cardia into the mediastinum;

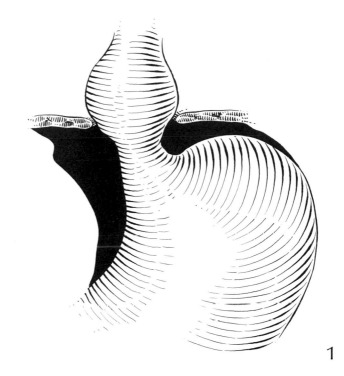

1

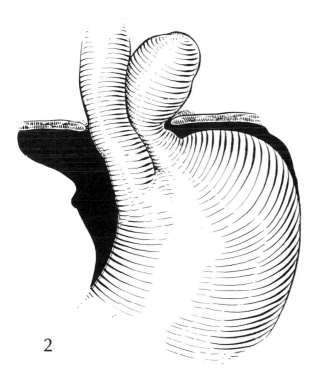

2

# 2

Paraoesophageal or rolling hernia, in which the gastro-oesophageal junction remains in the abdomen while part of the gastric fundus prolapses through the oesophageal hiatus into the mediastinum.

The sliding hernia is frequently associated with reflux, while gastric stasis in the paraoesophageal hernia predisposes to peptic ulceration, perforation or haemorrhage.

## NORMAL MECHANISMS PREVENTING REFLUX

Physiological control of reflux is dependent upon the following factors:

1. Lower oesophageal sphincter;
2. The intra-abdominal segment of the oesophagus;
3. The gastro-oesophageal angle (angle of His);
4. The lower oesophageal mucosal rosette;
5. The phreno-oesophageal membrane;
6. The diaphragmatic hiatal pinchcock effect.

## PATHOPHYSIOLOGY OF REFLUX

The squamous epithelium of the oesophagus is unable to resist the irritant effect of gastric juices. The acid-pepsin causes a chemical inflammation with erythema of the mucosa. With continued reflux, the mucosa becomes friable and bleeds easily on contact. Later, frank ulceration develops which, with repeated attempts at repair and relapse, eventually leads to stricture formation.

Acid-pepsin reflux

↓

Erythema of mucosa

↓                          } Reversible

Friability and contact haemorrhage
Continued reflux

↓

Ulcerative oesophagitis
Potentially reversible

↓

Stricture formation.

## INVESTIGATIONS

1. Barium oesophagogram with particular attention to:
   (a) anatomy of the oesophagus – presence of strictures, ulcerative oesophagitis, abnormal narrowing or displacement;
   (b) presence of a hiatus hernia;
   (c) peristaltic activity of the oesophagus and rate of clearance of contrast material;
   (d) degree of gastro-oesophageal reflux:
       Grade I   – distal oesophagus;
       Grade II  – proximal/thoracic oesophagus;
       Grade III – cervical oesophagus;
       Grade IV  – continuous reflux;
       Grade V   – aspiration into tracheobronchial tree;
   (e) evidence of gastric outlet obstruction.
2. Oesophageal pH monitoring. Continuous 24-hour monitoring of the pH in the distal oesophagus is the most accurate method of documenting reflux. Levels below pH 4 are regarded as significant, and during the 24-hour recording the following parameters are examined:
   (a) number of episodes where the pH falls below pH 4;
   (b) duration of each reflux episode;
   (c) number of episodes lasting more than 5 minutes;
   (d) total duration of reflux expressed as a percentage of recording time.
3. Oesophageal manometry. Pressure recordings are made with continuously perfused open-tipped catheters. A high-pressure zone is normally present in the distal oesophagus. Individual pressure values are unreliable diagnostic indicators of reflux but may be useful in predicting cases which will eventually require surgical treatment.
4. Endoscopy and biopsy. Endoscopy will determine the degree of oesophagitis, while histology of the biopsy will provide pathological grading of inflammatory cell infiltration. Four grades of oesophagitis are recognized at endoscopy.
   Grade I   – erythema of mucosa;
   Grade II  – friability of mucosa;
   Grade III – ulcerative oesophagitis;
   Grade IV – stricture.
5. Scintiscanning. Technetium ($Tc^{99}$) sulphur colloid scans are useful in documenting pulmonary aspiration.

## MEDICAL MANAGEMENT

1. Small, frequent, thickened feeds should be given.
2. A 30° head-elevated, prone position is the most suitable posture.
3. Antacids–alkalis with or without alginic acid (Gaviscon) should be administered.
4. Histamine receptor antagonists (cimetidine, ranitidine) will suppress acid secretion and allow healing of severe oesophagitis.
5. Metoclopramide and bethanechol are drugs which increase lower oesophageal pressure and stimulate gastric emptying.

## INDICATIONS FOR ANTIREFLUX SURGERY

1. An established oesophageal stricture.
2. Failure of conservative measures:
   (a) in the presence of an anatomical anomaly, e.g. oesophageal atresia, malrotation, exomphalos;
   (b) in the presence of associated neurological damage where the response to conservative measures is notoriously poor;
   (c) apnoeic episodes and repeated respiratory infections due to aspiration of refluxed material;
   (d) failure to thrive in spite of adequate therapy.

The Nissen fundoplication is the most reliable procedure in the prevention of gastro-oesophageal reflux.

# Nissen fundoplication

## Anaesthesia

General endotracheal anaesthesia with the patient supine on the operation table. Most surgeons insist on a large-calibre bougie in the oesophagus during the construction of the fundoplication to ensure that the wrap is not too tight. The author prefers a regular size nasogastric tube and constructs a very loose wrap.

# 3

## Incision

In the majority of cases the ideal approach is via a midline upper abdominal incision extending from the xiphisternum to the umbilicus. This incision may be extended caudally to one side of the umbilicus. Where there has been extensive previous abdominal surgery, a lateral thoracic approach via the bed of the seventh or eighth rib may be more appropriate.

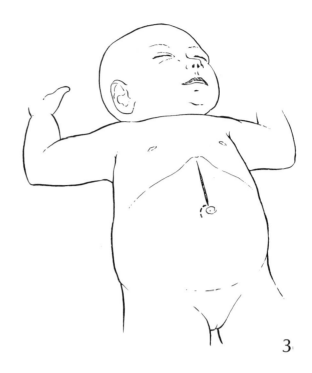

3

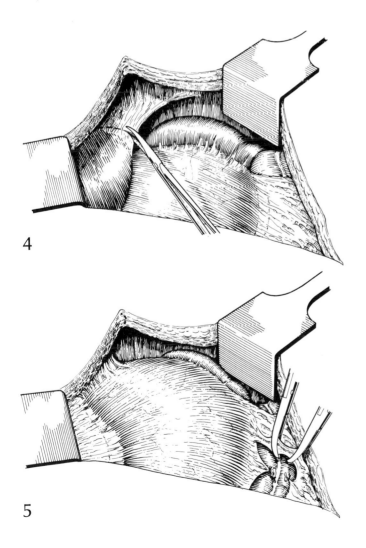

4

5

# 4 & 5

## Exposure

In most cases adequate exposure of the gastro-oesophageal junction can be obtained by retracting the left lobe of the liver anterosuperiorly with a Morris retractor. If required, additional exposure may be attained by dividing the left triangular ligament in the avascular plane and then retracting the left lobe of the liver to the right.

# 6 & 7

## Mobilization of the fundus of the stomach

The proximal one-third of the greater curvature of the stomach is liberated from its attachment to the spleen by ligating and dividing the short gastric vessels in the gastrosplenic ligament. This is accomplished most safely using a right-angled clamp passed around each vessel in turn and ligating the vessel on the gastric and splenic side before dividing it.

When all the vessels in the gastrosplenic ligament have been divided, the spleen should be allowed to fall back into the posterior peritoneum thereby avoiding inadvertent trauma. Splenectomy should rarely be necessary in this procedure. The fundus is now sufficiently free to allow a loose ('floppy') fundoplication.

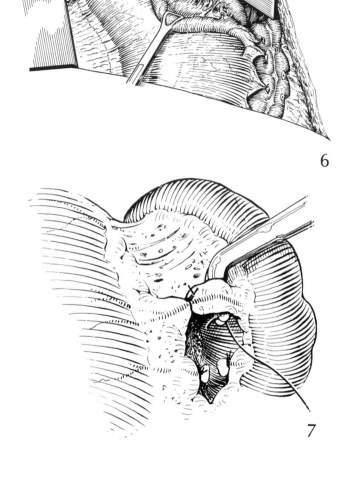

6

7

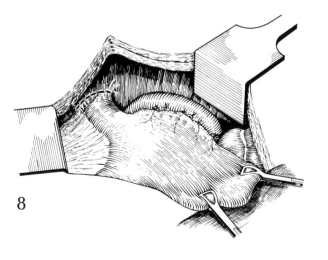

8

# 8

## Exposure of the oesophageal hiatus

The phreno-oesophageal membrane is placed on stretch by downward traction on the stomach while the diaphragmatic muscle is held anteriorly. The avascular membrane is incised with scissors and the musculature of the oesophagus displayed. The anterior vagus nerve will be seen coursing on the surface of the oesophagus. It should be carefully protected and preserved.

# 9

## Mobilization of the distal oesophagus

Using a combination of sharp and blunt dissection, the lower end of the oesophagus is encircled taking care not to injure the posterior vagus nerve. A rubber sling is placed around the oesophagus. The lower 3 or 4 cm of oesophagus is now mobilized using blunt dissection with either a pledget or right-angle forceps. The oesophageal hiatus is completely exposed by dividing the upper part of the gastrohepatic omentum above the left gastric vessels.

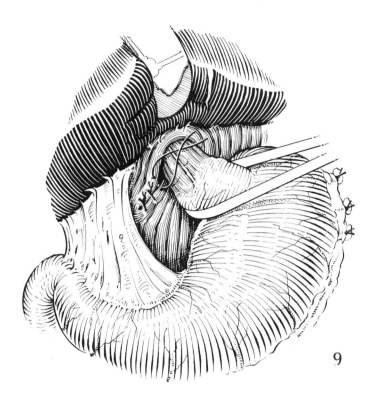

9

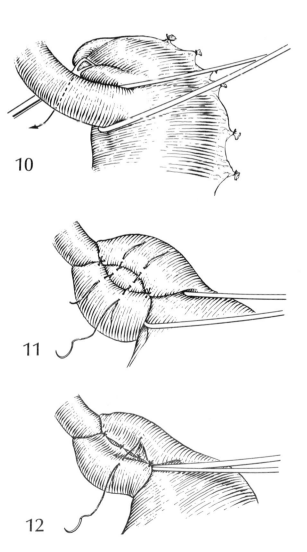

10

11

12

## Narrowing of the hiatus

The oesophageal hiatus is narrowed posterior to the oesophagus by placing deep sutures through the two limbs of the left crus of the diaphragm. The sutures are tied loosely to prevent them from cutting through, but leaving sufficient space alongside the oesophagus to allow passage of the tip of a finger. Two or three sutures may be required for this purpose.

# 10–12

## Construction of the fundoplication

The mobilized fundus of the stomach is folded behind the oesophagus so that the invaginated part of the stomach appears on the right side of the oesophagus. It is important not to twist the stomach during this manoeuvre and to ensure that there has been sufficient mobilization to be able to fashion a loose wrap.

# 13

Sutures of non-absorbable material (000 braided poly-propylene) are placed through the gastric and oesophageal muscle commencing at the gastro-oesophageal junction. The length of the wrap varies from 1.5 to 2.5 cm depending on the age of the patient. A second layer of sutures including only the seromuscular surface of the stomach will prevent subsequent disruption of the wrap. A few sutures are placed between the diaphragmatic hiatus and the fundoplication to prevent migration of the fundoplication into the posterior mediastinum.

A feeding gastrostomy may be added if the child is severely neurologically damaged and is unable to swallow.

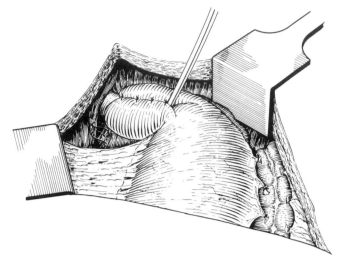

**13**

## Closure

The wound is closed either in layers or with interrupted en-masse sutures. A subcuticular suture approximates the skin edges.

# Postoperative care

Nasogastric decompression and intravenous fluids are continued until postoperative ileus has resolved (2–4 days on average).

## COMPLICATIONS

1. Too tight a wrap – leads to dysphagia;
2. A twisted wrap also causes dysphagia;
3. Wrapping the stomach rather than the lower oesophagus leads to recurrent reflux;
4. Prolapse of the fundoplication through the oesophageal hiatus into the posterior mediastinum causes dysphagia;
5. Paraoesophageal herniation due to inadequate hiatal narrowing;
6. Adhesive intestinal obstruction (10 per cent incidence);
7. Gas bloat, if the wrap is too long;
8. Dumping syndrome.

## Further Reading

Johnson, D. G. (1986) The Nissen fundoplication. In Pediatric Esophageal Surgery, T. M. Holder, K. W. Ashcraft (eds.) Orlando: Grune and Stratton.

Leape, L. L., Ramenofsky, M. L. (1980) Surgical treatment of gastro-esophageal reflux in children. Results of Nissen fundoplication in 100 children. American Journal of Diseases in Children, 134, 935–938

Randolph, J. (1983) Experience with the Nissen fundoplication for correction of gastroesophageal reflux in infants. Annals of Surgery, 198, 579–584

Tunnel, W. P., Smith, E. I., Carson, J. A. (1983) Gastroesophageal reflux in childhood: the dilemma of surgical success. Annals of Surgery, 197, 560–565

Spitz, L., Kirtane, J. (1985) Results and complications of surgery for gastroesophageal reflux. Archives of Disease in Childhood, 60, 743–747

Illustrations by Kevin Marks

# Gastrostomy in the newborn

**N. A. Myers** AM, FRCS, FRACS
Senior Surgeon, Royal Children's Hospital, Melbourne, Australia
Professorial Associate, University of Melbourne, Victoria, Australia

Gastrostomy has come to play an increasing role in the management of many different neonatal disorders and is now a frequently performed operation. Careful attention to technique and an awareness of the many specific needs in the newborn period make this a safe and beneficial procedure in many conditions as well as being life-saving in others. In these young patients special care must be taken:

1. to maintain fluid and electrolyte balance;
2. to avoid sepsis, hypothermia, hypoglycaemia and hypocalcaemia; and
3. to recognize and treat problems associated with deficiencies in the blood coagulation mechanisms – specifically hypothrombinaemia, which is so common as to demand routine administration of vitamin $K_1$ to all babies undergoing operation in the newborn period.

## Indications

Gastrostomy may be indicated in newborn babies with any of the following diseases.

1. Oesophageal atresia – with or without tracheo-oesophageal fistula.
2. High small bowel obstruction, particularly duodenal or jejunal atresia (as an adjunct).
3. Unusual problems such as stricture of the oesophagus, neonatal rupture of the oesophagus. It may also be indicated in some babies with pharyngeal, laryngeal or other cervical problems (e.g. laryngo-oesophageal cleft) and occasionally in babies with the Pierre Robin syndrome or where there is gross extrinsic obstruction as a result of a large cervical hamartoma (haemangiomatous or lymphangiomatous).

Gastrostomy was frequently used in babies with diaphragmatic hernia and gastroschisis, but is now rarely employed for these conditions.

The basic objects of gastrostomy are: (1) to provide a means of alimentation where the normal route is either impossible, e.g. oesophageal atresia not immediately amenable to surgical repair, or where alimentation is associated with regurgitation into the respiratory tract with the complication of aspiration pneumonitis, e.g. in laryngo-oesophageal cleft or nasopharyngeal incoordination; and (2) to provide more effective gastric decompression when nasogastric decompression is considered inadequate, e.g. in certain babies with diaphragmatic hernia or gastroschisis.

It is clear that it is impossible for gastrostomy to serve both of these functions at the same time, and for this reason attention is drawn to the value of combining routine gastrostomy with the introduction of a transpyloric jejunal feeding tube. For some time this has been a well-recognized technique after duodenoduodenostomy or duodenojejunostomy and many would advocate that this procedure should always be combined with a gastrostomy and a transanastomotic tube.

As an extension of this principle, the combination has proved to be extremely useful in many babies with oesophageal atresia and distal tracheo-oesophageal fistula, permitting early alimentation with its obvious beneficial anabolic effects on oesophageal healing to be combined with the advantages of adequate gastric decompression. Another advantage of this combined procedure is that prolonged intravenous infusions can be avoided.

In babies with oesophageal atresia – the most frequent indication for gastrostomy in the newborn period – this procedure may be performed (1) routinely, either as a preliminary to repair or at the same time as repair; or (2) as an essential part of a staged procedure, both in babies with a distal fistula and also in those with oesophageal atresia unaccompanied by tracheo-oesophageal fistula. (3) It may also be required in the management of postoperative complications, e.g. anastomotic leak, stricture, or recurrent tracheo-oesophageal fistula.

In babies with a tracheo-oesophageal fistula without atresia (H-fistula), our policy for some time was to combine gastrostomy with fistula division but, as with diaphragmatic hernia and gastroschisis, gastrostomy is no longer universally advocated.

## Preoperative

Appropriate management of the umbilical cord is necessary, including adequate ligation as close as possible to the abdominal wall followed by excision of the distal cord stump. If bacteriological examination has not already been carried out, cultures should be taken at this time. As a further precaution to avoid contamination of the peritoneal cavity from the umbilicus, an occlusive skin drape with a circular hole can be used at the time of operation (No. 1020 Steridrape is suitable for this).

Preoperatively, a full blood count should be obtained and, although blood transfusion is unlikely to be required, availability of one unit of blood is a wise precaution.

In the presence of an intact oesophagus (i.e. in patients other than those with oesophageal atresia) a nasogastric tube should have been passed and the stomach aspirated. The tube is left *in situ* during the operation.

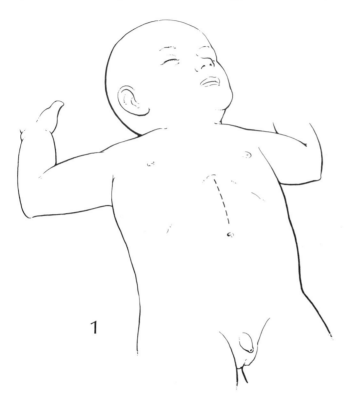

## The operation

### 1

An upper midline incision is made and the peritoneal cavity entered via the linea alba and underlying peritoneum.

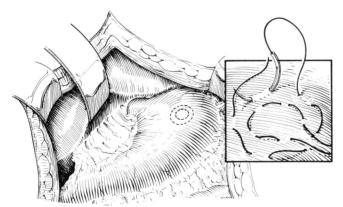

### 2

Two circumferential silk sutures are placed in the gastric wall as far to the left as possible. Ideally, these should be inserted some distance from the greater curvature.

# 3

A self-retaining Malecot catheter of appropriate size (about 12 Fr) is introduced into the stomach and the sutures are tied. The patency of the catheter and its position can be tested by syringing air into the stomach via the catheter at this stage.

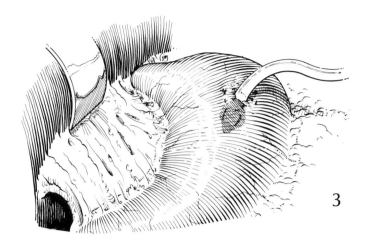

3

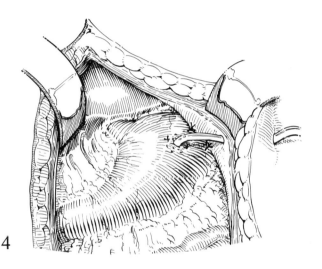

4

# 4

The catheter is brought out through a stab incision and the stomach anchored to the deeper aspect of the peritoneum.

# 5

The midline incision is closed routinely and the catheter anchored securely.

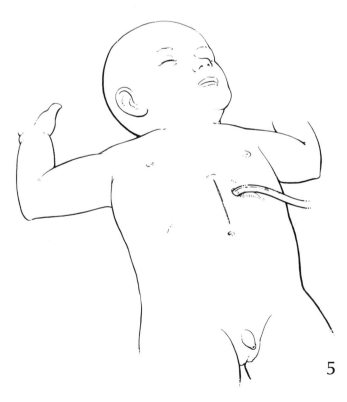

5

# 6

## Combined gastrostomy and transpyloric feeding tube

The Malecot catheter is introduced as described above. Circumferential silk sutures are then inserted immediately to the left of the pylorus and a Silastic feeding tube is fed via these through the duodenum and advanced towards the duodenojejunal flexure. Ideally, the tip of this tube should lie a short distance distal to the duodenojejunal flexure.

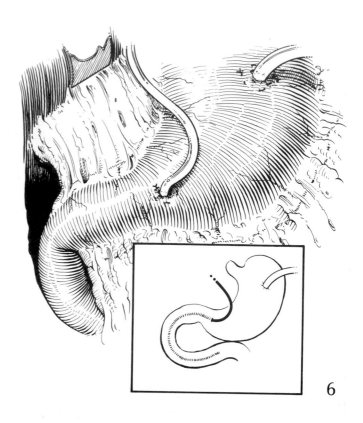

6

# 7

The gastrostomy tube (to be used for drainage purposes) is brought out through a left-sided stab incision and the transpyloric jejunal feeding tube through a right-sided stab incision. The midline incision is closed in layers.

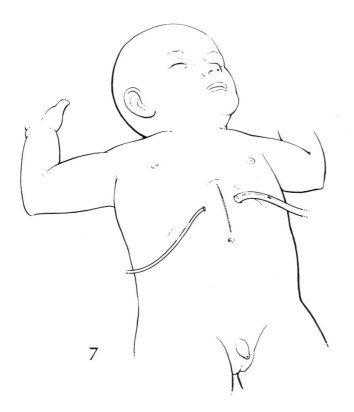

7

# Postoperative care

## Drainage

The gastrostomy tube must be on 'free drainage'. If drainage is nil, the tube should be aspirated. Occasionally it may be necessary to syringe 1–2 ml of water into the tube to maintain patency; this should be done slowly and with extreme caution.

It is vital to avoid any traction on the tube and to ensure that it does not become dislodged

## Feeding

When the tube is used for feeding purposes, small volumes of clear fluids are given initially, commencing 36 hours after operation. Milk is then introduced. Ideally this should be fresh breast milk; there is some evidence to suggest that this significantly lessens the risk of necrotizing enterocolitis. If the stomach is of normal size, appropriate volumes of milk can usually be given within 24–36 hours of commencing feeding.

In babies with 'pure' oesophageal atresia the stomach is very small, and it is wise to perform X-ray studies with barium before feeding is commenced. This will usually give some information about the distal oesophagus as a result of gastro-oesophageal reflux and also exclude distal obstruction. Hourly feedings should continue in this group for one week. Thereafter, the interval can be gradually increased to 2 and later to 3 hours between feeds. The ultimate result of giving large volumes into the stomach will be to increase gastro-oesophageal reflux and consequently growth of the lower oesophageal segment. This of course is particularly important when a staged anastomosis is planned.

## Prevention of infection

The presence of an indwelling foreign body predisposes to secondary fungal infection and therefore an appropriate antifungal agent (e.g. nystatin) should be given. This should be continued more or less indefinitely. Part of the medication is given orally and part via the gastrostomy tube.

The dressings should remain undisturbed for at least one week. Ideally the first dressing change should be performed by the surgeon who carried out the operation and is familiar with the method of fixation of the gastrostomy tube.

# Complications

These occur rarely but can be serious. The most serious is perforation of the stomach, which is occasionally seen and no doubt results from ulceration of the gastric wall by the gastrostomy tube. Spontaneous perforation can of course occur in the stomach and is probably best described by the term 'necrosing gastritis'.

Another serious complication is tube dislodgement. If this occurs early, operative replacement will be required. Later, for example during the period 1–4 weeks after gastrostomy, the tube can usually be safely replaced using an appropriate introducer. However, even when replacement is achieved readily, it is essential to check the position of the tube radiologically in order to avoid the risk of 'intraperitoneal feeding' with an inevitable peritonitis.

A minor complication is the formation of granulation tissue at the site of exit of the gastrostomy tube from the abdominal wall. Low-grade sepsis accompanies this but measures such as application of silver nitrate usually suffice to control the granuloma.

Although the operation itself may be associated with sepsis, reactionary or secondary haemorrhage, or wound disruption, these complications are rare.

When the gastrostomy tube is no longer required it is removed and, by 'pleating' the skin at the site of the stoma, spontaneous closure usually occurs. Occasionally, however, gastrostomy fistula (a gastrocutaneous fistula) may persist and require surgical closure.

# Results of surgery

Chevalier Jackson once stated that 'there is no contraindication to tracheostomy'. The same could be said of gastrostomy. Although there may be operative difficulties and/or postoperative complications, both are unusual and the results of surgery are usually excellent. The procedure is simple and effective and rarely leaves any permanent aftermath except a small midline scar and a smaller scar at the site of exit of the tube.

Illustrations by Gillian Oliver

# Oesophagogastroduodenoscopy

**Stephen L. Gans**  MD, FACS, FAAP
Clinical Professor of Surgery (Pediatric), University of California at Los Angeles; Chairman, Subdivision of Pediatric Surgery, Cedars Sinai Medical Center, Los Angeles, California, USA

**Edward Austin**  MD
Attending in Surgery (Pediatric), Cedars Sinai Medical Center; Consultant in Pediatric Surgery, Olive View Medical Center (UCLA), Los Angeles, California, USA

For more than one hundred years oesophagoscopy has been performed with an open tube, available in a wide variety of shapes and sizes, and using proximal or distal lighting. In recent years newly designed rigid endoscopes using rod-lens telescopes have provided a superior bright, clear, wide-angle view, and have sufficient extra space in the lumen to permit additional procedures. Small, flexible endoscopes have been developed for use in infants and children, which give an added dimension to the examination of the alimentary tract and also facilitate the performance of a variety of instrumental manipulations. Second- and third-generation flexible endoscopes have improved this method and their use has been firmly established in paediatric patients. An extended dimension is the technique of cannulating the ampulla of Vater for endoscopic retrograde cholangiopancreatography (ERCP).

# Indications

## Oesophagoscopy

The indications for *Oesophagoscopy* are headed by dysphagia, pain, and bleeding.

*Dysphagia* may be due to mechanical obstruction, neurogenic abnormalities, or pain. Mechanical obstructions are caused by congenital stenosis or are acquired after oesophageal surgery or follow peptic or corrosive ingestion. In order to treat chemical burns of the oesophagus it is necessary to evaluate early the nature and extent of the injury.

The role of oesophagoscopy in neurological or physiological dysphagia is to rule out mechanical obstruction. When the diagnosis of achalasia is established, treatment varies from simple dilatation or forceful stretching with a balloon or mechanical device to oesophagogastric surgery.

*Pain* may be due to foreign-body impaction, cyst, tumour, cardiospasm or oesophagitis. Foreign-body removal may be carried out in a variety of ways, with a wide assortment of instruments. The diagnosis of oesophagitis is made by demonstrating abnormal redness, friability and bleeding, ulceration, and stricture in the lower oesophagus.

*Bleeding lesions* include hiatus hernia, oesophagitis or ulcer, oesophageal varices, or a bleeding tumour. Their presence or absence will usually be demonstrated rapidly and accurately by oesophagoscopy. For this purpose the flexible fibrescope has the advantage of allowing continuation of the investigation into the stomach and duodenum if the oesophagus is found to be clear.

## Gastroduodenoscopy

Indications for gastroduodenoscopy are haematemesis and/or melaena, unexplained abdominal pain or vomiting, evaluation and biopsy of a tumour, and removal of foreign bodies.

Bleeding may be due to oesophageal varices, oesophagitis, Mallory–Weiss syndrome, acute gastritis and duodenitis, peptic ulcer of the stomach or duodenum, angiomata, polyps, and tumours such as lymphoma. Most of these lesions produce mucosal defects and are more accurately diagnosed (and biopsied when necessary) by endoscopy than by contrast radiological studies.

When the diagnosis of the cause of abdominal pain and/or vomiting cannot be made by the usual examinations and studies, endoscopy may demonstrate a missed peptic ulcer or one of the other lesions mentioned above.

The importance of evaluation and biopsy of a tumour is self-evident. Most foreign bodies will pass spontaneously, but when one produces abdominal pain or bleeding it can sometimes be removed effectively with an endoscope.

## Endoscopic retrograde cholangiopancreatography

ERCP should only be considered if other diagnostic studies have been inconclusive. The procedure is most commonly performed for difficult biliary-tract diagnosis and obstructive jaundice, for acute recurrent and chronic pancreatitis, for the suspicion of haemobilia, and for the diagnosis of pancreatic anomalies or rupture (from blunt abdominal trauma). It is contraindicated in patients with acute pancreatitis, pseudocysts of the pancreas, and acute cholangitis.

# Preoperative preparation

General evaluation of the patient and appropriate investigation of the region or abnormality are carried out as indicated.

Radiology and endoscopy are complementary techniques, the former demonstrating better the topographic relationship of the organs under almost physiological conditions, and the latter providing a more accurate assessment of mucosal lesions and also the operative capability. The sequence priority or choice of method depends upon the problem being investigated. For example, patients with bleeding problems should first undergo endoscopy.

## SEDATION AND ANAESTHESIA

# 1

*Oesophagoscopy with the rigid endoscope* is performed with greater safety and better results in the operating room or a special endoscopy room which has adequate space, availability of accessory equipment, and facilities for resuscitation.

In most instances general anaesthesia is preferred because it eliminates the need for co-operation, and thus minimizes psychiatric trauma, as well as reducing instrumental trauma due to unexpected movements. Exceptions to the use of general anaesthesia are the tiny neonate who can be well immobilized and controlled, and the well-sedated and co-operative older child (carefully selected).

In addition to the endoscopist and anaesthetist, a most important member of the team is an experienced 'head-holder' who can follow the instructions and movements of the operator in a gentle and smooth manner and maintain complete control of the head at all times.

*In using the flexible endoscope* for diagnosis in small *infants,* no sedation or light sedation may be adequate. However, as in all endoscopy, complete resuscitation equipment must be on hand should any problem such as reflex apnoea develop. Many procedures in well-selected *children* may also be done with sedation only. The surroundings should be pleasant. Parents are permitted to stand nearby and the patient is well prepared psychologically and completely informed about the procedure. He may even assist in passing the scope, and may like to look into the eyepiece of a teaching attachment.

General anaesthesia is preferred in some centres for almost all gastrointestinal endoscopy, and the final choice may depend on the availability of adequate instruments, the training and experience of the endoscopist, and the personal preference of the physician or patient. Almost all agree that painful or delicate procedures should be done under general anaesthesia.

## CHOICE OF INSTRUMENTS

The conventional open-tube oesophagoscope is frequently indicated for dilatation after a stricture or stenosis has been identified. Larger dilators can pass through its lumen. For almost all other procedures and manipulations, the newer instruments have superior capabilities and safety.

The Storz rigid oesophagoscope with the Hopkins rod-lens telescope is the standard to which all other telescopic endoscopes should be compared. It provides a brilliant, wide-angle view for examination and evaluation of the oesophagus and facilitates a wide variety of manipulations in the direct magnified field of the telescope. These include suction, irrigation, biopsy, electrocoagulation, dilatation, grasping, injection, and the use of lasers.

Flexible endoscopes are indicated where the oesophagus (or its surgical replacement) may be tortuous in shape,

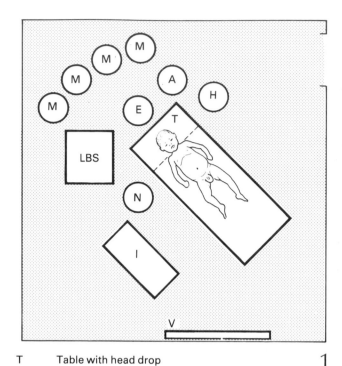

| T | Table with head drop |
| V | X-ray view box |
| E | Endoscopist |
| A | Anaesthetist |
| H | Head-holder (seated) |
| LBS | Light source, air blower, suction apparatus |
| N | Nurse technician |
| I | Instrument table |
| M | Circulating nurse, assistant, paediatrician, observer, student (? parent) |

1

or when general anaesthesia is undesirable. They are further indicated for the investigation of bleeding of the alimentary tract, because oesophagoscopy can then be extended to gastroduodenoscopy if required. They are provided with channels for suction, irrigation, and biopsy, and the grasping of foreign bodies. Injection of tissue can be readily accomplished. Clinical investigation of the use of lasers through the instrument channel has already been carried out. The view has been significantly improved in later models.

There are a large number of flexible fibre-endoscopes with varying capabilities and advantages. Selection is particularly important for paediatric endoscopy because the limitation in the outer diameter of the instrument poses problems in the versatility needed for this purpose. In addition to the outer diameter, attention should be paid to flexibility and weight. The bending tip is provided with two-way or four-way control and the facility for directing it is an important factor. The bending angle and length of the bending segment affect both retrograde vision and the adaptability to the narrow curves in an infant's stomach and duodenum. The sharpness of vision is directly related to the quality and number of fibres. The ease and capability of aspiration, insufflation, irrigation, biopsy, and the use of other accessories can make the difference between a short, successful procedure and a long, frustrating one.

## Technique

### INTRODUCTION OF THE OESOPHAGOSCOPE

When using a rigid oesophagoscope, the patient is placed supine on the table with the shoulders propped by a sandbag or blanket roll. The head-rest is dropped completely or the child's head is moved over the end of the table, into the hands of the head-holder. The head is extended on the neck, and the upper alveolar ridge or the upper teeth are retracted with the fingers of the left hand. The distal end of the oesophagoscope is controlled with the left thumb and forefinger while the proximal part is manipulated with the right hand, holding it as one would a pen or pencil.

# 2a–c

The tip of the scope is advanced along the right lateral border of the tongue and passed laterally to the epiglottis and into the right piriform sinus. Under direct vision the larynx is lifted forward by the lip of the advancing oesophagoscope to reveal the entrance of the oesophagus. This may be clearly visualized after a few moments of observation, and the scope is then inserted into the cervical oesophagus. If this anatomy is not clearly demonstrated *very* gentle probing with the tip may reveal it and allow introduction. Use of the laryngoscope may facilitate this exposure, but care must be taken not to obstruct the endotracheal tube.

If this exposure and introduction are not readily accomplished, it may be helpful to pass a rubber or plastic catheter through the oesophagoscope, through the cricopharyngeal sphincter, and then into the oesophagus. The scope is then advanced over this 'lumen finder' under direct vision, and as the oesophagus is entered the guide is removed.

Inspection is carried out, keeping the lumen in view by manipulation of both the scope and the head. Passage of the oesophagoscope into the lower third of the oesophagus is sometimes facilitated by having an assistant straighten out the dorsal curve by placing his hands beneath the lower chest and elevating the dorsal spine.

The same position and a similar but simpler technique may be used to introduce the flexible endoscope. The lateral position is also satisfactory. A bite protector should always be used with the flexible scope.

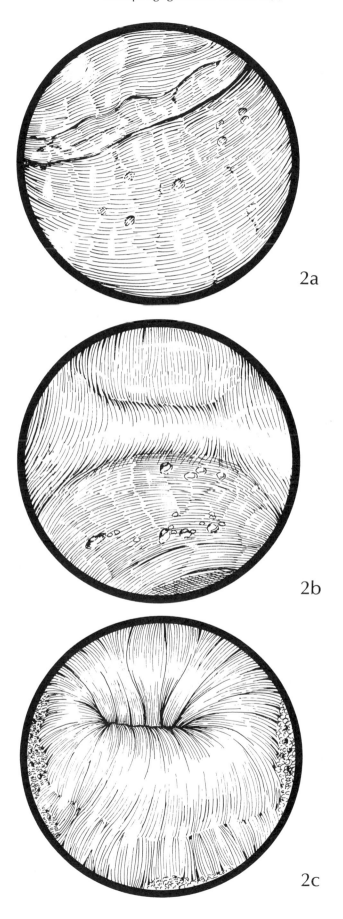

2a

2b

2c

## GASTRODUODENOSCOPY

### 3

A bite mouthpiece is inserted between the teeth and the tip of the endoscope is introduced smoothly and gently under visual control into the oesophagus (see above). After examination of the entire length of the oesophagus passage into the stomach is carried out with caution, using air insufflation to guide and assist the manoeuvre.

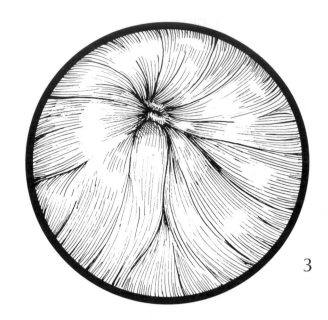

3

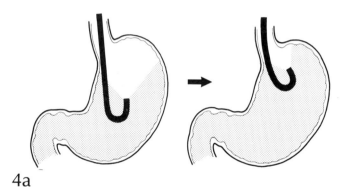

4a

### 4a–e

After retrograde vision of the cardia and oesophageal entrance, the stomach is systematically examined throughout, down to the antrum. With the pylorus in view the instrument is advanced through it into the duodenum. Knowledge of gastroduodenal anatomy allows appropriate orientation and manipulation around the bends and curves of these organs. Biopsy and photography are done for documentation of lesions as needed, and re-examination can be carried out during withdrawal of the instrument.

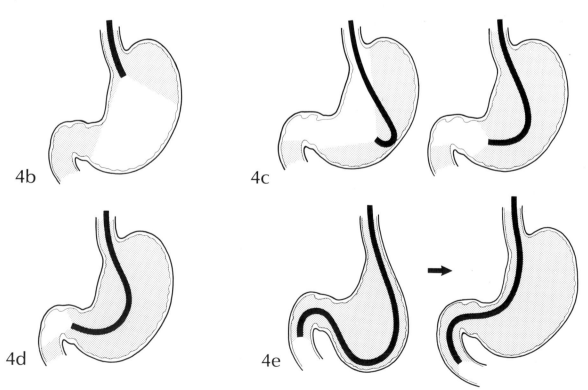

4b

4c

4d

4e

## ENDOSCOPIC RETROGRADE CHOLANGIOPANCREATOGRAPHY (ERCP)

This is best performed with a side-viewing endoscope. Because such an instrument is not yet available in paediatric sizes, experience in this field is somewhat limited, and the procedure is most often carried out in older children. Whichever endoscope is used, the instrument is advanced into the duodenum as above, the papilla is located, identified and cannulated. If the opening is too small to be cannulated, the catheter is placed on to it. The contrast medium is instilled, while the examiner watches the screen continuously. Manipulation and probing is helpful in filling the bile duct or pancreatic duct. With improvement of instruments, this procedure will become more feasible in the smaller patients.

## Manipulations

### STENOSES

# 5a & b

Congenital stenosis may require dilatation under direct vision through a rigid scope, or even an electrocautery incision in the case of a web.

Postoperative acquired stenosis is most often a complication of surgery for oesophageal malformations and is usually managed by dilatation with endoscopic assistance and monitoring. This can be done by an antegrade approach under direct vision, with a variety of dilators. At times this can be more safely started by passing a well-lubricated Fogarty catheter through the tiny opening, gradually inflating the balloon, and withdrawing it through the narrow area. With the now enlarged opening dilators can be readily passed.

Retrograde dilatation is possible and appropriate when a gastrostomy is present. The infant is fed a string (suture) to swallow, and one end of this is subsequently fished out of the stomach. Graduated Tucker dilators are attached to the gastric end of the string and drawn through the stricture. This is a relatively safe and effective procedure, which can be repeated at later intervals by retaining the string. If the infant is unable to swallow the string, oesophagoscopy may be used to start the dilatation and pass the string into the stomach, where it is picked up with a clamp, or with an endoscope passed through the gastrostomy. It is then tied to the retrograde dilators. It is also possible to treat persistent strictures by injection of steroids under direct vision, followed by dilatation.

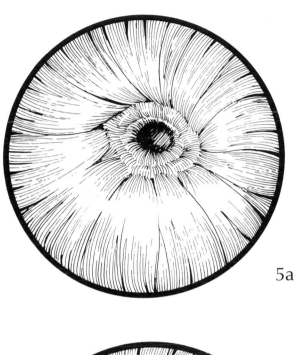

5a

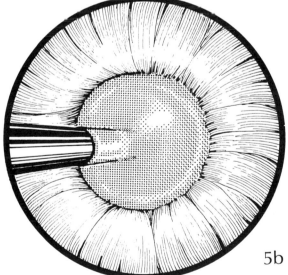

5b

# 6

## EXTRACTION OF A FOREIGN BODY

When a hollow tube endoscope is used to remove a foreign body from the oesophagus, the extracting instrument itself fills a good portion of the lumen necessary for viewing, and grasping is done in a semi-blind manner. With the telescopic oesophagoscope, however, the object can be located more quickly and less traumatically, and a variety of grasping instruments can be used in full view of the telescope. Hard and smooth objects may be difficult to grasp, but may be successfully and quickly removed by directing a well-lubricated Fogarty catheter beyond the object and, after slight inflation, drawing the catheter, object and endoscope out together.

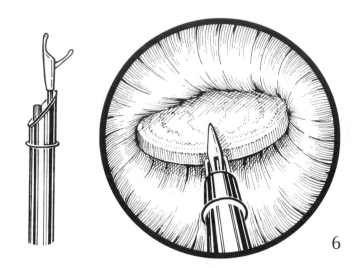

6

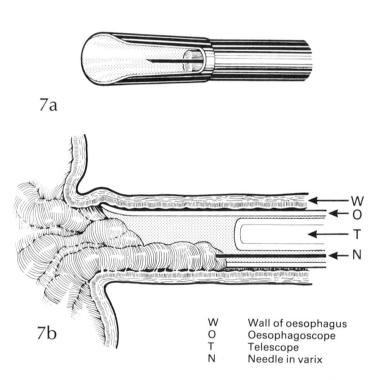

7a

7b

| W | Wall of oesophagus |
|---|---|
| O | Oesophagoscope |
| T | Telescope |
| N | Needle in varix |

# 7a & b

## OESOPHAGEAL VARICES

Injection of oesophageal varices with a sclerosing solution is a valuable adjunct in the treatment of this disease. We use a rigid, slotted oesophagoscope sheath for injection in direct view of the telescope. The varix enters the slot and injection is made accurately into it. Five per cent sodium morrhuate, sodium tetradecyl sulphate or sodium psylliate are used as sclerosing agents. After injection, the scope is rotated somewhat to compress and tamponade the injection site. It may be advantageous to compress the cardio-oesophageal junction with the inflated bag of a Foley catheter passed into the stomach alongside the oesophagoscope, in order to prevent the too rapid escape of the sclerosant from the varix.

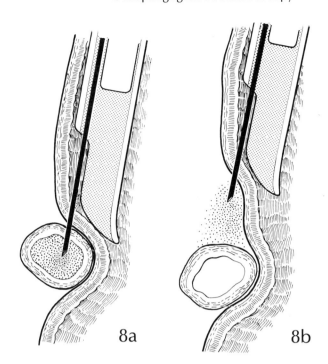

# 8a & b

Some prefer the flexible fibrescope for injection treatment, and others report that good results are obtained by injecting just outside the lumen of the varix.

## BIOPSY

Oesophageal biopsy is done with a biopsy forceps passed through the instrument channel of the scope. Small, superficial bites are obtained with the flexible instrument, and deeper, larger ones with the rigid one. In the stomach or duodenum the flexible scope is used.

## Postoperative care

Periods of observation and withholding of feeding are indicated according to the general condition of the patient and the nature of the procedure, bearing in mind the possible complications noted below.

## Complications

Laceration and perforation are the greatest hazards of endoscopy but should be extremely rare with examination alone. They may occur more frequently with blind instrumentation, vigorous dilatation, or other operative manoeuvres. No doubt the incidence of these problems is reduced by better vision and by procedures carried out in direct sight through the telescope. Bleeding may be a problem after biopsy, or after injection of varices.

### Further reading

Cadranel, S., Rodesch, P. (1983) Fiberendoscopy of the upper gastrointestinal tract. In: Pediatric Endoscopy, S. L. Gans (ed.), p. 67–86. New York: Grune and Stratton

Gans, S. L., Berci, G. (1971) Advances in endoscopy of infants and children. Journal of Pediatric Surgery, 6, 199–233

Gans, S. L., Ament, A., Christie, D. L., Liebman, W. M. (1975) Pediatric endoscopy with flexible fiberscopes. Journal of Pediatric Surgery, 10, 375–380

Gans, S. L. (1983) Esophagoscopy. In: Pediatric Endoscopy, S. L. Gans (ed.), pp. 55–66. New York: Grune and Stratton

Holder, T. M., Ashcraft, K. W., Leape, L. (1969) The treatment of patients with esophageal strictures by local steroid injection. Journal of Pediatric Surgery, 4, 646–653

Howard, E. R., Stamatakis, J. D., Mowat, A. P. (1984) Management of esophageal varices in children by injection sclerotherapy. Journal of Pediatric Surgery, 19, 2–5

Huchzermeyer, H. (1983) Endoscopic retrograde cholangiopancreatography (ERCP). In: Pediatric Endoscopy, S. L. Gans (ed.), p. 87–102. New York: Grune and Stratton

Lilly, J. R. (1981) Endoscopic sclerosis of esophageal varices in children. Surgery, Gynecology and Obstetrics, 152, 513–514

Paquet, K.-J. (1985) Ten years experience with paravariceal injection sclerotherapy of oesophageal varices in children. Journal of Pediatric Surgery, 20, 109–112

Peterson, W. L. (1982) Laser therapy for bleeding peptic ulcer – a burning issue. Gastroenterology, 83, 485–488

Illustrations by Gillian Oliver

# Laparoscopy in infants and children

**Stephen L. Gans**  MD, FACS, FAAP
Clinical Professor of Surgery (Pediatric), University of California at Los Angeles; Chairman, Subdivision of Pediatric Surgery, Cedars Sinai Medical Center, Los Angeles, California, USA

**Edward Austin**  MD
Attending in Surgery (Pediatric), Cedars Sinai Medical Center; Consultant in Pediatric Surgery, Olive View Medical Center (UCLA), Los Angeles, California, USA

The use of laparoscopy in infants and children was virtually unknown until we investigated the procedure and reported our initial methods and results in 1971, and our further experience in 1973. Since that time other investigators have confirmed our early results, and laparoscopy is now an established method of investigation and treatment in a wide variety of conditions in infants and children.

## Indications and contraindications

Laparoscopy is indicated for *diagnosis* only when more simple studies are not adequate and when exploratory laparotomy would therefore be considered. It is indicated for *therapy* only when such a procedure can be carried out safely without laparotomy. Table 1 lists indications from our experience. Details of its use for these conditions will be found later in this chapter.

In general, laparoscopy is contraindicated in infants and children for whom general anaesthesia is contraindicated. It is further contraindicated in conditions where puncture of the abdominal wall might be hazardous. Such situations are peritonitis, intestinal obstruction, or where extensive scarring or adhesions are present from previous surgery.

## Preoperative preparation and anaesthesia

The stomach is emptied if the upper organs are to be examined and the bladder and colon are emptied if the lower organs or pelvis are to be examined.

Although in adults laparoscopy can sometimes be done under local anaesthesia, general anaesthesia with controlled respiration is necessary in infants and children, because pneumoperitoneum significantly inhibits diaphragmatic movement. A possible exception is the patient with multiple-system trauma.

## Choice of instruments

The Storz laparoscopy instruments are the standard to which all other arrangements should be compared. An insufflating device is necessary through which carbon dioxide is introduced, and which automatically controls the flow and pressure of the gas. A good light source with enough illuminating power for photography and video is an important component. Also needed is a special needle for establishing pneumoperitoneum. Most commonly used is the Veress needle with a spring-controlled stylet; also available is a modification which combines this needle with a cannula, the Gans–Austin single-puncture needle.

Cannulas with trocars, appropriate telescopes, other trocars and cannulas for introduction of instruments applicable for grasping, biopsy, suction, electrocoagulation, palpation, and dissection (scissors) complete the basic set. The use of lasers through the laparoscope is a recent addition.

Teaching attachments and video cameras for projection on to a screen or for recording, and X-ray facilities, are all desirable accessories.

**Table 1. Indications for laparoscopy**

I.  HEPATOBILIARY CONDITIONS
    1. Metabolic or inflammatory disease
    2. Hepatomegaly
    3. Hepatosplenomegaly
    4. Jaundice
        Newborns
        Infants and children

II.  ASCITES

III.  ABDOMINAL CYSTS AND TUMOURS
    1. Primary
    2. Metabolic
    3. 'Second look'

IV.  STATUS OF PELVIC GENITALIA
    1. Intersexuality
    2. Precocious puberty
    3. Primary and secondary amenorrhoea
    4. Gonadal dysplasia
    5. Ovarian cysts and tumours
    6. Congenital virilizing adrenal hyperplasia
    7. Presence and site of clinically impalpable testes

V  OCCULT ABDOMINAL PAIN

VI.  MANIPULATION OF V-P SHUNTS

VII.  ABDOMINAL TRAUMA

# Technique

## CARBON DIOXIDE INSUFFLATION

# 1

With the patient in the supine position on the operating table, and under satisfactory endotracheal anaesthesia, the operating team and equipment are appropriately positioned. The skin of the abdomen is prepared and draped.

A stab wound is made in the skin with a pointed knife blade. This puncture is usually made in the rim of the umbilicus where the abdominal wall is thin; this central location permits examination of the entire peritoneal cavity, and it leaves an almost invisible scar. In the small or malnourished infant the tissues around the umbilicus may be too thin and air may leak out. In these patients the puncture is made over the medial portion of one of the rectus muscles, above or below the level of the umbilicus, mindful of the presence of the epigastric vessels.

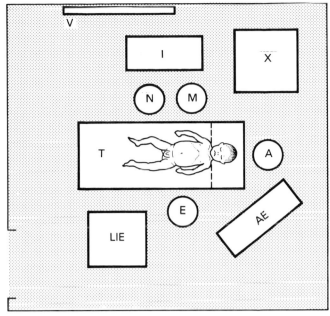

| | | | |
|---|---|---|---|
| V | X-ray view box | T | Table |
| I | Instrument table | A | Anaesthetist |
| X | X-ray equipment | AE | Anaesthesia equipment |
| N | Nurse | E | Endoscopist |
| M | Assistant | | |
| LIE | Light source, Insufflation, electrocoagulation | | |

1

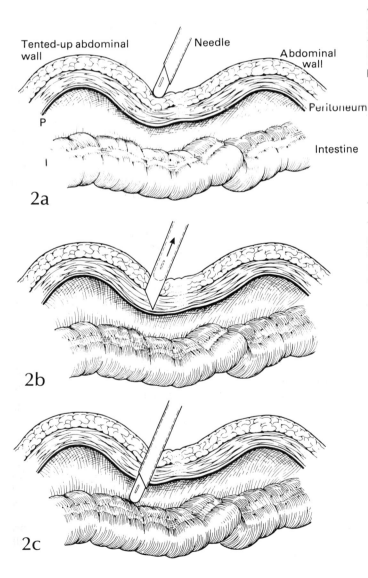

**2a**

**2b**

**2c**

# 2a–c

The abdominal wall is tented upwards by the operator and assistant by grasping it above and below, using a sponge between the fingers to aid in maintaining traction, and the needle with the spring-controlled blunt stylet is introduced into the peritoneal cavity. As the needle pierces the peritoneum the blunt stylet springs out, thus protecting the abdominal contents from injury.

The needle is tested by side-to-side motion to see if the intra-abdominal portion moves freely. A 10 ml syringe is connected to the needle and aspiration is carried out to ensure that no bowel contents are present in the needle. Saline (5–10 ml) is then injected to demonstrate free flow.

## 3

Pneumoperitoneum is accomplished by connecting this needle to a carbon dioxide cylinder through the insufflating device so that flow and pressure can be controlled as desired or set automatically. Abdominal pressure in the infant should not exceed 10–15 mmHg.

During the insufflation the abdomen is gently percussed and palpated, and when the pneumoperitoneum is considered adequate the needle is removed. The skin puncture is enlarged by spreading it with a haemostat until it can admit the trocar and cannula snugly.

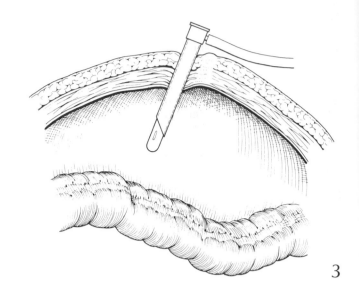

3

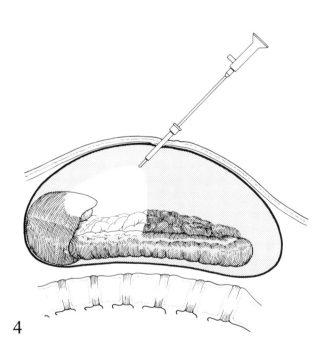

4

## 4

The abdominal wall is again tented up by the operator and the assistant by grasping it above and below the puncture, and the cannula with a pointed trocar is then directed with a twisting motion through the abdominal wall and into the intra-abdominal air cushion. The trocar is then removed and replaced by the appropriate telescope. The viscera underlying the puncture are inspected first to confirm that no injury has been produced.

An alternative method, with only a single puncture, is to use the Gans–Austin needle, a somewhat larger diameter needle of the Veress type which is combined with a cannula. It is introduced in the same way as the Veress needle, and after the pneumoperitoneum is established this needle is removed and the telescope introduced through the cannula which is already in place. This procedure eliminates the need for a second blind puncture with a pointed trocar.

Inspection of the peritoneal contents may then begin. Should fogging of the telescope occur it may be simply and easily cleared by gently touching the bowel wall with the telescope end. Needles for biopsy or injection may be inserted through the abdominal wall in direct view through the telescope.

# 5

For more involved manipulations a second, smaller cannula is introduced separately through the abdominal wall, observing its entrance through the telescope. Through this second cannula all the accessory instruments listed earlier may be introduced under direct vision.

In certain unstable patients laparoscopy can be safely performed in the emergency room or intensive-care unit using local anaesthesia. The entire instrument set including the light source may be quickly and easily moved anywhere for immediate use. The procedure may be completed in a few minutes by an experienced laparoscopist with a nurse assisting.

While the assistant is preparing the skin of the abdomen with a suitable antiseptic solution the instrument tray is opened and checked. Sterile drapes are placed, leaving the entire abdominal wall exposed. A local anaesthetic is injected just below the umbilicus in the midline. A stab wound is made as previously described with the scalpel and bluntly spread down to the midline fascia with a small haemostat. The skin is tented upward and the single-puncture needle-cannula is advanced through the fascia and the peritoneum into the abdominal cavity. A noticeable snap is felt and heard as the blunt stylet springs forward upon puncturing the peritoneum. The cannula is moved and saline injected and aspirated as before to confirm that the bowel has not been entered. Air can be insufflated with a rubber bulb connected to the cannula until sufficient pneumoperitoneum is present for examination. The needle component is removed from the cannula and replaced by the telescope. Examination and evaluation are then carried out and more air is insufflated as needed.

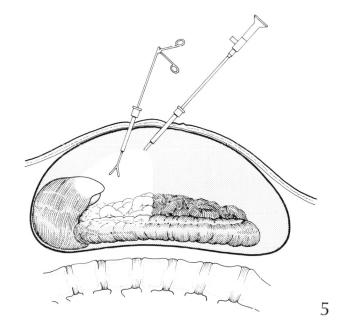

5

# Investigative procedures

The most common use of this method is inspection of the intraperitoneal contents. Through one tiny puncture all four quadrants of the abdominal cavity may be inspected. This procedure fulfils the needs for the majority of indications listed previously. Additional procedures and manipulations are described below.

### LIVER BIOPSY

Hepatobiliary conditions include a wide variety of patients, who, after thorough study, may still require a piece of liver tissue for accurate diagnosis. Undoubtedly the simplest method of liver biopsy is with a percutaneous needle. Occasionally the results are not satisfactory and

open operation for liver biopsy is considered. Our experience has shown that laparoscopic examination and biopsy has distinct advantages.

The colour, size, structure and feel can be evaluated and the presence of cysts, haemangiomas, nodules, tumours, or diffuse hepatic processes can be noted before the biopsy needle or forceps is directed under vision into the most promising areas. Focal or nodular lesions can be missed by blind needling and direct observation is a safety factor in preventing penetration of vascular or other potentially harmful targets. If bleeding or leakage of bile persists after biopsy, it is readily observed and controlled by electrocoagulation. The advantages of laparoscopy over laparotomy for liver biopsy are numerous. One can obtain a better view of the liver and even of the spleen. There is less chance of adhesion formation and other surgical complications. The operating time is shorter, the hospital stay is less, and there is no abdominal scar.

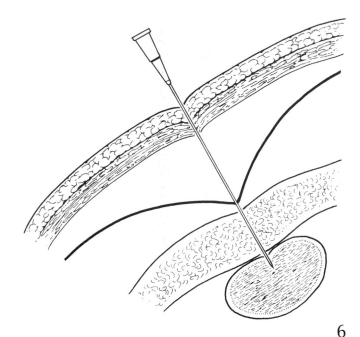

6

## CHOLANGIOGRAPHY

# 6 & 7

Percutaneous transhepatic cholangiography can be performed as illustrated in well-selected cases. It is not an
easy manoeuvre, but when successful it is quite definitive.
A plastic needle with metal trocar is introduced through
the abdominal wall and peritoneum (shown tented
inward), then through the liver and gall bladder bed into
the gall bladder. The liver acts as a tamponade to prevent
bile leakage. Under direct vision, radio-opaque dye is
injected, and films are made with fluoroscopic guidance.

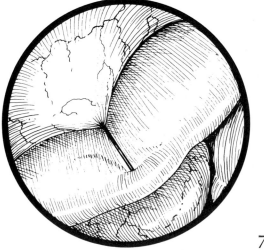

7

# 8

We have found this method useful in distinguishing neonatal hepatitis from biliary atresia. If on inspection the gall bladder is found to be absent, this is sufficient evidence to indicate exploration for biliary anomalies. If the gall bladder is present, cholangiography can demonstrate either a normal biliary duct system as in illustration 6, or an obstructed one, which would be an indication for open exploration.

In the older infant or child with jaundice a small number of cases remain after the usual investigations, in which laparoscopy is considered. Again, the appearance of the liver and gall bladder are significant, and biopsy and percutaneous transhepatic cholangiography can be done with acceptable safety, frequently avoiding open surgery, or in some cases providing a definite indication for operation.

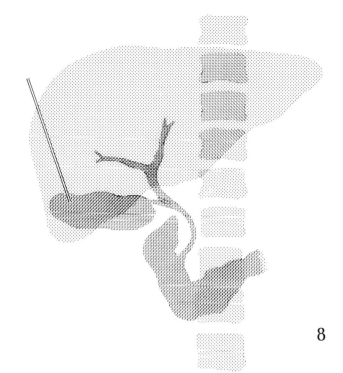

8

## ASCITES

In the investigation of ascites, removal of the ascitic fluid, replacing it with carbon dioxide, followed by laparoscopy, can sometimes reveal the aetiology of the condition.

## CYSTS AND TUMOURS

In the investigation of abdominal cysts and tumours, a clear view and biopsy can sometimes surpass other procedures in providing necessary information for indications for surgery, or for the avoidance of open surgery when scattered metastases are seen. This is particularly true for tumours of the liver. In selected situations, 'second look' procedures may be appropriate.

# Pelvic procedures

When there is a question as to the anatomical or metabolic status involving the uterus, tubes and ovaries, laparoscopy will find its greatest application in three different age ranges: in the newborn with ambiguous genitalia, in the child with pain or precocious puberty, and in the postpubertal adolescent.

In addition to inspection, ovarian tumours may be biopsied, ovarian cysts may be aspirated, and adhesions may be separated by electrocoagulation or with the tiny scissors.

## OCCULT PAIN

Occult abdominal pain is a category which consists of infants and children with recurrent, bizarre, or chronic abdominal pain in whom a satisfactory diagnosis cannot be established by the usual methods and laparotomy is now being considered. If by laparoscopy, a surgically treatable lesion such as an inflamed appendix or ovarian cyst is found, operation can be carried out immediately under the same anaesthetic. Non-surgical causes of such pain, for example regional enteritis and salpingitis, may be identified and the appropriate medical therapy given, thus avoiding a laparotomy. It is also helpful, when no pathology is found by laparoscopy, in providing reassurance that the organs are normal and no disease entity is present.

## VENTRICULOPERITONEAL SHUNT

Correction of malfunctions of ventriculoperitoneal shunts with the laparoscope is one of the most rewarding of its capabilities. Entrapment or encystation of the peritoneal catheter can be corrected by shifting its position to an appropriate site. Peritoneal fluid and tissue are easily obtained for culture. The entire peritoneal cavity is visualized and a region most suitable for repositioning of the shunt catheter is determined. Finally, the use of laparoscopy rather than laparotomy avoids formation of new adhesions within the abdominal cavity and may therefore reduce the likelihood of recurrent problems.

## TRAUMA

In abdominal trauma the non-operative treatment for a ruptured spleen or liver is now the preferred treatment. When laparotomy is being considered, however, even when a considerable amount of blood is present in the peritoneal cavity, laparoscopy can determine by direct vision whether or not *active* bleeding is still taking place, and which organ is bleeding. Furthermore, the infant or child with severe multiple organ system trauma, who is frequently unconscious, requires rapid and accurate assessment, urgent respiratory and circulatory resuscitation and maintenance, and prompt therapeutic intervention. When a child has sustained significant head, chest, and extremity trauma the possibility of serious intra-abdominal injury must be ruled out before the priority of any particular regional or organ intervention is determined. Laparoscopy can be carried out in the emergency room, intensive-care unit, or in the operating room in a short time with portable equipment and will help provide surgeons with an appropriate priority decision.

Indications for emergency laparoscopy are multiple organ system trauma, impaired sensorium, unexplained falling haemoglobin, equivocal abdominal examination, or a stab wound with questionable abdominal-wall penetration.

# Postoperative care and complications

At the conclusion of laparoscopy, the carbon dioxide is allowed to escape from the peritoneal cavity through a cannula. Postoperative care consists only in observation for possible complications of the procedure itself or from the condition for which it was performed. Two serious complications occur rarely and indicate laparotomy for correction. One is perforation of the bowel during blind puncture of the abdominal wall or in the use of manipulating instruments. The other is uncontrollable bleeding from a biopsy site. Both of these complications are readily identified through the laparoscope at the time of occurrence, and appropriate treatment can be immediately instituted.

The incidence of these complications is not accurately known, but it must be very small, being entirely absent from several large series. When one considers that laparoscopy is only done when laparotomy is the alternative, and that such laparoscopy very often avoids laparotomy, the low risk of this procedure is acceptable when proper indications and precautions are followed.

To appreciate this method fully one must gain one's own experience. It is difficult at first, as with any new technique, but as the method becomes comfortable and easy, one will delight in the clear view of the peritoneal contents which can be obtained safely, and in the many manipulations which can be performed under direct vision.

## Further reading

Austin, E., Gans, S. L. (1983) Laparoscopy for trauma. In Pediatric Endoscopy, S. L. Gans (ed.), pp. 189–194. New York: Grune and Stratton

Gans, S. L., Berci, G. (1971) Advances in endoscopy of infants and children. Journal of Pediatric Surgery, 6, 199–233

Gans, S. L., Berci, G. (1973) Peritoneoscopy in infants and children. Journal of Pediatric Surgery, 8, 399–405

Gans, S. L., Austin, E. (1983) The technique of laparoscopy. In Pediatric Endoscopy, S. L. Gans (ed.), pp. 151–160. New York: Grune and Stratton

Rodgers, B. M., Vries, J. K., Talbert, J. L. (1983) Laparoscopy in the diagnosis and treatment of malfunctioning ventriculoperitoneal shunts. In Pediatric Endoscopy, S. L. Gans (ed.), pp. 179–187. New York: Grune and Stratton

Stauffer, U. G. (1983) Laparoscopy in hepatology and hepatobiliary diseases. In Pediatric Endoscopy, S. L. Gans (ed.), pp. 161–168. New York: Grune and Stratton

Illustrations by Kevin Marks

# Pyloromyotomy

**Lewis Spitz**   MB, ChB, PhD, FRCS(Eng), FRCS(Ed), FAAP(Hon)
Nuffield Professor of Paediatric Surgery, Institute of Child Health, University of London; Consultant Paediatric Surgeon, Hospital for Sick Children, Great Ormond Street, London, UK

## Historical background

Fabricius Hildanus first described pyloric stenosis in 1646. Harold Hirschsprung described the clinical presentation and pathology of the condition in 1888. At this stage the preferred treatment was medical, using a combination of gastric lavage, antispasmodic drugs, dietary manipulations and the application of local heat, as the surgical mortality rate was almost 100 per cent. Fredet in 1908 advocated longitudinal submucosal division of the thickened pyloric muscle, but in addition attempted to suture the defect transversely. Ramstedt (1912) later simplified the Fredet procedure by omitting the transverse suturing, leaving the mucosa exposed in the defect created by longitudinal splitting of the hypertrophied muscle. The procedure was an unqualified success and has remained virtually unmodified since 1912. Surgery has totally replaced medical measures in the treatment of pyloric stenosis.

## Incidence

The incidence of pyloric stenosis among Caucasians is 2–3 per 1000 live births. Black races are less frequently affected. The male to female ratio is 4:1. There is a strong familial pattern of inheritance.

## Diagnosis

Symptoms usually commence between 2 and 4 weeks of age and consist of (1) projectile vomiting of non-bilious material, (2) constipation, and (3) failure to thrive. In 10–15 per cent of cases, haematemesis has been documented.

Physical signs are (1) variable degrees of dehydration, (2) visible gastric peristalsis, and (3) palpation of the pyloric 'tumour'.

The diagnosis can be made on clinical examination in over 90 per cent of cases.

## Special investigations

## 1

*Barium meal*

—The following features are diagnostic.

1. 'String sign' of the narrow elongated pyloric canal.
2. 'Double track' in the pyloric canal due to infolding mucosa.
3. Delayed gastric emptying.
4. Gastric hyperperistalsis.
5. Mushroom effect in the duodenal cap due to indenting by the pyloric tumour.

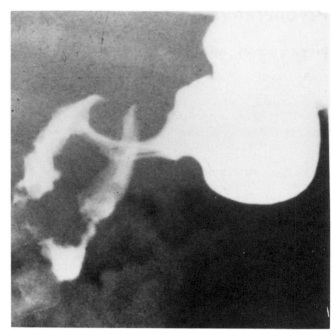

1

## 2

*Ultrasonography*

This typically shows a thickened pyloric musculature with a central sonolucent area representing the lumen of the pyloric canal.

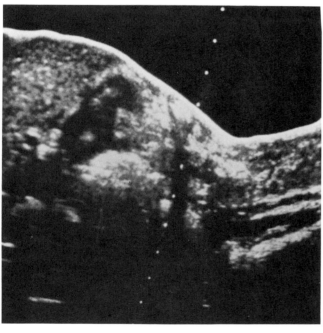

2

# Preoperative

## Preparation of patient

The operation of pyloromyotomy is *never* an emergency. Correction of dehydration and acid-base imbalance takes precedence. Mildly dehydrated infants may be rehydrated with oral glucose-saline solution (5 per cent glucose in isotonic saline), omitting milk feeds. Rehydration will usually be complete in 12–24 hours. For more severely dehydrated infants, parenteral correction of the imbalances is safer and more accurate. An intravenous infusion of isotonic saline or plasma (20 ml/kg) is administered over 60 minutes. Once urinary output has been established, potassium chloride (20–30 mmol/l) is added to the infusate of 5 per cent glucose in 0.9 per cent saline. The infusion is given at a rate of 150–180 ml/kg body weight per 24 hours. It may take as long as 48–72 hours for rehydration to be complete and for the infant to be ready for surgery.

Evacuation of retained contents in the stomach by gastric lavage with warm isotonic saline is also recommended.

## Anaesthesia

Although local anaesthesia has been used successfully, general endotracheal anaesthesia is now preferred. The stomach should be emptied immediately before induction to avoid vomiting and aspiration. An intravenous infusion is set up for administration of perioperative fluids and for delivery of muscle relaxants.

## Position of patient

The patient is placed supine on the operating table with the head turned to the left side. A rolled towel under the thoracic vertebra facilitates delivery of the pyloric tumour into the incision.

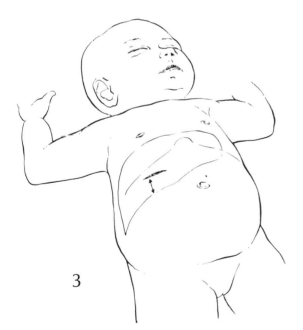

3

# The operation

## The incision

# 3

A transverse incision 3–4 cm long is made in the right upper quadrant of the abdomen, one finger's breadth below the costal margin and starting immediately lateral to the lateral border of the rectus abdominis muscle. The incision is deepened through the subcutaneous tissues, and the underlying external oblique, internal oblique and transversus abdominis muscles are divided in the line of the incision, using cutting diathermy and coagulating bleeding vessels. The peritoneum is opened transversely in the line of the incision.

An alternative approach is to enter the peritoneal cavity by splitting the muscles of the anterior abdominal wall in the direction of their fibres. This approach has the disadvantage of exposing unnecessarily wide tissue planes but is claimed to be associated with a lower incidence of dehiscence.

A vertical incision – midline or paramedian – leaves a cosmetically unacceptable scar.

## Identification of stomach

### 4

With the peritoneum opened, the liver covers the opening into the peritoneal cavity. The edge of the liver is gently retracted cranially using a malleable retractor protected by a moist gauze swab.

No attempt should be made to grasp the pyloric tumour directly, as this only leads to serosal tears and haemorrhage. The greater curvature of the stomach is identified and grasped in a moist gauze swab. This step may be facilitated by the anaesthetist instilling 20–30 ml of air into the stomach via the nasogastric tube. The stomach is thereby distended and appears in the wound. If the stomach is not readily found, traction on the transverse mesocolon will draw the greater curvature of the stomach into the wound.

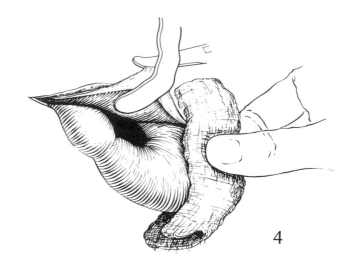

4

## Delivery of pyloric tumour

With the greater curvature of the stomach firmly drawn across to the left and exerting traction on the antrum, the pyloric tumour is delivered out of the incision by applying a gentle to and fro rocking traction on the pylorus.

### 5

The distal extent of the tumour is marked by the pyloric vein of Mayo. Proximally the tumour is less obvious where it merges with the hypertrophied stomach musculature. The tumour has a glistening greyish appearance and is firm to palpation. There is a relatively avascular plane in the middle of the anterior surface where the vessels entering the pylorus superiorly and inferiorly merge.

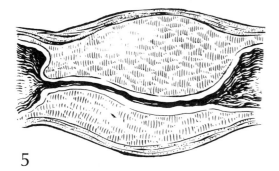

5

## Incision of pylorus

### 6

An incision is then made through the serosa of the pylorus in the avascular area on the anterior surface of the tumour. It is carried distally as far as the pyloric vein of Mayo, which marks the pyloroduodenal junction, while proximally it extends well on to the anterior surface of the antrum of the stomach. The length of the incision is 2–3 cm. Protrusion of the pyloric tumour into the lumen of the duodenum creates a critical zone of folded duodenal mucosa in a very superficial position at the distal end of the incision (see Illustration 5). It is in this area that perforation of the mucosa most commonly occurs.

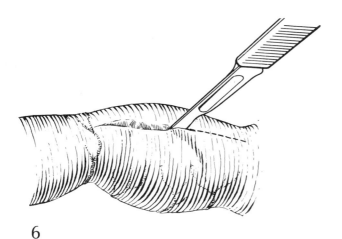

6

## Splitting of pyloric musculature

# 7

Pressure with a blunt instrument (handle of a scalpel, MacDonald dissector) into the incision, with counter-pressure by a finger placed behind the tumour, allows splitting of the hypertrophied muscle fibres down to the submucosa. This appears as a white glistening membrane in the depth of the incision in the pylorus. A twisting movement on the blunt instrument produces an extension of the split proximally and distally and widens the incision.

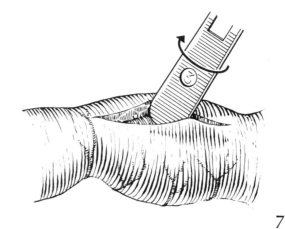

7

# 8 & 9

In order to ensure that all muscle fibres have been divided throughout the length of the incision, the edges of the split muscle are spread apart with either a blunt artery forceps (ensuring that the points are held well away from the mucosa) or a pyloric spreader (Denis Browne or Benson and Lloyd) so that the mucosa bulges into the incision. Special care must be taken at the pyloroduodenal junction to avoid entering the lumen of the duodenum, which is particularly vulnerable because of the protrusion of the pyloric tumour into the duodenal lumen.

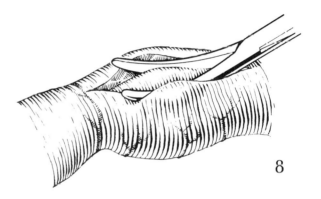

8

## Testing for perforation

About 20–30 ml of air is introduced into the stomach via the nasogastric tube and then gently milked through the pylorus into the duodenum. Any perforation of the mucosa will become obvious at this juncture and should be closed by direct suture with 4/0 chromic catgut or polyglycolic acid.

Slight haemorrhage from the edges of the pyloro-myotomy will cease once the tumour has been replaced into the peritoneal cavity and hence venous congestion relieved.

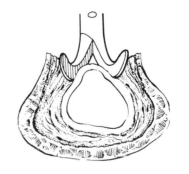

## Closure

The wound is closed with an interrupted *en masse* suture of 4/0 polyglycolic acid. The subcutaneous fat layer is closed with a continuous 4/0 polyglycolic acid suture and the skin edges are approximated with a 5/0 polyglycolic acid subcuticular suture.

9

# Postoperative care

The nasogastric tube is left *in situ* on free drainage until the infant is fully recovered from the anaesthetic. In the event of a perforation the tube is left on free drainage for 24 hours.

Many feeding regimens have been advocated, varying from commencing oral feeds within 2–4 hours of surgery to delaying feeds for 24 hours. It has been demonstrated that gastric peristalsis is abolished for 12–24 hours after operation and that early introduction of feeds is associated with a high incidence of postoperative vomiting, which may delay discharge from hospital. The regimen shown in the table has been found to be most acceptable.

**Table 1   Feeding schedule after pyloromyotomy**

| Stage | Volume of feed | Type of feed | Interval |
|-------|---------------|--------------|----------|
| I | 15 ml | Glucose-saline | 3 hours |
| II | 30 ml | Half-strength formula or breast | 3 hours |
| III | 60 ml | Half-strength formula or breast | 3 hours |
| IV | 90 ml | Full-strength formula or breast | 4 hours |

Introduction of the first feed is delayed for 12 hours but progression from one stage to the next proceeds rapidly as feeds are tolerated. The majority of infants are ready for discharge within 48–72 hours of the operation.

# Complications

The operation is associated with few complications and operative mortality is extremely rare. Wound sepsis occurs in less than 5 per cent of cases and wound dehiscence in less than 2 per cent. Recurrence is rare and is usually due to either inadequate separation of muscle fibres (to allow mucosa to bulge to the surface) or failure to divide muscle far enough proximally on to the antrum of the stomach.

## Further reading

Benson, C. D. (1970) Infantile pyloric stenosis. Historical aspects and current surgical concepts. Progress in Paediatric Surgery, 1, 63–88

Carter, C. O., Evans, K. A. (1969) Inheritance of congenital pyloric stenosis. Journal of Medical Genetics, 6, 223–254

Schärli, A. F., Leditschke, J. F. (1968) Gastric motility after pyloromyotomy in infants. Reappraisal of postoperative feeding. Surgery, 64, 1133–1137

Spicer, R. D. (1982) Infantile hypertrophic pyloric stenosis: a review. British Journal of Surgery, 69, 128–135

Spitz, L. (1979) Vomiting after pyloromyotomy for infantile hypertrophic pyloric stenosis. Archives of Disease in Childhood, 54, 886–889

# Duodenoduodenostomy

**U. G. Stauffer**
Director, Department of Surgery, University Children's Hospital, Zürich; Professor of Paediatric Surgery, University of Zürich, Switzerland

## Preoperative

Because of the early onset of symptoms, newborn infants with complete intrinsic duodenal obstruction are usually admitted within the first two days of life. In most cases early bilious vomiting indicates an obstruction below the entry of the bile duct; less frequently the obstruction may occur at or above the ampulla of Vater. A partial intrinsic duodenal obstruction may not cause symptoms for weeks, months or even years. Occasional cases have even been described in adults.

Children admitted within the first two days of life are generally in good physical condition. They do not need prolonged preoperative treatment and it generally suffices to pass a small nasogastric tube into the stomach and strap the catheter to the nostril. The stomach is aspirated, and if contents are very thick, it is washed out with warm isotonic saline solution. An intravenous infusion should be started and blood should be cross-matched. One milligram of vitamin K is given intramuscularly. The infant is nursed in a surgical incubator.

In only a few cases with delayed diagnosis are prolonged resuscitation, gastric decompression and intravenous therapy necessary. These infants will be dehydrated, suffer from alkalosis and sodium, potassium and chloride depletion. Their blood chemistry must be investigated and the appropriate solutions infused. They may have partial pulmonary collapse and pneumonia secondary to inhalation of vomitus, and may, therefore, need bronchial toilet, postural drainage, and nursing in an oxygen-enriched atmosphere with a humidity of 100 per cent.

In more severe cases tracheal intubation and mechanical respiration may be necessary. If the infant's body temperature is subnormal on admission, operation must be postponed until normothermia is established.

Congenital anomalies in other organ systems are found in approximately half of the babies presenting with duodenal atresia or stenosis. Down's syndrome is present in approximately 20 per cent of cases. This association may raise one of the most difficult ethical problems for the family and the surgeon involved.

Intrinsic duodenal obstruction is never a surgical emergency. It must therefore be stressed that all patients should be checked carefully for other associated anomalies and possible metabolic and respiratory complications which have to be corrected prior to operation.

Malrotation and volvulus can present with features indistinguishable from duodenal atresia. This is a potentially lethal situation for which urgent surgery is essential.

273

# 1

## ANAESTHESIA

Endotracheal intubation with controlled ventilation is used.

*Pathological anatomy:* Figures 1a to 1c show various types of intrinsic duodenal obstructions:
1) Intestine still in continuity. There may be an additional duodenal membrane (*see Fig. 7*)
2) A fibrous cord is left between the two segments.
3) There is a gap between the two segments.

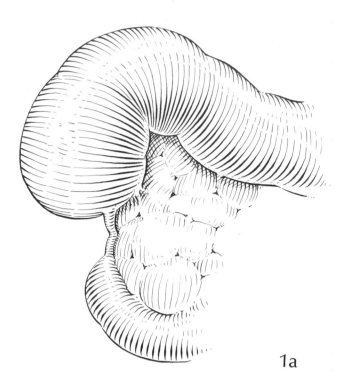

1a

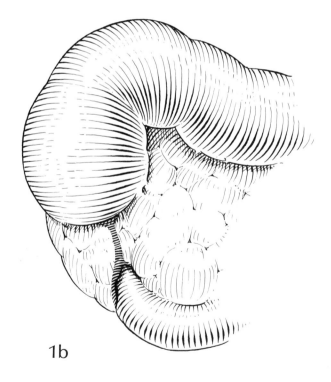

1b

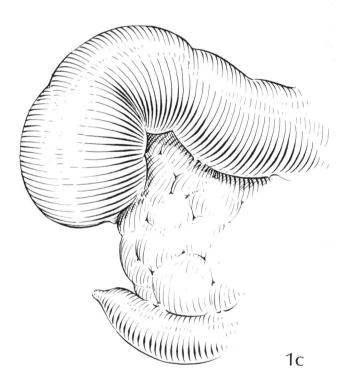

1c

## Position and preparation of patient

The infant is placed supine on the operating table on a thermostatically controlled warm water blanket. In newborns the umbilical cord is tied and cut flush with the surface, the abdominal skin is cleaned and a self-adherent plastic sheet may be fixed. This sheet should be big enough to cover the whole of the baby and will effectively protect him against too rapid heat loss. Body temperature is monitored by an endorectal probe. Blood loss is meticulously measured and replaced.

# The operation

In principle, there are three possible options in the surgical treatment of intrinsic duodenal obstruction: direct excision of an obstructive web, bypass of the obstruction with a duodenoduodenostomy, and bypass of the obstruction with a retrocolic duodenojejunostomy. In the following we will describe *duodenoduodenostomy*, which is the procedure of choice.

## 2

### The incision

A transverse abdominal incision is made 1 cm above the umbilicus, starting 1 cm to the left of the midline and running laterally in a skin crease for about 5–6 cm. The abdominal muscles are divided transversely with cutting diathermy and the peritoneal cavity is opened in the line of the incision.

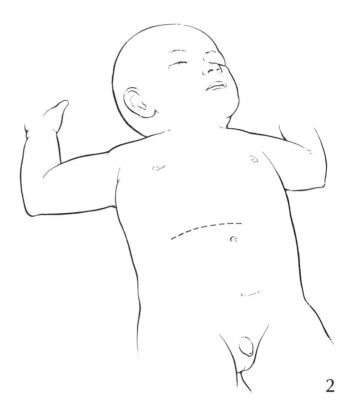

2

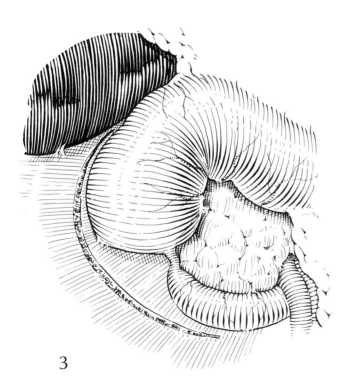

3

## 3

### Mobilization of second part of duodenum

The hepatic flexure of the colon is mobilized and the colon is displaced downwards and medially. The second part of the duodenum is now exposed and widely mobilized by Kocher's manoeuvre. The third and fourth parts of the duodenum must also be mobilized; this is usually quite easy even in those cases in which there is a gap or fibrous cord between the two segments of the duodenum. The distal duodenum is mobilized behind the superior mesenteric vessels and then drawn, together with the duodenojejunal junction, towards the right.

The grossly dilated proximal and narrow distal segments of the duodenum are now clearly visible. In cases with the so-called annular pancreas the segments are separated by a ring or wedge of pancreatic tissue. Whether an annular pancreas is present or not, whether we are dealing with duodenal atresia or stenosis or a duodenal membrane, the subsequent steps of the operation are identical.

## 4

### Approximation of duodenal segments

The upper and lower segments of the duodenum are approximated with two stay sutures and a few interrupted Lembert sutures, using 4/0 Dexon or Vicryl on a fully curved intestinal needle. Incisions are then made parallel to the line of approximation opening both duodenal segments. These incisions should be between 1.5 and 2 cm long.

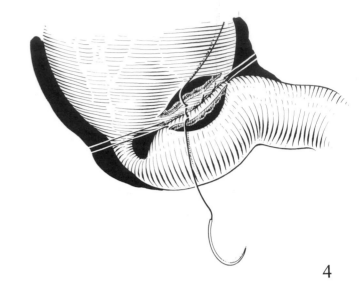

4

## 5

### Duodenoduodenal anastomosis

The two segments of duodenum are then anastomosed using 4/0 Dexon or Vicryl and interrupted mattress sutures through all the layers of the intestinal wall. The sutures should be placed about 2 mm apart and about 1 mm away from the cut edge of the intestine.

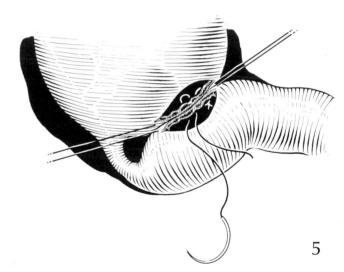

5

## 6

When the anterior layer of the interrupted mattress sutures has been completed it is reinforced with a few Lembert sutures.

6

# 7

## DUODENAL MEMBRANE

In cases with a duodenal membrane, which usually has a small central aperture, we usually adopt the procedure described above. However, some authorities recommend that the proximal duodenum should be opened and the membrane excised or incised. This procedure is potentially dangerous because in some cases the opening of the bile ducts (A) lies on the membrane close to the central hole (B) and may be injured by excision. This technique is therefore only permissible when the opening of the bile ducts has been clearly identified during surgery. There is a second potential hazard because a lax membrane may bulge downwards distally into the distended duodenum (the so-called windsock phenomenon) and may thus be missed completely at operation. This can be avoided if a temporary catheter is advanced by the anaesthetist into the stomach and is then guided by the surgeon until it appears in the opened proximal duodenum. Distal patency of the entire small intestine is then demonstrated by passing another catheter through the distal opening and by injecting air or saline. Although a second distal atresia is uncommon, the possibility should always be excluded.

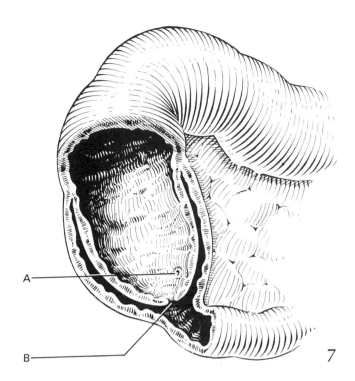

7

## Closure of the abdominal incision

The abdominal incision is now closed in layers, using interrupted absorbable sutures. The skin edges are approximated with a subcuticular suture of 4/0 or 5/0 polyglycolic acid.

# Postoperative care

The infant is returned to the incubator. Continuous gastric suction and intravenous feeding are continued until the stomach aspirate becomes clear, bowel sounds are audible, and stools are passed; this often takes 3–7 days. We have not used transanastomotic feeding tubes or gastrostomy for drainage. A narrow nasogastric tube provides adequate drainage and is free of complications. It can easily be removed and replaced if necessary. More recently, the additional insertion of a jejunostomy tube at the time of correction of duodenal obstruction has been recommended by some authors. The jejunostomy tube is inserted according to the technique of a gastrostomy tube, and allows enteral feeding to start immediately after surgery. With this technique, central or peripheral alimentation, which may otherwise be necessary, can be avoided.

Oral feeding must be introduced very gradually and, at first, only clear fluids (e.g. half strength normal saline diluted in 10 per cent glucose) should be given. Gradually increasing feeds are offered at two-hourly intervals and the stomach is aspirated before feeds if necessary. When it is possible to give 20 ml of clear fluids 2–3-hourly, milk feeding is commenced.

# Long-term prognosis

Long-term results are excellent in children with duodenal atresia and no other defects. These children have normal gastrointestinal function, normal growth and psychomotor development.

Illustrations by Kevin Marks

# Achalasia

**L. Spitz**   MB, ChB, PhD, FRCS(Ed), FRCS(Eng), FAAP(Hon)
Nuffield Professor of Paediatric Surgery, Institute of Child Health; Consultant Paediatric Surgeon, Hospital for Sick Children, Great Ormond Street, London, UK

## Introduction

Achalasia is a motility disorder of the oesophagus characterized by an absence of peristalsis and a failure of relaxation of the lower oesophageal sphincter. The cardinal symptoms in childhood are vomiting, dysphagia, chest pains and recurrent respiratory infections, and weight loss.

# Diagnosis

## Radiological features

The plain chest X-ray may show a dilated food-filled oesophagus with an air-fluid level. There may be radiological signs of recurrent aspiration pneumonitis. The cardinal features of achalasia on barium swallow are a dilated oesophagus, absence of stripping waves, incoordinated contraction and obstruction at the oesophago-gastric junction with prolonged retention of barium in the oesophagus. Failure of relaxation of the lower oesophageal sphincter gives rise to the classical 'rat-tail' deformity of funnelling and narrowing of the distal oesophagus.

## Endoscopy

The main value of oesophagoscopy is to exclude an organic cause for the abnormality.

## Oesophageal manometry

The criteria for diagnosis include (1) a high pressure (> 30 mmHg) lower oesophageal sphincter zone; (2) failure of the lower oesophagus to relax in response to swallowing; (3) absence of propulsive peristalsis; and (4) incoordinated tertiary contractions in the body of the oesophagus.

# Treatment

## Forceful dilatation

The aim of this treatment is to physically disrupt the muscle fibres of the lower oesophageal sphincter by means of pneumatic dilatation. A fluid- (Plummer) or air-filled (Browne–McHardy, Rider–Moeller, angioplasty catheter) bag of fixed diameter is radiologically positioned in the distal oesophagus and gently inflated. Relief of symptoms may only be temporary.

## Surgical treatment

The basis of all surgical procedures is the cardiomyotomy described in 1914 by Heller. Controversies concern the length of the myotomy, the extent to which the myotomy extends onto the stomach and the necessity for an antireflux procedure.

The author's preference is for a transabdominal oesophagogastric myotomy supplemented by a Nissen fundoplication.

# The operation

## Anaesthesia

General endotracheal anaesthesia is administered, with the patient supine on the operating table. Preoperative oesophagoscopy is recommended to ensure complete evacuation of retained food and secretions from the oesophagus. A medium-calibre nasogastric tube is passed into the stomach.

## Incision

The approach is via an upper abdominal midline incision extending from the xiphisternum to the umbilicus.

## Exposure

In most cases adequate exposure of the abdominal oesophagus can be obtained by retracting the left lobe of the liver anterosuperiorly with a wide retractor. If necessary, additional exposure may be attained by dividing the left triangular ligament in the avascular plane and retracting the left lobe of the liver towards the midline.

## Mobilization of the fundus of the stomach

As a Nissen fundoplication will be performed after completing the extended oesophagogastric myotomy, the operative procedure for fundoplication should be followed at an early stage.

The proximal one-third of the greater curvature of the stomach is liberated from its attachment to the spleen by ligating and dividing the short gastric vessels in the gastrosplenic ligament. This is accomplished most safely using a right-angled clamp passed around each vessel in turn and ligating the vessel on the gastric and splenic side before dividing it. When all the vessels in the gastrosplenic ligament have been divided, the spleen should be allowed to fall back into the posterior peritoneum, thereby avoiding inadvertent trauma. Splenectomy should never be necessary in this procedure. The fundus is now sufficiently free to allow a loose ('floppy') fundoplication.

## Exposure of the oesophageal hiatus

The phreno-oesophageal membrane is placed on stretch by downward traction on the stomach while the diaphragmatic muscle is held anteriorly. The avascular membrane is incised with scissors and the musculature of the oesophagus displayed. The anterior vagal nerve will be seen coursing on the surface of the oesophagus. It should be carefully protected and preserved.

# 1

## Mobilization of the distal oesophagus

Using a combination of sharp and blunt dissection, the lower end of the oesophagus is encircled, taking care not to injure the posterior vagal nerve. A rubber sling is placed around the oesophagus. The lower 5–8 cm of oesophagus is now mobilized through the oesophageal hiatus via the posterior mediastinum by blunt dissection with either a moist pledget or right-angled forceps.

The oesophageal hiatus is completely exposed by dividing the upper part of the gastrohepatic omentum above the left gastric vessels.

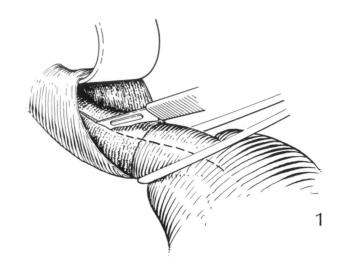

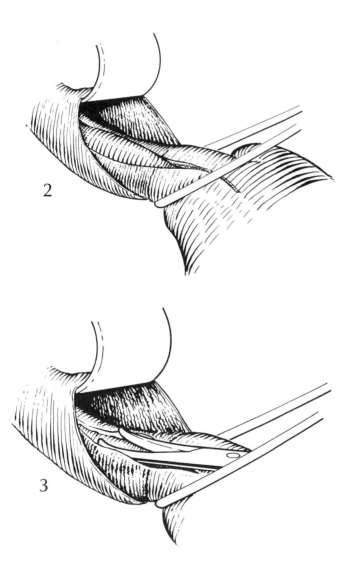

## Oesophagogastric myotomy

# 2 & 3

The myotomy is performed on the anterior wall of the oesophagus, extending for 2–3 cm onto the fundus of the stomach. A superficial incision (1–2 mm in depth) is made in the musculature of the distal 3–4 cm of the oesophagus. The divided muscle is gently parted with a blunt haemostat until the underlying mucosa of the oesophagus is encountered. The thickness of the muscle of the lower oesophagus varies from a few millimetres to half a centimetre or more. Great care must be taken to avoid opening into the lumen of the oesophagus.

# 4a & b

The divided muscle is now separated from the underlying mucosa by blunt pledget dissection in the submucosal plane. The dissection is continued until at least 50 per cent of the circumference of the oesophagus is free of the constricting muscle.

The myotomy is extended through the gastro-oesophageal junction for 2–3 cm onto the fundus of the stomach and the musculature similarly elevated from the underlying mucosa.

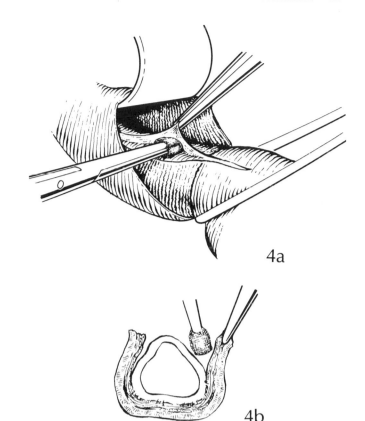

4a

4b

## Testing for oesophageal perforation

The stomach and oesophagus are distended with air introduced through the nasogastric tube, and the exposed mucosa carefully inspected for perforation. A mucosal defect should be carefully closed with fine polyglycolic acid sutures.

## Narrowing of the hiatus

The oesophageal hiatus is narrowed posterior to the oesophagus by placing deep sutures through the two sides of the left crus of the diaphragm. The sutures are tied loosely to prevent them from cutting through, but leaving sufficient space alongside the oesophagus to allow passage of the tip of a finger. Two or three sutures may be required for this purpose.

## The fundoplication

A loose ('floppy') Nissen fundoplication is now constructed over the distal 1.5–2.0 cm of the oesophagus. The sutures are only placed through one side of the divided oesophageal muscle in order to prevent reapproximation of the edges of the myotomy (see Fundoplication section).

## Closure

The wound is closed either in layers or with interrupted *en masse* sutures of 000 polyglycolic acid. A subcuticular suture approximates the skin edges.

# Postoperative care

Nasogastric decompression and intravenous fluids are continued until the postoperative ileus has resolved (average of 3–4 days).

# Complications

1. Mediastinitis due to failure to detect a mucosal perforation.
2. Recurrence of symptoms if the muscle is not separated from the underlying mucosa for at least half the circumference of the oesophagus.
3. Gastro-oesophageal reflux due to an inadequate fundoplication.
4. Dysphagia for solids due to too tight a fundoplication.

## Further Reading

Donahue, P. E., Schlesinger, P. K., Bombeck, C. T., Samelson, S., Nyhus, L. M. (1986) Achalasia of the esophagus: treatment, controversies and the method of choice. Annals of Surgery, 203, 505–511

Vantrappen, G., Janssens, J. (1983) To dilate or to operate? That is the question. Gut, 24, 1013–1019

Berquist, W. E., Byrne, W. J., Ament, M. E., Fonkalsrud, E. W., Euler, A. R. (1983) Achalasia: Diagnosis, management and clinical course in 16 children. Pediatrics, 71, 798–805

Ellis, F. H., Gibb, S. P., Crozier, R. E. (1980) Esophagomyotomy for achalasia of the esophagus. Annals of Surgery, 192, 157–161

Buick, R. G., Spitz, L. (1985) Achalasia of the cardia in children. British Journal of Surgery, 72, 341–343

Illustrations by Kevin Marks

# Malrotation

**Daniel G. Young**   MB, ChB, FRCS(Ed), FRCS(Glas), DTM&H
Reader in Paediatric Surgery and Honorary Consultant Paediatric Surgeon, Royal Hospital for Sick Children, Glasgow, UK

## Introduction

Malrotation is the term widely used for the condition in which the bowel returning to the abdominal cavity in the fetus fails to rotate to the normal extent. This incomplete rotation or malrotation leaves the midgut loop more mobile than normal, as the dorsal attachments of the peritoneum or mesentery are not fully developed. Rarely, the gut may twist in the opposite direction from the usual anticlockwise rotation, giving rise to another form of malrotation. The complete reversal which occurs with situs inversus does not cause symptoms and will not be discussed.

On return to the abdomen the midgut loop undergoes rotation so that the distal duodenum crosses the midline from the right side of the vertebrae to the left paraverte-bral region, where the ligament of Treitz develops, fixing the duodenojejunal flexure. At the same time the distal part of the midgut loop also rotates in an anticlockwise direction. This rotation brings the caecum and proximal colon across the upper abdomen and then down the right side where the caecum becomes relatively fixed in the right iliac fossa. The hindgut remains relatively fixed at the splenic flexure. This change is effected by the differential growth of the enveloping peritoneum over the midgut loop. The process may not be completed at birth, and it is well recognized, particularly by paediatric radiologists, that a high caecum in the neonate is not necessarily of any pathological significance but simply a stage in development.

## Pathological anatomy

Failure of the bowel to undergo or to complete the rotation process leaves the duodenum in the shape of a 'reversed comma' rather than the normal 'C' configuration. The distal duodenum passes down the right side of the abdomen and fails to extend behind the superior mesenteric vessels to a more craniad duodenojejunal junction in the left upper abdomen. The caecum lies in the midline of the upper abdomen with peritoneal folds running posteriorly from it across the duodenum to the posterior abdominal wall in the right upper quadrant of the abdomen, and often to the undersurface of the liver and gall bladder area (Ladd's bands).

## Clinical features

Malrotation may be detected.

1. Being an incidental finding.
2. Causing extrinsic duodenal obstruction which may be intermittent and requires operative intervention.
3. When complicated by volvulus, it is a serious life-threatening state requiring emergency operation.

The surgeon lacking experience with malrotation should beware of initiating treatment simply because the infant's caecum has not fully descended on the right side of the abdomen to reach the right iliac fossa. The gradual fixation of the large bowel in its inverted 'U' shape continues to occur in early postnatal life and even into childhood.

Malrotation may coexist with a number of other serious anomalies. Two classical examples are left-sided congenital diaphragmatic hernia and exomphalos. In these conditions some degree of malrotation is invariable. With diaphragmatic hernia the gut, on return to the abdominal cavity in early fetal life, passes through a pleuroperitoneal defect into the left chest and this interferes with the normal process of rotation and fixation. In exomphalos the gut has not completely returned to the abdominal cavity. In both these conditions the malrotation is incidental, and as the peritoneal folds are greatly elongated and may not cause extrinsic duodenal obstruction, no operative action is considered necessary by some paediatric surgeons.

Clinical problems from malrotation causing extrinsic duodenal obstruction usually arise in the first week of life but may be delayed for weeks or months. Postnatally, with feeding, the infant's gut becomes more active and the peritoneal bands crossing the duodenum compress it to cause extrinsic duodenal obstruction. The clinical sign of this obstruction is bile-stained vomiting. The infant has usually passed normal meconium and has often passed changing stool. For some unexplained reason, extrinsic duodenal obstruction is more common in males than females, with the ratio of approximately 4:1. These infants are usually in good general condition and rarely have other major anomalies. The bile-stained vomiting usually results in the parents or attending staff seeking early expert advice.

Malrotation complicated by volvulus of the midgut loop is a serious and potentially lethal condition. The lack of rotation results in failure of development of the root of mesentery, which should extend from the upper left to the lower right side of the posterior abdominal wall, leaving a narrow base around which the midgut twists, usually in a clockwise direction. The dangerous aspect for the infant is that in addition to the extrinsic duodenal obstruction caused by this volvulus, the superior mesenteric venous drainage or the arterial inflow may be obstructed by compression at the base of the mesentery.

Volvulus sometimes occurs during intrauterine life, with infarction of the midgut loop. Reabsorption of part or all of the affected midgut loop may occur. After birth the serious consequences of this are apparent, when the infant presents with signs of an intestinal atresia.

Volvulus of the midgut loop is not necessarily a static condition and in the postnatal period it may give rise to intermittent symptoms, which resolve each time the bowel twists back to relieve the compression. The infant may appear normal for days or months until volvulus recurs.

## Presentation

Symptomatic malrotation usually occurs in otherwise normal infants. Bile-stained vomiting is always present, whether the duodenal obstruction is caused by the peritoneal bands or a volvulus. Commonly the infant has progressed satisfactorily at first and then develops the bile-stained vomiting. The obstruction may be intermittent or incomplete, but the presence of bile in the vomit should always alert the clinician. With volvulus superimposed the infant may pass blood per rectum. Abdominal examination is often unrewarding as there may be no clinical signs. On occasion there may be abdominal distension or the gut may be palpable as a vague mass in the centre of the abdomen, with relatively empty flanks.

## Diagnosis

# 1

As the clinical signs are not diagnostic of malrotation, further investigations of the infant are necessary. X-ray of the abdomen may show signs of duodenal obstruction or it may show the small bowel, if visible, on the left. The presence of air in the gut, which is a feature of infants, often serves as a contrast medium, allowing definition of the position of the bowel.

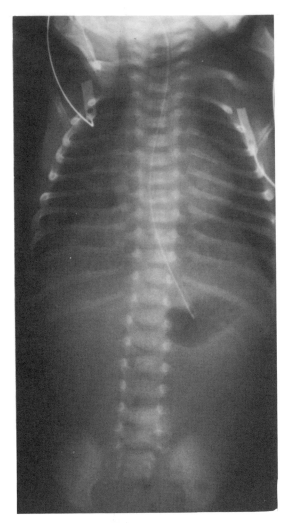

1

**2**

Contrast studies may be necessary and a barium meal will show the contrast passing down the duodenum either to the obstruction or, usually because the obstruction is incomplete, demonstrating the rotation of the duodenum described above. Upper gastrointestinal studies are preferred to barium enema because they demonstrate the malrotation of the duodenum and obstruction, whereas the enema may only show the caecum to be high or near to midline, a matter which is not necessarily clinically significant.

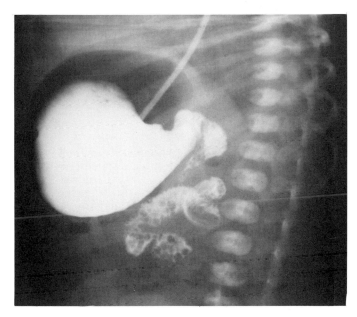

2

## Preoperative management

Provided that the diagnosis has been made promptly, preoperative preparation is simply the routine for any infant, and the setting up of an intravenous infusion line. Where there is delay in diagnosis, fluid and electrolyte loss may necessitate a short period of intensive resuscitation with intravenous fluid administration. Laparotomy should be performed within a few hours of the diagnosis of malrotation being established, since it is not possible to predict when volvulus might supervene, with the danger of midgut infarction.

Where volvulus tight enough to impair the blood supply to the midgut exists, it is necessary to replace lost intravascular fluid quickly before proceeding to laparotomy. Intravenous administration of fluid and electrolytes suffices for the infant without abdominal tenderness, but if the abdomen is tender, plasma replacement and sometimes blood may be required. A simple guide is to measure the peripheral temperature, e.g. from the foot or toe, and infuse at 20 ml/kg per hour until the temperature rises above 32°C. The drip rate is then halved, any premedication required by the anaesthetist is given, and laparotomy is then performed.

## The operation

# 3 & 4

Through a transverse supraumbilical incision which extends across both rectus muscles, the peritoneal cavity is opened. The umbilical vein is divided and the hepatic end ligated. Any free fluid is mopped out of the peritoneal cavity. The presence of blood-stained peritoneal fluid indicates the existence of a volvulus.

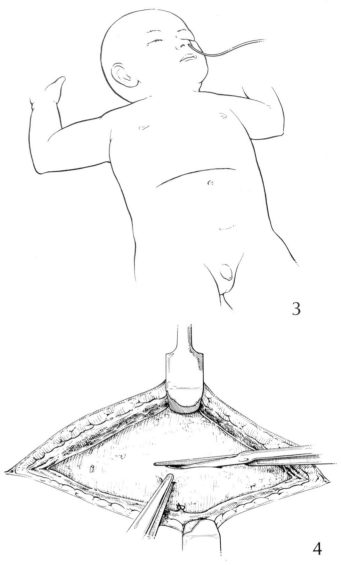

3

4

# 5

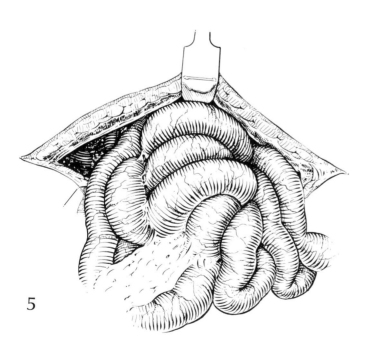

5

The midgut loop is brought out of the abdominal cavity and the position defined. If volvulus is present it is undone by anticlockwise rotation by as many 180° turns as needed.

# 6 & 7

The peritoneal folds which extend from the caecum and ascending colon laterally are then divided. Division of these folds in front of the lateral border of the duodenum allows the caecum to be displaced to the left. After incision of the right-sided layer of peritoneum at the root of the mesentery blunt dissection is continued. The distal duodenum and proximal jejunum are gently mobilized from the superior mesenteric vessels and can be displaced to the right.

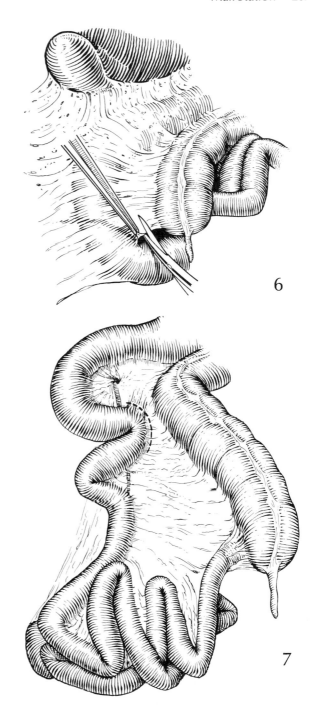

6

7

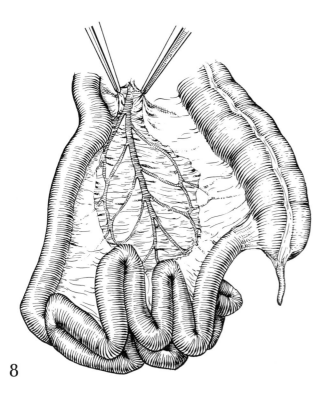

8

# 8

The superior mesenteric vessels are exposed centrally, and the large bowel is freed sufficiently to form a minimum of a 5 cm base to the mesentery.

# 9

The appendix is then removed if the viability of the gut is not impaired. This is done because the appendix would otherwise need to be replaced in the left upper abdomen, and this may give rise to considerable diagnostic difficulty should appendicitis supervene later. The proximal small bowel is then replaced in the right side of the abdomen, the remainder of the small bowel in the lower abdomen, and the caecum in the left hypochondrium.

If on untwisting the volvulus some of the gut has impaired viability, though still intact and not frankly gangrenous, the root of the mesentery is mobilized in the fashion described, sufficiently to ensure that the superior mesenteric vessels are running freely into the midgut loop. The gut is then replaced in the peritoneal cavity. The abdomen is closed and after 24 hours repeat laparotomy is performed to reassess the viability of the bowel. Clear demarcation will have become apparent, and resection with end-to-end anastomosis can be performed.

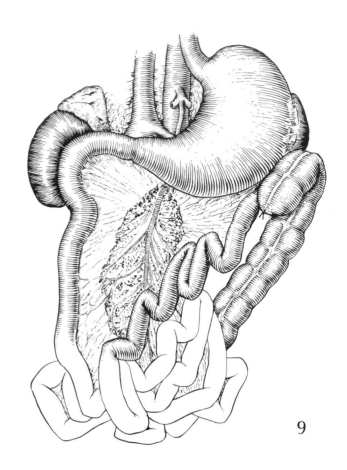

9

# 10

10

The dissection of the root of the mesentery as described above is then completed at this second laparotomy, and the abdomen closed in layers.

If gangrene with perforation of gut has occurred before the first laparotomy and involves only a very small local area, the perforation may be repaired and oversewn. The above Ladd's procedure is then performed and the laparotomy closed. When a more extensive area of small bowel is gangrenous, but provided that more than 100 cm of small bowel remains viable, resection of the gangrenous bowel and anastomosis of the viable bowel is performed. Where less than 100 cm of bowel is clearly viable, only the frankly gangrenous bowel is exteriorized after untwisting the volvulus. The remainder is replaced for a second laparotomy 24 to 36 hours later for appropriate resection and anastomosis. On occasions a further delay of 24 hours may be indicated before a third laparotomy, to allow maximal redevelopment of circulation to the strangulated loops. Ultimately, resection with end-to-end anastomosis of viable bowel is performed.

# Postoperative management

Postoperative management consists of nasogastric aspiration and intravenous fluid support until gut function returns, which is usually after 48 hours. The nasogastric tube of adequate size, e.g. 12 FG, is aspirated hourly for 24 hours and then 2-hourly until the gastric aspirate ceases to be bile-stained and its volume is decreasing. Oral feeds are then recommenced and graduated up to normal feeding over 48 hours. Blood transfusion may not have been necessary initially at operation, but postoperatively there is loss of fluid from the handled gut and the raw area on the posterior abdominal wall. Hence, alternating plasma with dextrose 10 per cent/saline 0.225 per cent at 150 ml/kg per 24 hours over the first 12 hours will maintain an adequate intravascular volume. After 24 hours potassium chloride is added to the intravenous fluids to give the infant 3–4 mmol/kg per day. As oral feeding increases, the infusion rate is reduced.

# Results

As infants with symptomatic malrotation are usually otherwise normal, recovery is frequently prompt and the outcome excellent, except in the infant who has suffered delayed diagnosis of volvulus with consequent infarction of the midgut. In the most severe cases of infarction, the infant or child may be dependent on parenteral nutrition for maintenance of life and growth. With lesser lengths of midgut involved, parenteral nutrition may still be necessary over weeks or even months.

The great majority of infants with malrotation have an uninterrupted recovery following Ladd's procedure, and the only complication likely in the future is adhesion obstruction, which affects approximately 5 per cent over the succeeding 10 years. This complication is usually relieved by simple freeing of the bowel at laparotomy.

Illustrations by Gillian Oliver

# Congenital atresia and stenosis of the small intestine

**S. Cywes**  MMed(Surg), FACS, FRCS(Eng)
Professor of Paediatric Surgery, University of Cape Town; Chief Surgeon, Red Cross War Memorial Children's Hospital, Cape Town, S. Africa

## History

In 1911 Fockens[1] of Rotterdam reported the first successfully treated case of small-bowel atresia. However, up to 1952 the mortality of atresia of the small bowel remained prohibitive even at the best paediatric surgical centres in the world, for example 84 per cent at the Children's Medical Center in Boston[2] and 88 per cent at the Hospital for Sick Children, Great Ormond Street in London[3]. In a comprehensive review of the world literature up to 1950, Evans[4] could find reports of only 39 successfully treated cases of jejunoileal atresia.

In 1952 Louw[3] published the results of an investigation of 79 patients treated at Great Ormond Street, London, and suggested that jejunoileal atresia was probably due to a vascular accident rather than the result of inadequate recanalization as had previously been the commonly accepted hypothesis. At his instigation, Barnard perfected the experimental model in pregnant mongrel bitches[5]. This not only confirmed the hypothesis and supported changes in the surgical procedure, but also paved the way for further fetal experiments.

Since then there has been a steady improvement in the results of treatment of atresia and stenoses of the small intestine[6,7,8]. More recently Tibboel et al., in chick-embryo studies, showed that intrauterine perforation of the small intestine may also produce atresia[9].

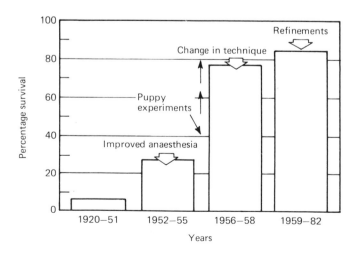

Figure 1   Operative results in congenital atresia and stenosis of the small intestine

# Preoperative

## Indications

Many cases of intestinal atresia are now being diagnosed prenatally by ultrasonographic investigation of the fetus, showing dilated and obstructed fetal intestine. Postnatally, atresia or severe stenosis of the small intestine present as neonatal intestinal obstruction with persistent bilious (green) vomiting dating from the first or second day of life, varying degrees of abdominal distension, and perhaps some abnormality in evacuating meconium. Erect and supine abdominal radiographs will reveal distended small-bowel loops and air–fluid levels. An inverted radiograph is useful to distinguish between low small-bowel and colonic obstruction.

In some cases the first abdominal radiograph reveals a completely opaque abdomen due to a fluid-filled, obstructed bowel. Emptying of the stomach by means of a nasogastric tube and the injection of a bolus of air will demonstrate the level of the obstruction. When intestinal stenosis is present, an abnormal differentiation in calibre of the proximal obstructed intestine and the distal tract will be evident. When the radiograph suggests a complete low obstruction, a contrast enema is performed to rule out an associated colonic atresia or functional obstruction such as total colonic aganglionosis or meconium ileus, which may be confused with an atresia of the distal ileum. When an incomplete small-bowel obstruction is diagnosed, an upper gastrointestinal contrast study is indicated to demonstrate the site and nature of the obstruction. In congenital stenosis of the small intestine the proximal bowel is usually more dilated than in malrotation with volvulus.

## Preparation

The newborn baby tolerates operative intervention all the better after a few hours of preoperative preparation, especially if diagnosis has been delayed. This preparation should pay particular attention to hypothermia, hypoxia, hypovolaemia, hypoglycaemia and hypoprothrombinaemia.

The baby is nursed in a warmed, well-humidified incubator. A nasogastric tube is passed to decompress the stomach and prevent aspiration of vomitus. The aspirate is cultured. Blood gas levels are monitored and the fractionated inspired oxygen level is adjusted as required. An intravenous infusion is set up by means of a 'push in' into a vein of the scalp, or dorsum of the hand or foot, to re-establish fluid and electrolyte balances, to correct any acid–base abnormality and to facilitate blood transfusion during operation. A unit of fresh blood is cross-matched in readiness. One-fifth normal saline plus added potassium in a 10 per cent dextrose solution is used to correct fluid and electrolyte deficits, and is given at a rate of 2 ml/kg per hour.

In neglected cases more energetic therapy is required. If there has been perforation of the bowel with shock, colloid solutions, stabilized human serum and/or fresh blood 10–20 ml/kg must be added. Hyperbilirubinaemia when present is treated by phototherapy, but if severe may demand preoperative exchange transfusion. Regular testing with Dextrostix is done to ensure adequate sugar levels.

The baby is washed with chlorhexidine, and vitamin $K_1$ is given to counteract prothrombin deficiency. The lungs are kept clear by nasopharyngeal aspiration. When respiration is impeded by severe abdominal distension and/or pulmonary infection, intermittent positive-pressure respiration is often life saving.

Prophylactic broad-spectrum antibiotics are given immediately before operation, if not already administered for an associated complication.

## Temperature regulation

Heat is conserved by having the theatre comfortably warm (24°C), and by placing the baby supine on a warming blanket through which water at 40°C is circulated. Further heating can be achieved by an infrared lamp. The baby is well covered with Gamgee tissue until anaesthetized and connected up to all the monitoring devices such as rectal thermometer, ECG, oesophageal stethoscope and flow detector, and blood pressure cuff.

## Anaesthesia

Endotracheal anaesthesia with nitrous oxide, oxygen and halothane, and intermittent positive-pressure ventilation is used, and is supplemented with a non-depolarizing relaxant (alcuronium). The anaesthetic gases are passed over a heated humidifier.

## Sterilization of skin and draping

The umbilical cord is cleansed with 70 per cent alcohol and is transected flush with the abdominal wall. The abdominal skin is prepared by cleansing with prewarmed povidone iodine 2 per cent in 70 per cent alcohol. Sterile, warm Gamgee rolls are placed alongside the baby, who is then draped with towels, and a sterile, transparent adhesive drape is applied over the operative field.

## Perioperative supportive care

During the operative procedure the baby is given a balanced electrolyte solution containing 10 per cent dextrose, by slow intravenous infusion, to provide about 15 ml/kg during the first hour of surgery and 8 ml/kg during the second hour. Blood lost during the operation is carefully measured colorimetrically and replaced volume for volume plus 10 per cent. The blood tubing is warmed by immersion in water heated to 37°C.

# The operation

### The incision

An adequate incision is required. Exposure is obtained by a supraumbilical transverse incision transecting the rectus muscles 2–3 cm above the umbilicus.

# 1

### Exploration

If free gas escapes on opening the peritoneum, or if there is contamination of the peritoneal cavity, the perforation should be sought immediately and closed before further exploration. The bowel proximal to the obstruction is distended, while the bowel distal to the obstruction is collapsed, tiny and worm-like. All the bowel is exteriorized to determine the site and type of obstruction and to exclude other areas of atresia or stenosis, as well as associated lesions such as incomplete intestinal rotation or meconium ileus.

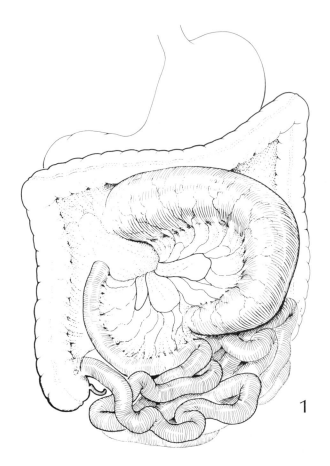

### Appearance of atretic segment

This depends upon the type of occlusion but in all cases the maximal dilatation and enlargement of the proximal bowel occurs at the point of obstruction, and this segment is often aperistaltic and of questionable viability.

# 2

### Stenosis

The proximal dilated bowel and distal bowel are in continuity with an intact mesentery, but at the point of junction there is a short, narrow, somewhat rigid segment with a minute lumen. The small intestine is of normal length.

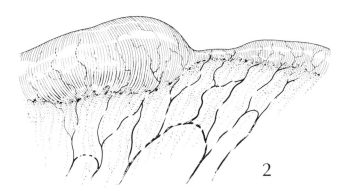

# 3

## Atresia type I (membrane)

The dilated proximal and collapsed distal bowel are in continuity and the mesentery is intact. The pressure in the proximal bowel tends to bulge the membrane into the distal intestine so that the transition from distended to collapsed bowel is conical in appearance: the 'windsock' effect. The distal bowel is completely collapsed.

The small intestine is of normal length.

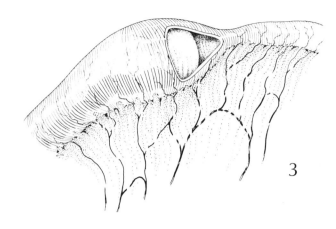

# 4

## Atresia type II (blind ends joined by a band)

The proximal bowel terminates in a bulbous, blind end which is grossly distended and hypertrophied for several centimetres. This blind end is often aperistaltic and cyanosed, and may be necrotic with a perforation. The bowel proximal to this is usually considerably distended and hypertrophied for a further 5–10 cm, but more proximally the distension is less marked and the walls become thinner. The distal, completely collapsed bowel commences as a blind end which is occasionally bulbous, owing to remains of a fetal intussusception. The two blind ends are joined by a thin, fibrous band. The corresponding intestinal mesentery is usually normal but may occasionally be absent, leaving a V-shaped gap. The small intestine length is usually normal.

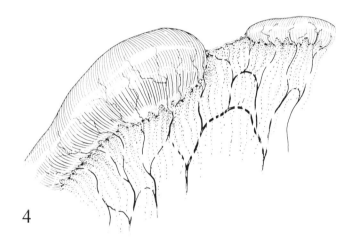

# 5

## Atresia type IIIa (disconnected blind ends)

The appearance is similar to that in type II but the blind ends are completely separate. There is always a gap in the mesentery and the total length of bowel is reduced to a varying extent.

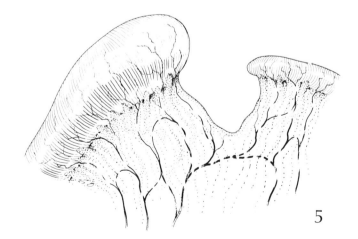

# 6

### Atresia type IIIb ('apple peel' atresia)

As in IIIa the blind ends are unconnected, but the mesenteric defect is gross. This type is due to an extensive infarction of the midgut following a proximal superior mesenteric artery occlusion. The distal ileum remains viable, receiving its blood supply from an abnormal arterial collateral from the arterial supply to the right colon, around which vessel the ileum appears to be coiled. There is always a significant reduction in intestinal length.

### Atresia type IV (multiple atresia)

Multiple atresias can be combinations of types I to III. The bowel length is always reduced.

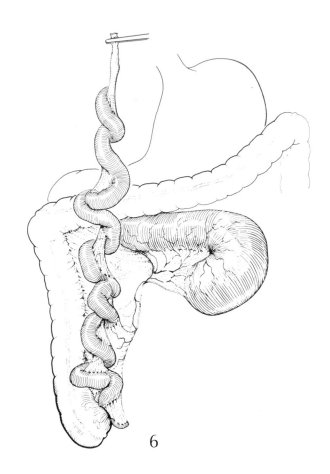

6

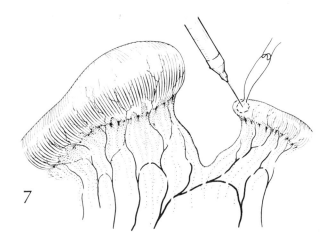

7

# 7

### Detection of other atretic areas

After the location and type of lesion have been identified, the distal bowel is carefully examined to untwist any volvulus present, and to exclude other atretic segments, which occur in 10–15 per cent of cases. Intraluminal membranes are best detected and localized by injecting half-normal saline into the lumen of the collapsed bowel and milking it down to the caecum. The total length of small bowel is measured. The normal length at birth is approximately 250 cm.

# 8

## Distension of distal end

After complete patency of the distal small bowel has been established, the next task is to splice the disproportionate proximal and distal blind ends. This is facilitated by applying a bulldog clamp about 6–8 cm from the distal blind end and distending the intervening segment with half-normal saline, taking care not to split the serosa. The needle puncture is closed with an encircling 5/0 silk suture to prevent leakage.

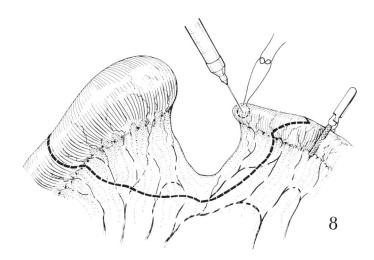

# 9

## Resection

The atretic area and adjacent distended and collapsed loops of bowel are isolated by replacing the rest of the bowel and walling off the rest of the abdominal cavity with moist packs. To ensure adequate postoperative function *the proximal distended and hypertrophied bowel must be liberally resected*, even if it appears viable. Usually 10–15 cm are removed. After milking the intestinal contents into the proximal bulbous end, a bulldog clamp is applied across the bowel a few centimetres proximal to the site selected for transection. The mesentery adjoining the portion to be resected is clamped, divided and ligated up to the proposed lines of section of proximal and distal bowel. A clamp is then applied to the proximal bowel which is transected between this and the bulldog clamp. The blood supply at this point should be excellent, and therefore the bowel is divided at right angles, leaving an opening of about 1.5 cm in width. Some 4–5 cm of the distal bowel are then removed. This bowel is transected slightly obliquely and the incision is continued along the antimesenteric border to create a 'fish-mouth' which renders the opening about equal to that of the proximal bowel.

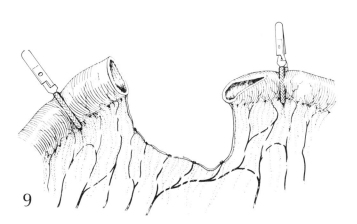

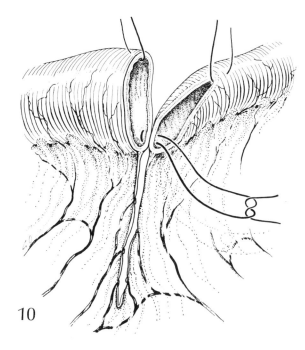

# 10

## Uniting the mesenteric borders

An inverting mattress 5/0 silk or other non-absorbable suture unites the mesenteric borders of the divided ends, and temporary stay sutures are inserted at the antimesenteric angles to facilitate accurate approximation.

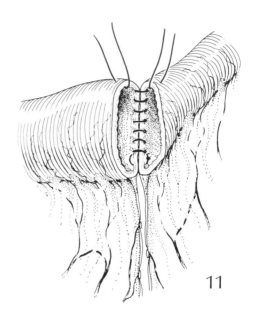

# 11

### The 'posterior' sutures

The 'posterior' edges of the loops are united with interrupted through-and-through silk sutures tied on the mucosal aspect.

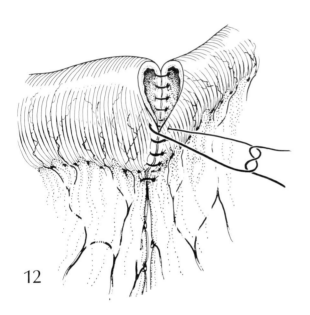

# 12

### The 'anterior' sutures

The 'anterior' edges are joined by similar through-and-through sutures tied on the serosal surface.

# 13

### Completion of anastomosis and closure of mesenteric gap

The completed anastomosis is not strictly end-to-end but a modification of Denis Browne's 'end-to-back' method. The suture line is tested for leakage, and reinforcing sutures inserted as required. The defect in the mesentery is repaired by approximating (and overlapping if necessary) the divided edges with interrupted 5/0 silk or other non-absorbable sutures. Thereafter the intestines, well moistened with warm saline, are returned to the peritoneal cavity.

A similar technique is used for stenosis and intraluminal membranes. Procedures such as simple enteroplasties, excision of membranes, and bypassing techniques are not recommended because they fail to remove the abnormal segment of bowel. Side-to-side anastomosis is avoided because of the increased risk of creating blind loops.

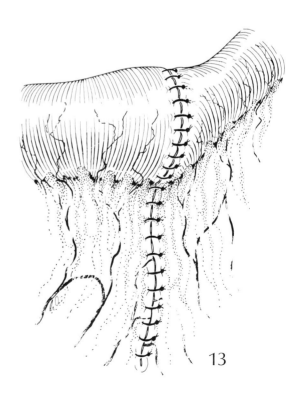

# 14

## GASTROSTOMY

In babies with high jejunal atresias just beyond the duodenojejunal flexure, it is advisable to perform a gastrostomy, and the trimmed DePezzer gastrostomy tube is used as a conduit for a transanastomotic Silastic feeding tube. The tube should be passed into the small bowel distal to the anastomosis before completing the anterior layer of sutures; it is stabilized at the anastomotic site by a single tethering stitch which prevents its retrograde displacement into the stomach.

## Closure of abdominal wound

If the peritoneal cavity has been soiled from a perforation, the abdominal cavity is irrigated with copious amounts of saline or a 0.01 per cent aqueous solution of povidone iodine.

The abdominal wound is closed in layers, using continuous 3/0 chromic catgut or synthetic absorbable sutures for the peritoneum, and interrupted 3/0 catgut, synthetic absorbable, or monofilament non-absorbable sutures, according to preference, for the anterior rectus sheath. Before closing the skin the wound is irrigated with a 0.01 per cent povidone iodine solution. The skin is approximated with a continuous subcuticular synthetic absorbable suture or interrupted 4/0 Dermalon or silk sutures. The wound is dressed with sterile plastic skin spray and a thin strip of sterile Micropore.

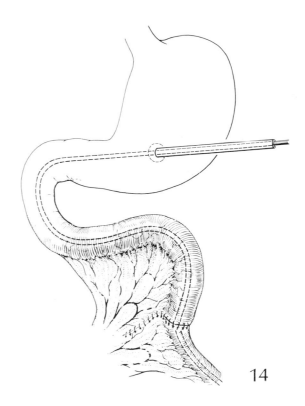

14

# Postoperative care

The baby is transferred from the operating table to the warmed incubator and moved to the neonatal surgical unit for continuous intensive care. Oxygen is given to produce a 40 per cent saturation in a head box placed in the incubator. The pulse, respiratory rate and temperature are monitored. The position of the baby is changed from side to back to side and the nasopharynx is cleared of secretions. Nasogastric (or gastrostomy) decompression is maintained to prevent gastric distension and vomiting and inhalation of secretions. The urinary output is carefully recorded.

Intravenous maintenance fluids and electrolytes are kept at a minimum but not over-restricted, aiming at 120 ml/kg body weight per day of a balanced electrolyte maintenance solution containing 10 per cent dextrose. Losses from gastric suction are measured at 4-hourly intervals and replaced volume for volume with half-normal saline solution. Postoperative acid-base and gas studies are done regularly and any acidosis is corrected with 8.5 per cent sodium bicarbonate. The antibiotics commenced preoperatively are continued. An oral anti-fungal agent is given prophylactically in the immediate postoperative period.

Where colloid loss is anticipated due to intraperitoneal inflammation or much tissue handling at surgery, stabilized human serum 10 ml/kg body weight should be given. The serum bilirubin should be repeatedly checked and phototherapy continued or exchange transfusion performed if necessary. Nasogastric decompression is usually required for 3 or 4 days postoperatively (longer in high jejunal atresias). After 24–36 hours insertion of a finger into the rectum or a small half-normal saline enema is useful for promoting expansion of the distal bowel, the passage of meconium, and the establishment of peristalsis. The nasogastric tube is removed and graduated feeding is commenced when the gastric aspirate is no longer bile stained, the abdomen is not distended, peristalsis is present, and meconium has been passed. The antibiotics are discontinued on the fifth postoperative day if there is no evidence of infection. The baby is removed from the incubator when stabilized on oral feeds and weighing over 2 kg. When necessary the sutures are removed on the tenth postoperative day.

If at any time there is suspicion of a leak at the anastomosis (suggested by sudden collapse, abdominal distension and vomiting) a plain erect radiograph of the abdomen should be taken. If this should reveal free air in the abdomen more than 24 hours after operation laparotomy should be performed immediately and the leaking site sutured.

In babies with less than 75 cm of small bowel remaining, diarrhoea and excessive water loss may pose a problem. In these and in every instance where normal enteral alimentation is not expected to be established within 5 postoperative days, parenteral feeding is indicated. Intravenous carbohydrate, amino acid and fat-containing solutions are introduced in a graduated manner over a period of 4 days. Peripheral venous push-in lines are used in preference to central, surgically placed venous catheters. The aim is to have the baby on a complete parenteral feeding regimen by the 5th postoperative day. Once intestinal function has been re-established, the baby is gradually weaned from parenteral to enteral feeding. Careful tailoring of the diet is required, as each patient has different tolerance thresholds.

Predictions of the degree of intestinal hypofunction are based upon the known residual length of small intestine. When gross intestinal insufficiency is expected, a hypo-osmolar elemental diet is introduced in accurately titrated volumes. Regular monitoring for clinical signs and/or biochemical evidence of intestinal overload is required. Disaccharide intolerance and the rare monosaccharide intolerance, indications of gross brush-border malfunction of the intestine, should be detected by regular biochemical assessment of samples of stool fluid before severe clinical signs become manifest.

A falling pH and an associated increasing level of reducing substances denote unsatisfactory carbohydrate assimilation. The patient's oral intake is gradually increased in volume and in energy content, while the small intestine is allowed time to adapt, until maximum intake tolerance is reached. This can take up to a month or more. Pharmacological control of intestinal peristaltic activity has been achieved more effectively since the introduction of loperamide hydrochloride. Vitamin $B_{12}$ should be given if the terminal ileum has been resected.

In predicting the ultimate functional outcome the following factors must be taken into consideration. The ileum adapts to a greater degree than the jejunum; the neonatal small intestine still has a period of maturation and growth ahead of it; and the actual residual small intestinal length is difficult to determine accurately. The proximal obstructed bowel segment is dilated and its length may be overestimated, while the distal, unused, collapsed bowel should have its measured length at least doubled when calculating the residual small intestine.

# Results

Before 1952 the mortality rate for congenital atresias of the small intestine in Cape Town was 90 per cent. Between 1952 and 1955, 28 per cent of the babies survived. At that stage most were treated by primary anastomosis without resection. With liberal resection of the blind ends and end-to-end anastomosis the survival rate increased to 78 per cent during the period 1955–1958.

During the 24-year period 1959–1982, 114 patients with jejunoileal atresias and stenoses were admitted to the paediatric surgical service at the Red Cross War Memorial Children's Hospital. There were 16 deaths, giving an overall survival rate of 86 per cent (*Figure 1*). One of these deaths was due to aspiration during induction of anaesthesia. One death occurred soon after admission in a moribund baby with a perforation in whom resuscitation proved unsuccessful, one was in a patient with a duodenal atresia plus multiple small intestinal atresias and associated mongolism (the only patient in this series with a duodenal and small intestinal atresia) and two babies had a midgut volvulus with gangrene of the whole of the midgut and a jejunal atresia at laparotomy, in whom the abdomen was closed without resection. One baby with multiple atresias and 30 cm residual bowel after surgery died 7 months afterwards because of septicaemia from a central venous catheter for parenteral nutrition. Eight of the deaths occurred in babies with type IIIb or type IV atresias.

The survival in relation to birth weight and associated anomalies is shown in Table 1 and the survival in relation to the risk group is outlined in Table 2.

**Table 1    Survival in relation to weight and associated abnormalities**

|  | Patients (N) | Survivors (N) | Survival rate (%) |
|---|---|---|---|
| *Weight* | | | |
| >2300 g | 61 | 57 | 93 |
| 1800–2200 g | 37 | 30 | 81 |
| <1800 g | 16 | 11 | 69 |
| *Associated abnormalities* | | | |
| Insignificant or nil | 69 | 66 | 96 |
| Moderate | 27 | 21 | 78 |
| Severe | 18 | 11 | 61 |

**Table 2    Survival in relation to risk group**

| Risk Group | Patients (N) | Survivors (N) | Survival rate (%) |
|---|---|---|---|
| A | 42 | 40 | 95 |
| B | 39 | 35 | 90 |
| C | 33 | 23 | 70 |
| **Total** | **114** | **98** | **86** |

## References

1. Fockens, P. (1911) Ein operativ geheilter Fall von kongenitaler Dünndarmatresie. Zentralblatt für Chirurgie, 38, 532–535

2. Ladd, W. E., Gross, R. E. (1941) Abdominal Surgery of Infancy and Childhood. Philadelphia: W. B. Saunders

3. Louw, J. H. (1952) Congenital intestinal atresia and severe stenosis in the newborn: report on 79 consecutive cases. South African Journal of Clinical Science, 3, 109–129

4. Evans, C. H. (1951) Atresias of the gastrointestinal tract. International Abstracts of Surgery, 92, 1–8

5. Louw, J. H., Barnard, C. N. (1955) Congenital intestinal atresia: observations on its origin. Lancet, 2, 1065–1067

6. Nixon, H. H. (1960) An experimental study of propulsion in isolated small intestine, and applications to surgery in the newborn. Annals of the Royal College of Surgeons of England, 27, 105–124

7. Benson, C. D., Lloyd, J. R., Smith, J. D. (1960) Resection and primary anastomosis in the management of stenosis and atresia of the jejunum and ileum. Pediatrics, 26, 265–272

8. Cywes, S., Davies, M. R., Rode, H. (1980) Congenital jejuno-ileal atresia and stenosis. South African Medical Journal, 57, 630–639

9. Tibboel, D., Molenaar, J. C., Nie, C. J. (1979) New perspectives in fetal surgery: the chicken embryo. Journal of Pediatric Surgery, 14, 438–440

Illustrations by Kevin Marks

# Meconium ileus

**Harry C. Bishop**   MD, FACS, FAAP
Professor of Pediatric Surgery, The Children's Hospital of Philadelphia, The University of Pennsylvania School of Medicine, Philadelphia, Pennsylvania, USA

**Moritz M. Ziegler**   MD, FACS, FAAP
Associate Professor of Pediatric Surgery, The Children's Hospital of Philadelphia, The University of Pennsylvania School of Medicine, Philadelphia, Pennsylvania, USA

## Preoperative

### Aetiology

Meconium ileus, an intraluminal obstruction due to inspissated meconium, is one of the rare causes of intestinal obstruction in the newborn, occurring in 5–15 per cent of infants afflicted with cystic fibrosis of the pancreas (mucoviscidosis). Cystic fibrosis is a generalized disease involving not only the pancreas but most of the exocrine glands of the body, and occurs once in 2500 live births. Since it is a genetically determined disease other family members may be afflicted, a fact which may help in the initial diagnosis. The familial incidence is due to its autosomal recessive inheritance.

These infants have an abnormal, obstructing meconium due to a deficiency of pancreatic secretions and abnormal mucus secreted by the intestinal glands. The obstruction is complete and requires urgent attention.

# UNCOMPLICATED MECONIUM ILEUS

## 1 & 2

### Appearance of the intestinal tract

The gross appearance of the intestinal tract is characterized by a tremendously dilated loop of lower jejunum or upper ileum containing soft, semi-liquid meconium (a). The ileum just beyond the massive loop measures 2–4 cm in diameter and is firmly packed with a viscid, putty-like meconium, dark in colour and quite adherent to the mucosal lining (b and *see Illustration 2*). Both these segments are hypertrophied due to an overly active *in utero* peristalsis attempting to relieve the obstruction. The distal ileum and occasionally the ascending colon appear beaded, and the thin bowel wall conforms over the individual pellets of abnormal meconium (c). These individual pellets are firm, yellow, green or black in colour, and have a waxy consistency. The colon beyond appears normal, although smaller in diameter than expected, since it has not as yet been used to transport meconium down into the rectum (d).

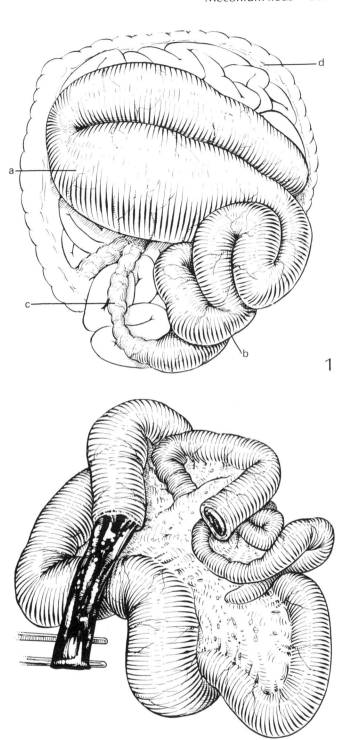

1

2

## DIAGNOSIS

The infant has a distended abdomen at birth. Dilated loops and peristaltic waves may be seen through the thin abdominal wall. Finger pressure over a firm loop of bowel may hold the indentation, the so-called 'putty' sign. Vomiting occurs early and is bile-stained. If a nasogastric tube is passed there is an increased quantity of gastric fluid, which is bile-stained since the duodenal content readily refluxes back into the stomach. There may or may not be a small amount of abnormal meconium passed per rectum, usually in the form of pellets.

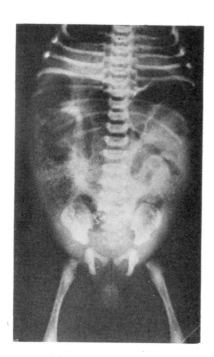

3a

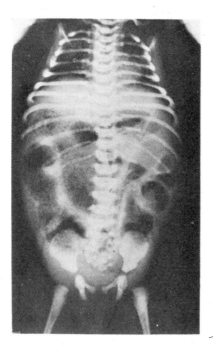

3b

# 3a & b

### Radiographic findings

Radiographs of the abdomen may be diagnostic with the erect film (a) varying little from the supine film (b). Characteristic findings are: (1) great disparity in the size of the intestinal loops due to the configuration of the different segments of the gastrointestinal tract; (2) absent or greatly diminished fluid levels on the upright film, since the swallowed air cannot layer above the thickened inspissated meconium; (3) granular appearance, so-called 'soap bubbles', is frequently seen in the right half of the abdomen and is strongly suggestive of meconium ileus, but can occasionally be seen in intestinal obstruction from other causes. This finding would be seen only after the newborn infant swallows enough air to force the bubbles into the sticky meconium.

## IMMEDIATE MANAGEMENT

*The stomach must be kept empty*  To avoid further distension and aspiration pneumonitis due to vomiting, a multi-holed tube, no smaller than 8 Fr, should be passed through the nose into the stomach, and irrigated and aspirated as necessary to the keep the stomach empty.

*Vitamin K*  One or two milligrams of a vitamin $K_1$ preparation should be given to avoid hypoprothrombinaemia, which might lead to excessive bleeding if laparotomy is necessary.

*Antibiotics*  Antibiotics may help to avoid the early pulmonary complications that so frequently occur in fibrocystic disease, or may be necessary to treat aspiration pneumonia if this has occurred before the baby is decompressed.

*Intravenous catheter*  A reliable route for fluid and electrolyte replacement is essential. This catheter can usually be placed percutaneously without resorting to an open cut-down and can be used continuously until oral feeding is possible.

Fresh frozen plasma, albumin, and type-specific blood should be available and used if necessary.

## NON-OPERATIVE MANAGEMENT OF UNCOMPLICATED MECONIUM ILEUS

Uncomplicated meconium ileus, as diagnosed by the clinical and X-ray findings, may be relieved by the use of Gastrografin enemas. Gastrografin (meglumine diatrizoate) contains a wetting agent, Tween-80 (polyoxyethylene sorbitan mono-oleate). When used as an enema it is capable of separating the very viscid, tenacious meconium from the mucosal wall. Gastrografin has a high osmolarity (1900 mosmol/l); thus, fluid is pulled into the intestinal tract, which further aids in the evacuation of the abnormal meconium.

The contraindications for the use of Gastrografin are discussed under Complicated meconium ileus.

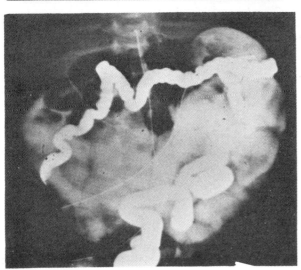

4a

4b

# 4a & b

### Gastrografin enema method

With a well-functioning nasogastric tube in place, ensuring an empty stomach and with a well-functioning intravenous line, a small rectal catheter is passed and the buttocks are strapped together. Under fluoroscopy, the Gastrografin solution is slowly injected by means of a hand syringe, outlining the small and as yet unused colon. Great patience and care must be exercised as the Gastrografin slowly progresses through the entire colon, around the pellets in the terminal ileum, and up into the segment of ileum containing the most inspissated meconium. Hopefully, the Gastrografin can be gradually worked through this obstructing segment and up into the maximally dilated loop. This is the end point of the fluoroscopically controlled enema and the Gastrografin is allowed to remain, separating the inspissated meconium from the surrounding mucosa and liquefying the meconium at the interface.

The rectal catheter is removed and the infant is returned to his incubator; the volume of intravenous fluid is increased in anticipation of the excessive fluid loss due to the hyperosmolarity of the Gastrografin. Over the next few hours, first the obstructing pellets from the terminal ileum and later semi-liquid meconium are evacuated. A second or even third Gastrografin enema may be necessary 6–8 hours later if the first enema failed to reach the proper height in the small bowel or if the amount of meconium evacuated was not adequate to relieve the obstruction.

If this non-operative enema technique fails to relieve the obstruction, or if there are contraindications to its use, laparotomy should not be delayed.

# Operation for uncomplicated meconium ileus

### RESECTION WITH ROUX-EN-Y ILEOSTOMY (BISHOP–KOOP PROCEDURE)

## 5

An endotracheal tube is passed while the infant is awake. The infant is then anaesthetized. This avoids any chance of aspiration during induction. A right transverse incision starting slightly above the level of the umbilicus and extending from the mid-rectus laterally is made. The lateral half of the rectus is transected and the external oblique and internal oblique muscles are divided. The peritoneal cavity is entered by opening the transversalis and posterior rectus fascia and peritoneum as a single layer.

If exploration of the abdomen finds no complications, the following operation is our procedure of choice.

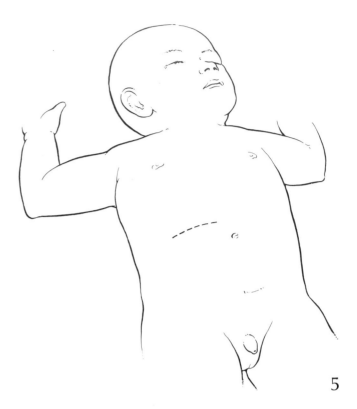

5

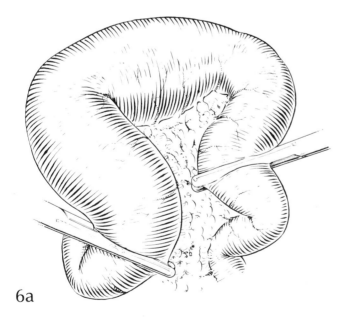

6a

## 6a

Without attempting to empty any of the bowel content, the large dilated loop is resected between intestinal clamps as a means of lessening the volume of the abdominal contents, which will allow an easier, safer abdominal closure, and removes a segment of bowel in which recovery of peristalsis may be delayed. The proximal *end* of the transected ileum is then anastomosed to the *side* of the distal and still obstructed ileum by a Roux-en-Y technique. The anastomosis uses segments of bowel that have been dilated and are thickened, and hence it can be easily accomplished, producing a large, fluid-tight anastomosis.

# 6b & c

The end-to-side anastomosis is fashioned with a continuous 5/0 atraumatic chromic catgut suture placed through all layers as the first inverting layer. A second layer, using interrupted 5/0 silk on atraumatic needles, approximates the seromuscular coats. The mesenteric defect is closed.

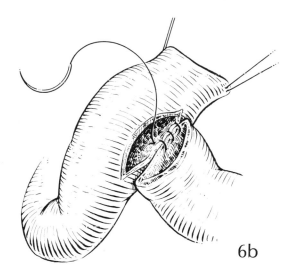

6b

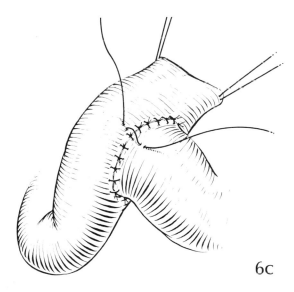

6c

# 6d

The limb of the ileum, 3–4 cm in length, is brought out through the lateral end of the abdominal incision or preferably through a separate stab wound slightly more inferior.

Interrupted seromuscular sutures of atraumatic 5/0 silk are then used to approximate the peritoneum to the full circumference of the exteriorized ileal limb. Several similar sutures are taken at the level of the deep fascia to prevent postoperative dehiscence around the exteriorized limb. It is usually possible to aspirate the meconium from the most exterior portion of the exteriorized limb and frequently down to the level of the end-to-side anastomosis. At this point a soft 8 Fr red rubber catheter, or soft plastic catheter, with multiple holes in the tip is passed down through the exteriorized limb, past, but not through the anastomosis into the lower ileum, and into the still obstructing meconium distal to the anastomosis. A small metal probe positioned in the end hole of the catheter aids its placement 6–8 cm beyond the anastomosis. This catheter should be sutured to the rim of the open end of the ileostomy to prevent inadvertent withdrawal.

The peritoneum is closed with a continuous 3/0 chromic or Vicryl suture, and interrupted sutures of the same materials are used to approximate the internal and external oblique muscles and the anterior rectus fascia. The subcutaneous tissue is closed with 5/0 Vicryl and the same suture is used to close the primary wound with subcuticular interrupted sutures. No additional sutures are placed between the exteriorized ileum and the skin.

When the operation has been completed the infant has a patent intestinal tract from mouth to exteriorized ileostomy. The residual intestinal obstruction is only in the small bowel distal to the anastomosis, and the catheter gives access for postoperative irrigation of this still obstructing meconium.

Once the abdomen is closed, Viokase powder, 2.5 ml in 30 ml of saline or a 10 per cent solution of acetylcysteine, is gently injected through the catheter, 5–8 ml at a time, and this is repeated every 2–3 hours. The meconium gradually liquefies and initially passes back out through the ileostomy. Eventually the obstruction is completely relieved and the meconium then passes down and out of the anus. It is helpful to instil the liquefying enzyme or Gastrografin rectally during the postoperative period, but these solutions should not be placed in the stomach for fear of vomiting and aspiration. It is important to remove the ileostomy irrigating catheter as soon as possible and this can be done on the second, or at the latest, the third postoperative day.

As soon as the distal bowel is free of obstructing meconium the small bowel content will no longer be lost through the ileostomy, since the peristaltic stream is downward and the ileostomy will remain as a non-functioning mucous fistula. There is no urgency to close this and the dangers of an early second operation are therefore avoided. Occasionally the ileostomy will close spontaneously, particularly if it has been trimmed down to just below the skin level with cautery, avoiding a second surgical procedure altogether.

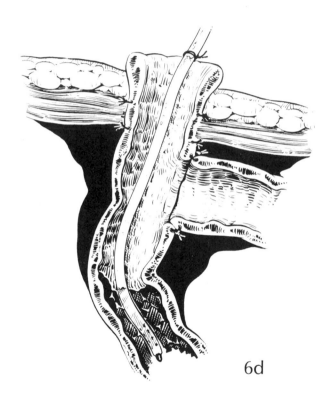

6d

## ALTERNATIVE OPERATIVE PROCEDURES FOR UNCOMPLICATED MECONIUM ILEUS

# 7a & b

### Resection and ileo-ascending colostomy (Swenson procedure)

If the segment of obstruction is short, the entire segment can be excised and ileo-ascending colostomy performed. Rarely is this possible without too great a sacrifice of small bowel.

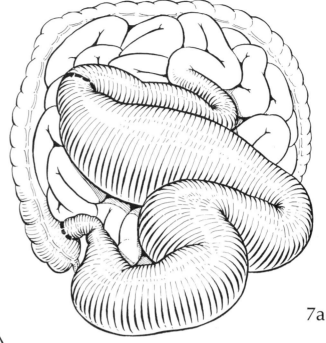

7a

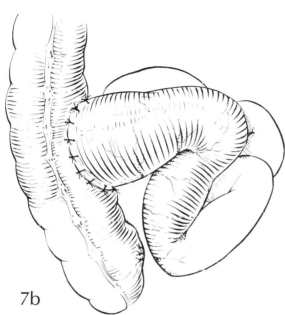

7b

# 8

### Multiple ileostomies and irrigation

Attempts to remove the obstructing meconium through one or more ileostomies while the infant's abdomen is open, although occasionally successful, generally should not be attempted. With this procedure, 'milking' is necessary, since saline or a Viokase solution or Gastrografin will not liquefy meconium on contact but merely loosen it from the mucosa. This leads to contamination of the abdominal cavity and may result in irreversible shock.

Although acetylcysteine liquefies meconium more readily than the solutions mentioned above, the use of an exteriorization procedure seems safer and more reliable. If the lower ileum is merely emptied of inspissated meconium through an ileotomy there is a possibility of recurrence of the obstruction as the more liquid meconium comes down from above and becomes inspissated in the lower intestines.

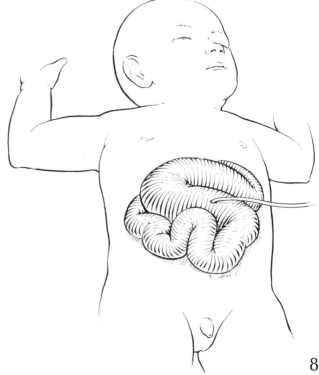

8

# 9a–c

## Mikulicz ileostomy (Gross procedure)

An alternative procedure of great merit is the construction of a double-barrelled Mikulicz ileostomy with resection of the large dilated loop after the abdomen is closed, which avoids any intra-abdominal contamination (*Figure 9a*). This double-barrelled ileostomy avoids the slight danger of an intra-abdominal anastomosis but still offers a route for the instillation of enzymes that will relieve the obstruction in the distal bowel (*Figure 9b*). At the completion of the operation the proximal bowel from mouth to proximal ileostomy is patent. This procedure has the disadvantage that the double-barrelled ileostomy must be closed early in order to eliminate the fluid and electrolyte losses from the small bowel. Even though this closure can be done extraperitoneally after a spur-crushing clamp has created a common lumen for the two limbs (*Figure 9c*), an early second operation is undesirable.

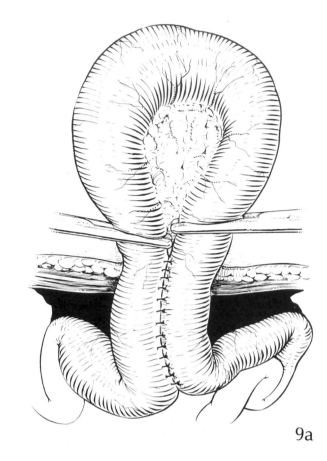

9a

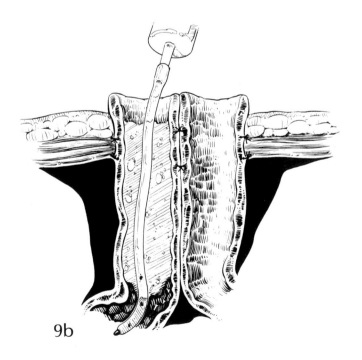

9b

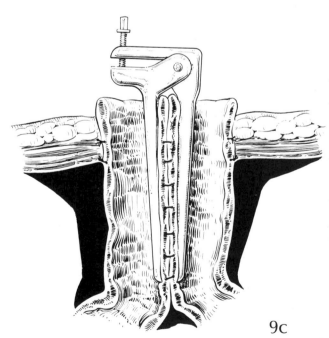

9c

# COMPLICATED MECONIUM ILEUS

Meconium ileus can, unfortunately, develop complications *in utero*. The most common is a volvulus of the massively dilated loop of small bowel, resulting in necrosis and perforation, which leads to meconium peritonitis. The affected segment may undergo gradual absorption producing an atresia of the small bowel at the proximal end of the twist.

These complications can usually be suspected or diagnosed by X-ray examination. Calcification within the peritoneal cavity suggests an *in utero* perforation with soilage of the peritoneal cavity by meconium. Such perforations occasionally seal spontaneously and are not apparent at the time of subsequent laparotomy. Infants with atresia usually show a dilated air-filled loop proximal to the intraluminal obstruction, so that the 'soap bubbling' effect is not as obvious as in the simple cases when the bowel gas has been forced down into the intraluminal meconium. If bowel perforation persists a loculated intraperitoneal pseudocystic type of meconium peritonitis may be present, with or without calcifications.

Gastrografin enema reduction should not be attempted when any one of these complications of meconium ileus is suspected. These infants should be prepared and operated upon without delay.

The procedure used depends on the findings at laparotomy. If there is an atresia with intraluminal obstruction of the distal bowel, a Roux-en-Y anastomosis and single-limb ileostomy for postoperative irrigation may be used. If there is meconium peritonitis with a sealed perforation, the peritonitis is sterile and an intra-abdominal anastomosis with a Roux-en-Y exteriorized limb may be the procedure of choice, since there is no bacterial contamination. If there is free air in the abdominal cavity, suggesting a contaminated meconium peritonitis, a double-barrelled exteriorization as with the Mikulicz procedure may be the procedure of choice, since bacterial contamination might have occurred after delivery.

An alternative method of managing meconium ileus which is unresponsive to Gastrografin enema is to resect the grossly dilated ileum or, in the event of complicated disease, to resect the atretic, perforated, volvulated, or gangrenous intestine. The proximal and distal intestine is cleared of inspissated meconium or mucous plugs by gentle irrigation with Tween-80, sterile Gastrografin, or acetylcysteine, followed by warm isotonic saline washouts until the entire bowel from the duodenojejunal flexure to the anus is completely patent and emptied of meconium. This procedure is time-consuming, and unless handling of the intestine is gentle, serosal tears can occur. Reconstitution of intestinal continuity is achieved by an end-to-end seromuscular anastomosis.

## Postoperative complications

### Delayed relief of remaining obstruction

As has been stated, when using a Roux-en-Y anastomosis and ileostomy (see *Illustration 6a–d*) it is important to irrigate the catheter early and repeatedly during the postoperative period in order to relieve the obstructing meconium in the first two or three days following surgery. On one occasion in our experience the catheter produced a perforation of the ileum when left unused for five days.

### Return of recurrent obstruction

Recurrent obstruction can occur if multiple ileotomies and irrigation (see *Illustration 8*) have been used or if there has been a local resection of the bowel (*Illustration 7*). This is particularly likely to occur if the remaining semi-liquid meconium becomes more inspissated after the operative procedure has been completed.

### Unrelenting pulmonary disease

This is the greatest cause of concern, and early use of humidity, chest physiotherapy, and even tracheal aspiration may be necessary to prevent or treat the pulmonary complications resulting from the thickened and tenacious bronchial secretions.

### Later intestinal obstruction

This may occur due to intra-abdominal adhesions but these are less likely to form if intra-peritoneal contamination from the chemically irritating spilled meconium is avoided.

# Cystic fibrosis: later manifestations and care

After meconium ileus obstruction is relieved, the patient should have laboratory confirmation of the generalized disease. The most common confirmatory study is an analysis of the skin sweat electrolytes, but it is difficult to obtain enough sweat from the infant under two weeks of age. The sweat glands secrete a high concentration of sodium and chloride and levels over 60 mmol/l are, if confirmed twice, considered diagnostic. Duodenal aspirate will reveal a decrease of trypsin, lipase, and amylase in the succus entericus. Since these patients have diminished pancreatic secretions, they require continued substitution animal enzymes in the diet to avoid the malnutrition and steatorrhoea seen in the untreated patient.

Pathological changes also occur in the liver in some patients, leading eventually to cirrhosis and secondary portal hypertension. The male, either at the time of a herniorrhaphy or at autopsy, is often found to have absence of the vas deferens on both sides, which explains the high incidence of infertility in the male patient. Occasionally rectal prolapse is seen in an individual not yet recognized to be fibrocystic, or one who has received inadequate enzyme substitution therapy.

The most common later problems, however, are pulmonary. The abnormal bronchial secretions lead to inspissation of the bronchial mucus, with areas of atelectasis and compensatory emphysema with progressive chronic pulmonary disease.

The management of the generalized disease, therefore, requires prolonged and comprehensive medical care by a practitioner particularly interested in the complications of this disease. The pulmonary problems remain the most demanding. All siblings should be checked for unsuspected fibrocystic disease.

## RESULTS OF TREATMENT OF MECONIUM ILEUS

The results of both medical and surgical management of meconium ileus at The Children's Hospital of Philadelphia have recently been reviewed for the period 1960–1984. During this time 40 patients were admitted. Ten patients died, giving an overall survival of 75 per cent, including both the complicated and the uncomplicated cases. The following charts show a breakdown of the cases into two periods, 1960–1970 and then 1970–1984. For the uncomplicated cases of meconium ileus there were eight cases in the first period, with four survivors, and in the second period there were ten cases, with nine survivors. When reviewing the complicated meconium ileus cases in the first period, there were five cases with no survivors and in the second there were 17 cases with 17 survivors. From 1960–1970 there was, therefore, a 31 per cent overall survival rate whereas from 1970–1984 there was a 96 per cent survival. The one death was not due to the surgical problems but to unrelenting pulmonary disease.

### 1960–1984

| | |
|---|---|
| Uncomplicated meconium ileus | 18 patients: 5 deaths |
| Complicated meconium ileus | 22 patients: 5 deaths |
| | 40 patients: 10 deaths |
| | Survival of 75 per cent |

#### Uncomplicated meconium ileus

| | 1960–70 | 1970–84 |
|---|---|---|
| Enema reduction | 0 | 3/3 survive |
| Bishop-Koop procedure | 6/3 | 6/5 |
| Enterostomy + irrigation | 2/1 | 0 |
| Resection with 1° anastomosis | 0 | 1/1 |
| | 8/4 | 10/9 |

#### Complicated meconium ileus

| | 1960–70 | 1970–84 |
|---|---|---|
| Bishop-Koop procedure | 3/0 | 8/8 survive |
| Mikulicz resection | 1/0 | 2/2 |
| Resection – 1° anastomosis | 0 | 6/6 |
| Resection – stoma | 0 | 1/1 |
| Laparotomy only | 1/0 | 0 |
| | 5/0 | 17/17 |

In summary, we recommend that Gastrografin enema reduction be tried in the uncomplicated cases. The Bishop-Koop procedure, our procedure of choice, has been proven by the test of time. There were 13 survivors of the 14 patients seen during the 1970–1984 period. It must be remembered that those listed as survivors survived 30 days following relief of the intestinal obstruction. Undoubtedly there were some patients who later succumbed to the ravages of the generalized disease.

## Further reading

Bishop, H. C., Koop, C. E. (1957) Management of meconium ileus: resection Roux-en-Y anastomosis and ileostomy irrigation with pancreatic enzymes. Annals of Surgery, 145, 410–414

Gross, R. E. (1953) The Surgery of Infancy and Childhood, p. 175–191. Philadelphia: Saunders

Holsclaw, D. S., Eckstein, H. B., Nixon, H. H. (1965) Meconium ileus: a 20 year review of 109 cases. American Journal of Diseases of Children, 109, 101–113

Neuhauser, E. B. D. (1946) Roentgen changes associated with pancreatic insufficiency in early life. Radiology, 46, 319–328

Noblett, H. R. (1969) Treatment of uncomplicated meconium ileus by Gastrografin enema: a preliminary report. Journal of Pediatric Surgery, 4, 190–197

Lloyd, D. A. (1986) Pediatric Surgery, Vol, 2, K. J. Welsh et al. (eds.), p. 849–858. Chicago: Year Book Medical Publishers

Swenson, O. (1958) Pediatric Surgery, p. 319–324. New York: Appleton-Century-Crofts

Wagget, J., Bishop, H. C., Koop, C. E. (1970) Experience with Gastrografin enema in the treatment of meconium ileus. Journal of Pediatric Surgery, 5, 649–654

Wagget, J., Johnson, D. G., Borns, P., Bishop, H. C. (1970) The non-operative treatment of meconium ileus by Gastrografin enema. Journal of Pediatrics, 77, 407–411

# Meckel's diverticulectomy

**H. Homewood Nixon**   MA, MB, BChir, FRCS(Eng), Hon. FAAP
Honorary Consulting Surgeon, The Hospital for Sick Children, Great Ormond Street, and St. Mary's Hospital, Paddington, London, UK

# Introduction

Meckel's diverticula may have diverse clinical presentations or remain quiescent throughout life. An assessment by Soltero and Bill[1] suggests that the chances of clinical developments do not in general justify the operative risks of 'en passant' removal when the structure is observed during operation for some other reason.

## Presentation

### Acute

1. Inflammation (imitating appendicitis).
2. Haemorrhage (as a result of containing ectopic gastric mucosa producing a peptic ulcer at the base).
3. Perforation (of such an ulcer).
4. Obstruction (a) by invagination of the diverticulum as the apex of an intussusception; (b) by volvulus around a cord from its apex to the umbilicus; (c) by incarceration of a loop of bowel between the diverticulum with a persistent vitelline vessel and the ileal mesentery.

All these forms are potentially *strangulating* obstructions.

### Elective

The commonest presentation is a history of bleeding from the rectum. This is typically profuse, dark red but fluid blood and usually causes anaemia sufficient to require transfusion. Meckel's diverticulum does not produce frequent small bleeds over a long period. After perhaps a small initial bleed there is usually a profuse one.

Such a history merits: (a) exclusion of blood dyscrasia; (b) barium enema, then sigmoidoscopy for polyps. If negative, proceed to exploration for Meckel's diverticulum.

Barium series is of no value in demonstrating the diverticulum but a good intubation barium meal can diagnose a diverticulum if performed by a radiologist skilled in this technique. A technetium radioscan has recently been shown to demonstrate such a diverticulum by concentration in ectopic gastric mucosa. In the author's view, until more experience is gained, the possibility of false negatives would not yet justify failing to explore on negative findings.

## Forms of Meckel's diverticulum

# 1

This shows the typical form which may contain ectopic gastric mucosa – a firm nodule may represent ectopic pancreatic tissue.

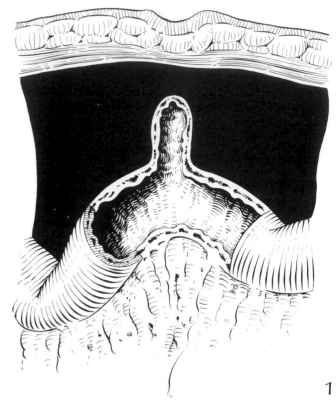

1

# 2

This form has a cord to umbilicus.

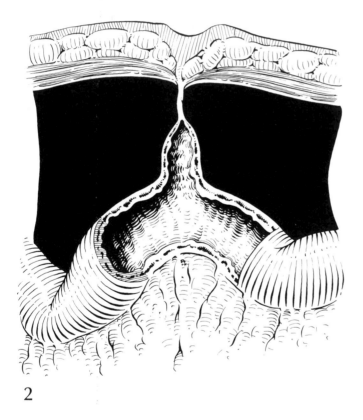

2

# 3

This form has a cord containing a cystic remnant.

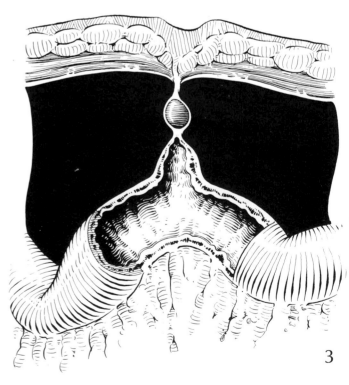

3

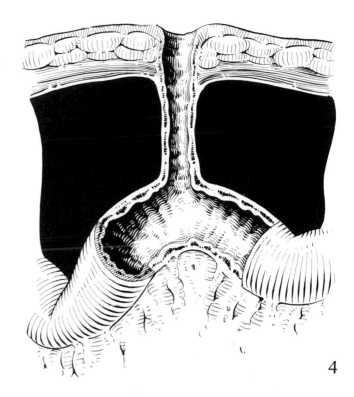

4

# 4 & 5

This form is patent as an umbilical fistula (illustration 4) which may allow prolapse of ileum as a 'pair of horns' (illustration 5).

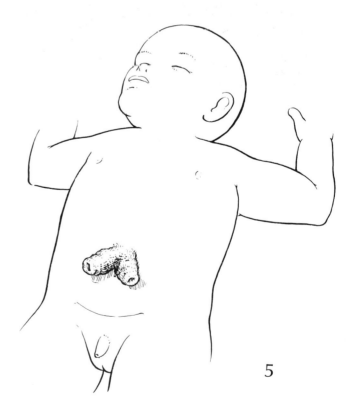

5

# 6

This form is bound down by vitelline vessels from its apex and adherent to ileal mesentery, giving a false appearance of a mesenteric origin. (Division of vessel at apex and of peritoneal fold reveals typical antimesenteric origin).

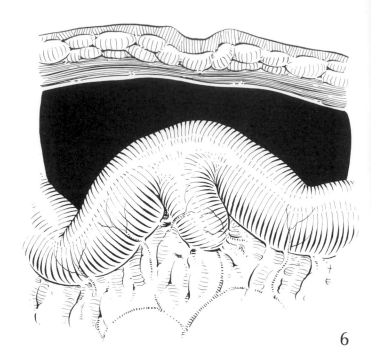

6

# 7

This form presents with a mucosal remnant at the umbilicus. A weeping, minor annoyance, but a reminder that there may (or may not) be a diverticulum within the abdomen.

7

# The operations

### Resection of the diverticulum

The surgical approach is through a high right iliac fossa, muscle-splitting incision. This can be extended medially by retracting the rectus towards the midline, or even dividing the muscle if necessary.

## 8

A crushing clamp is placed across the base of the diverticulum at 45° to the long axis of the ileum. This avoids the narrowing which may be caused by longitudinal incision, or the kinking which may be caused by a transverse one. (It is *essential* that the entire base of the diverticulum is removed, because the ulcer which may be caused by the secretions of ectopic gastric mucosa will arise in the adjacent ileal mucosa. Hence a remnant left at the base of the diverticulum could continue to cause ulceration.)

Mattress sutures of 3/0 catgut are placed under the clamp, tied and the diverticulum cut away at the distal border of the clamp.

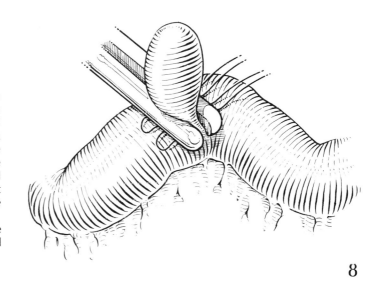

8

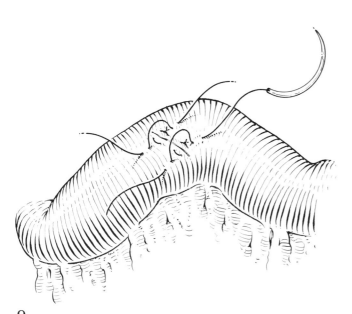

9

## 9

The clamp is then removed and the line of section is buried by a second layer of 3/0 silk Halsted sutures.

# 10

### Alternative method for a broad-based diverticulum

The adjacent ileum is emptied and kept so by application of non-crushing clamps. A stay suture is placed proximal and distal to the diverticulum to control the bowel. The diverticulum is then excised with a wedge of adjacent ileum from the antimesenteric border, leaving the mesenteric border intact. The bowel is closed with a single layer of invaginating mattress sutures of 3/0 silk as for the orthodox end-to-end anastomosis. The last suture is placed from outside the bowel as a Halsted suture.

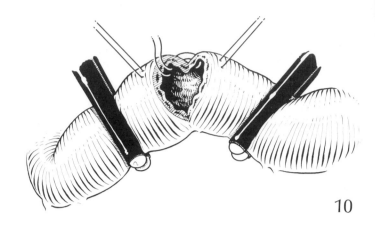

10

# Postoperative care

The only variation from aftercare for a routine abdominal operation is the advisability of the slower introduction of a fluid diet for the first 3 or 4 days after operation. Otherwise there is a tendency for distension and vomiting to develop on about the fourth postoperative day – apparently as a result of the poor peristaltic activity of this weakest muscled part of the small intestine rather than to any organic narrowing, for it soon settles on ceasing feeds.

## References

1. Williams, R. S. (1981) Management of Meckel's diverticulum. British Journal of Surgery, 68, 477–481

# Duplication of the alimentary tract

**James Lister**  MD, FRCS(Ed), FRCS(Glas), FRCS(Eng), FAAP(Hon)
Formerly Professor of Paediatric Surgery, University of Liverpool; Consultant Paediatric Surgeon, Alder Hey Children's Hospital, Liverpool, UK

**George C. Vaos**  MD
Formerly Research Fellow, Department of Paediatric Surgery, University of Liverpool, Alder Hey Children's Hospital, Liverpool, UK

## Introduction

Duplications of the alimentary tract may occur anywhere from the base of the tongue to the rectum. Many terms are used in their description, such as enteric, enterogenous or inclusion cyst and giant diverticulum, but their common derivation from the alimentary tract justifies their description under a common generic term. Whatever their size or shape, they have three common characteristics: they are closely attached to some part of the alimentary canal; they have a coat of smooth muscle; and their lining is of epithelium resembling the mucous membrane of some part of the alimentary tract.

## Aetiology

# 1

There does not appear to be a single explanation for all varieties of duplication. Cystic duplications may result from the persistence of transitory intestinal diverticula which are known to occur in human and animal embryos[1]. They may also result from errors of recanalization in the development of the gut in those areas – duodenum and oesophagus – where the lumen is known to be virtually obliterated at a certain stage of development[2]. Long tubular duplications and some cystic duplications have been explained by the 'notochord theory', suggesting a failure of separation of the roof of the primitive gut from the notochord and the 'tenting' out of a band of endodermal cells, as the ectodermal elements extend cranially early in the fourth week of development. If the endodermal cells remain intact, a tube will be formed running from abdominal gut, passing through the diaphragm and reaching the dorsal spine, which may show vertebral anomalies (butterfly vertebrae). If the tube breaks, a cystic duplication in the mesentery could result[3,4].

The rare cases of duplication of the colon, with two tubes lying side by side rather than anteriorly and posteriorly, may involve the whole of the hind gut and have duplication of the genitourinary tract, as well as doubling of the spine, spina bifida and even doubling of the lower extremities; these probably represent a degree of caudal twinning[5].

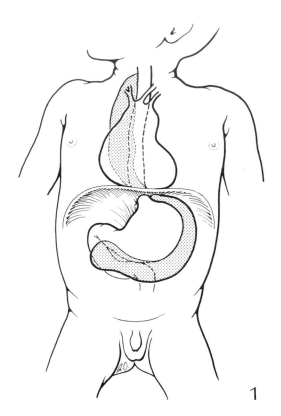

1

## Clinical picture

Duplications may be asymptomatic and found incidentally at laparotomy, but the majority of those which are symptomatic appear in children under 3 months of age. They may present because of their size alone, producing an abdominal mass, or because of pressure effect, for example respiratory distress resulting from lung compression by a large thoracic duplication or duodenal obstruction mimicking pyloric stenosis from quite a small duplication cyst. They may also act as the leading point for an intussusception or a volvulus, or cause perforation or severe haemorrhage from peptic ulceration due to the presence of ectopic gastric mucosa in the lining epithelium, particularly in tubular duplications.

X-ray studies may confirm the presence of a mass or show displacement of bowel or mediastinal structures. Ultrasound scanning may reveal a cystic mass, which is increasingly likely to be detected at antenatal screening. Prenatal aspiration of such cystic lesions should be avoided.

# Preoperative

Some duplications are discovered incidentally at laparotomy. Most, however, will require operation because there have been complications. If intestinal obstruction is present, nasogastric decompression and fluid and electrolyte replacement is indicated. Prophylactic antibiotics may be administered because of presumed inflammatory reaction around the duplication and in anticipation of bowel resection. Cross-matched blood must be available since the duplication may already have bled and dissection of the lesion, particularly dissection of the mucosa alone, may involve considerable blood loss.

# The operations

The surgical approach is determined not only by the site of the lesion but also by its shape and its relation to surrounding structures, particularly blood vessels. These are benign lesions and minimal interference with normal organs is essential.

## CYSTIC DUPLICATION

# 2

Complete removal of a cyst without damage to adjacent organs is rarely possible. Exceptions are the non-communicating thoracic lesions commonly related to the oesophagus on the right side, which can be approached transpleurally through a posterolateral mid-thoracotomy, and the small perianal cysts lined with bowel mucosa.

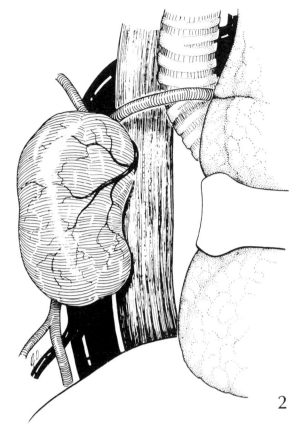

2

# 3, 4 & 5

In cystic duplication of ileum or jejunum, the muscular coats of normal bowel and duplication are often continuous, making excision of the cyst alone very difficult. Even if the muscle coats are separate, enucleation of the cyst may endanger the blood supply of the remaining intestine since the cyst lies between the leaves of the mesentery. It is therefore necessary to resect a loop of bowel together with the cyst and approximate the ends with an end-to-end anastomosis using a single layer of interrupted inverting horizontal mattress sutures of 4/0 silk through all coats.

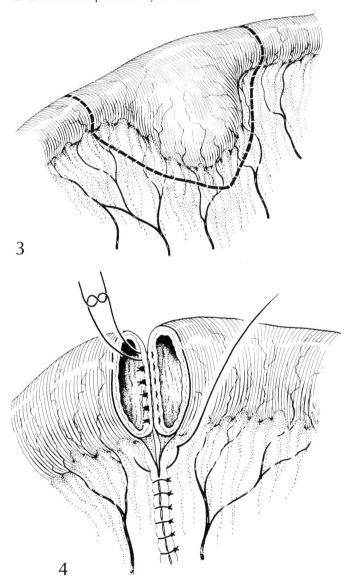

3

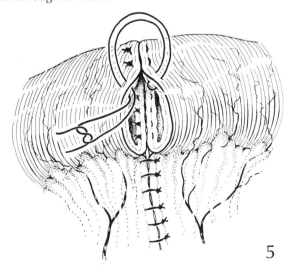

4

5

# 6

A similar technique can be used for small duplications of the stomach. A wedge of stomach is excised together with the cyst which is usually on the greater curvature, and the gap closed with a single layer of through-and-through inverting mattress sutures.

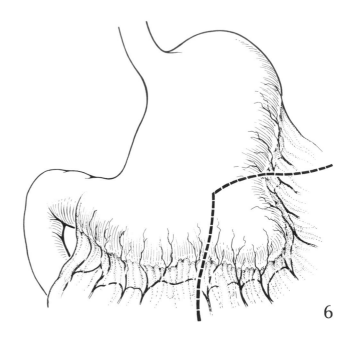

6

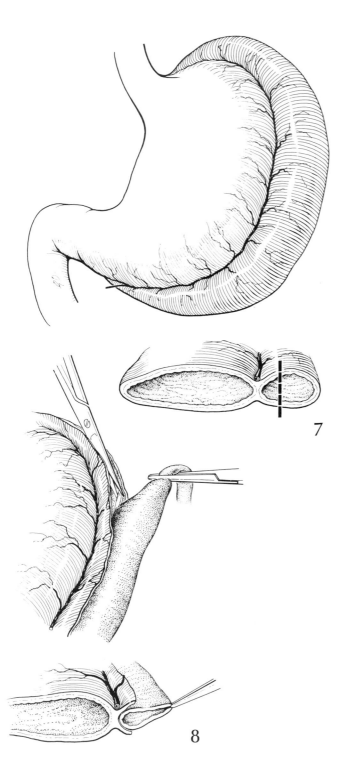

7

# 7, 8 & 9

When resection of the adjoining normal gut is impracticable, as in duplications involving the whole of the greater curvature of the stomach or duodenal duplications close to the ampulla of Vater, the main part of the duplication may be excised and the remaining mucosa at the point of contact with normal stomach or duodenum stripped off. The fringe of seromuscular coat can then be sutured over the denuded area after closing any communication with the adjacent organ.

8

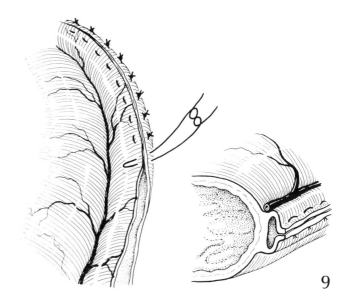

9

## TUBULAR DUPLICATION

# 10a & b

Tubular duplications of the small intestine may occasionally be relatively short and can then be treated in the same way as cystic dilatations (*see Illustrations 3 and 4*). More commonly, however, they involve a considerable length of intestine. Unlike cystic duplications, they usually communicate with the normal bowel. If the communication is only at the distal end, the duplication remains tubular (*a*), but if the distal end is blind and the communication is at the proximal end, there is likely to be considerable distension distally (*b*). The duplication may be closely related to the adjacent small bowel for its entire length, sharing its muscle coat, or it may deviate from the normal bowel, passing between the leaves of the mesentery. Most of these tubular duplications contain gastric mucosa, which is responsible for the pathological features of ulceration and bleeding or perforation. It is mandatory that formal segmental resection of the junction of the duplication and the normal bowel should be carried out with an end-to-end anastomosis. This resection must include 3–4 cm of normal bowel distal to the junction because there may be peptic ulceration in the normal bowel mucosa at this level. Total extirpation of the remainder of the tubular duplication together with the normal adjacent bowel may involve an unacceptably major intestinal resection.

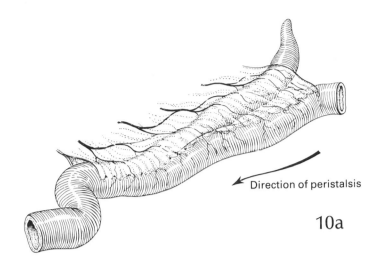

Direction of peristalsis

**10a**

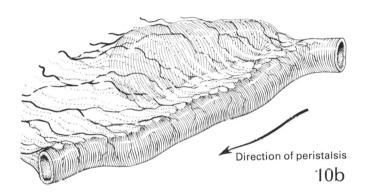

Direction of peristalsis

**10b**

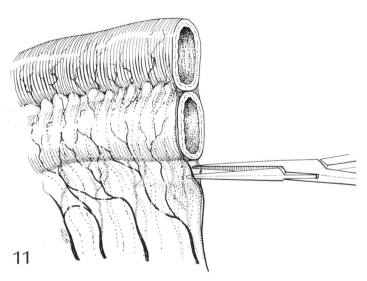

**11**

# 11

In some instances, especially when the duplication deviates from the normal bowel (*see Illustration 10a*), it may be possible to take advantage of the anatomical arrangement of the superior mesenteric artery whose terminal branches tend to run alternatively to either side of the gut between muscle and serosa. Bianchi[6] showed experimentally that it was possible, by careful separation of the peritoneal leaves of the mesentery, to separate these two groups of arteries so that division of the vessels on one side allows enucleation of the duplication without jeopardizing the blood supply of the adjacent normal bowel.

**12**

Alternatively, a submucosal resection as described by Wrenn[7] can be carried out. The mucosal lining is stripped out using several longitudinal incisions through the seromuscular coat if necessary. This can be done by blunt dissection after submucosal injection of saline to help define the line of cleavage. A varicose vein stripper may help in this procedure. The remainder of the seromuscular sleeve of the duplication may be safely left *in situ*. Bleeding from the raw muscle surface almost always stops spontaneously.

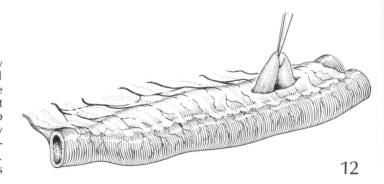

**12**

## THORACOABDOMINAL DUPLICATIONS
(see *Illustration 1*)

When it is known that the patient has a thoracoabdominal duplication, the thoracic portion is dealt with first unless there are complications related to the abdominal portion. Through a mid-posterolateral thoracotomy (usually on the right) the duplication is freed transpleurally. At the upper extremity of the duplication there is likely to be a deep attachment to bone, especially if there is an abnormal vertebral body. This extension must be separated from bone with a gouge or chisel, since infection of any residual communication may result in meningitis. The duplication is followed downwards where it lies free in the mediastinum and usually passes behind the diaphragm to communicate with duodenum or small bowel. Rarely it may pass through the oesophageal hiatus and end in relation to the stomach. The duplication is pulled up into the chest and divided between ligatures. The upper part is removed and the lower end dropped into the abdomen. The chest is closed with drainage.

The abdominal portion of the duplication can be approached at a later stage or at the same operation. Most commonly it appears as a tubular duplication communicating with the jejunum and is dealt with as such. Occasionally it ends blindly, passing through the leaves of the gastrosplenic ligament and around the greater curvature of the stomach. This portion may be dealt with similarly to the large duplication of the stomach.

Thoracoabdominal duplication may present as an emergency. The thoracic element may develop peptic ulceration and erode into the oesophagus or more commonly the lung, causing haematemesis or haemoptysis. Excision of the duplication may involve lobectomy in such cases; the abdominal extension may be closed and dealt with at a later stage. If the emergency procedure has been a laparotomy for exsanguinating gastrointestinal bleeding, and a tubular duplication with a thoracic extension has been found, the upper extension of the lesion can be closed in a similar way. However, in this case, the thoracic stage of the operation must not be delayed for more than a day or two because secretions and possibly bleeding into the undrained thoracic part could result in the development of a large cystic lesion with possible respiratory embarrassment.

## COLONIC DUPLICATIONS

Colonic duplications usually involve the whole length of the colon and are complicated by abnormalities of the lumbosacral spine and urogenital system. Both colons communicate with the faecal stream proximally. Distally they may both open on the perineum, or one or both may terminate blindly in the pelvis or by a fistula into the genitourinary tract. The principal aim of management is to end up with the two colons draining through one anal orifice. If one or both already reach the perineum, then one colon is divided across and anastomosed to the other, the mucous membrane of the detached distal part being excised and any fistula closed. If neither colon reaches the perineum, then a similar anastomosis is carried out after treating one colon by a pull-through procedure as for a high anorectal anomaly. In either case a preliminary colostomy is made to drain both colons.

# Results

In the 15 years from 1969 to 1983 in Alder Hey Children's Hospital, 32 duplications were treated in 29 patients (*see* Table 1).

**Table 1 Site and morphology of duplications of the alimentary tract treated in Alder Hey Children's Hospital, 1969–1983**

| Site | Cystic | Tubular | Total |
|------|--------|---------|-------|
| Oesophagus | 3 | 0 | 3 |
| Stomach | 1* | 0 | 1 |
| Jejunum | 3† | 2§ | 5 |
| Ileum and ileocaecal | 11** | 4 | 15 |
| Colon | 2 | 3†† | 5 |
| Rectum | 3 | 0 | 3 |
| Total | 23 | 9 | 32 |

\* This patient also had a separate cystic duplication of the oesophagus.
† One of these patients had a separate cystic duplication of the oesophagus and another also had a tubular ileal duplication.
§ One patient also had a tubular ileal duplication.
** All these were in the distal ileum or ileocaecal region.
†† Two of these were complete hindgut duplications.

Only 5 of the 29 patients were over one year old on admission. Eighteen presented in the neonatal period, three between 1 and 6 months of age and another three from 7 to 12 months. The tubular hindgut duplications presented in the neonatal period because of their associated anorectal anomalies. The majority of the cystic jejunoileal lesions were recognized as a palpable mass shortly after birth, and more than half of the tubular jejunoileal duplications caused gastrointestinal haemorrhage very early in life.

Three children were investigated for rectal bleeding on one or more occasions before a duplication was diagnosed – diagnosis was delayed for up to one year. Another child had an ileocaecal intussusception reduced by barium enema at the age of 8 years, and 4 years later had a recurrent ileocaecal intussusception resected with an ileocaecal cystic duplication at its apex.

Operative treatment was by excision in almost every case. The mucosal stripping technique (*see Illustrations 7, 8 and 9*) was used only once, for a para-oesophageal cyst. Postoperative complications were few. One child with an oesophageal duplication developed a chylothorax after excision and another developed Horner's syndrome. One boy with jejunal tubular duplication had recurrent bleeding 9 months after resection: this was found at reoperation to be due to ectopic gastric mucosa related to a small duplication at a higher level in the jejunum. Two patients had an anastomotic leak and wound dehiscence following excision of tubular jejunoileal duplications with end-to-end bowel anastomosis; in each case there had been preoperative perforation of a peptic ulcer.

Only one patient died. This was a neonate who had undergone reduction of a volvulus and resection with end-to-end anastomosis for ileal atresia. He subsequently developed a leak from the anastomosis as a result of which he eventually died. Post mortem examination revealed a previously undetected cystic rectal duplication causing partial large bowel obstruction.

The following conclusions may be drawn:

1. Unexplained, significant gastrointestinal bleeding in children, particularly those under 1 year of age, should suggest the possibility of duplication. Investigation should include isotope scanning for ectopic gastric mucosa.
2. Intussusception in children over the age of 2 years should be viewed with suspicion; it is unlikely to be of the idiopathic type and a cystic duplication is among the possible causes. Should it be reduced by hydrostatic pressure, an ultrasound study of the terminal ileum should be carried out a few days later when the oedema has subsided. A small cystic duplication might still remain undetected.
3. When one duplication has been found, the presence of others should be suspected and excluded by preoperative investigations where possible and adequate exposure during operation.
4. In most cases, it will be possible to remove the entire duplication. However, when total extirpation might endanger neighbouring normal structures or when a hazardous dissection seems likely, the possibility of stripping the mucosa, leaving a seromuscular sleeve or cuff should be considered. This would seem to be particularly important in mediastinal duplications, where the thoracic duct or sympathetic trunk may be at risk.

## References

1. Lewis, F. T., Thyng, F. W. (1907) The regular occurrence of intestinal diverticula in embryos of the pig, rabbit and man. American Journal of Anatomy, 7, 505–519

2. Bremer, J. L. (1944) Diverticula and duplications of the intestinal tract. Archives of Pathology, 38, 132–140

3. Fallon, M., Gordon, A. R. G., Lendrum, A. C. (1954) Mediastinal cysts of foregut origin associated with vertebral abnormalities. British Journal of Surgery, 41, 520–533

4. Bentley, J. F. R., Smith, J. R. (1960) Developmental posterior enteric remnants and spinal malformations: the split notochord syndrome. Archives of Disease in Childhood, 35, 76–86

5. Ravitch, M. M. (1953) Hindgut duplications: doubling of the colon and genital urinary tracts. Annals of Surgery, 137, 588–601

6. Bianchi, A. (1980) Intestinal loop lengthening – a technique for increasing small intestinal length. Journal of Paediatric Surgery, 15, 145–151

7. Wrenn, E. L., Jr. (1962) Tubular duplication of the small intestine. Surgery, 52, 494–498

# Intussusception

**Vanessa M. Wright**  FRCS, FRACS
Consultant Paediatric Surgeon, Queen Elizabeth Hospital for Children, and University College Hospital, London, UK

An intussusception is an invagination of proximal bowel into the lumen of the distal bowel. The leading point or apex of an intussusception in children is typically a Peyer's patch in the terminal ileum, the ileocaecal valve itself or the caecal wall. The apex commonly reaches the midtransverse colon but can proceed distally sufficiently far to be palpable on rectal examination and on rare occasions may even present at the anal margin. The incidence is highest in infants between 4 and 10 months of age but earlier and later (up to 2 years) presentation is not unusual.

## Aetiology

There is very often a preceding history of upper respiratory tract infection, gastroenteritis or a significant change in diet (i.e. weaning). The finding at operation of an oedematous Peyers patch as the leading point and of enlarged mesenteric lymph nodes suggests 'irritation' of the intestinal lymphoid tissue. There is some serological evidence for adenovirus infection but to date no single aetiological factor predominates and the term 'idiopathic' remains appropriate. Occasionally a Meckel's diverticulum, polyp, intramural cyst or solid tumour may initiate an intussusception. A pathological leading point should always be suspected when the child is outside the usual age range and the intussusception has occurred away from the terminal ileal and caecal region.

## Clinical presentation

Sudden onset of spasmodic pain is characteristic, the episodes of pain occurring with remarkable regularity. Initially the child may behave normally between the spasms but after some hours lethargy and pallor occur. Vomiting is common but is rarely bile-stained in the first few hours. Overt rectal bleeding is not a consistent finding; in many cases blood in the rectum only becomes apparent on rectal examination. A palpable abdominal mass, most easily felt in the right upper quadrant, is the cardinal sign of an intussusception and may be present in the absence of all the typical symptoms. There may be a feeling of emptiness in the right iliac fossa. Tenderness and guarding over the mass may preclude easy palpation but is sufficient to justify further investigation.

The characteristic radiological features of a low small bowel obstruction usually occur late. More often the bowel gas pattern is not particularly abnormal although a paucity of gas in the bowel is not unusual. The soft tissue mass of the intussusception may be visible as an opacity. Where doubt exists, a barium enema will confirm or exclude the diagnosis.

# BARIUM ENEMA REDUCTION

Hydrostatic reduction of an intussusception by barium enema under fluoroscopic control is possible in the vast majority of cases. It is widely accepted, however, that this procedure is contraindicated in seriously ill children requiring intensive resuscitation and in those with signs of peritonitis. Some radiologists may add a history of more than 48 hours, passage of blood per rectum and radiological evidence of a bowel obstruction to the list of contraindications.

## The technique

Adequate sedation and analgesia are essential. Pethidine compound in appropriate dosage is effective. Ideally an intravenous infusion and a nasogastric tube should be in position before starting the enema but this is not essential in early cases if the child is well.

Barium is instilled through a well-secured wide-bore tube from a reservoir no more than 90 cmH$_2$O above the patient and its progress is monitored on the fluoroscope. Initial reduction of the intussusception is often rapid and may be complete, with filling of several loops of ileum. Frequently, however, the barium is held up in the caecum. If there is no further progress after 3–4 minutes, the hydrostatic pressure is reduced and some of the barium evacuated. Two further attempts are then made to reduce the remaining bowel. Occasionally there is doubt whether the persistent filling defect in the caecum is unreduced terminal ileum or an oedematous ileocaecal valve. In these circumstances it may be reasonable to return the child to the ward and take a plain abdominal X-ray an hour or so later. This may show the barium to have refluxed into the ileum or may demonstrate the persisting intussusception.

The radiological criterion for reduction is reflux of barium into the ileum. If this does not occur, laparotomy is mandatory. Occasionally the colon is extremely irritable and there is difficulty retaining the barium. Hyoscine (Buscopan) or glucagon may then be used. If the barium is diluted, physiological saline should be used, not water, to avoid the possibility of excessive water absorption leading to water intoxication. Oral fluids can be introduced a few hours after successful reduction. The child should be observed in hospital for 48 hours after reduction.

# SURGICAL REDUCTION AND RESECTION

## Preoperative

Many children, particularly if barium enema reduction is not available as an alternative, will require little preoperative resuscitation. Those considered unfit for barium enema will usually benefit from intravenous fluids, including plasma or blood, antibiotics and gastric decompression with a nasogastric tube. Optimal resuscitation is usually achieved within 2–4 hours and no benefit will accrue from delaying surgery beyond this time since this is a strangulating obstruction.

### Anaesthesia

General anaesthesia with endotracheal intubation and relaxation is essential. Antibiotics are advisable after induction of anaesthesia because appendicectomy is likely to be carried out and bowel resection may be necessary.

# The operation

## The incision

### 1

A right transverse skin incision is made above the umbilicus. The lateral abdominal muscles, anterior rectus sheath, and rectus muscle are divided, the extent of division being dictated by the exposure required to reach the apex of the intussusception

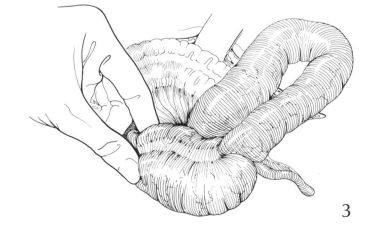

1

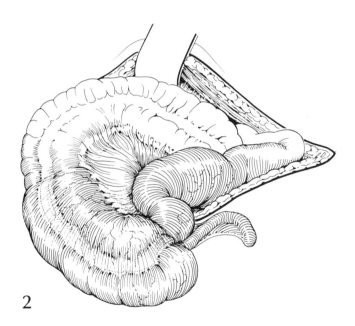

2

## Reduction of intussusception

### 2

Delivery of the bowel involved in the intussusception, particularly the right colon, facilitates reduction and reduces manipulation of the remainder of the proximal bowel. To achieve this the bands between right colon and lateral abdominal wall are divided by a combination of sharp dissection and sweeping with a pledget.

### 3

Once the affected section of bowel has been delivered, packs are positioned to absorb any fluid which escapes from the space between intussusceptum and intussuscipiens during the reduction. Reduction is achieved by squeezing the bowel distal to the apex as though squeezing a tube of toothpaste. Placing a layer of gauze between the bowel and fingers may facilitate manipulation. Traction on the intussuscepted bowel should be avoided but a gentle pull may establish the direction in which to apply the reducing push.

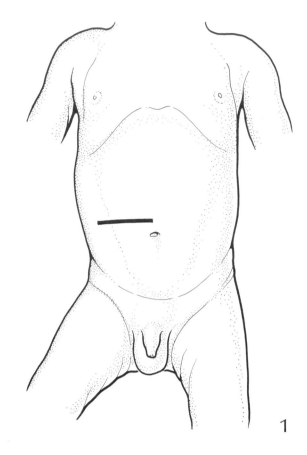

3

## 4

Reduction of ileum through the ileocaecal valve requires patience. Using both thumbs to push on the apex while using the fingers to pull back the caecal wall is usually effective.

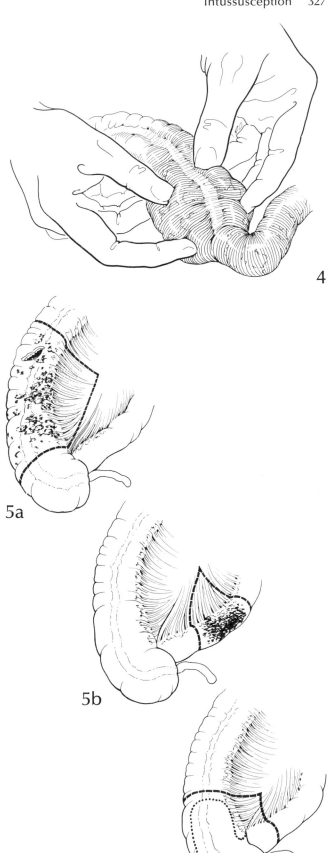

**4**

**Resection**

# 5a, b & c

Resection is necessary if the intussusception cannot be reduced, or if after reduction there is necrotic bowel or a pathological lead point, e.g. a Meckel's diverticulum or a duplication cyst. It is occasionally necessary if reduction has caused serious trauma and perforation of the ascending colon or caecal wall which has already been stretched by the contained intussusception. Even if resection is necessary the intussusception should be reduced as far as possible and only the minimum of bowel compatible with a good blood supply to the two ends should be removed. Formal right hemicolectomy is rarely required. An oedematous ileocaecal valve or Peyers patch can mimic an intraluminal mass – careful palpation and a knowledge of the likely aetiology of this condition, particularly in the young infant, should prevent unnecessary resection. Appendicectomy is not contraindicated if the adjacent caecal wall is normal.

**5a**

**5b**

**5c**

### Anastomosis

## 6

Care should be taken when using bowel clamps on the intestine of young infants because of the risk of trauma. If the contents of the proximal bowel are sucked out, the need for a clamp may be avoided. A single layer of 4/0 black silk mattress sutures is used for the anastomosis, tying the knots on the inside to ensure good serosal apposition. Any mesenteric defect must be closed. In seriously ill infants requiring resection it may be wiser to bring the ends of the bowel out through the wound as ostomies. Closure is then postponed until the child's general condition has improved and the proximal ileostomy is working – usually after 36–48 hours.

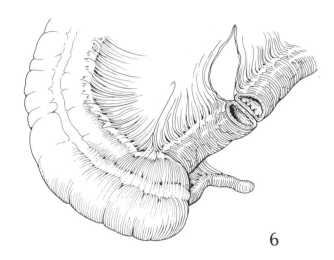

6

## Postoperative care

Appropriate intravenous fluids are continued until oral feeds are tolerated. A nasogastric tube decompresses the stomach, and is left on free drainage and regular aspiration initially. Return of satisfactory bowel function is indicated by the absence of abdominal distension, minimal nasogastric aspirate and the passage of stools. Antibiotics may be continued if necessary for a maximum of 48 hours after operation. A high temperature is common in the first 24–48 hours and usually subsides without specific measures.

## Prognosis

About 2–4 per cent of children will have a recurrence of intussusception.

Death following an intussusception is rare unless there has been a significant delay in diagnosis.

If an extensive length of ileum has been resected, the child will require long-term follow-up to monitor vitamin $B_{12}$ absorption. Loss of the ileocaecal valve may also affect absorption and transit time.

## References

1. Hoy, G. R., Dunbar, D., Boles, E. T. (1977) The use of glucagon in the diagnosis and management of ileocolic intussusception. Journal of Pediatric Surgery, 12, 939–944

2. Ein, S. H., Stephens, C. A. (1971) Intussusception: 354 cases in 10 years. Journal of Pediatric Surgery, 6, 16–27

3. Man, D. W. K., Heath, A. L., Eckstein, H. B. E. (1983) Intussusception in infancy and childhood – a thirteen year review of 75 patients. Zeitschrift für Kinderchirurgie, 38, 383–386

Illustrations by Kevin Marks

# Appendicectomy

**Barry O'Donnell** MCh, FRCSI, FRCS
Professor of Paediatric Surgery, Royal College of Surgeons in Ireland, Consultant Paediatric Surgeon, Children's Research Centre, Our Lady's Hospital for Sick Children, Dublin, Ireland

## History

It seems likely that appendix abscesses, or appendix masses, were drained from time to time before formal appendicectomy was first carried out. Reginald Fitz, a Boston surgeon (1843–1913), coined the word 'appendicitis'. Although T. G. Morton of Philadelphia carried out the first deliberate appendicectomy for ruptured appendicitis in 1887, the name of Charles McBurney (1845–1913) of New York is most closely associated with appendicitis because of his accurate and careful description of the point of maximum tenderness. He used the expression 'the seat of greatest pain'. In the United Kingdom, the best known name in appendicitis is that of Sir Frederick Treves (1853–1923), whose name is attached to the not always bloodless fold between the caecum and ileum. The dramatic circumstances, and the safe outcome, of King Edward VII's appendicectomy in Buckingham Palace, London, two days before the date proposed for his Coronation in 1902, did much to popularise the operation.

The initial mortality and morbidity of appendicitis was high, particularly if perforation and other complications had occurred. Because of this, appendicectomy was advised and carried out in a great number of patients (on slender indications) between 1910 and 1950. Significant postoperative complications are now uncommon. Adequate intravenous fluids and effective antibiotics have reduced the mortality in childhood to almost zero so that a more rational and expectant approach can now be used safely in patients in whom the diagnosis is in doubt.

The single most important recent advance has been the introduction of metronidazole, which, in combination with other new antimicrobials, has greatly reduced the rate of complications.

# Preoperative

## Indications

Appendicectomy is indicated if the diagnosis of appendicitis is made. Operation is usually advisable within a few hours. The most serious forms of appendicitis result from obstruction of the lumen, and in these cases it is usually a progressive condition. In time, the obstruction will result in increased permeability of the appendix, allowing microorganisms to escape into the peritoneum; a gradual attenuation of the wall; and eventually gangrene and rupture with local spillage of the appendix contents (pus and faeces). The timescale of these events is influenced by many factors, including the resistance of the wall (which may be less in early childhood), contents of the lumen, site of the obstruction and, significantly, the completeness or otherwise of the luminal obstruction. It follows that the operation is usually advisable within a matter of hours particularly if it is considered that the appendix is unperforated. Paradoxically, if the appendix is considered to be perforated there is less urgency, and preparation for up to 12 hours may be necessary in an ill child with generalized peritonitis. Surgery for an appendix mass may be deferred for weeks. Appendicectomy should also be considered during any elective laparotomy in childhood, particularly large bowel surgery. Removal is also advised during laparotomy for tumours and splenectomy, where the future immune response may be compromised. We routinely remove it during abdominal operations such as those for hiatus hernia and intussusception, and advise its removal during laparotomy in the newborn unless there is generalized peritonitis. In our experience there have been no complications as a result of this policy.

## Contraindications

The commonest contraindication to appendicectomy is an appendix mass or abscess. Operation should be deferred until this has resolved.

Vigorous conservative management of the appendix mass, even if it is discovered only when the patient is anaesthetized and on the operating table, is effective in terms of both hospital stay and morbidity.

## Preparation of patient

In appendicitis without perforation, no preparation is required other than passing of a nasogastric tube and appropriate anaesthetic premedication. An intravenous infusion is set up routinely, partly to facilitate the administration of anaesthetic agents.

If there is evidence of perforation of the appendix, such as abdominal distension, generalized tenderness, a rapid pulse of over 120/min and a pyrexia above 38.5°C, the operation should be deferred until the temperature and pulse have been controlled. If anaesthesia is induced before this, the pulse may accelerate further (this may be accompanied by peripheral circulatory shutdown) and the temperature may rise steeply to hyperpyrexia. This combination is the real cause of what used to be known as 'ether convulsions'. Hyperpyrexia remains a common cause of an uncommon event – death from appendicitis in childhood. Temperature control is achieved by sedation, intravenous fluids and antibiotics in *adequate* dosage. If the operation is delayed to prepare the child for surgery, sedation with morphine 1 mg/5 kg body weight is indicated. If intravenous fluids are required, a 4-year-old child with a perforated appendix will need about 1000 ml of half-strength isotonic saline given over 1–2 hours, while a 12-year-old may require double this volume.

If there is any possibility that the appendix is perforated, intravenous antibiotics active against Gram-negative bacilli and bacteroides are given. The introduction of metronidazole has been a turning point in the battle against the bacteroides. Oral, intravenous and rectal forms are all effective. Rectal suppositories providing a dose of 0.5 g or 1.0 g are well tolerated. The dose of intravenous metronidazole is 15 mg/kg infused over one hour, followed by a maintenance dose of 7.5 mg/kg every six hours. Blood concentrations after intravenous injections approximate those after rectal administration, indicating nearly complete absorption from mucosal surfaces.

An aminoglycoside (e.g. gentamicin) is administered routinely because of its effectiveness against Gram-negative bacilli. In patients with normal renal function, it is given eight-hourly to a total of 8 mg/kg per day. In life-threatening infections the amount may be increased and adjusted according to the results of serum assays. Higher doses are also necessary in infants. If possible, its concentration in the blood stream should be monitored to ensure that it is present in adequate minimum inhibitory concentration (MIC). Overdosage or renal shutdown can cause ototoxicity and nephrotoxicity if there is any renal tubular damage.

If the patient is dehydrated, a urethral catheter should be passed to assess the response to rehydration. As indicated earlier, operation should not be undertaken until the pulse is below 120/min and the temperature below 38.5°C.

## Special equipment

A bowel-holding forceps, e.g. Denis Browne's, is useful. The author tries to use diathermy as little as possible. Suction is essential when perforation has occurred, though multiple moist packs probably pick up as much pus. All packs used within the abdomen should be wet so as not to abrade the fragile serosa of the bowel.

## Anaesthesia

Rectal premedication with pentothal is reliable. Morphine 1 mg/5 kg body weight or Omnopon with an appropriate dose of atropine sulphate is the usual premedication in older children but the atropine is omitted if the temperature is high.

General anaesthesia is essential and an endotracheal tube adds to safety. Halothane, Ethrane (enflurane) or nitrous oxide and oxygen with muscle relaxants are usually used.

## Position of patient

The child should be supine and placed towards the right side of the table if an adult table is being used. Chlorhexidine solution is a suitable antiseptic for skin preparation.

Four towels surround the generous area of exposed abdomen. They are placed (1) well above the umbilicus, (2) well to the left of the umbilicus, (3) lateral to the right anterior superior iliac spine and (4) horizontal across the pubic bones.

# The operation

## The incision

# 1

Before proceeding with the operation it is most important to palpate the abdomen of the fully anaesthetized patient. An inflamed appendix or small mass can frequently be felt, which helps greatly in siting the incision. If a large mass is palpated even at this late stage, operation should be deferred.

McBurney's incision with the various modifications and extensions available is the *only* incision required in childhood appendicitis. Even if there is doubt about the diagnosis, unless there is a palpable mass, it covers almost all diagnostic errors. In practice the great majority of patients operated on for appendicitis in whom the appendix is not inflamed require no further surgery. Meckel's diverticulum occurs in about 1 per cent of normal children whether or not the appendix is inflamed, but complications of the diverticulum are much less common and can be dealt with through a gridiron incision.

The siting and direction of the incision requires particular care in the podgy abdominal wall of the toddler or plump child. The presence of a small palpable mass obviously influences the site but in a child it is always wise to make the incision too high rather than too low and too lateral rather than too medial. If nothing abnormal is palpated at the preliminary examination the incision is planned as follows.

McBurney's point is marked one-third of the way from the anterior superior iliac spine to the umbilicus. The incision above it is almost transverse, with two-thirds extending lateral to this point and one-third medial. A common mistake is to make the incision too medial and too low.

Small 'keyhole' incisions are only suitable for interval appendicectomy. An adequate incision will make the operation safer and quicker, and if there is any periappendicular infection it will also reduce the likelihood of wound infection.

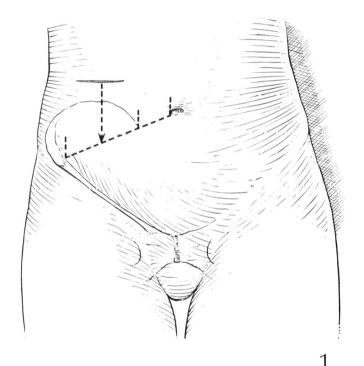

1

## 2

The external oblique muscle, which is muscular in its upper part and aponeurotic in the lower, is divided generously along the line of its fibres from the right flank down towards the pubis. It is this layer that determines the adequacy of the exposure.

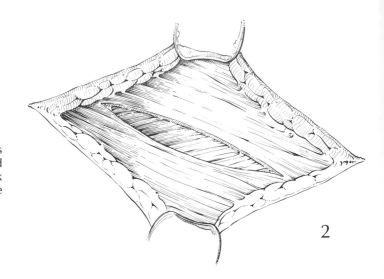

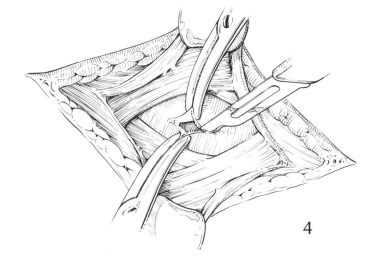

## 3

The internal oblique is entirely muscular in this region and its fibres are best separated by passing blunt-tipped scissors through the muscle. The thinner underlying transversus abdominis can be separated along with it since the fibres of both muscles run almost transversely and slightly upwards from the flank. First the left and then the right forefinger is put into the hole and the fibres are pulled apart.

## 4

The peritoneum is now grasped with an artery forceps, taking care not to include any bowel. Another artery forceps is placed 5 mm away. The peritoneum is incised transversely with a knife and the opening enlarged with scissors. If free pus is found, it is advisable to take a specimen and put a gentle sucker into the wound. The sump variety with many holes is the least traumatic.

# 5

The caecum is then delivered out of the wound by passing the right forefinger into the opening as far laterally as possible, crooking the finger to engage a taenia coli. It should now be possible to lift the caecum into the wound so that the actual appendicectomy can be performed under complete control. If the caecum is adherent to the posterior abdominal wall (either by congenital or in-flammatory adhesions), the lateral peritoneal fold will have to be divided, usually with the fingertip, until it can be delivered out of the wound. The difficulties of this step are compounded by an incision that is either too small or too low and medial.

If necessary, the incision can be enlarged by extending the external oblique incision in both directions and then cutting the internal oblique and transversus first upwards and laterally. If still further enlargement is required, these two muscles should be cut downwards and medially. Alternatively the wound may be enlarged by dividing the anterior and posterior rectus sheaths and retracting the muscle medially. The inferior epigastric vessel near the lateral edge of the posterior sheath must be controlled.

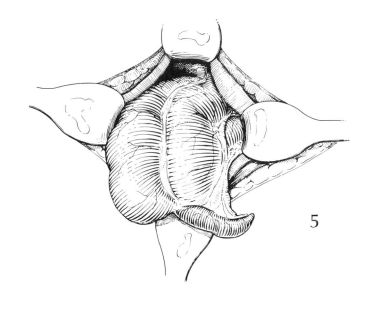

5

# 6

To remove the appendix, a haemostat is put on the free edge of its mesentery, which is then divided in two or three bites of tissue; the vessels are tied. When the appendix is free of its mesentery, a haemostat is applied transversely about 8 mm from its junction with the caecum. Retrograde appendicectomy, i.e. beginning at the base by dividing the appendix itself and then dividing the mesentery from the base to the tip should rarely be necessary in children.

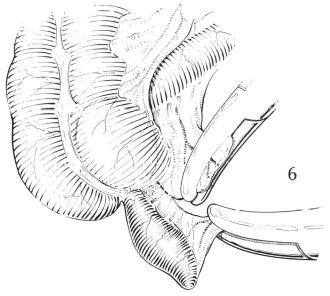

6

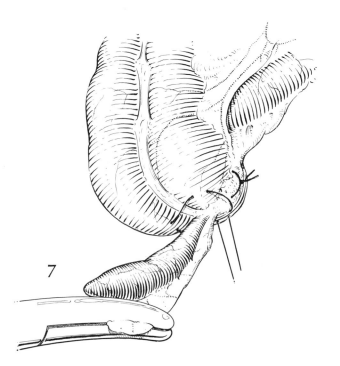

7

# 7

A purse-string suture of catgut is placed in the seromuscular layer of the caecum at the base of the appendix. Particular care should be taken in the area of the divided appendix mesentery, as failure to include this part of the caecum may allow the stump to escape the purse-string. If any of the sutures of the purse-string cut through when it is tied, burying of the stump will be difficult. Meticulous technique is essential, as perforation of a vein can cause haematoma, which can lead to other complications such as infection. If a haematoma occurs, it should be pricked with a scalpel and the purse-string suture tied as soon as possible to reduce further bleeding. A carelessly inserted purse-string is as likely to cause a blown stump as a necrotic gangrenous organ.

# 8, 9 & 10

A catgut ligature is then placed around the base of the appendix, which is transected below the proximally applied haemostat. The stump is then inverted. Occasionally this is not possible. In this case, it must be tied with a non-absorbable suture such as silk, linen, cotton or a synthetic material.

The use of carbolic on the stump is not recommended.

If the appendix is not perforated, a search should be made for Meckel's diverticulum. It should be within 75 cm of the caecum and occurs in about 1 per cent of children undergoing appendicectomy. If found, it should be removed.

All free pus from a perforated appendix should be carefully mopped out with swabs soaked in saline. The use of intraperitoneal antibacterials or antibiotics is controversial. If there has been gross contamination, the author instils ampicillin 0.5 g in 20 ml of water.

Replacing the caecum into the peritoneal cavity can be difficult, as it may well have filled with gas during the operation which cannot easily be pushed onwards into the ascending colon. Careless handling at this stage may be the beginning of a blown appendix stump.

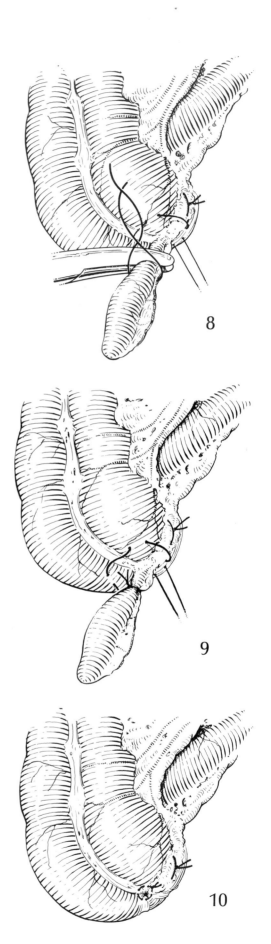

8

9

10

### Closing of wound

The peritoneum is closed first with a continuous suture. The fibres of the transversus and internal oblique muscles are brought together with two or three interrupted sutures. The external oblique is closed with a continuous suture along the line of the incision. Fat children should have a subcutaneous layer of 4/0 catgut. The skin is closed with a subcuticular 5/0 polyglycolic acid (Dexon) suture even if there has been peritonitis and gross contamination of the wound.

Although not necessary, a dressing will probably reduce the child's fears and his temptation to interfere with the wound. No drainage of the wound or peritoneal cavity is required. This policy has been followed in all of our 3000 patients with appendicitis over the past 25 years.

# Postoperative care

If antibiotics are needed, the first dose should be administered on the table. If intravenous antibiotics are required, the patient usually also requires an intravenous infusion. As the wound will be painful if there has been much retraction, regular postoperative sedation should be prescribed for at least the first 24 hours and administered at 6-hourly intervals.

A nasogastric tube is rarely needed for more than 48 hours. Intravenous fluid requirements should be assessed twice daily and the infusion discontinued as soon as possible. If the appendix was not perforated, intravenous therapy may not be required at all and certainly not for more than 24 hours.

# Complications

## Wound infection

Wound infection occurs in about 5 per cent of patients. Unduly heavy suture materials employed in the closure of the superficial layers may contribute to sinus formation. The first sign of an infection may be that the child is unwilling to walk or straighten up or is walking with a tilt to the right to minimize discomfort. The most effective treatment is early probing of the wound. If possible, this should be carried out in the outpatient department.

## Intra-abdominal abscess

This usually occurs in the pelvis. Antibiotics may not cure a large intra-abdominal abscess but they may help to localize it. Once it is localized, the patient should be examined under anaesthesia and the abscess, if sufficiently large, drained through the point of maximum convexity (this is often between the umbilicus and the symphysis pubis). A bladder catheter is inserted. A 1 cm transverse opening in the skin and linea alba or rectus muscles, followed by insertion of a sinus or artery forceps, is satisfactory if the abscess has first been accurately delineated. A soft rubber drain (Paul's tubing) keeps the sinus open for the first 5 days.

*Pelvic abscess*, palpable on rectal but not abdominal examination, often disappears with time and chemotherapy. Early evacuation into the rectum is not necessary. If a fluctuant bulge develops later, vigorous rectal examination may produce a gush of pus.

*Subphrenic abscess* occurs in about 1 in 200 cases of childhood appendicitis. It is important to localize the abscess with chemotherapy and to delineate it by imaging before attempting to drain it. Treatment requires a combined radiological and surgical approach. A catheter passed under some form of screening (usually ultrasound) to drain the cavity will often avoid open surgery.

## Unresolved abscess

If complications have not subsided after 10 days of antibiotics, they are unlikely to do so. In such cases it is usually best to allow a 'ripening' process to take place. Antibiotics are withdrawn and the patient is supported by intravenous fluids, and total parenteral nutrition if necessary. This allows the abscess to grow in size so that it can be drained. The temperature chart is a useful guide to progress. Ultrasound and, if necessary, an examination under anaesthesia may be of considerable assistance in determining tactics.

# Results

The following are hospital results from Our Lady's Hospital for Sick Children, Dublin, where 80 per cent or more of all appendicectomies are carried out by resident doctors in training. Safe precedents and practices have evolved over the years.

A recent (1984) review of 500 consecutive appendicectomies revealed that 56 per cent of appendices were acute, suppurative or gangrenous but unperforated, 22 per cent were perforated, 13 per cent presented as a mass, and 9 per cent were normal.

Antibiotics were used in 20 per cent of those with unperforated appendices to treat gangrene or near-gangrene. All perforations were treated with antibiotics for an average of 7–8 days and 85 per cent of these patients were discharged in under 10 days.

All patients with an appendix mass were treated conservatively for an average of 7–8 days. Vigorous antibiotic therapy was effective in 90 per cent of these patients. The remaining 10 per cent required drainage of pus following a trial period of 5–7 days on full chemotherapy. Interval appendicectomy was planned for a month later and 77 per cent of these patients were discharged by the fourth day.

Wound infection occurred in 3 per cent of patients although all wounds were closed with a subcuticular suture of 5/0 polyglycolic acid. Infection was no more common in perforated than in unperforated appendices. Pelvic and other intra-abdominal abscesses were rare (less than one per cent) and only one of the 500 patients required relaparotomy for adhesions. Peritonitis and pelvic abscess following appendicitis in girls is no longer a significant cause of infertility.

# Necrotizing enterocolitis

**J. A. S. Dickson**   MB, ChB, FRCS, FRCS(Ed)
Consultant Paediatric Surgeon, Children's Hospital, Sheffield, UK

Necrotizing enterocolitis[1] may be defined as 'a condition in which there is diffuse or patchy necrosis of the mucosa and submucosa of the large and/or small bowel. The process can spread longitudinally to involve long segments of gut or progress transmurally leading to perforation'[2]. Although there have been sporadic accounts of babies presenting with this disease since the turn of the century, the first of the present series of mini epidemics[3] was reported from New York in 1965. Outbreaks have since been recognized in many Special Care Baby Units. A special group occurs after exchange transfusion[4], and it is likely that most recorded instances of neonatal appendicitis[5] were in fact cases of necrotizing enterocolitis.

A histologically similar condition is recognized as a complication of Hirschsprung's disease[6]. This has been shown to be associated with colonization with *Clostridium difficile*[7]. Another similar condition, 'necrotising jejunitis', is seen in children in the tropics. This appears very similar to 'Pig-bel' enteritis of New Guinea which has been shown to be due to *Clostridium perfringens*[8]. Many organisms, including *Cl. perfringens*, *Cl. butyricum* and *Cl. difficile*, *Bacteroides fragilis*, coliforms, klebsiellae, and salmonellae[9], have been cultured from the blood or the intestine in this disease.

## 1a

The original description of a 'syndrome of lethargy in preterm infants'[3] implied that this was predominantly a disease of small and preterm infants. Despite this, in the early series about half the babies had a birth weight of over 2.5 kg. More recently, half the babies have weighed 1.5 kg or less; thus, half the cases come from one per cent of babies born[10]. The preterm infant is at risk for a longer period of time after birth – the condition is very rare after the third week of life in term babies, whereas first presentations or recurrences may be seen in the preterm for six weeks.

In the orally-fed preterm infant, due to a relative deficiency of enzymes and antibodies, organisms can multiply rapidly in the incompletely digested intestinal contents[11]. As a result of haemorrhage or ischaemia associated with vascular instability[12] these organisms penetrate through breaches in the mucosa and gain access to the submucosa where the damage is initiated.

The clinical presentation[13] varies from sudden collapse associated with perforation of a small ischaemic area to the more typical progressive disease, which may lead to obstruction, perforation, septicaemia, disseminated intravascular coagulation, or uncontrollable metabolic acidosis. The baby at risk is typically a preterm infant, with gross distension, dilated abdominal veins, and peripheral cyanosis.

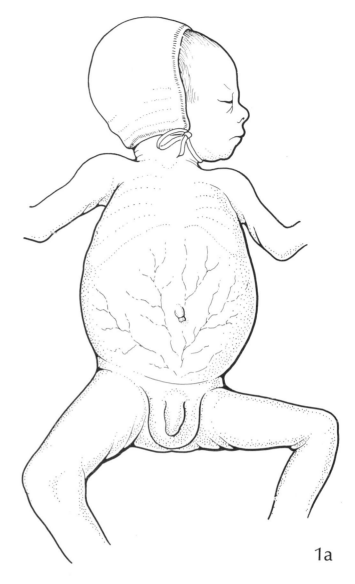

1a

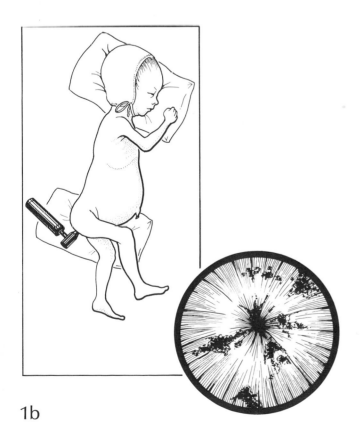

1b

## 1b

The criteria for diagnosis[14] are a typical history of sudden deterioration of an at risk infant, with pallor, lethargy, temperature instability, gastric retention and bile-stained vomit or nasogastric aspirate, abdominal distension and tenderness, the passage of blood per rectum, or blood on the finger after rectal examination, and evidence of inflammation and bleeding mucosa on proctoscopy[15]. There is typically a low platelet count with a low plasma fibrinogen level.

# 2a–f

X-ray signs are the mainstay of diagnosis[16, 17]. They are:

1. (a) Gaseous distension and fluid levels on the plain X-ray of the abdomen (2a);
   (b) evidence of oedematous gut;
   (c) a fluffy mucosal pattern (2b).
2. Evidence of submucosal gas producing a 'tramline' or 'signet ring' appearance when the bowel is seen in longitudinal or transverse view, respectively (2b).
3. (a) Free gas under diaphragm (2b, 2c).
   (b) free gas under the liver, outlining the falciform ligament (2c).
4. Gas outlining the portal venous system in the liver (2e).

Two conditions may cause diagnostic difficulty:

1. Volvulus neonatorum. The relatively gasless abdomen and the position of the duodenum on a limited type gastrointestinal contrast study will assist in establishing this diagnosis.
2. Hirschsprung's colitis. The history of delayed passage of meconium, the demonstration of a 'cone' at the transition between aganglionic and ganglionic colon, and the histopathological and histochemical appearances on suction rectal biopsy will confirm the diagnosis of Hirschsprung's disease. Pneumatosis intestinalis is rare in Hirschsprung's colitis but usual in necrotizing enterocolitis.

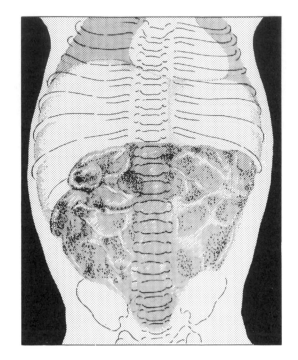

2a

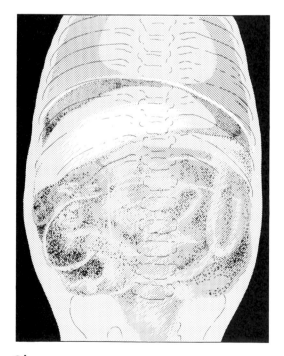

2b

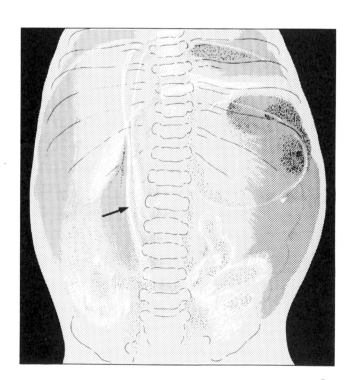

2c

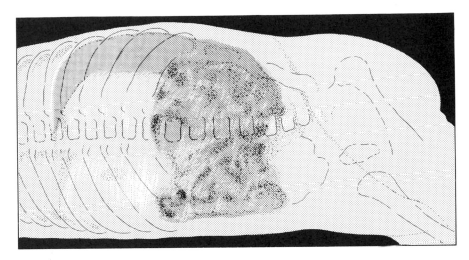

2d

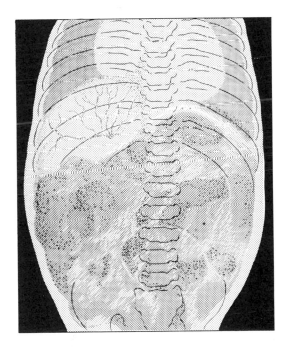

2e

2f

## PLAN OF MANAGEMENT

### Medical treatment[18]

1. Nothing by mouth.
2. Nasogastric tube decompression.
3. Antibiotics[19]. Penicillin with an aminoglycoside or third-generation cephalosporin and metronidazole or lincomycin.
4. Parenteral nutrition until the intestinal mucosa has recovered sufficiently for the infant to tolerate oral feeds, i.e. 10–14 days.

The infant is monitored closely in the acute phase of the illness, with regular observation of temperature, pulse, respiration, abdominal girth, haemoglobin, platelets, urea, electrolytes, and blood gases. Abdominal X-rays are taken every 6–8 hours for two days and then daily until the infant's condition is stable.

Oral feeds may be introduced one week after the infant's condition has stabilized and the pathological features on abdominal X-ray have resolved.

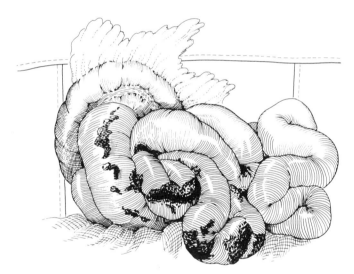

3

### Surgical treatment

## 3

Operation is reserved for the complications of necrotizing enterocolitis. These include[20]:

#### *Absolute*

1. Free perforation, with meconium escaping from perforations;
2. Deterioration or failure to improve on intensive medical therapy.

#### *Relative*

1. Localized perforation;
2. Obstruction;
3. Uncontrolled acidosis;
4. Uncontrolled disseminated intravascular coagulation.

At operation the principles of management are:
1. Minimal handling of intestine.
2. Resect all frankly necrotic intestine.
3. Preserve intestine of doubtful viability, provided there is a proximal defunctioning stoma.
4. Never anastomose intestine in the acute phase.
5. Fashion as many stomas as necessary, preferably exteriorizing adjoining ends together as 'double-barrelled' stomas.
6. If the rectum is irreversibly damaged down to the pelvic floor, it may be necessary to close and oversew the rectal stump, but if possible the distal end should be brought out to the abdominal wall, as this facilitates later reconstruction.

## INCISION

For the laparotomy the standard transverse supra-umbilical muscle-cutting incision is recommended. The poor collagen development in the extremely preterm infant (28 weeks and under) demands even more delicate surgical technique in handling and suturing tissues than that required for term neonates.

## PROCEDURE

The ascending colon, terminal ileum, and splenic flexure are most frequently affected. The transverse colon often remains relatively uninvolved. Lines of resection are shown for terminal ileum and ascending colon.

Where extensive areas of the intestine are affected, ample peritoneal drainage combined with the fashioning of a proximal stoma will permit survival of the maximal length of intestine. This course of action is preferable to immediate radical resection, when the length of excision could approach the limit for normal viability, leaving only 20–50 cm of small intestine.

When all the intestine from the duodenum to the rectum is involved, simple drainage with a second look after 24–48 hours is recommended.

## Excision of affected intestine

# 4a,b

Lines of resection where the terminal ileum, caecum and ascending colon are affected, and fashioning of a double-barrelled ileostomy-colostomy in the epigastrium.

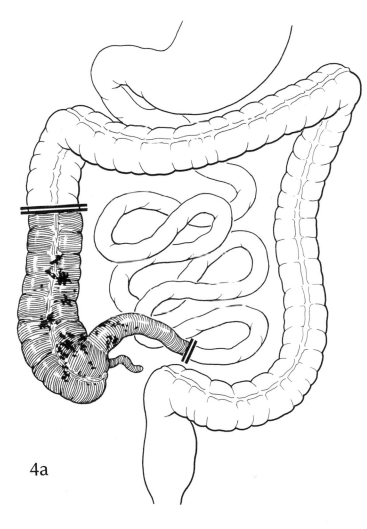

4a

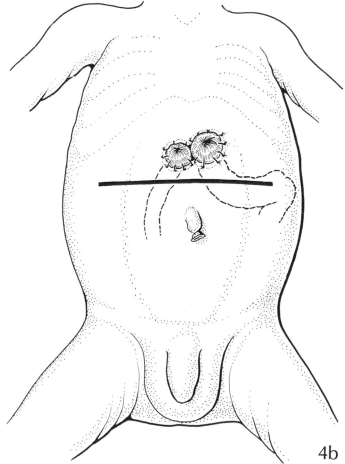

4b

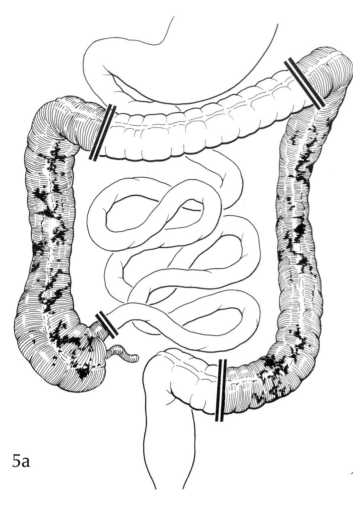

5a

# 5a,b

Excision of the ascending and descending colon, and preservation of the transverse colon, with construction of an ileostomy-colostomy, a distal transverse colon colostomy, and a sigmoid mucus fistula.

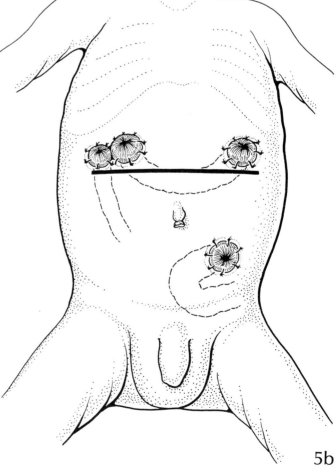

5b

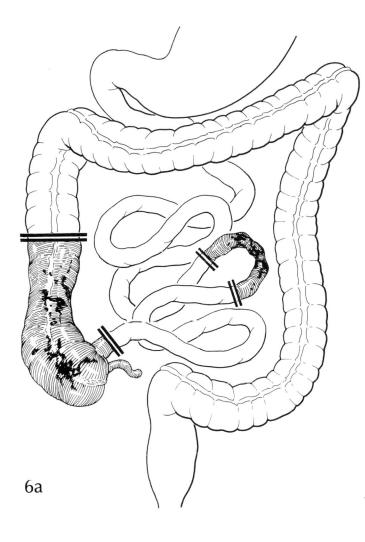

6a

## 6a, b

Resection of part of small bowel and part of ascending colon, with an ileostomy-colostomy and a double ileostomy.

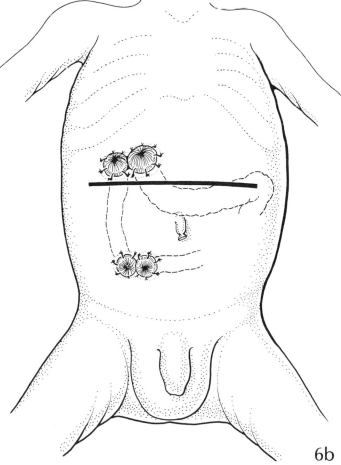

6b

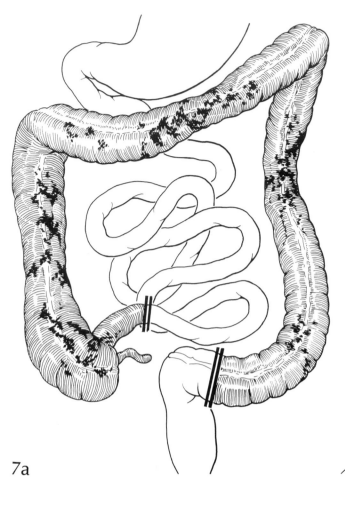

7a

# 7a,b

Excision of entire colon, and construction of an ileostomy and a sigmoid colostomy.

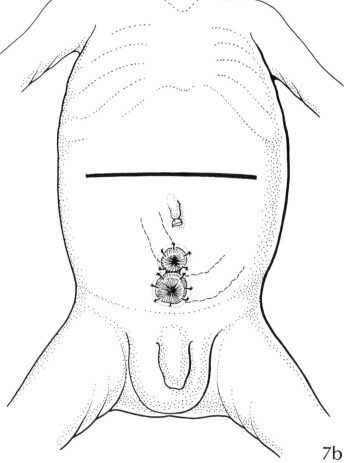

7b

## 8

Multiple perforations from major intestinal damage may be treated with simple drainage either after laparotomy or without operation, using infant intercostal drainage tubes.

### CLOSURE OF STOMAS

The *timing* of closure is dictated by healing of the retained intestine. This is usually secure after two weeks. The final decision depends on the general condition of the infant. In a preterm baby with only a colonic or a minimal ileal resection, it is usually safe and wise to delay closure until the infant weighs 2500 g. Many infants with proximal stomas causing severe malabsorption will require an earlier closure to permit enteral feeding[21].

Before closure it is essential:
1. To check patency of all the distal intestine by contrast studies, which must clearly demonstrate patency between the most distal stoma and the anal canal.
2. If there has been any suggestion in the history of Hirschsprung's disease, a suction rectal biopsy should be performed to demonstrate the presence or absence of ganglion cells in the submucosa.

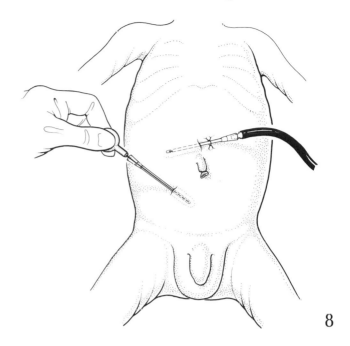

8

## 9

### Technique of closure

A double stoma has the advantage that it can be circumcised and a full end-to-end intraperitoneal closure performed without an extensive laparotomy. It is essential to resect the intestine intra-abdominally until healthy ends free from fibrous tissue are obtained. There is often quite severe scarring at the distal end. Both two-layer and one-layer anastomotic techniques are satisfactory. It is unnecessary to drain the wound.

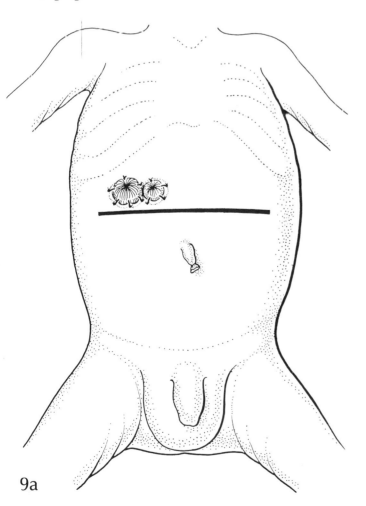

9a

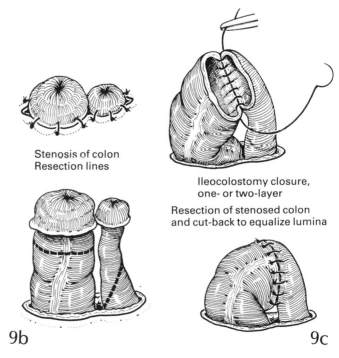

Stenosis of colon
Resection lines

Ileocolostomy closure,
one- or two-layer

Resection of stenosed colon
and cut-back to equalize lumina

9b                                                    9c

# 10a,b,c

### LATE STRICTURE FORMATION

In 20–40 per cent of cases following conservative treatment, or even after a surgical resection, late strictures may form from 2 to 3 months after the onset of the disease[22]. Difficulty with feeds should lead to suspicion of stricture formation. Frank vomiting, abdominal distension, and constipation or diarrhoea may develop later. The diagnosis is confirmed on contrast studies – barium meal and/or enema – which will identify the level of obstruction. Illustration 10a shows a barium enema demonstrating a long stricture in the ascending colon, with dilated loops of ileum. Some strictures recover spontaneously over 2–3 weeks. Many, however, require resection (see Illustration 10b). A primary anastomosis is usually safe at this stage (see Illustration 10c).

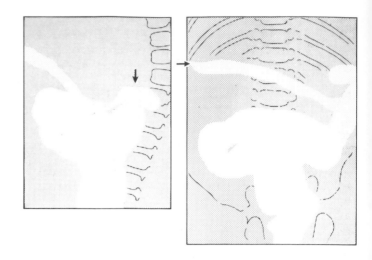

10a

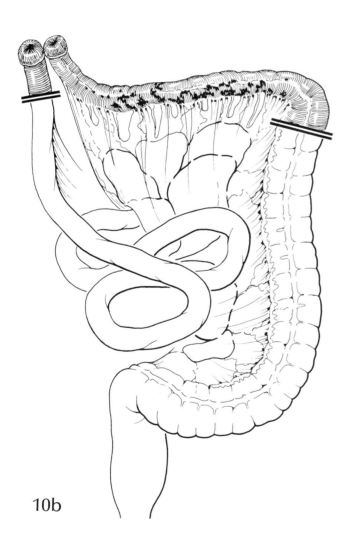

10b

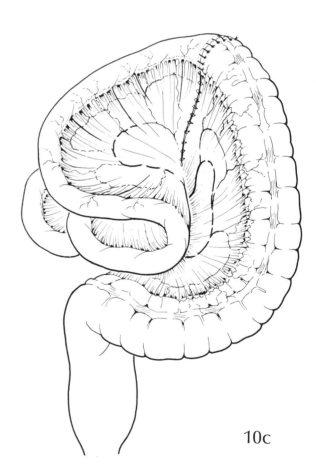

10c

## RESULTS

Because of the varying degrees of severity of the condition, with lesser degrees recognized earlier in some series and only more severe cases in others, it is difficult to give clear indications of the results to be expected.

In the Clinical Diseases Surveillance Committee Study in the UK, the disease was grouped into four categories: confirmed and unconfirmed, with severity grade I or grade II for each group. To be a *confirmed* case the infant must have positive X-ray findings or the disease be demonstrated at operation or post mortem. *Unconfirmed* cases had a history and findings suggestive of the disease, but none of the other factors were present. To be graded as *grade I severity* two of the following signs must be present: (a) pneumatosis, (b) abdominal distension or an X-ray with a fluffy mucosal pattern, (c) blood in the stool, (d) lethargy, hypotonia or apnoea. For *severity grade II* one or more of the following signs must be present: (a) Abdominal tenderness or rigidity; tissue in the stool. (b) Abnormal bleeding with trauma; spontaneous bleeding. (c) A peripheral white count $<6 \times 10^6/l$; a peripheral platelet count $<100 \times 10^6/l$. (d) Portal venous gas or free gas in the peritoneum.

For confirmed cases the death rate was 5/42 in grade I and 24/50 for grade II severity. Correlated with the birth weight, the results were:

All cases

| Birthweight | Confirmed | Unconfirmed |
| --- | --- | --- |
| >2.5 kg | 2/20 | 0/10 |
| 1.5–2.5 kg | 4/27 | 0/18 |
| <1.5 kg | 23/44 | 5/32 |

Infants with confirmed disease weighing over 1500 g had a survival rate of around 87 per cent, whereas for infants under 1500 g, the survival rate was only 48 per cent.

Despite surgical success, the long-term outcome in many of these severely ill preterm infants may be unsatisfactory due to neurological impairment[23].

## References

1. Dickson, J. A. S. (1975) Necrotizing enterocolitis in the newborn infant. Proceedings of the 68th Ross Conference on Pediatric Research. pp. 13–18. Columbus, Ohio: Ross Laboratories

2. Thelander, H. E. (1939) Perforation of the gastrointestinal tract of the newborn infant. American Journal of Diseases of Children, 58, 371–393

3. Mizrahi, A., Barlow, O., Berdon, W., Blanc, W. A., Silverman, W. A. (1965) Necrotizing enterocolitis in premature infants. Journal of Pediatrics, 66, 697–706

4. Corkery, J. J., Dubowitz, V., Lister, J., Moosa, A. (1968) Colonic perforation after exchange transfusion. British Medical Journal, 4, 345–349

5. Bax, N. M. A., Pearse, R. G., Dommering, N., Molenaar, J. C. (1980) Perforation of the appendix in the neonatal period. Journal of Pediatric Surgery, 15, 200–202

6. Berry, C. L., Fraser, G. C. (1968) The experimental production of colitis in the rabbit with particular reference to Hirschsprung's disease. Journal of Pediatric Surgery, 3, 36–42

7. Thomas, D. F. M., Fernie, D. S., Bayston, R., Spitz, L., Nixon, H. H. (1986) Enterocolitis in Hirschsprung's disease: a controlled study of the etiologic role of Clostridium difficile. Journal of Pediatric Surgery, 21, 22–25

8. Murrell, T. G. C., Roth, L., Egerton, J., Samels, J., Walker, P. D. (1966) Pig-bel: enteritis necroticans. Lancet, 1, 217–222

9. Brown, E. G., Ainbender, E., Henley, W. L., Hodes, H. L. (1980) Etiologic role of bacteria and intestinal function. In: Neonatal Necrotizing Enterocolitis. E. G. Brown and A. Y. Sweet (eds.), pp. 69–100. New York: Grune & Stratton

10. Yu, V. Y. H., Joseph, R., Bajuk, B., Orgill, A., Astbury, J. (1984) Perinatal risk factors for necrotizing enterocolitis. Archives of Disease in Childhood, 59, 430–434

11. Touloukian, R. J. (1980) Etiologic role of the circulation. In Neonatal Necrotizing Enterocolitis. E. G. Brown and A. Y. Sweet (eds.), pp. 41–56. New York: Grune & Stratton

12. Bell, E. F., Warburton, D., Stonestreet, B. S., Oh, W. (1980) Effect of fluid administration on the development of symptomatic patent ductus arteriosus and congestive heart failure in premature infants. New England Journal of Medicine, 302, 598–604

13. Herbst, J. J., Book, L. S. (1980) Clinical characteristics. In Neonatal Necrotizing Enterocolitis. E. G. Brown, A. Y. Sweet (eds.), pp. 25–39. New York: Grune & Stratton

14. British Association for Perinatal Paediatrics and the Public Health Laboratory Service Communicable Disease Surveillance Centre (1983) Surveillance of necrotizing enterocolitis, 1981–1982. British Medical Journal, 287, 824–826

15. Fenton, T. R., Walker-Smith, J. A., Harvey, D. R. (1981) Proctoscopy in infancy with reference to its use in necrotising enterocolitis. Archives of Disease in Childhood, 56, 121–124

16. Berdon, W. E., Grossman, H., Baker, D. H., Mizrahi, A., Badow, A., Blanc, W. A. (1964) Necrotizing enterocolitis in the premature infant. Radiology, 83, 879–887

17. Rabinowitz, J. G. (1980) Radiographic manifestations. In Neonatal Necrotizing Enterocolitis. E. G. Brown and A. Y. Sweet (eds.), pp. 101–128. New York: Grune & Stratton

18. Sweet, A. Y. (1980) Medical management. In Neonatal Necrotizing Enterocolitis. E. G. Brown and A. Y. Sweet (eds.), pp. 143–165. New York: Grune and Stratton

19. Khan, O., Nixon, H. H. (1978) The management of neonatal necrotising enterocolitis 1977: A preliminary report. Zeitschrift für Kinderchirurgie, 25(3), 196–205

20. Kosloske, A. M., Papile, Lu-A., Burstein, J. (1980) Indications for operation in acute necrotizing enterocolitis of the neonate. Surgery, 87, 502–508

21. Rothstein, F. C., Halpin, T. C. Jr., Kliegman, R. J., Izant, R. J. Jr. (1982) Importance of early ileostomy closure to prevent chronic salt and water losses after necrotizing enterocolitis. Pediatrics, 70, 249–253

22. Schwartz, M. Z., Richardson, C. J., Hayden, C. K., Swischuk, L. E., Tyson, K. R. T. (1980) Intestinal stenosis following successful medical management of necrotizing enterocolitis. Journal of Pediatric Surgery, 15, 890–899

23. Stevenson, D. K., Kerner, J. A., Malachowski, N., Sunshine, P. (1980) Late morbidity among survivors of necrotizing enterocolitis. Pediatrics, 66, 925–927

Illustrations by Kevin Marks

# Anorectal malformations: neonatal management

**R. C. M. Cook**  MA, BM, FRCS
Consultant Paediatric Surgeon, Alder Hey Children's Hospital, Liverpool, UK

## Introduction

'The child who is so unfortunate as to be born with an imperforate anus may be saved from a lifetime of misery and social seclusion by the surgeon who with skill, diligence and judgement performs the first operation'[1].

The infant born with an 'imperforate anus' has a complex malformation that presents a considerable challenge, not only to the skill of the surgeon who performs the first operation, but also, and more importantly, to the diligence and judgement needed to arrive at an exact anatomical diagnosis. Only then can the most appropriate mode of management be selected. The most useful classification of the pathological anatomy, based on the relationship of the lowest normal portion of bowel to the functionally vital puborectalis sling, was the internationally agreed Melbourne classification[2,3], that has recently been simplified and clarified as the Wingspread Classification[4].

The avoidance of disaster depends on distinguishing infants with a 'low' lesion (where the normal bowel extends through the puborectalis sling) from those with an 'intermediate' or 'high' lesion. The low, or infralevator, lesion can be safely corrected by a primary perineal operation. In all others a sacroperineal or sacroperineoabdominal approach is essential, and usually done at a few months of age following a colostomy in the neonatal period (see chapter on 'Anorectal malformations: posterior sagittal anorectoplasty', pp. 356–362). The construction of a colostomy not only relieves intestinal obstruction and allows reconstructive surgery to be carried out in a clean field, but also enables the surgeon to make a full assessment of the distal bowel and its relationships and to carry out the essential search for other malformations, which will be found in well over 60 per cent of such infants[5].

# Neonatal assessment

The infant's weight and gestational age must be noted and other major anomalies (e.g. oesophageal atresia) excluded. A correct primary diagnosis can nearly always be made by careful inspection of the perineum and by probing any visible orifice of the bowel. Radiography is occasionally needed to clarify the level of the lesion.

## Male infants

A perineal opening exuding meconium is found in both ectopic anus and anocutaneous fistula.

The *ectopic anus* always lies anterior to the normal site and is often stenotic. No treatment is necessary unless there is a posterior shelf or it is stenosed, in which case daily dilatation is required.

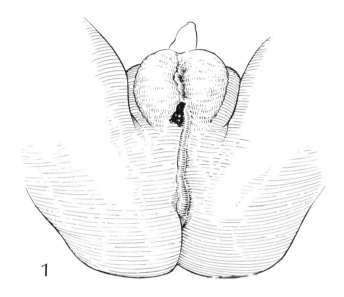

# 1

In *anocutaneous fistula* the anal canal is covered by hypertrophied perineal tissues while a fistula runs forward subcutaneously along the median raphe for a variable distance. 'Pearls' of epithelial debris may lie in the fistulous track distal to the point where it leaks meconium. A cutback procedure is indicated (see *Illustrations 7–10*).

An anal dimple without meconium being passed signifies rectal atresia or covered anus. In *rectal atresia* the anus appears normal but the anal canal is short and blind. An initial colostomy is needed (see *Illustrations 11–14*).

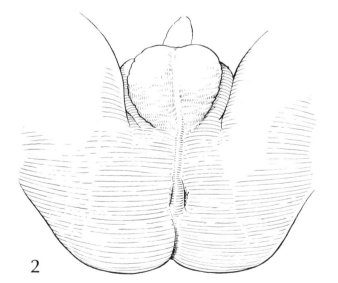

# 2

In *covered anus* a thick median bar covers the anus completely and is flanked by two dimples, through the thin base of which meconium may be visible. The anus is deroofed and mucocutaneous sutures are inserted (see *Illustrations 7–10*).

If there is no perineal opening and no visible meconium, but the urine contains meconium or squamous cells, or meconium is passed per urethram between acts of micturition, the child has *anorectal agenesis with either a rectourethral or a rectovesical fistula*. This is a high lesion requiring colostomy (see *Illustrations 11–14*).

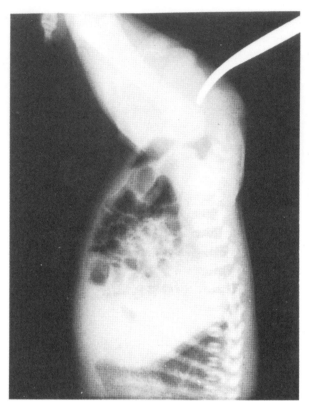

3a

# 3a & b

If there is no perineal opening, no meconium visible and none found in the urine, further investigation is necessary. When the child is at least 24 hours old a lateral radiograph is taken, centred on the trochanters, with the child held inverted with extended hips and with a marker on the anal site[6].

A satisfactory alternative is to nurse the infant prone and head down for 24 hours, and then, with the infant in the knee-elbow position, take a true lateral 'shoot-through' radiograph, again centred on the trochanters[7].

The position of the rectal gas shadow in relation to the bony points of the pelvis is assessed. Air in the urinary bladder indicates *anorectal agenesis with rectourinary fistula,* which is treated by colostomy as above. Rectal air still proximal to the pubococcygeal line may signify *anorectal agenesis with or without rectourinary fistula.* A colostomy is indicated before further evaluation.

Rectal air below the shadow of the ischium and very close to the marker resting on the presumed site of the anus is seen in *covered anus (complete).* A perineal approach as shown in *Illustrations 7–10* is indicated.

## Female infants

The abnormalities may be grouped according to the number of identifiable orifices.

### Three identifiable orifices

In *ectopic anus* urethra, vagina and an anteriorly placed anus can be identified. As in the male infant, no treatment is required unless there is stenosis or a posterior shelf.

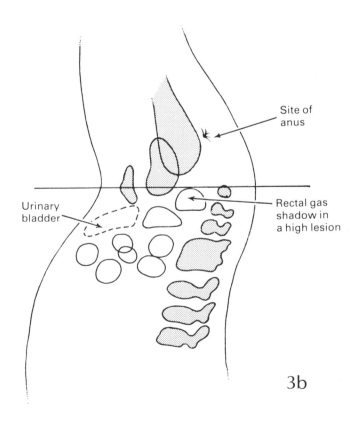

Site of anus

Urinary bladder

Rectal gas shadow in a high lesion

3b

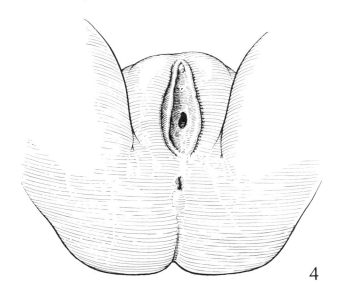

**4**

# 4 & 5

If the third orifice is a fistula and gentle probing confirms that the fistulous track lies just deep to the perineal skin, the infant has *covered anus with an anocutaneous, anovulvar or anovestibular fistula*. A cutback operation is indicated (see *Illustrations 7–10*).

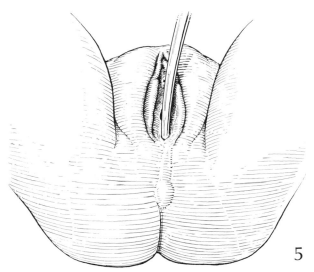

**5**

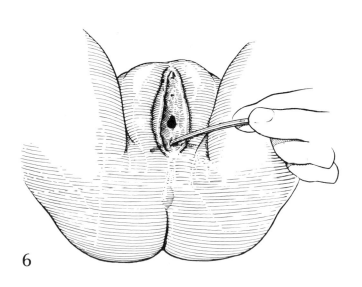

**6**

# 6

If the fistula lies in the vestibule and a probe shows that it runs upwards, parallel to the vaginal wall, the infant has *anal agenesis with a rectovestibular fistula*. This is an intermediate lesion and requires a colostomy.

## Two identifiable orifices

If only the urethra and vagina are identifiable there is *anal or anorectal agenesis with a rectovaginal fistula*. This is an intermediate or high lesion and a colostomy is indicated.

## Only one identifiable orifice

This indicates *anorectal agenesis with a rectocloacal* or, rarely, *rectovesical fistula*. A colostomy is indicated.

# The operations

## CUTBACK OPERATION

# 7

### Male infant

The anaesthetized infant is held in the lithotomy position by a nurse sitting alongside the operating table. The fistula is laid open to the posterior margin of the anus, by incising on to a probe. The operative field is kept clear of meconium by suction (or by inserting a small gauze pack into the now open anal canal).

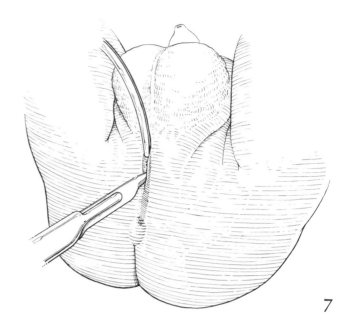

7

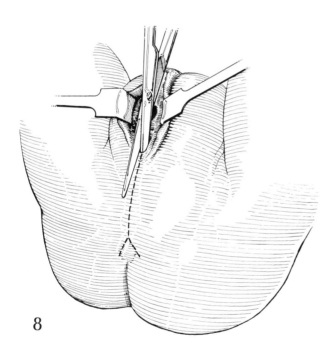

8

# 8

### Female infant

An alternative method is to insert one blade of a pair of pointed straight scissors along the length of the fistula. The posterior end of the skin incision can be made Y-shaped to allow a flap to be turned up into the sagittally opened anal canal.

# 9

Care must be taken to cut far enough back by either method and to avoid leaving a posterior shelf.

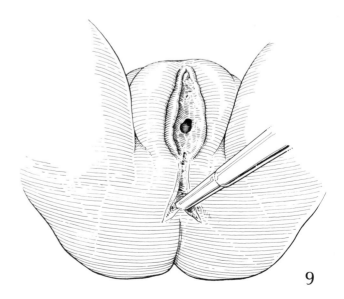

9

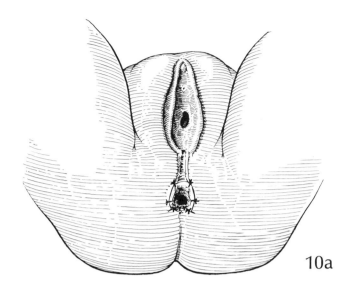

10a

## 10a & b

The mucous membrane and skin edges are approximated with fine interrupted sutures of silk or an absorbable material such as Vicryl (polyglactin 910; Ethicon).

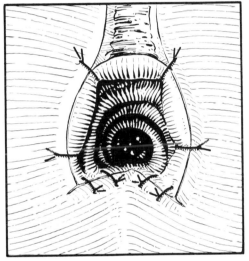

10b

### Postoperative care

Normal cleansing of the nappy (diaper) area is carried out as often as necessary, and dilatations are begun on the eighth postoperative day. This is best done with graduated Hegar's dilators in hospital but continued digitally at home by the mother until the anal margin is soft and easily dilated. This may take 2–3 months. Intermittent medical supervision is essential for several years, with attention being given to the prescription of aperients, such as Lactulose, and the encouragement of an appropriate diet to avoid constipation.

### Results

Mortality in a child with a 'low' lesion is rare, and usually due to associated urinary or cardiac anomalies.

Normal continence should be anticipated unless the child is allowed to become severely constipated, when overflow around a hard faecal mass will occur.

Hygiene is not difficult in the girls, and, although the anus may lie rather anteriorly in the infant, a perineal body develops as she grows older and normal vaginal delivery is not contraindicated in adult life. The risk of recurrence of a low lesion in the next generation is small, but a few families with multiple affected members have been described, inheritance apparently following an autosomal recessive pattern in most.

## COLOSTOMY CONSTRUCTION

A pelvic loop colostomy has been found entirely satisfactory by the author. Some surgeons prefer to use the transverse colon. This leaves ample bowel distal to the colostomy for the definitive procedure, but cleansing of the defunctioned loop is not easy, and looser stools make skin care more difficult and may lead to serious fluid balance problems. A separated, completely defunctioning colostomy has also been advocated with the aim of protecting the urinary tract. However, good care of a pelvic loop colostomy, even in a child with a rectourinary fistula, will prevent urinary infection unless there is an associated obstructive urinary tract anomaly[3].

General anaesthesia is usually preferable, but local anaesthesia may in certain circumstances be necessary and has proved satisfactory[8]. Antimicrobial therapy should be started immediately before surgery and continued for 48 hours. Metronidazole with gentamicin or cefuroxime is an appropriate combination.

## The incision

## 11

A broad M-shaped incision is made in the left iliac fossa, and the lateral and medial triangles of skin are excised. The external oblique aponeurosis is split and the internal oblique and transversus abdominis muscles are divided with diathermy in the same direction. The peritoneum is opened. An extensive exploratory laparotomy is unnecessary, but in female infants the intestines should be gently retracted so that the uterus and ovaries can be inspected. Genital anomalies are common[9]. The most proximal part of the sigmoid colon is pulled out.

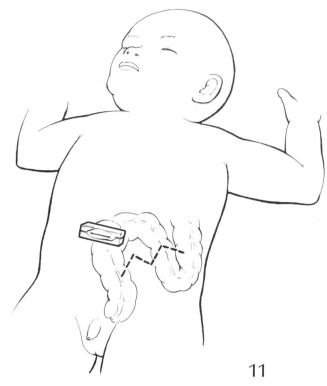

11

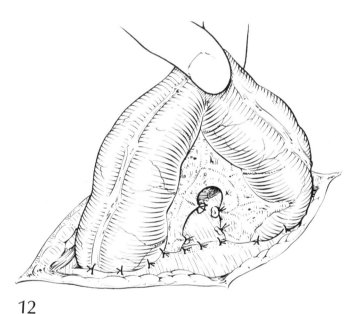

12

## 12

An opening is made in the mesocolon so that the ultimate opening of the colostomy will be *as proximal as possible*. This will leave sufficient bowel to mobilize from the sacral route in the children with an intermediate anomaly, without the need for further laparotomy. One or two small vessels may need to be divided between ligatures, but the marginal vessels must be preserved. The parietal peritoneum is approximated between the exteriorized limbs of the colon and sutured to the serosa of the bowel, taking care not to perforate the colon and not to constrict its channel through the abdominal wall. The muscle is approximated through the mesocolic defect also.

## 13

The skin flap is passed through the mesocolic defect and sutured to the opposite skin edge. The colon is opened immediately with diathermy by an extensive longitudinal incision on the antimesocolic border.

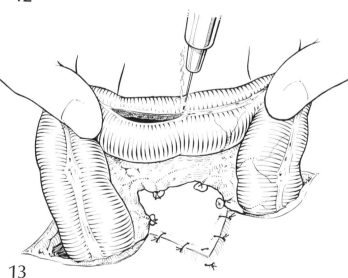

13

## 14

The bowel edge is sutured to the skin with interrupted silk sutures. Both the proximal and distal stomas should accept a No. 8 Hegar dilator. Meconium should be washed out of the distal loop by gentle irrigation with warm saline solution at the completion of the operation.

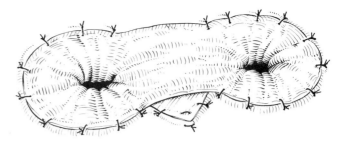

14

### References

1. Potts, W. J. (1959) The Surgeon and the Child. Philadelphia: W. B. Saunders

2. Santulli, T. V., Kiesewetter, W. B., Bill, A. H. (1970) Ano-rectal anomalies: a suggested international classification. Journal of Pediatric Surgery, 5, 281–287

3. Stephens, F. D., Smith, E. D. (1971) Ano-rectal Malformations in Children. Chicago: Year Book Medical Publishers

4. Stephens, F. D., Smith, E. D. (1986) Classification, identification and assessment of surgical treatment of anorectal anomalies. Pediatric Surgery International, 1, 200–205

5. Cook, R. C. M. (1978) Anorectal malformations. In: Neonatal Surgery, 2nd ed., Rickham, P. P., Lister, J., Irving, I. M. (eds.), pp. 457–481. London: Butterworths

6. Wangensteen, O. H., Rice, C. O. (1930) Imperforate anus: method of determining surgical approach. Annals of Surgery, 92, 77–81

7. Narasimharao, K. L., Prasad, G. R., Katariya, S., Yadar, K., Mitra, S. K., Pathak, I. C. (1983) Prone cross-table lateral view: an alternative to the invertogram in imperforate anus. American Journal of Roentgenology, 140, 227–229

8. Adeyemi, S. D. (1982) Management of imperforate anus at the Lagos University Teaching Hospital, Nigeria: a review of 10 years' experience. Progress in Pediatric Surgery, 15, 187–194

9. Palken, M., Johnson, R. J., Derrick, W., Bill, A. H. (1972) Clinical aspects of female patients with high ano-rectal agenesis. Surgery, Gynecology and Obstetrics, 135, 411–416

Illustrations by Kevin Marks

# Anorectal malformations: posterior sagittal anorectoplasty

**R. C. M. Cook** MA, FRCS
Consultant Paediatric Surgeon, Alder Hey Children's Hospital, Liverpool, UK

## INTRODUCTION

This approach to high and intermediate anomalies offers some advantages over the Stephens' sacral operations. Complete division of the pelvic floor will reveal the full extent of available musculature. It is claimed that (1) the wider exposure will allow safer dissection of the terminal bowel from the posterior capsule of the prostate in the male child, (2) the dilated or ectatic bowel can be tapered, and (3) in the female child with a rectocloacal fistula the vaginal and urethral abnormalities can be visualized and corrected at the same operation[1,2].

De Vries and Peña's concept of the anatomy is that the external sphincter muscle is a functionally useful element, and with the thick ventral portion of the pubococcygeus forms a 'striated muscle complex', external to and continuous with the levator ani muscle.

## PREOPERATIVE PREPARATION

Surgery is carried out when the child is 8–12 months of age. The distal loop of the colostomy is washed out to ensure that it is free from solid debris, and in the operating theatre it is irrigated with aqueous povidone-iodine solution.

## The operation

## 1

The anal site is identified by transcutaneous electrical stimulation. A self-retaining catheter or a metal urethral sound is inserted into the urethra, and the child placed prone in the jack-knife position. An incision is made in the midline from the midsacrum, through the anal site to the perineum.

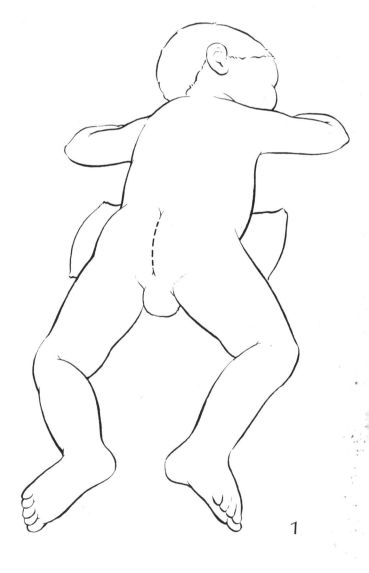

1

# 2a & b

Keeping strictly to the midline, the coccyx is split and all the musculature of the pelvic floor divided. The use of a nerve stimulator may help to identify these muscle layers and to ensure that they are divided in a sagittal plane. The rectum is exposed.

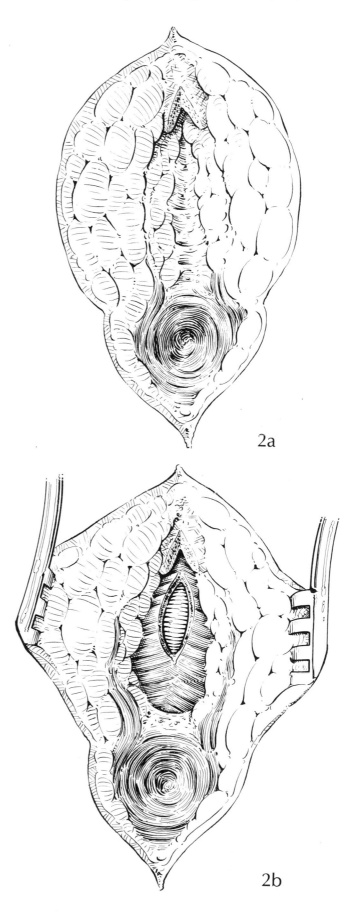

2a

2b

# 3

Deep to the levator muscle, and keeping very close to the bowel wall, the rectum is mobilized laterally by sharp dissection; the distal end is then opened longitudinally and in the midline, between stay sutures. The recto-urethral fistula (if present) is then easily identified.

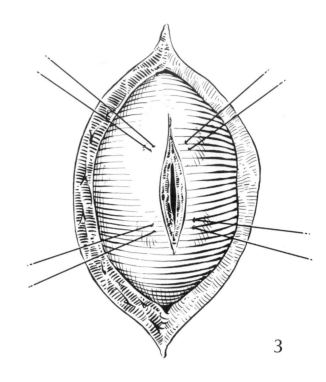

3

4

# 4

Fine stay sutures are placed just above the fistula, to pick up the rectal mucosa. The rectum is then dissected off the prostate gland, leaving a cuff of rectal muscle attached to the posterior capsule.

## 5a

At the upper border of the prostate the full thickness of the bowel is divided and lifted off the seminal vesicles and the bladder neck.

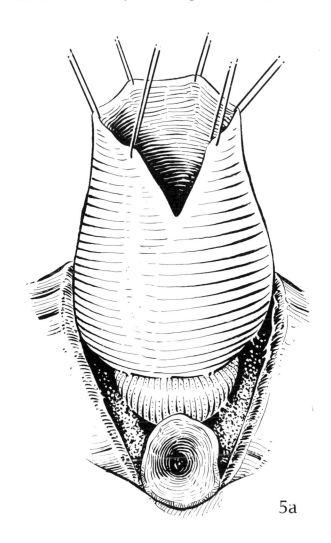

5a

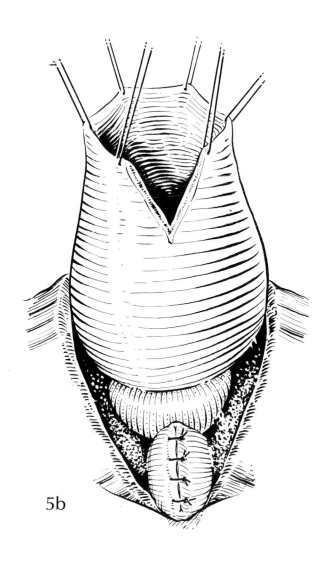

5b

## 5b

The fistula is closed with interrupted absorbable sutures.

# 6

By traction the rectum is mobilized further, any small vascular bands being cauterized and divided. Peritoneum may be met ventral to the rectum. A greater length of bowel can be obtained, if necessary, by sweeping this off the anterior rectal wall.

(In rare instances, usually when there is no fistula and the bowel terminates very high, it is only possible to obtain a sufficient length of rectum by turning the child over at this stage and performing a laparotomy.)

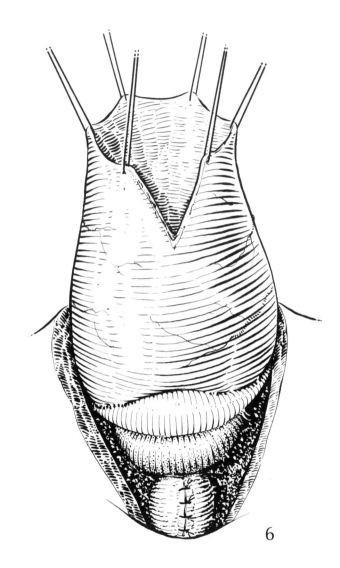

6

# 7a & b

A longitudinal wedge is then resected from the dorsal aspect in order to taper the dilated and ectatic terminal rectum. It is repaired with continuous absorbable sutures to the mucosa, and non-absorbable to the muscle, around a number 10 Hegar dilator.

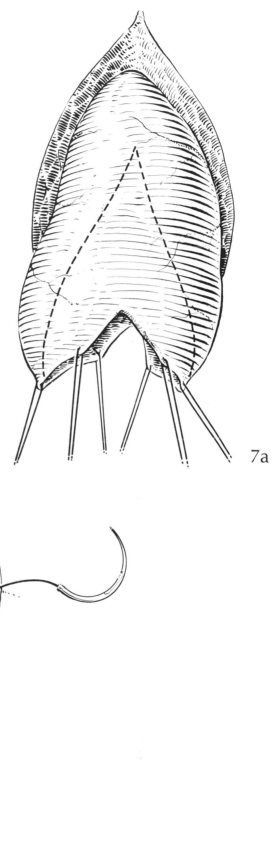

7a

7b

## 8

In the perineum, immediately dorsal to the urethra, the terminal portion of the bowel is fixed to the ventral part of the 'striated muscle complex', and then further sutures wrap the muscle around the new anal canal.

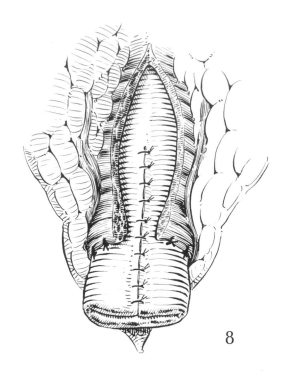

8

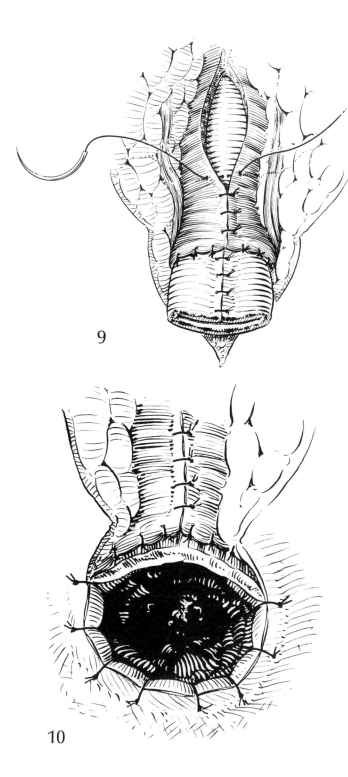

9

## 9

Working from the ventral end dorsally, the striated muscle complex and the levator muscles are sutured to the bowel wall and joined together again in the midline.

## 10

The anal orifice is formed after trimming the end of the bowel. The muscle coat is sutured circumferentially to the external sphincter muscles, and the mucosa/submucosa is sutured to the skin at the previously identified centre of contraction of the superficial external sphincter muscle.

The rest of the incision is closed, bringing the fatty tissue (with its strands of fibrous and muscle tissue that run from the external sphincter to the coccyx) together with non-absorbable interrupted sutures. The skin is closed.
   Postoperatively, oral fluids and feeds can begin promptly provided the peritoneum has not been opened. Gentle anal dilatations are begun after 4 weeks and continued daily until a supple anus of adequate calibre has developed. This is usually achieved, and the colostomy closed, in 3 months.

### References

1. De Vries, P. A., Peña, A. (1982) Posterior sagittal anorectoplasty. Journal of Pediatric Surgery, 17, 638–643

2. Peña, A., De Vries, P. A. (1982) Posterior sagittal anorectoplasty: important technical considerations and new applications. Journal of Pediatric Surgery, 17, 796–811

10

Illustrations by Kevin Marks

# Anorectal malformations: Stephen's sacral approach

**R. C. M. Cook**  MA, BM, FRCS
Consultant Paediatric Surgeon, Alder Hey Children's Hospital, Liverpool, UK

## Introduction

Following the construction of a colostomy in the neonate with a high or intermediate anorectal malformation, the distal colon is irrigated from the fifth postoperative day onwards until it is free of meconium. If a rectourinary fistula is present the wash-out should be repeated weekly to minimize the risks of urinary tract infection[1].

Investigations to exclude other anomalies and to clarify the rectal anatomy should include intravenous urography (or DMSA scan), cystourethrography and distal colonography, but these should not be allowed to delay the early return of the infant to its mother. Definitive surgery is usually postponed until the infant is thriving and growing well at 6–9 months of age, but construction of a new anus as early as 3 or 4 months may be advantageous to the learning of bowel control. In some cultures a colostomy may be unacceptable and definitive surgery may then be advanced to a few weeks of age.

If colonograms show the rectal pouch to be between the pubococcygeus and the ischium a sacroperineal approach is possible. If the rectal pouch is above the pubococcygeal line, a sacroperineoabdominal approach will be needed.

## Preoperative

The distal limb of the colostomy is washed out daily in the immediate preoperative period and neomycin and metronidazole may be given. Blood should be cross-matched, but it is unlikely to be used during the simpler sacroperineal approach.

# The operations

### Sacroperineal pull-through

## 1

The entire lower trunk, perineum and thighs are cleaned. A metal sound is put in the urethra (in the male) or the vagina. The child is placed prone on sterile towels, either in the jack-knife position with the pelvis supported or, often much more easily, kneeling. A vertical incision is made from the level of the fourth sacral vertebra to just below the tip of the coccyx.

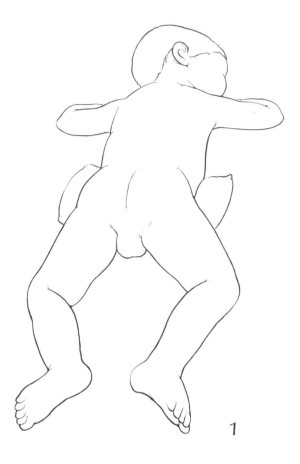

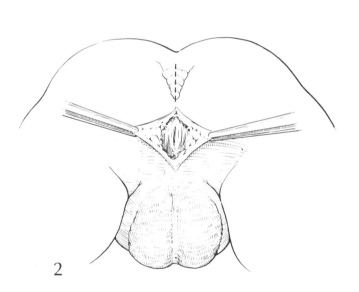

## 2

A cruciate incision is made over the site of the external anal sphincter muscle, which has been located by pin prick or a faradic stimulator. The skin flaps are raised and the centre of the muscle is identified, although its fibres often run longitudinally rather than in a circle. The external sphincter muscle may be poorly developed, and extensive dissection to search for it is not warranted.

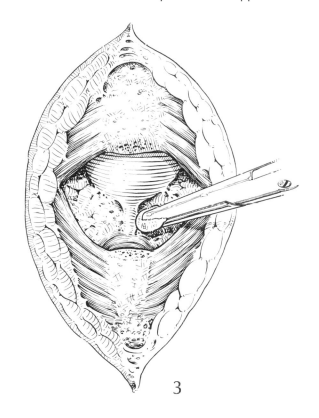

## 3

Through the sacral incision the coccyx is separated from the fifth sacral vertebra by a transverse incision that is extended laterally for no more than 1 cm on each side. Exposure may be increased by excising the coccyx or splitting it in the sagittal plane. The pelvic floor is then followed by blunt dissection, strictly in the midline, until the urethra (or vagina) is identified as it is embraced by the puborectalis sling.

3

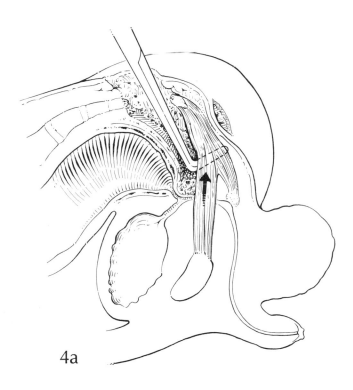

4a

## 4a, b & c

The urethra (or vagina) is gently separated from the muscle, which is stretched enough to pass the tip of a right-angled forceps down to the anal incision. The tip of the forceps is guided through the centre of the sphincter muscle here, and a 2 cm wide Latex Penrose drain is pulled through into the sacral wound.

If the lesion is high rather than intermediate, the sacral wound is now closed with the upper end of this drain left inside above the pelvic floor. The infant is then turned over for the abdominal part of the operation (see *Illustrations 10–12*).

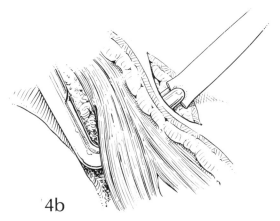

4b

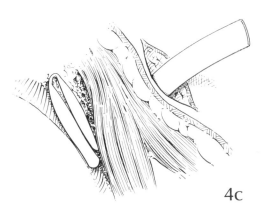

4c

# 5a & b

For an intermediate lesion, the child is kept in the jack-knife position and the rectal pouch is opened through the sacral wound to identify and isolate the fistula, if present. Keeping close to the rectal wall, the lower part of the pouch is dissected free and opened in the sagittal plane. The incision is extended forwards and around the fistula, which is transfixed and/or ligated.

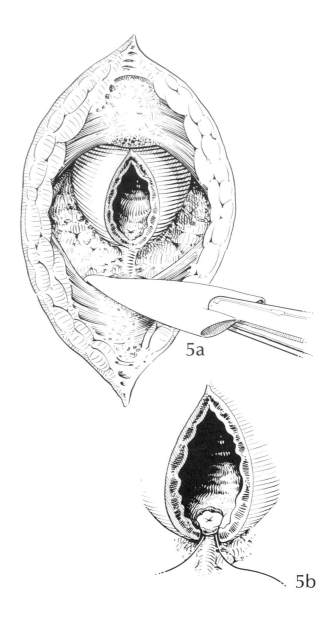

5a

5b

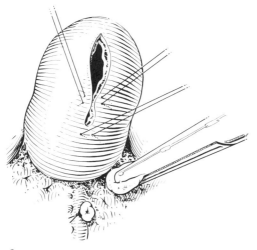

6

# 6

With stay sutures helping to pull on the anterior edge of the opened rectum, dissection is continued upwards between rectum and vagina (or urethra and seminal vesicles). Again it is important to keep close to the rectal wall. Traction on the rectum helps to define the attachments, particularly laterally, which can then be successively divided to free it from the bladder or cervix. When enough has been mobilized to pull down to the new anus, it should be possible to lift several centimetres of rectum out of the sacral wound.

## 7

The route through the puborectalis sling is now dilated just enough to pull the rectum through it. This is best done by passing Hegar's dilators (well lubricated with liquid paraffin) up inside the Penrose drain, to avoid damaging the fibres of the muscle or creating false passages.

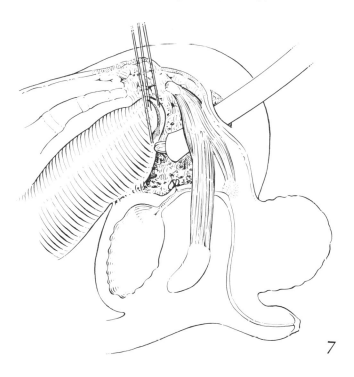

7

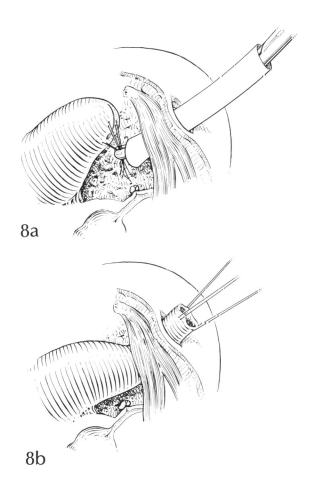

8a

8b

## 8a & b

A slim artery forceps is then passed up (again inside the Penrose drain), and the stay sutures on the cut edge of the rectum are grasped and gently guided through the anal incision. The Penrose drain will fall out at the same time.

## 9

The distal rectum is trimmed to accept the four skin flaps of the cruciate incision and skin and rectal wall are apposed with interrupted sutures. The sacral wound is closed with drainage.

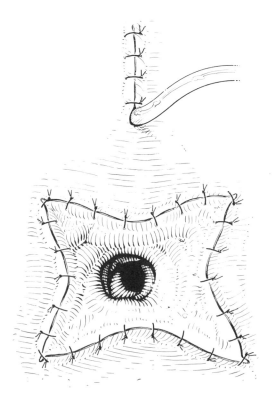

9

## SACROPERINEOABDOMINAL PULL-THROUGH

In infants with a high lesion, the initial four steps are the same as for the sacroperineal pull-through (*see Illustrations 1–4*) so that the correct route through the puborectalismuscle is marked by the tubular drain, and this channel is gently dilated (*see Illustration 7*). The sacral wound is then closed, the child turned over and the abdomen opened by mobilizing the colostomy and extending the incision medially.

The colostomy is excised and the proximal colon is mobilized, dividing the inferior mesenteric vessels if necessary so that its end can be pulled down to form the new anus without tension.

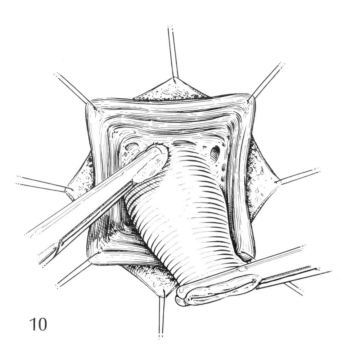

10

# 10

The distal bowel is divided 1 cm above the pelvic reflection, the superior rectal artery being preserved to supply the rectal muscle. The mucosa is stripped away from the muscular wall of the rectum. Stay sutures drawing on the muscle layer and saline injected into the submucosa help. The small bleeding vessels passing to the mucosa are controlled by compression with gauze or with diathermy.

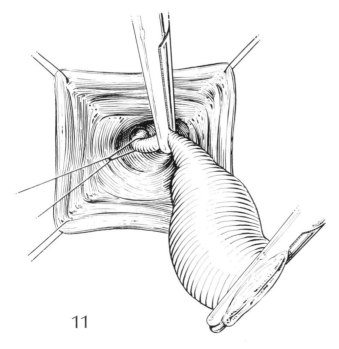

11

# 11

The mucosa funnelling into the fistula is ligated and the rectal mucosa removed.

## 12

A fine artery forceps is now passed up from the new anus through the Penrose drain and pushed against the floor of the muscular rectal pouch. By cutting down onto this an adequate channel is made for the colon to be pulled through.

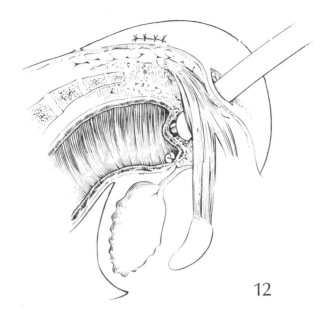

12

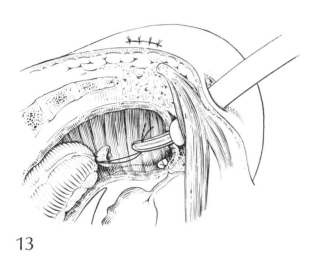

13

## 13

The colon is pulled down through the sleeve of the rectal muscle and the puborectalis sling. Its distal end is trimmed and sutured to the skin flaps of the anal incision (compare *Illustrations 7 and 8*). A new loop colostomy is made in the transverse colon.

## Postoperative care

The infant is nursed with the perineum exposed, if possible, so that the anal and sacral wounds can be kept clean and dry. After the simple sacroperineal operation, normal feeding can be resumed after full recovery from the anaesthetic, but the abdominal operation will necessitate a few days of nasogastric suction and intravenous infusion.

Daily dilatation of the puborectalis sling through the new anus is begun on the seventh postoperative day and continued daily, slowly increasing the dilator size over a period of 8–12 weeks before colostomy closure. Thereafter daily dilatations must continue for 2 or 3 months, together with the use of aperients and the adjustment of diet to produce soft, but not watery stools and to prevent the insidious development of constipation and a 'terminal reservoir syndrome'. Periodic supervision will be required until adolescence.

## Results

Anorectal anomalies are so frequently associated with major malformations of other systems that the high overall mortality rates (20–30 per cent) are not surprising, death most often being due to the other anomalies – of renal tract, heart or oesophagus.

In terms of absolute continence, results are disappointing and the pre-school child usually appears to have little voluntary control. Some faecal soiling often persists to early adolescence, when stronger motivation, attention to diet and prompt response to the often faint premonitory signs of a bowel movement will usually produce a socially acceptable degree of continence.

Later revision, with re-routing of the bowel if the bulk of the puborectalis sling has not been utilized, may be worthwhile, but the occasional child willingly abandons an uncontrollable anus for a manageable permanent colostomy.

### Reference

1. Stephens, F. D., Smith, E. D. (1971) Anorectal malformations in children. Chicago: Year Book Medical Publishers

Illustrations by Kevin Marks

# Minimal mobilization inversion proctoplasty

**H. Homewood Nixon**  MA, MB, BChir, FRCS(Eng), FRCSI(Hon), FACS(Hon), FAAP(Hon)
Honorary Consulting Paediatric Surgeon, The Hospital for Sick Children, Great Ormond Street, London and St. Mary's Hospital, Paddington, London, UK

## Introduction

The normal anorectum has an ectodermal lining of modified skin up to the level of the dentate line and is surrounded by striated muscle sphincter contiguous with the puborectalis sling. In so-called anorectal agenesis the modified skin is present with the same reflex sensitivity at the normal site or a little anterior to it. The muscle is present beneath, i.e. there is an everted proctodaeum rather than agenesis (admittedly developed to a varying degree).

The operation aims to minimize mobilization of the rectum to reduce the risk of destroying the recto-striated sphincteric reflex which is congenitally present.

This is achieved by invagination of the 'proctodaeum' to reach the 'fistula', which is used to construct the anus and which appears to have some internal sphincter potential.

Neonatal operation is performed so that the defaecatory response can be learned at the normal time. Magnifying spectacles are invaluable for this simple but precise procedure. The operation can, however, be carried out later in infancy if special circumstances such as associated anomalies (e.g. congenital heart disease) make this necessary.

Preliminary colostomy is performed, preferably of the low sigmoid, and full investigation is then required to assess the condition and exclude associated anomalies. This should include a clinical examination, spine X-ray (including the sacrum), ultrasound of the kidney, ureter and bladder, voiding cystourethrography, distal loopography and routine blood and urine examinations.

# The operation

## 1

The patient is placed in the semilithotomy position on a suitable baby table. In a newborn baby it may be preferable to flex the thighs completely and strap them across the abdomen, provided the colostomy is in the preferred left iliac fossa and the surgeon will not need to open the abdomen for colotomy.

A urethral sound is inserted so that the position of the bulb can be determined by palpation. (If preferred this sound can be introduced from above via a cystotomy. This would avoid its handle obstructing the operator, and can be used for placement of the suprapubic catheter at the end of the procedure.) A semicircular incision is then made with its apex just behind the bulb of the urethra and its base between the ischial tuberosities at the level of the normal anal site. (In these patients the modified skin representing the proctodeal site is usually a little anterior.)

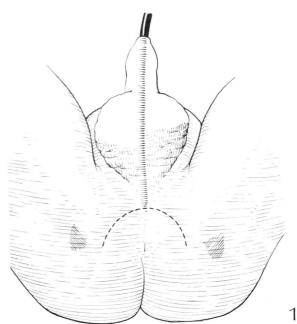

## 2 & 3

The flap is turned back after placing an artery forceps on the superficial fibres of the external sphincter where they join the perineal body. The subcutaneous fat is divided by diathermy to turn back the flap. Using blunt dissection immediately behind the urethra, the lower border of the puborectalis sling is identified and gently eased back.

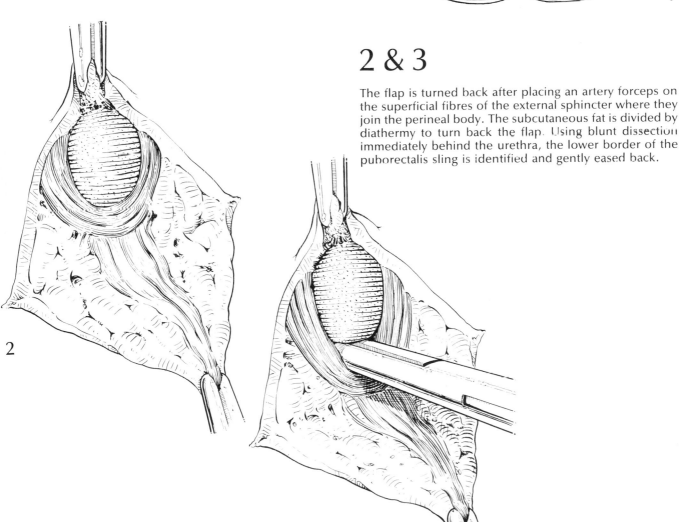

# 4

A Hegar dilator is then passed from the left iliac colostomy to thrust the lower end of the bowel into this space behind the bulb. If a right transverse colostomy has been performed, it may be necessary to make a limited opening of the abdomen to form a low sigmoid colotomy for this purpose.

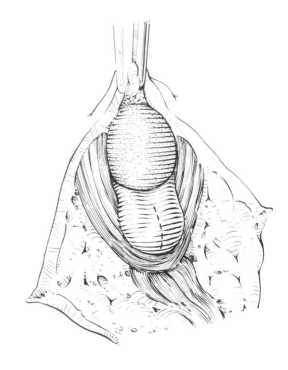

4

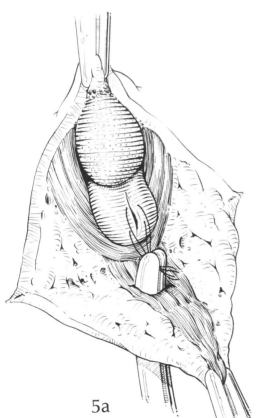

5a

# 5a & b

The end of the bowel is held with stay sutures and incised. The incision is carried cautiously around the fistula, using palpation of the urethral and bowel sounds to maintain the correct plane, and avoid damage to the urethra. A continuous 5/0 Dexon suture is inserted on the urethral side as the division proceeds. (Although preferred, this closure is not essential, provided a urethral catheter is inserted for the next 7 days.) The bowel is usually wide, with a thickened muscular wall right up to the urethra, but sometimes tapers terminally.

In the occasional anorectal agenesis without a patent fistula the bowel is very similarly attached to the urethra and can then be separated from it in a similar fashion, but more easily.

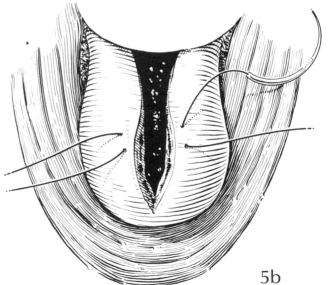

5b

## 6

The flap is now held forward again while cruciate skin flaps are prepared at the site of the modified skin, which is usually a little anterior to the normal anal site.

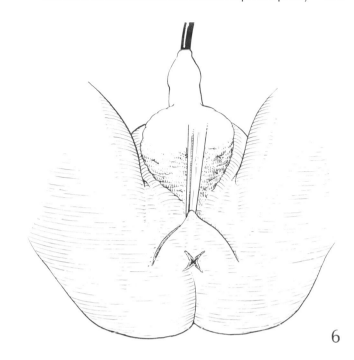

6

## 7

As the flaps are reflected a 'knot' is usually seen in the external sphincter fibres through which a tunnel is easily made with the tips of mosquito forceps. Electrostimulation is used to confirm the path as required.

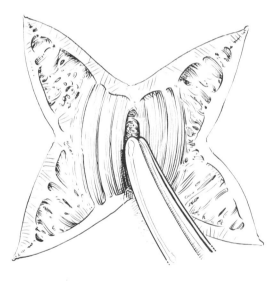

7

## 8

Having made this track through the external sphincter, the flap is again turned back so that the stay sutures on the fistula (which is used as the anus) can be drawn down through the flap.

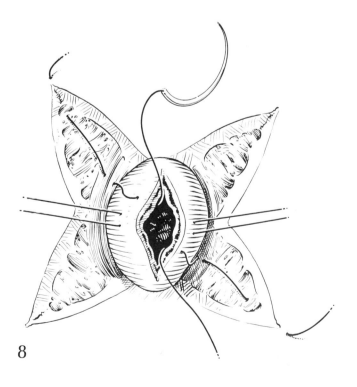

8

## 9

With the flap held forward again the opening in the bowel is lengthened if necessary to match the skin and is then sutured with one layer of 5/0 Dexon to the cruciate skin flaps, passing through skin, muscle and end of bowel. Sutures must be tied *very* slackly to avoid cutting out. No formal interdigitation is needed. Since the rectal ampulla has scarcely been mobilized, the suture line retracts upwards when the stay sutures are removed.

The flap is closed with subcutaneous and subcuticular 4/0 or 5/0 Dexon or catgut sutures without drainage

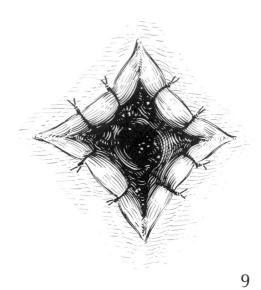

9

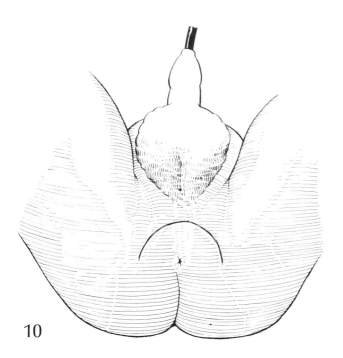

10

## 10

A suprapubic catheter is placed in addition to the urethral indwelling catheter to minimize the risk of postoperative blockage. A formal suprapubic placement of a Malecot catheter is preferred to percutaneous procedures such as Bonano drainage.

## Postoperative care

The urethral catheter is removed on the 7th day. A descending voiding cystourethrogram is obtained through the suprapubic catheter on the 10th day. If all is well a sound is then passed to calibrate the rectum on the 14th day and closure of the colostomy is considered from 3 weeks after the operation or later. In neonates the anus should take a No. 8 Hegar dilator before closure. Although routine dilatation is not usually needed, it is essential to continue checks since early stenosis is much easier to treat than a tightly formed stricture.

(*Note:* in the unlikely event of the operator not being able to coax the end of the bowel through the intact sling, the perineal dissection constitutes the first phase of a standard Mollard endorectal pullthrough. The author has experienced this on only one occasion.)

## References

1. Frenckner, B. (1985) Use of the recto-urethral fistula for reconstruction of the anal canal in high anal atresia. Zeitschrift für Kinderchirurgie, 40, 312–314

2. Keith, Sir A. (1908) Malformations of the hind end of the body. 1. Specimens illustrating malformations of the rectum and anus. British Medical Journal, 2, 1736–1740

3. Mollard, P., Marechal, J. M., de Beaujeu, M. J. (1978) Surgical treatment of high imperforate anus with definition of the puborectalis sling by an anterior perineal approach. Journal of Paediatric Surgery, 13, 499–504

4. Nixon, H. H., Callaghan, R. P. (1964) Anorectal anomalies: physiological considerations. Archives of Diseases in Childhood, 39, 158–160

Illustrations by Kevin Marks

# Hirschsprung's disease

**H. Homewood Nixon**  MA, MB, BChir, FRCS(Eng), FRCSI(Hon), FACS(Hon), FAAP(Hon)
Honorary Consulting Paediatric Surgeon, The Hospital for Sick Children, Great Ormond Street, London and St Mary's Hospital, Paddington, London, UK

## Introduction

Most patients now present in the first weeks or months of life when a colostomy is the usual primary treatment. Should the baby have a complicating enterocolitis, treatment may be a matter of great urgency. The signs and symptoms are basically those of low intestinal obstruction of varying severity, from intractable constipation to complete obstruction, but are commonly subacute and recurrent. Ninety per cent fail to pass meconium in the first 24 hours of life. This may be followed by days, weeks or even months of remission before signs and symptoms recur. Thus careful observation is justified in the absence of other obvious causes such as prematurity or stressful delivery, this observation usually leading to rectal suction biopsy.

About 30 per cent present with paradoxical 'diarrhoea' caused by enterocolitis. This is the commonest cause of death in Hirschsprung's disease, particularly in the first months of life where mortality has reached over 20 per cent . 'Diarrhoea with distension of the abdomen' should be treated urgently by intravenous fluid, wide-spectrum antibiotics (including vancomycin), and deflation by rectal saline irrigation. Colostomy should then follow, with frozen-section biopsy to assess the level of ganglionosis.

Right transverse colostomy is preferred in the usual cases. Ileostomy may be necessary if a long aganglionic segment is present. Should unrelieved obstruction or enterocolitis necessitate colostomy in the first days of life, the author prefers Swenson's plan of colostomy immediately above the transition to ganglionic bowel, so that all the normal bowel continues to function, develop and lengthen its mesenteric vessels. This facilitates the later pull-through procedure; an end-colostomy is less prone to prolapse. The distal end is brought out as a mucus fistula through the lower end of the midline incision.

Patients diagnosed when older may sometimes be maintained in good health by daily rectal irrigations before primary definitive operation, at which time the author now always performs a covering colostomy, although some believe this to be unnecessary. Colostomy cover does not reduce the incidence of anastomotic complications, but virtually eliminates serious consequences which may otherwise become irreversible or fatal. (A carefully managed caecostomy, of which this author has little experience, may be a suitable alternative.)

Four main operations are extant (see Illustrations 1–9). The Duhamel operation modified by the use of the mechanical stapler is found more convenient in infancy, but there is little to choose between it and the Swenson operation except for long-segment cases. In these the extra 'reservoir' of the Duhamel neorectum seems to make convalescence easier.

When total colectomy is necessary a period of several months with an ileostomy to allow colonization of the ileum appears more useful than the construction of a longer neorectum in avoiding later fluid-balance problems. Both the Swenson and the Duhamel operations have been found satisfactory over long periods of follow-up. The urine should be monitored for sodium chloride, since the greater losses after total colectomy may require supplements.

Whilst the results of Soave's operation have also been good, the need for postoperative dilatations can be troublesome. The 'sutured Soave' (Denda/Scott Boley operation) avoids this necessity, but requires care in suturing to avoid retraction of the colon within the muscular cuff. It gives equally good results.

On theoretical grounds the author has not used Rehbein's operation of low anterior resection, but good results are reported in large, carefully followed series.

For secondary treatment after an inadequate resection the Duhamel operation is usually preferred, since the second eversion of the anal canal for a Swenson operation may jeopardize its blood supply. The colon is brought down to one side of the midline to avoid crushing the marginal vessels to the bowel, which has been brought down at the previous operation.

For those cases requiring secondary operation for rectovaginal or rectourethral fistula following unsatisfactory earlier surgery, the Soave procedure is preferred. It avoids a difficult dissection which may damage the nerve supply to the bladder.

For those rare instances with a significant extent of aganglionosis into the small intestine, some form of extended lateral anastomosis to retain colon is needed (Lester–Martin, Kimura, Shandling).

Definitive surgery has been carried out in patients from 6 weeks old onwards. If colostomy has been performed, delay for 6–9 months is usual. Toddlers are more likely to be upset by operation and may be difficult to train afterwards.

The present-day availability of intravenous nutrition and antibiotics against anaerobes offers significantly increased benefits which are difficult to quantify.

375

# Preoperative preparation

If a neonatal colostomy has been made, a weekly rectal digital examination and distal-loop irrigation should be carried out until definitive surgery is undertaken. This minimizes disuse contracture of the anus and avoids inspissation of mucus and retention of any overflow faeces in the bowel.

Those without a colostomy have daily rectal irrigations of normal saline (using up to 1.5 litres in small quantities in older children) until thoroughly clear. This may take 1 or even 2 weeks. A liquid diet is instituted for at least 24 hours before operation.

Flucloxacillin, gentamicin, and metronidazole are used to cover the operation, in addition to the thorough mechanical cleansing. A dose of metronidazole immediately *before* operation to obtain an adequate tissue concentration during surgery is a most important factor.

## TYPES OF OPERATION

# 1–4

### Swenson's operation

This comprises a resection of the aganglionic segment and pull-through abdominoanal anastomosis. Dissection is *on the muscle coat* to avoid pelvic splanchnic-nerve damage.

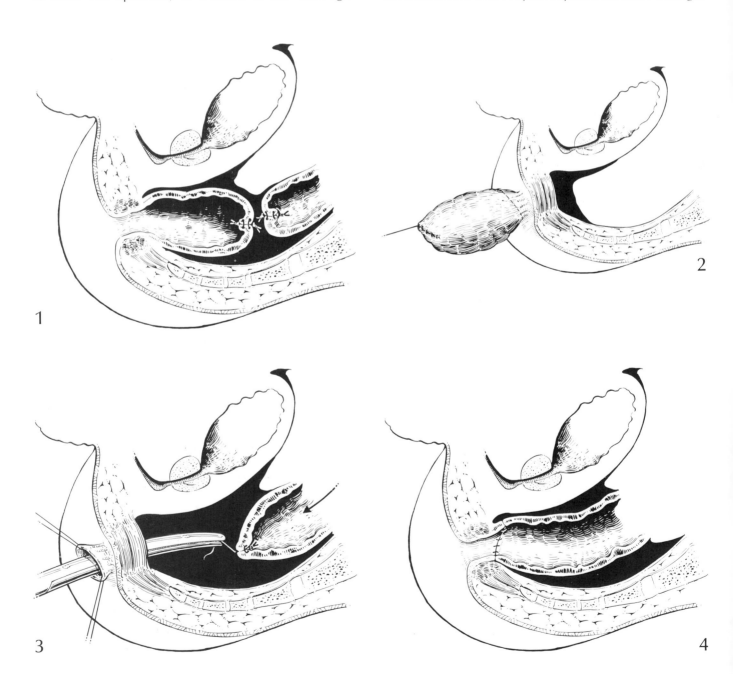

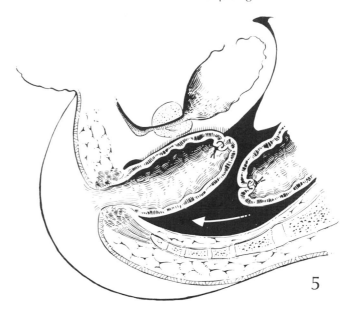

5

# 5–7

**Duhamel's operation**

This is a retrorectal transanal pull-through.

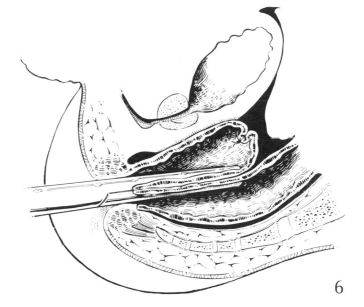

6

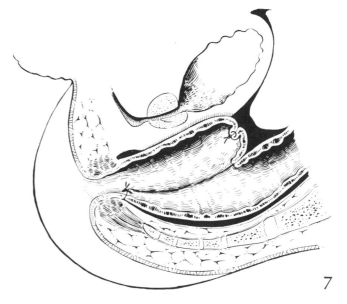

7

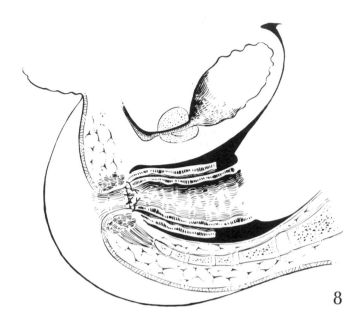

8

# 8 & 9

### Soave's operation

Submucous endorectal pull-through with sutured anastomosis as commonly practised, or with the original non-sutured anastomosis and secondary trimming of excess.

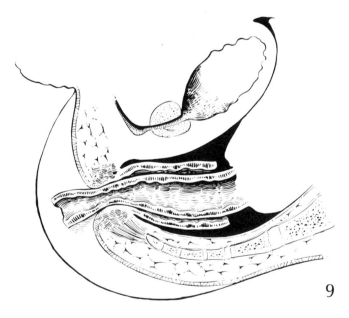

9

# The operations

## SWENSON'S OPERATION

# 10

### Position of patient

The patient is placed in the semilithotomy position. The sacrum is extended over the table end, falling back to allow a direct view down the pelvis, since all the dissection is from the abdomen. The catheter in the bladder is left open to drain during the operation.

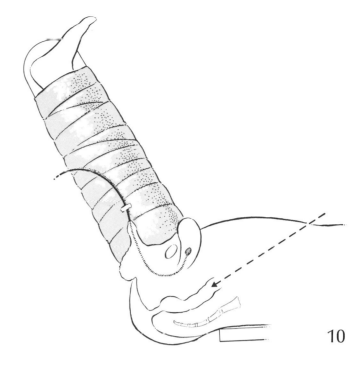

10

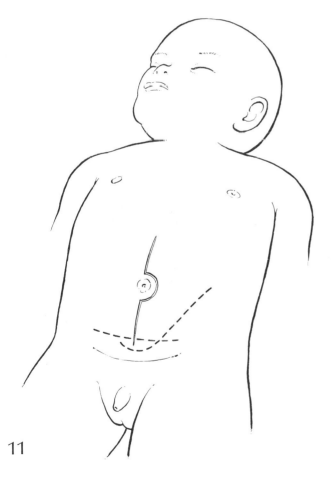

# 11

### The incision

The author prefers a midline incision. If there is a left iliac fossa colostomy a hockey-stick incision may be preferred to include this.

11

## 12

### Placing of the Denis Browne retractor

The retractor is positioned and the bladder is drawn forward out of the pelvis by stay sutures. Extramucosal frozen-section muscle biopsy confirms the safe level for resection (arrowed). The position of sigmoid vessels is demonstrated by transmitted light after division of the lateral 'congenital' adhesion to the sigmoid mesentery.

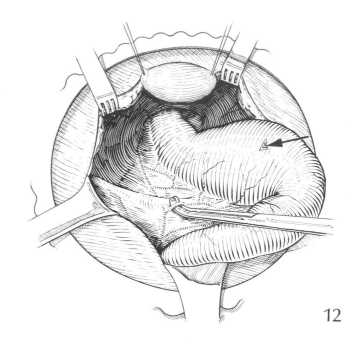

12

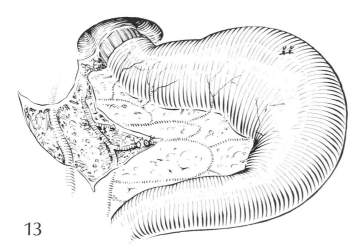

13

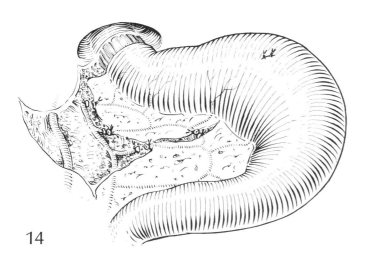

14

## 13 & 14

### Mobilization of the sigmoid

The sigmoid vessels are divided individually, retaining the marginal vessels. A marker stitch is placed at the level of good blood supply. The superior rectal artery is ligated in continuity to reduce bleeding during pelvic dissection. The peritoneal incision is carried around the bowel high above the pelvic reflection and deepened to expose the longitudinal muscle layer of the upper part of the rectum.

# 15

### Dissection on the muscle coat of the rectum down to the upper end of the anal canal

Individual terminal branches of vessels are tied or electrocoagulated as the assistant demonstrates them by traction on the rectum upwards and away from each quadrant in turn. Tonsil forceps with their angled handles are invaluable in enabling the assistant to exercise traction to demonstrate each quadrant without his hand obstructing the field. The muscular plane is *crucial* to preservation of the pelvic splanchnics.

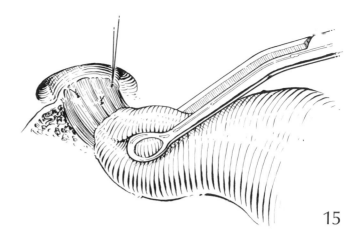

15

# 16

A fingertip rocking the coccyx indicates that the correct level is reached. It can be confirmed if necessary by putting a second glove over that on the left hand and by manual palpation with a finger in the anus.

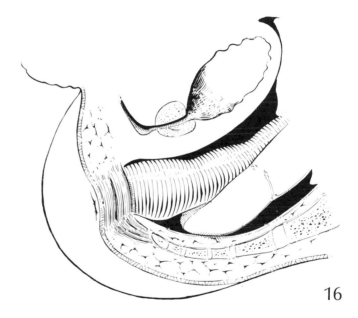

16

# 17

### Resection of the segment of bowel

The segment of bowel between the rectum and the site confirmed by biopsy and blood supply as suitable for pull-through is resected, and the ends oversewn or stapled. At this stage time is saved if the team divides, with an anal and an abdominal operator.

17

## ANAL PHASE

### Prolapse of rectum and pull-through anastomosis

The mobilized rectum is prolapsed outside the anus by passing a forceps from the anus up its lumen, grasping its upper end and withdrawing it. The mucosal surface is cleansed with antiseptic. (If freeing is found to be incomplete the rectum can be returned to the abdomen for further mobilization.) Ideally the mobilization should allow complete eversion of the anal canal when traction is exerted on the rectum, but with spontaneous re-inversion of the anal canal when traction is released.

# 18 & 19

One-half of the rectum is transected from a level 1 to 2 cm above the dentate line anteriorly (depending on the size of the patient) and extending obliquely down to the dentate line posteriorly (this should therefore include an upper partial internal sphincterectomy). The colon is drawn down to this incision and an outer layer of 3/0 silk sutures is placed. The same side of the end of the pull-through colon is then opened and an inner layer of 3/0 chromic catgut sutures is placed.

   The other half of the anastomosis is then made similarly and it is then allowed to retract within the anus.

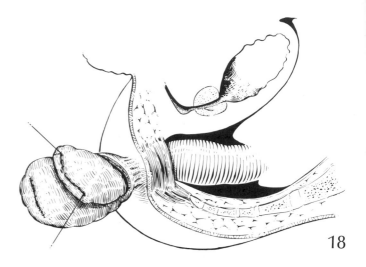

18

## FURTHER ABDOMINAL PHASE

The pulled-through colon is attached to the posterior abdominal wall by a few sutures to close the potential gap behind the mesenteric vessels. These attach the bowel to the edge of the peritoneum; attempts to suture the mesentery may damage the vessels close to its edge.

   A soft drain is laid in the pelvis and the upper end brought out through a stab wound in the left iliac fossa. Low-pressure suction drainage is applied for 48 hours.

   A proximal covering colostomy is made if one is not already present. The author's personal experience is limited, but with the antibiotics now available a carefully nurtured caecostomy is probably an adequate alternative, avoiding a further operation for colostomy closure.

   The wound is closed in layers.

# Postoperative care

The urethral catheter is removed after 24 hours. The abdomen should remain flat, and the colostomy usually acts in 48 hours. No routine rectal examination is carried out for 7 days. A radiographic 'distal loopogram' is performed 10 days after operation. If satisfactory, the colostomy is closed 14 days after operation. If a radiological leak' is revealed, closure is delayed.

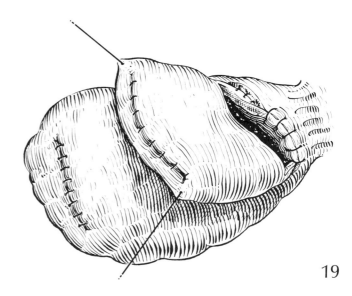

19

## VARIATIONS IN PARTICULAR CIRCUMSTANCES

# 20 & 21

### Presence of preliminary colostomy at the transition site

If a preliminary colostomy has been made just above the aganglionic colon, this is taken down and both ends of the bowel are closed by suture. The bowel distal to the colostomy is then mobilized in the usual way for resection, and that proximal to it is mobilized for the pull-through to the anal canal.

If a right transverse colostomy has been made for a usual-length segment it is left as a covering colostomy, to be closed 2 weeks later or when the anastomosis is soundly healed.

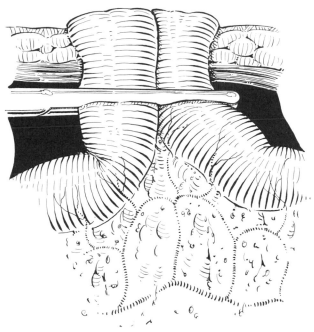

20

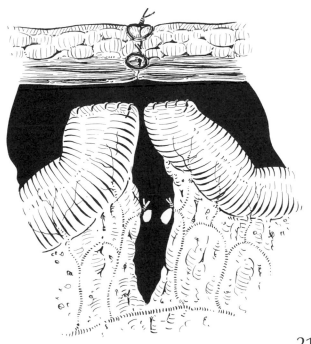

21

## Long-segment cases

# 22 & 23

If a long segment involves pull-through of the right colon, this is completely mobilized and rotated 180° down around the axis of the ileocolic vessels. Any attempt to achieve the usual course of the colon around the abdomen from right to left obstructs around the mesenteric root.

If only part of the ascending colon is ganglionic the author prefers to resect this and perform an ileorectal Duhamel procedure after at least 3 months with an ileostomy.

## Denis Browne modification

The advantage of this is that no bowel is opened or divided within the abdomen. The disadvantages are that (a) gross megacolon may overstretch the anus on prolapsing it, and (b) special (but easily constructed) instruments are needed: a very long 'knitting needle' and 'suture plugs' of plastic in three sizes.

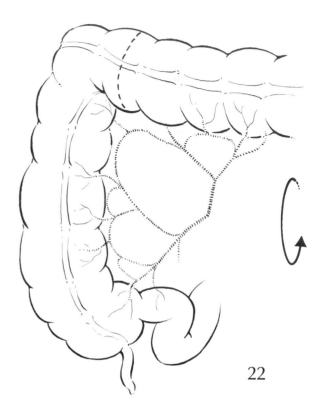

22

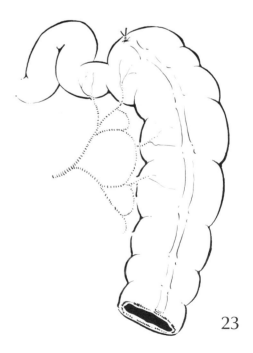

23

# 24

## Introduction of a sigmoidoscope

A sigmoidoscope is passed up to present its distal end above the pubis. A needle longer than the sigmoidoscope is threaded with a 1.5 m loop of thick plaited silk and passed around the mobilized bowel. The needle is then inserted through the bowel wall just proximal to the sigmoidoscope, withdrawn outside the anus and the silk snugged down at the distal end of the instrument. Traction on the silk and sigmoidoscope together prolapses the bowel.

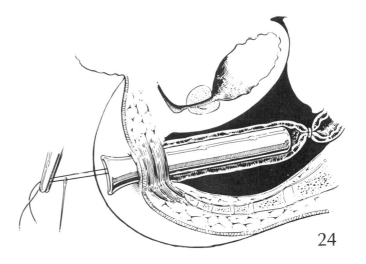

24

## Incision of outer layer

The outer layer is incised longitudinally down to just above the anal canal anteriorly, from 1 cm above the anal columns in the small infant to 2 cm above in an adolescent.

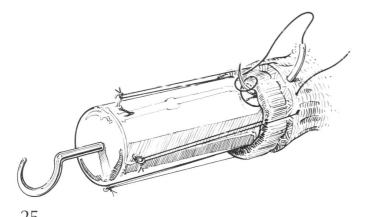

25

# 25

## Completion of bowel division

The inner layer is then withdrawn up to the marker stitch and is opened. A suture plug of suitable size is inserted and circumferential division of the bowel is completed in quadrants, attaching each in turn to the plug for control during the anastomosis. The anastomosis is made obliquely, reaching down almost to the dentate line posteriorly. Denis Browne mattress sutures are used and should be tied fairly loosely.

## DUHAMEL OPERATION WITH STAPLER

### Mobilization of the sigmoid

Exposure is obtained as in the Swenson operation; the sigmoid colon is mobilized in the same way but the superior rectal artery is preserved because part of the rectum is retained in this operation.

### Division of the colon

The bowel is divided for pull-through at a suitable point as confirmed by frozen-section biopsies.

### Retrorectal, transanal pull-through

The colon is drawn forward over the pubis, and the retrorectal space is easily opened by blunt dissection with the index finger.

The posterior half of the lower anal canal is exposed by an Allis clamp at each side, with one limb of the clamp on the para-anal skin and the other inside the anus so that the forceps grip around the superficial external sphincter and can be used to rotate the posterior anal wall outward.

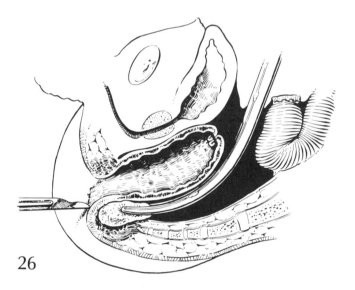

26

## 26

A small swab held in a long curved artery forceps is then thrust down the retrorectal space further to evert the posterior wall of the anal canal. An incision is made across the posterior wall of the canal a few millimetres above the dentate line, exposing the swab (this leaves the lower half of the internal sphincter intact).

The swab is grasped from below with another forceps and this forceps is guided up into the abdomen by traction on the upper forceps. The swab is released and sutures on the end of the colon are grasped in the forceps. The colon is then drawn down to the incision in the anal canal, sutured to this incision and its end opened.

## 27

### Application of the stapler

The GIA stapler is then inserted, one limb in the rectum and the other in the pulled-down colon. Activation of the stapler then divides the septum between colon and rectum over 5 cm, leaving two overlapping layers of staples on each side of the cut.

*Note:* The bowel wall in Hirschprung's disease is commonly so thickened that adult-size staples, rather than the paediatric size, may be needed for all but the very youngest infants.

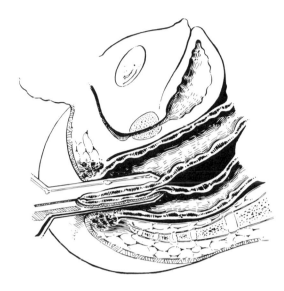

27

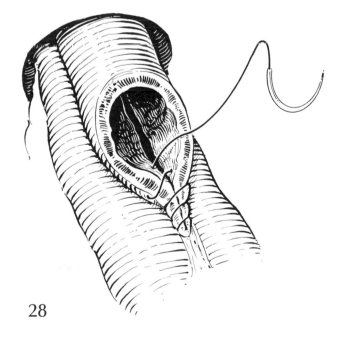

28

### Division of the rectum

## 28

The distal colon is drawn upwards and forward, demonstrating the upper end of the stapled lateral anastomosis. The rectum is divided at this level, cutting obliquely forwards and downwards. The open end is closed with a running 3/0 catgut suture and a second layer of interrupted 3/0 silks.

The TA stapler may be used if this rather bulky instrument can be fitted low enough in the small pelvis.
The author completes the operation with a proximal colostomy, although many believe this to be unnecessary. A drain is placed from the left iliac fossa before the abdomen is closed in layers.

## THE DUHAMEL OPERATION IN OLDER CHILDREN

In older children, the 5-cm division by the stapler does not reach the level of the peritoneal reflexion which is preferred for division of the rectum. In such cases a longer lateral anastomosis can be made by applying the stapler from above, within the abdomen. A stab wound is made in the rectum at the level of the peritoneal reflection and another in the adjacent anterior wall of the colon. The stapler is then placed with one limb in each and its action forms the upper part of the neorectum. The instrument is re-inserted from below to complete the division of the septum. The operation then continues as before. Indeed, by continuing the intra-abdominal applications the 'Lester-Martin' operation can be achieved, in which at least the entire left colon is retained, joined side-to-side to the ileum for cases of total colonic aganglionosis. This is intended to improve reabsorption of water and electrolytes.

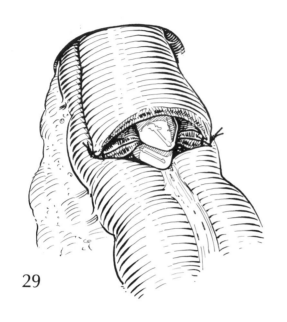

29

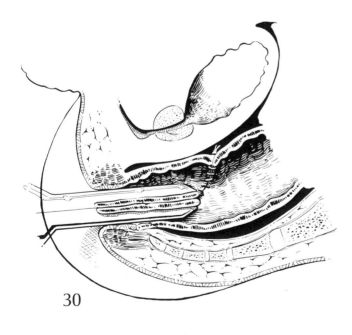

30

## DUHAMEL OPERATION WITHOUT THE STAPLER

# 29 & 30

### Martin's first modification

The upper end of the rectum is left open and sutured to an incision in the anterior surface of the colon at the same level. The modified Lloyd Davis or similar crushing clamp is placed with one blade in the rectum and the other in the pulled-down colon, under direct vision, before the anastomosis of the upper end of the rectum to the opening in the colon is completed. The clamps are tightened in the usual way, and separate in 4–5 days. This avoids the risk of any blind anterior pouch which sometimes followed the original Duhamel technique if the spur was not crushed right to its apex. Such a pouch could be the site of faecal impaction and hence troublesome soiling.

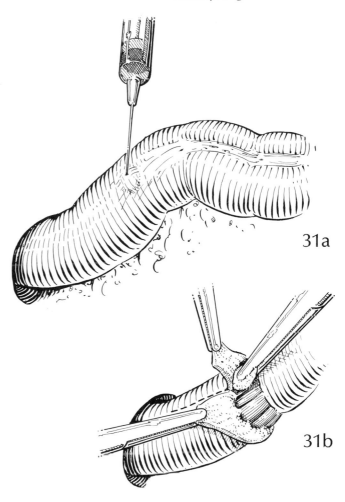

31a

31b

## SOAVE'S OPERATION

In this procedure also, care is taken to retain the superior rectal artery, because the muscle coat of the rectum is to be retained.

# 31a, b

### Submucosal resection

Saline injections help to find the submucous plane, in which blunt and forceps dissection is carried down to the anal canal. A few scissor snips may be required. Gauze pressure is sufficient to stop bleeding from the small vessels divided. The rectal muscle tube is slightly dilated.

### The 'non-suture' anastomosis

The anus is dilated and the mucosa is divided at the upper end of the anal canal. The colon is pulled through to the desired level and fixed with sutures to the upper end of the rectal muscle tube. A few loosely tied sutures also hold the bowel to the skin at the anal verge and a Penrose drain lies in the space between the colon and the rectal muscle tube.

# 32

About 5 cm of colon is left protruding. Twenty-one days later, when the colon is adherent to the rectal muscles, the external excess is cut off with diathermy. No covering colostomy is needed, since there is virtually an anal colostomy until the bowel is trimmed back. Daily dilatation of the non-suture anastomosis may be necessary for several weeks. At first the anastomosis feels very thick, not unlike a cervix, but this commonly causes little trouble and settles down surprisingly well.

32

## Denda technique ('Sutured Soave')

## 33

A similar procedure has been described by Scott Boley. The pulled-through colon is divided at the anus and sutured to the free edge of the mucosa at the upper end of the anal canal. Resection of the mucosal cylinder can be achieved by a prolapsing technique similar to that of the Swenson operation (see *Illustration 18*). These sutures are placed by everting each quadrant of the anal canal in turn with Allis forceps. It is *essential* also to place a few deep sutures through the full thickness of the lower rectal wall to avoid retraction within the rectal cuff.

A covering colostomy is constructed before wound closure.

## Author's personal variant

A midline incision down the muscle coats of the rectum eases the separation of the mucosal and submucosal layers from the muscle coats. The bowel is mainly held by the anastomosis at the anus after the pull-through, but a few sutures at the upper end give extra support. The muscular tube is not reconstituted, lessening the risk of a cuff abscess in a closed space, and of constriction of the pulled-through colon.

It is also possible to compromise between the non-suture anastomosis of Soave and the Denda/Scott Boley primary suture technique. The bowel is drawn down beyond the anus as in the Soave procedure and then a complete layer of sutures is placed between the sero-muscular coats of the bowel and the muscle coat and mucosa of the upper end of the anal canal. It is important to dilate the anus well to avoid premature separation of the pulled-through colon. Excision of the excess bowel is delayed for 21 days, as for the Soave operation. In children who are fit for definitive operation without a preliminary colostomy, this allows one to avoid a covering colostomy, since an anal colostomy virtually exists.

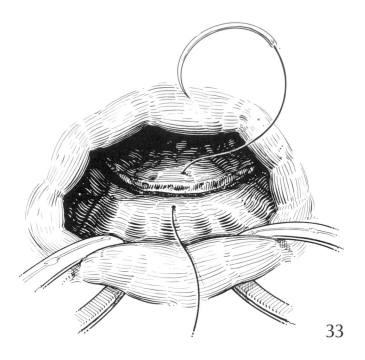

33

## Anorectal myectomy for ultra-short-segment Hirschsprung's disease

A syndrome with milder symptoms of constipation has been recognized in recent years and called ultra-short-segment disease. Barium enema may not demonstrate an unexpanded distal segment, but anorectal manometry and/or biopsy may be typical of aganglionosis. Anorectal myectomy to weaken the internal sphincter may be adequate treatment for these.

## 34

The anus is held open with a child-sized Goligher or Parks retractor, and a transverse incision is made across the posterior wall of the anal canal just above the dentate line. Adrenaline 1:200 000 is injected submucosally. The mucosa is elevated from the underlying muscle, largely by blunt dissection, and is held forward by stay sutures.

A strip of internal sphincter is excised 5–10 mm wide, depending on the size of the child, and the excision is extended as far proximally as can conveniently be reached, usually 5–8 cm.

The wound is then closed with a running suture of catgut, without drainage.

*Note:* Although these are called ultra-short-segment cases, sometimes the entire resected strip is aganglionic, even though the operation is clinically successful. It would be more precise to say that it is an uncommon mild variant presenting as chronic constipation without obstructive symptoms, and usually having a very short segment. The variation in the histological picture of aganglionic segments described by Garrett and Howard would explain this presentation.

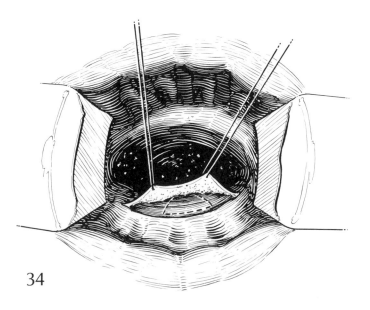

34

# Results

The long-term results of the three major types of operation, prolapse resection, retrorectal transanal resection and endorectal resection, are very similar in the usual forms of the disease. Minor soiling may persist for some time in childhood, but has usually resolved at puberty if not before. Major soiling is rare and probably due to technical shortcomings. Residual constipation may occasionally result from resection through transitional bowel which has some ganglia but is not fully normal.

The commonest cause of death remains enterocolitis and it is at its most serious in the early months of life. Vancomycin prescribed against *Clostridium difficile* is very effective in some but not all cases, so general management as described in the introduction remains important.

A 5–15 year follow-up of 276 of the author's patients treated by these operations revealed a combined early and late mortality of 12 per cent. Twenty-seven of the 34 deaths were related to enterocolitis, 19 being early and eight late, sometimes several years after apparent successful operations. Infectious complications of the operation (sometimes associated with enterocolitis) were next in frequency, and were the reason for reverting to a covering colostomy (or perhaps caecostomy).

## Further reading

Boley, S. J., Lafer, D. J., Kleinhaus, S., Cohn, B. D., Mestel, A. L., Kottmeier, P. K. (1968) Endorectal pullthrough procedure for Hirschprung's disease with and without primary anastomosis. Journal of Pediatric Surgery, 3, 258–262

Boley, S. J. (1984) A new operative approach to total aganglionosis of the colon. Surgery, Gynaecology and Obstetrics, 159, 481–484

Browne, D., (1949) Discussion on Hirschprung's disease. Proceedings of the Royal Society of Medicine, 42, 227–228

Denda, T., Katzumata, K. (1966) New techniques for Hirschprung's disease. Journal of Japanese Association of Pediatric Surgeons, 2, 37

Duhamel, B. (1956) Une nouvelle opération pour le mégacolon congénitale, l'abaissement retrorectale et trans-anal du colon et son application possible au traitement de quelques autres malformations. Presse Médicale, 64, 2249–2250

Kimura, K., Nishijima, E., Muraji, T., Tsugawa, C., Matsutmo, Y. (1988) Extensive aganglionosis: Further experience with the Colonic Patch Graft procedure and long term results. Journal of Pediatric Surgery, 23, 52–56

Kottmeier, P. K., Jonger, B., Velcek, A. Friedman, A., Klotz, D. H. (1981) Absorptive function of the aganglionic ileum. Journal of Pediatric Surgery, 16, 275–278

Lake, B. D., Puri, P., Nixon, H. H., Claireaux, A. E. (1978) Hirschprung's disease: an appraisal of histochemically demonstrated acetylcholinesterase activity in suction rectal biopsy specimens as an aid to diagnosis. Archives of Pathology and Laboratory Medicine, 102, 244–247

Nixon, H. H. (1985) Hirschprung's disease: Progress in management and diagnostics. World Journal of Surgery, 9, 189–202

Soave, F. (1960) A new surgical technique for treatment of Hirschprung's disease. Surgery, 56, 1007–1014

Stringel, G. (1986) Extensive intestinal aganglionosis including the ileum: a new surgical technique. Journal of Pediatric Surgery, 21, 667–670

Swenson, O., Sherman, J. O., Fisher, J. H., Cohen, E. (1978) The treatment and postoperative complications of congenital megacolon: a 25-year folow-up. Annals of Surgery, 182, 266–273

Thomas, D. F. M., Fernie, D. S., Bayston, R., Spitz, L., Nixon, H. H. (1986) Enterocolitis in Hirschprung's disease: a controlled study of the etiologic role of *Clostridium difficile*. Journal of Pediatric Surgery, 21, 22–25

Illustrations by Gillian Oliver

# Inflammatory bowel disease

**Eric W. Fonkalsrud** MD
Professor and Chief of Pediatric Surgery, and Vice-Chairman, Department of Surgery, University of California, Los Angeles School of Medicine, Los Angeles, California, USA

## PROCTOCOLECTOMY FOR INFLAMMATORY BOWEL DISEASE

## 1 & 2

The patient is placed on the operating table in the semi-lithotomy (Lloyd-Davis) position with the heels and popliteal fossa well padded. The site for the ileostomy stoma, which has been carefully selected by the stoma therapist preoperatively to avoid both skin creases and the belt line, is marked with a small superficial cross-incision. The abdomen is opened through an incision placed slightly to the left of the midline in order to provide more space for the ileostomy appliance, and extends from approximately 3 cm above the umbilicus to the pubic symphysis. The subcutaneous tissues are divided with electrocautery extending to the linea alba.

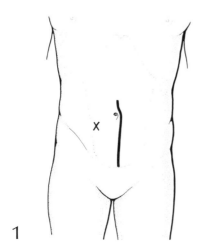

1

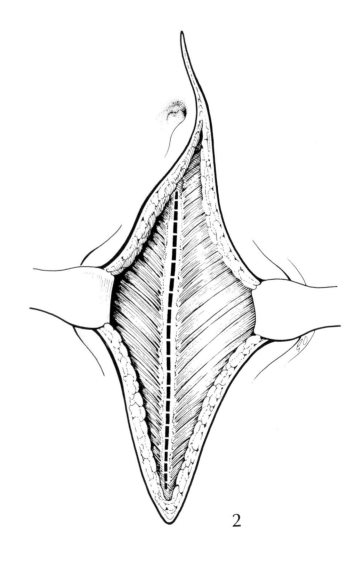

2

# 3

The intestine is carefully examined from the ligament of Treitz to the ileocaecal valve to exclude the possibility of Crohn's disease. The colon in most cases will be thickened, somewhat shortened, and be more extensively covered by fat than is normally seen. The gall-bladder, liver and pancreas are carefully inspected.

The ileum is divided approximately 2–4 cm proximal to the ileocaecal valve. It is rare that the terminal ileum is involved severely enough to warrant more extensive resection.

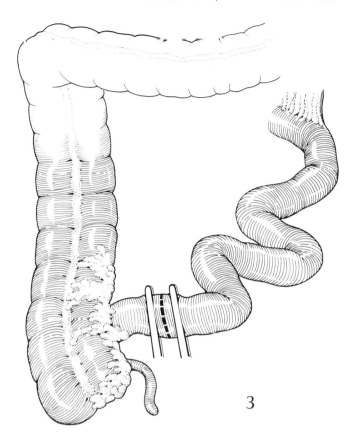

3

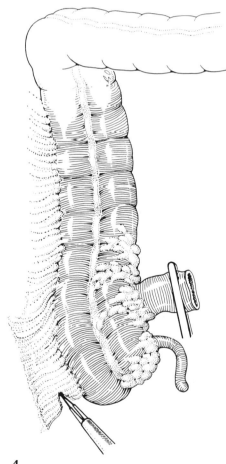

4

# 4

The ileocolic vessels are doubly ligated with silk and divided. The right colon is mobilized from the posterior abdomen with electrocautery, ligating larger vessels which are common with inflammatory bowel disease.

# 5

The hepatic flexure of the colon is mobilized and the major portion of the omentum is taken with the specimen. Blunt finger dissection is used to carefully separate the duodenum from the colon. The transverse mesocolon is divided near the base, with the middle colic vessels doubly ligated, and divided. The dissection is less extensive than for malignant lesions.

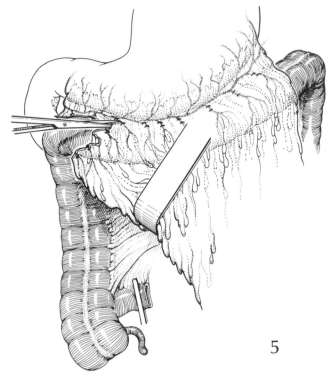

5

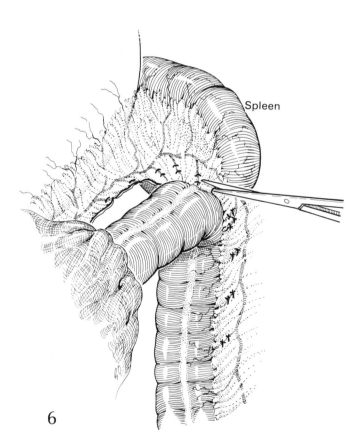

6

# 6

The splenic flexure of the colon is mobilized, with care taken to avoid injury to the spleen and pancreas. All vessels are ligated and divided. The left colon is mobilized by incising the peritoneum along the avascular line between mesentery and posterior peritoneum. The left colic vessels are doubly ligated and divided.

# 7

The sigmoid colon is transected approximately 6–10 cm above the peritoneal reflection, and the specimen submitted to the pathologist for examination. The sigmoid mesentery is divided, with the dissection carried progressively closer to the muscularis. The peritoneal reflection is incised circumferentially around the rectum with electrocautery.

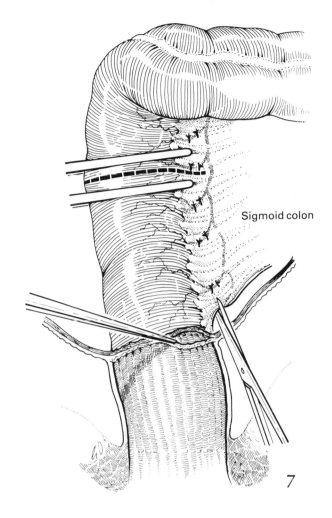

Sigmoid colon

7

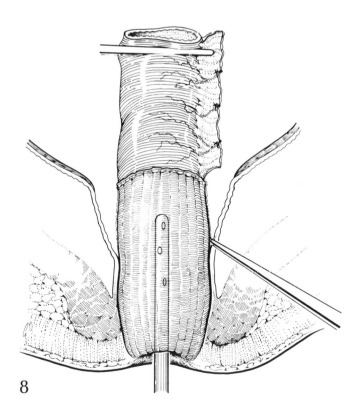

8

# 8

The rectal muscularis is dissected from the adjacent tissues with electrocautery, staying directly on the rectal muscularis or even leaving small segments of muscularis in the patient. A large rubber catheter (24 Fr) is inserted per rectum, which is then irrigated with antibiotic solution. The rectal muscularis is dissected free from the pelvic structures down to within 3–5 cm of the dentate line.

# 9

An elliptical incision is made around the anus with electrocautery and the dissection carried superiorly, staying very close to the rectal muscularis, leaving the striated sphincter mechanism in place.

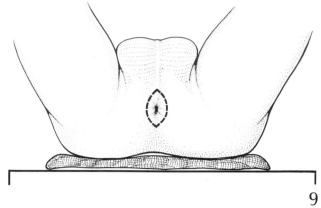

9

# 10

The rectal muscle is mobilized superiorly up to the level of dissection carried out from above. A finger placed into the rectum through the anus serves as a guide to ensure that the dissection is carried very close to the rectal muscle.

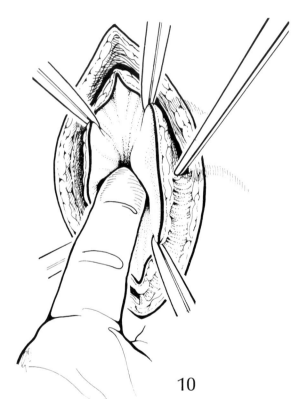

10

# 11

As the dissection is carried superiorly, vessels are cauterized, with care taken to avoid dissecting widely. The rectum and colon are then removed.

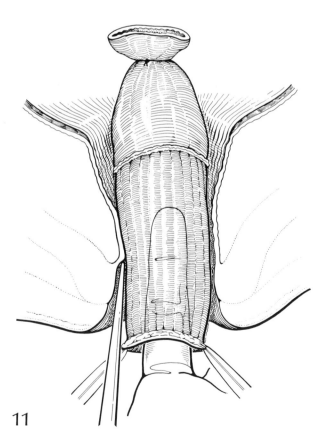

11

## 12

Following removal of the rectum and the sigmoid colon, the anal sphincter mechanism is divided posteriorly with electrocautery up to the level of the coccyx to ensure that the rectal space can be drained widely. Thorough haemostasis must be achieved.

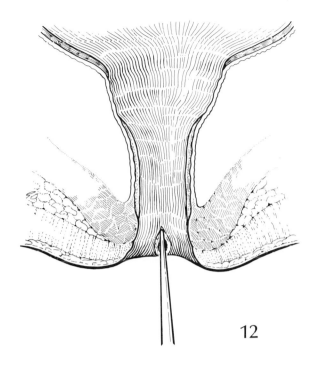

12

Peritoneal floor

13

## 13

A Silastic sump catheter is inserted into the rectal space from below and the space irrigated with antibiotic solution. The upper end of the rectal space is closed from above with several absorbable sutures, in layers in order to reduce the 'dead space'. The peritoneum is closed with a continuous row of absorbable sutures.

## 14

A disc of skin and underlying muscle is excised from the preselected site in the right lower abdominal wall to construct the ileostomy. The opening is made sufficiently large so that the surgeon's two index fingers may be snugly passed completely through the opening. The rectus muscle is retracted medially during construction of the ileostomy.

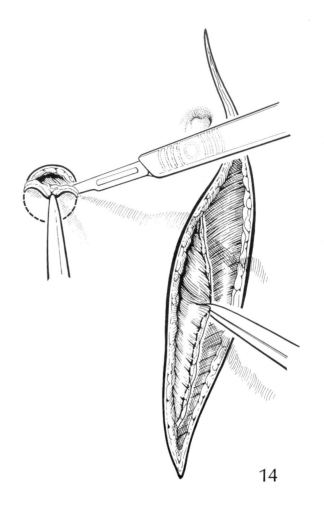

14

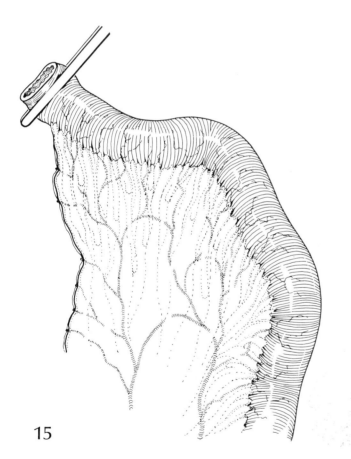

15

## 15

Mesenteric vessels of the terminal ileum are ligated to free sufficient length to construct the ileostomy stoma.

## 16

The terminal ileum is brought through the ileostomy opening in the abdominal wall and the posterior rectus sheath is attached to the muscularis of the ileum with four absorbable sutures. Approximately 3 cm of ileum are allowed to project from the surface of the abdominal skin. The anterior rectus sheath is attached to the intestine circumferentially with non-absorbable sutures. The end of the ileum is then matured by attaching the full thickness of the end of the ileum to the subcuticular tissue at the ileostomy site circumferentially with approximately 12 absorbable sutures.

In patients with a panniculus of more than 1 cm, the four quadrant sutures maturing the end of the stoma are attached to the ileum slightly exterior to the anterior rectus sheath as well as through the subcuticular tissues, to ensure than an adequate size stoma nipple projecting approximately 1 cm will be constructed. The ileal mesentery is attached to the peritoneum of the right lateral abdominal wall to prevent internal herniation.

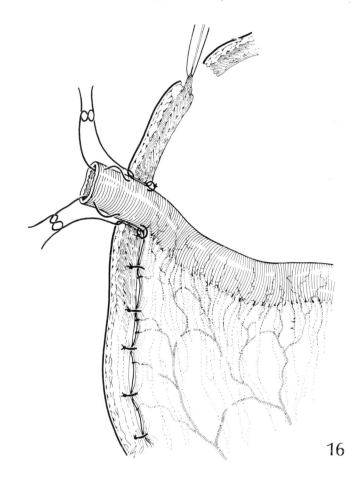

**16**

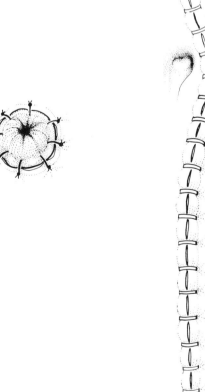

**17**

## 17

The abdomen is thoroughly irrigated with antibiotic solution. The rectus muscles are closed with interrupted absorbable sutures. The subcutaneous tissues are closed loosely with fine absorbable sutures, and the skin is closed with fine metal staples. A disposable ileostomy appliance is placed over the stoma.

# RESECTION OF TERMINAL ILEUM AND RIGHT COLON FOR CROHN'S DISEASE

## 18

With the patient in the supine position, a transverse right abdominal incision is made slightly inferior to the umbilicus.

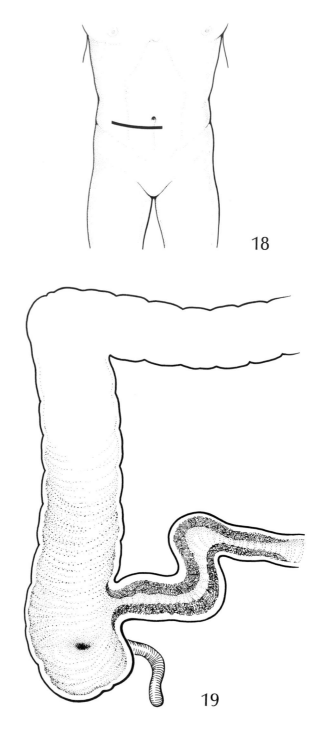

18

## 19

The abdomen is thoroughly explored, noting any areas of inflammation in the small intestine. The most frequent site of involvement is the terminal ileum and right colon which commonly produces obstruction and/or fistula formation. Areas of mild inflammation in the small or large intestines are not resected.

19

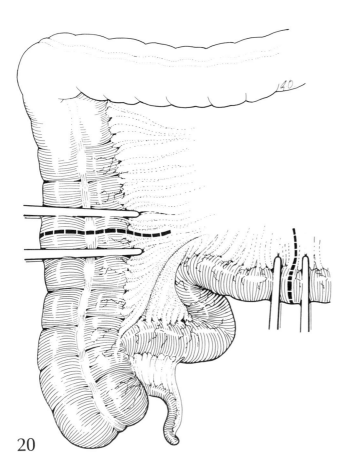

20

## 20

The ileum is divided approximately 3–5 cm proximal to the area of severe involvement in the terminal ileum. The site of resection need not be completely free of mild inflammatory disease. The site of distal resection can usually be placed just proximal to the hepatic flexure of the colon, or in some cases just distal to this point. The intestine is mobilized and divided both proximally and distally.

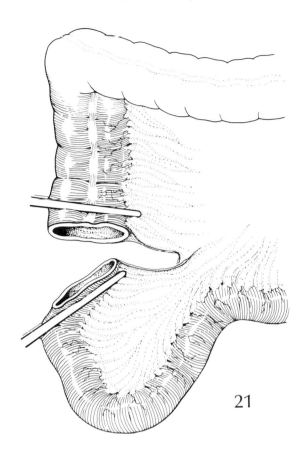

## 21 & 22

The ileocolic vessels are doubly ligated with silk and divided. The terminal ileum and right colon are resected. The end of the distal ileum is opened slightly along the antimesenteric border. An end-to-end anastomosis between terminal ileum and right colon is constructed, using continuous non-absorbable sutures to approximate the mucosa circumferentially.

21

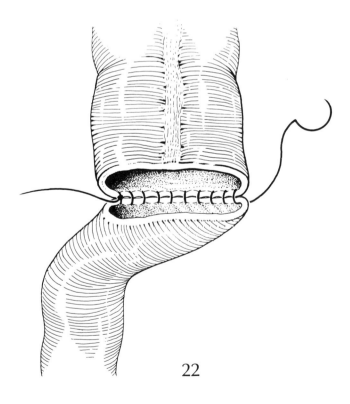

22

# 23

A second layer of seromuscular silk or Vicryl sutures is placed circumferentially about the mucosal repair. The mesenteric defect is closed with fine silk and the abdomen is closed with absorbable suture material.

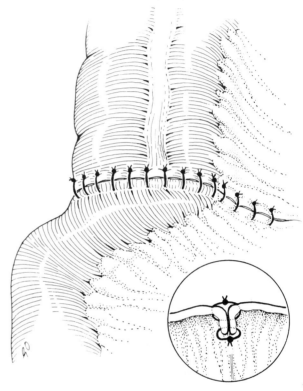

23

# ENDORECTAL ILEAL PULLTHROUGH WITH ILEAL RESERVOIR FOR COLITIS AND POLYPOSIS

## Introduction

During the past 15 years new operative techniques have become available for treating children with ulcerative colitis or familial polyposis which obviate the need for permanent ileostomy appliances. Since excellent clinical results have been obtained during the past two decades with proctocolectomy and standard Brooke cutaneous ileostomy, any new operative technique for treatment of ulcerative colitis must be carefully considered. Endorectal pullthrough operations have the attractive features of avoiding a permanent cutaneous stoma, obviating repeated stomal or rectal catheterizations as might be necessary with the Kock pouch, and eventually providing a near-normal pattern of defaecation. Moreover, patients who undergo mucosal proctectomy are almost certain to avoid complications of bladder dysfunction and impotence, both of which occasionally occur after standard proctocolectomy.

Children selected for proctocolectomy in most cases have chronic ulcerative colitis refractory to intensive medical therapy, including prednisone. If a child continues to have active symptoms when the steroids are tapered down on repeated occasions, it is highly unlikely that the disease will ever resolve without removal of the colon and rectum. Approximately 15 per cent of patients will present with major colorectal bleeding from colitis.

When the patient has been identified as refractory to medical therapy, the endorectal pullthrough procedure is preferred to standard proctocolectomy or Kock pouch if he or she is under the age of 55 years. Children recover from the pullthrough procedure extremely well compared to adults. A cutaneous ileostomy during childhood is somewhat limiting, both in athletics and in social activities, regardless of whether it is drained through a catheter as with the Kock pouch.

Patients selected for endorectal pullthrough should have biopsy-proven ulcerative colitis with definite absence of granulomatous disease. A normal small-bowel series is very helpful. Although haemorrhoids are common with ulcerative colitis, anal fistulae or abscesses should strongly suggest the presence of Crohn's disease, in which case an endorectal pullthrough procedure would be contraindicated.

During the past 6 years almost all surgeons performing the endorectal pullthrough procedure have utilized an ileal reservoir to reduce faecal urgency and frequency. The original S-shaped reservoir used clinically by Parks[1] does not provide peristaltic emptying and has a tendency to distend and develop pouchitis. None the less, many patients have had very good results with the S-shaped reservoir.

The J-shaped reservoir described by Utsonomiya and associates[2] has the lower end at the ileoanal anastomosis, and thus empties very readily. The greatest difficulty is achieving sufficient length on the ileal mesentery to allow the side of the ileum to extend to the anus for anastomosis. In addition, a long suture line is placed in the pelvis in an area which is particularly prone to infection after mucosal stripping. The J reservoir has been used with good success in a few large centres in the United States[3].

The lateral isoperistaltic ileal reservoir has the advantage of two isoperistaltic segments which form the reservoir emptying downward to the anus. Ideally, the lower end of the reservoir should be as close to the ileoanal anastomosis as possible, usually within 2–3 cm. The lateral reservoir may be performed in one or two stages depending upon the difficulty in removing the rectal mucosa[4].

During the past few years, certain features of the operation have become very apparent. The rectal muscle cuff need not be longer than approximately 5 cm. Longer muscle cuffs produce narrowing of the reservoir and partial obstruction. The reservoir should extend as close to the ileoanal anastomosis as technically feasible in order to assure proper emptying. The length of the reservoir for children rarely needs to exceed 12–15 cm, and in adults 14–16 cm. A completely diverting ileostomy is imperative to minimize contamination in the pelvis.

During the past ten years 180 patients in our hospital have undergone endorectal ileal pullthrough with ileal reservoir. The major complications were associated with infection in the rectal muscle cuff, leading to reservoir leak and pelvic abscess, and with eventual removal of the reservoir in four patients. A temporary diverting ileostomy was performed in 14 patients, in order to repair rectovulvar fistulae, relieve obstruction due to too long a rectal muscle cuff, or permit healing of a sinus tract between the ileal pullthrough segment and rectal muscle cuff. Eight of these ileostomies have subsequently been closed.

Fifty-six of the patients have undergone reoperation for release of adhesions causing obstruction, repair of internal hernias, or shortening of the ileal reservoir which was initially made too long. All the reservoirs removed, and all the patients undergoing ileostomy, as well as 23 of the patients requiring reoperation, were from the first 50 subjects to undergo the pullthrough procedure. Modifications in operative technique have markedly reduced complications. There was one death in the early postoperative period, related to steroid insuffiency and acute Addisonian crisis.

All the patients resumed near-normal physical activities within 2 or 3 months; 96 are vigorous athletes. None of the patients has experienced sexual or urinary-tract dysfunction. The incidence of faecal staining or occasional soiling 6 months postoperatively was 21 of 115 patients. At night, 27 of 115 patients experienced some soiling at 6 months. By 12 months only five of 90 patients experienced any staining or soiling. Nocturnal soiling occurred occasionally in nine of 90 patients.

Each of the patients in the present study indicated that they were minimally limited in any activities by the pullthrough operation, in contrast to the period between operations when each had an ileostomy; none would return to an ileostomy unless advised to do so because of complications. Greater consideration should be given to early operation for those with ulcerative colitis refractory to medical therapy. The endorectal ileal pullthrough operation is technically difficult; however, close attention to the many details of operative and postoperative care is likely to provide gratifying long-term results.

## The operation

## 24

Following removal of the colon to the sigmoid, as performed for total proctocolectomy, the peritoneal reflection is incised circumferentially around the rectum with electrocautery. The upper rectum is separated from the pelvic tissues by cautery dissection, staying as close to the rectal muscle as possible. This dissection is carried down approximately 5–7 cm below the peritoneal reflection. The rectum is irrigated extensively with antibiotic solution.

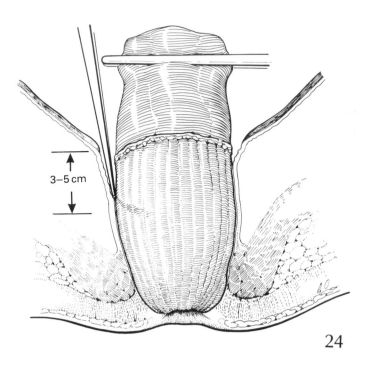

3–5 cm

24

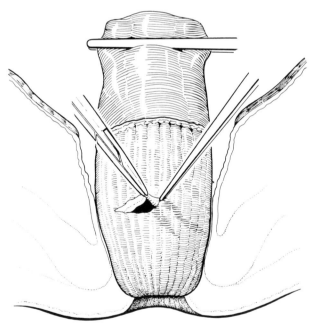

25

## 25

Using electrocautery, the rectal muscle and mucosa are incised circumferentially approximately 4–5 cm proximal to the dentate line.

## 26

The anus is dilated with the index fingers and a self-retaining anal retractor is inserted. Dilute adrenaline solution is injected beneath the mucosa circumferentially at the level of the dentate line to facilitate the initial dissection of the anorectal mucosa from the underlying muscularis.

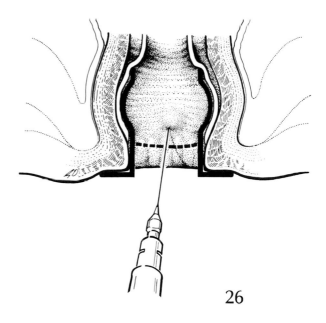

26

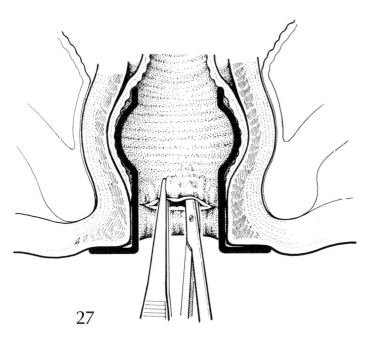

27

## 27

The mucosa is incised circumferentially at the level of the dentate line and the mucosa is elevated from the anal sphincter muscles using scissor dissection. The dissection is carried up to the plane of dissection established from above and the rectal mucosa is removed. Thorough haemostasis is achieved and the pelvis is thoroughly irrigated with antibiotic solution.

# 28

The end of the ileum is mobilized appropriately to provide sufficient length for the tip to be brought through the rectal muscularis down to the anus. The end of the ileum is oversewn loosely with fine silk to facilitate bringing it through the rectal muscular canal. The mesentery of the ileum is carefully placed posteriorly without twisting. The end of the full thickness of ileum is attached to the anal mucosa, taking bites of underlying muscularis using interrupted heavy absorbable suture material. A Silastic

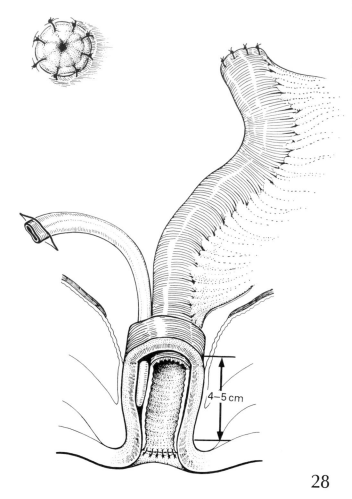

**28**

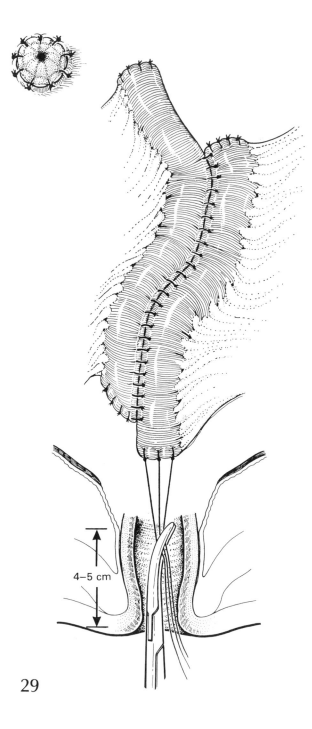

**29**

drain is placed between the ileal pullthrough segment and the rectal muscularis and brought through a separate incision in the left lower abdominal wall.

The ileum is divided approximately 12 cm above the peritoneal reflection and the distal end oversewn. The proximal end of the divided ileum is brought through the right lower abdominal wall as a cutaneous ileostomy. The mesentery of the ileum cannot be attached to the lateral abdominal wall in view of the close proximity to the pullthrough segment of ileum.

# 29

An isoperistaltic ileal reservoir 12–15 cm long is constructed after mucosal proctectomy in one stage. The reservoir is made with the GIA stapler. A second row of sutures is placed around the entire anastomosis. The spout at the end of the reservoir is brought through the rectal muscle canal and sutured to the anus. A temporary end ileostomy is used for diversion. This simplified technique of reservoir construction has been used successfully in our last 84 consecutive patients.

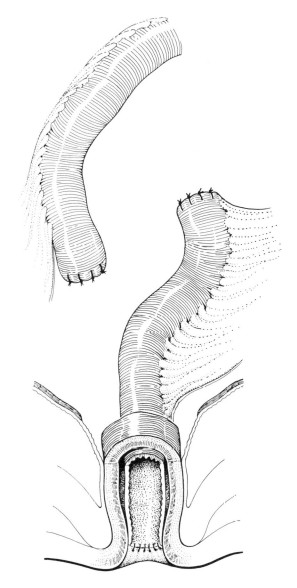

## 30

Approximately four months after the endorectal ileal pullthrough, the abdomen is entered through the previous surgical scar. The ileostomy is mobilized from the abdominal wall and the tip resected. The end of the ileum is oversewn with two layers of absorbable suture. The mesentery is mobilized appropriately so that the end extends into the pelvis. Any adhesions within the abdominal cavity are divided. The end of the distal segment of ileum extending to the pelvis is mobilized down to within 2–4 cm of the ileoanal anastomosis.

**30**

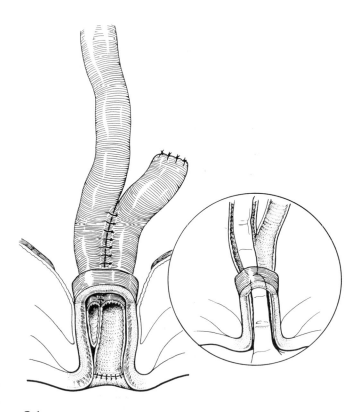

**31**

## 31

The end of the proximal ileum is brought down beside the pullthrough segment of ileum in such a manner that a side-to-side anti-mesenteric anastomosis can be constructed. A two-layer anastomosis is constructed using continuous absorbable sutures for the mucosa, interrupted every 3–5 cm, and interrupted Vicryl for seromuscular sutures. The lower end of the proximal ileum is brought sufficiently low into the pelvis so that the index finger from one hand can be placed into the anus from below and the index finger of the other hand placed through the site of the anastomosis; the two fingers should touch without stretching to ensure that the lower end of the proximal ileum is placed sufficiently low.

## 32

The two-layer anastomosis is continued superiorly almost to the end of the pullthrough segment of ileum.

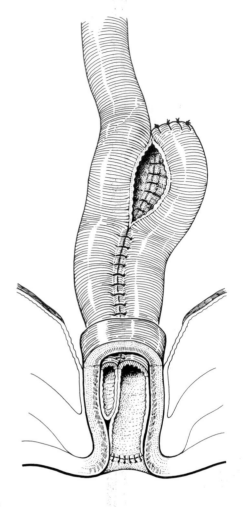

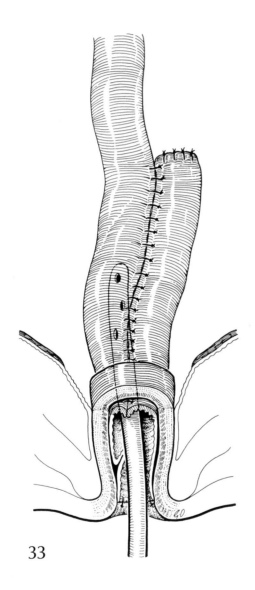

## 33

Following completion of this lateral isoperistaltic ileal reservoir, a Foley catheter (size 30) is placed through the end of the ileal pullthrough segment and brought through the anus. The mesentery of the ileal reservoir is attached to the posterior abdominal wall to prevent internal herniation. The ileostomy wound and the abdominal wound are closed as described for proctocolectomy (page 000).

## References

1. Parks, A. G., Nicholls, R. J. (1978) Proctocolectomy with ileostomy for ulcerative colitis. British Medical Journal, 2, 85–88

2. Utsunomiya, J., Iwama, T., Imajo, M., Matsuo, S., Sawai, S., Yaegashi, K. et al. (1980) Total colectomy, mucosal proctectomy and ileoanal anastomosis. Diseases of the Colon and Rectum, 23, 459–466

3. Kelley, K. A. (1985) Ileal pouch–anal anastomosis after proctocolectomy. Surgical Rounds, 8, 48–57

4. Fonkalsrud, E. W. (1985) Endorectal ileal pullthrough with isoperistaltic ileal reservoir for colitis and polyposis. Annals of Surgery, 202, 145–152

# Rectal polyps

**R. C. M. Cook**   MA, BM, FRCS
Consultant Paediatric Surgeon, Alder Hey Children's Hospital, Liverpool, UK

## Introduction

Juvenile polyps may present throughout childhood and adolescence; the peak incidence is at 4–5 years, and boys are affected a little more frequently than girls. While such polyps may develop in any part of the large bowel, the great majority are found in the rectum and rectosigmoid region, i.e. they are within reach of a standard sigmoidoscope. In about 25 per cent of these children, more than one polyp (but not diffuse polyposis) is found either at the initial examination or subsequently.

Juvenile polyps are hamartomas. They are usually 1–2 cm in diameter at presentation and have a smooth, ulcerated surface. The polyp is honeycombed with irregular cysts lined with mucus-secreting cells and separated by vascular connective tissue heavily infiltrated with inflammatory cells. Seventy per cent of polyps are situated in the rectum (usually on the posterior wall), 15 per cent occur in the sigmoid colon, and the remainder are scattered more proximally.

## Clinical features

Local abrasion by the passage of stools frequently leads to a little bright red bleeding at or after defaecation and a mucous secretion is often noticed. Polyps may also prolapse and be described by the mother as a 'dark red cherry' at the anus immediately after defaecation. Digital rectal examination may reveal the polyp, but being soft and mobile, it is not easy to feel.

Not uncommonly the history is given of several small bleeds, followed by a slightly larger one that precipitates a visit to the doctor. By the time of the hospital referral there has been no further sign of bleeding. Auto-amputation of the polyp may have occurred, with spontaneous cure. With such a clear history no investigation is warranted unless the symptoms recur.

## Differential diagnosis

The possibility of a fissure in ano, inflammatory bowel disease, or blood dyscrasia such as Henoch–Schönlein purpura, should be considered. A Meckel's diverticulum, duplication of the intestine, and intussusception may cause bleeding but it is generally more profuse, and the other related symptoms usually distinguish them from the simple polyp.

A solitary adenomatous polyp is rare in childhood, but if found, familial adenomatous polyposis should be considered, with appropriate examination of the rest of the colon.

Rectal polyps may occur in up to 30 per cent of patients with Peutz–Jeghers syndrome, and a rare condition in which there is diffuse polyposis with a mixture of juvenile and adenomatous polyps has also been described.

# Management

The child is admitted as a day case without any bowel preparation. A bisacodyl suppository is of value in evacuating the rectum. Suitable premedication is given and general anaesthesia induced. The child is turned into the left lateral position with the sacrum at the edge of the table and the pelvis raised on a small sandbag. The anus and perineum are inspected, the anus is lubricated, and digital rectal examination performed. It may be possible to remove the polyp at this stage (see *Illustration 1*).

A suitably sized (and lubricated) proctoscope or sigmoidoscope held in the left hand is inserted through the anus towards the umbilicus. As soon as the anal canal is felt to have been passed, the tip of the instrument is directed more posteriorly and the obturator removed and replaced with the glass window. Only the minimum amount of air is insufflated to distend the rectum enough to allow the instrument to be advanced gently up the rectum and into the sigmoid colon. Removal of faeces with a moistened cotton wool swab, or by suction, may be needed. The bowel wall is watched during all man-oeuvres, but a systematic search is easier on withdrawal rather than as the 'scope is being advanced. As soon as a polyp is found it may be removed and sigmoidoscopic inspection then completed.

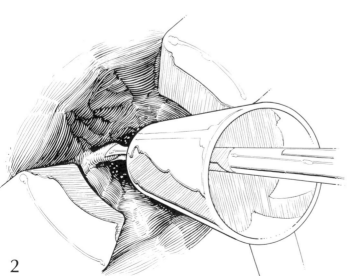

## 1

A polyp in the lower rectum can often be hooked out of the anus by the examining finger, and the stalk ligated with silk or cotton thread, before its removal. It often breaks off spontaneously. Such a simple deliberate avulsion is safely practised by some surgeons, since bleeding from the stalk is usually minimal and stops spontaneously. Persistent bleeding can be controlled by pressure from a cotton wool swab applied after identification of the site through the sigmoidoscope.

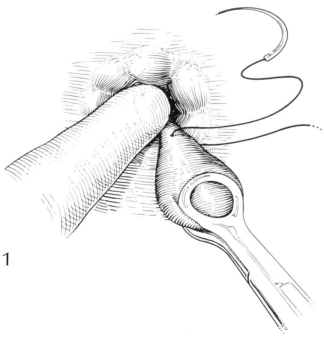

## 2

If bleeding is considerable, a Parks' or similar speculum is inserted. If the bleeding point is in view it can be grasped with an artery forceps and ligated or cauterized.

If not in view, the speculum is left in place and the sigmoidoscope passed into the rectum through it to locate the 'lost' pedicle. This is grasped with forceps. Traction on these while withdrawing the 'scope' will prolapse the mucosa into the view within the speculum where it is grasped with another pair of forceps held outside the sigmoidoscope which is then removed. The pedicle may then be securely ligated or cauterized under direct vision.

## 3

Polyps higher in the rectum are snared through the sigmoidoscope. A wire snare is looped over the polyp, and the polyp or the 'scope, or the patient is manipulated so that the stalk can be seen. It is not usually necessary to grasp the head of the polyp in order to snare it, but it may be helpful. The snare is tightened nearer to the head of the polyp than to the bowel wall. Using a suitably insulated snare, cautery can be used to coagulate and cut the stalk, but simple traction on the snare to cut it rarely causes significant haemorrhage. The polyp must be recovered for histological examination.

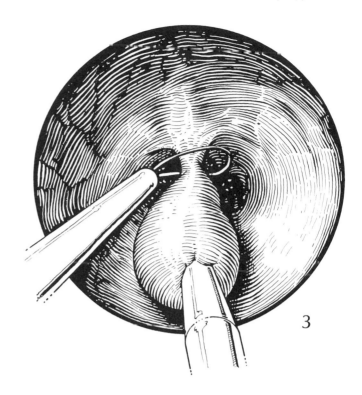

3

## Complications

Bacteraemia, perforation and haemorrhage are all possible, but are very rare. However, the surgeon should avoid rough handling, vigorous pulling on the polyp to tent the bowel wall, and excessive cauterization.

## Postoperative care

Most children can return home as soon as they have recovered from anaesthesia. Parents should be told to expect some old blood with the first bowel action, but warned to report any prolonged or large bleed. For solitary polyps a follow-up visit is not usually arranged, but parents should be asked to return if the symptoms recur, and the surgeon should not close the case until he has seen that histology confirms a hamartomatous juvenile polyp.

## Results

Between 3 and 25 per cent of children are said to get recurrent juvenile polyps at different sites. As this is a benign and self-limiting condition, a prolonged search for more proximal polyps is unwarranted, provided the histology of the distal removed polyp confirms the diagnosis. Such a search would involve full bowel preparation for double-contrast barium enema and colonoscopy. Easily accessible recurrent polyps should be removed as described, if symptomatic.

Illustrations by Kevin Marks

# Fissure in ano

**R. C. M. Cook**  MA, BM, FRCS
Consultant Paediatric Surgeon, Alder Hey Children's Hospital, Liverpool, UK

## Introduction

'The relatively trivial complaint of anal fissure can be a source of severe symptoms for many years. It is often misdiagnosed, yet proper treatment is almost always effective.'[1]

Fissures are not uncommon in childhood, with a peak incidence between 6 and 24 months. Some are short-lived and heal spontaneously. An acute fissure causes pain on defaecation, holding back when the call to defaecate comes, the development of a large and hard stool, further trauma to the fissure, increasing pain, and so on round the cycle. Unless this cycle is broken, intractable bowel problems will follow, with a profound influence on the child's life. Long after the fissure is forgotten the psychiatrist may be struggling to help a family recover from serious disturbances of the child's behaviour and of their relationships.

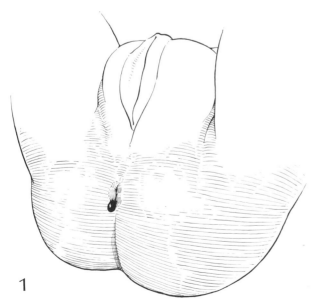

1

## Diagnosis

**1**

This history of pain on defaecation and of hard stools passed infrequently with a streak of blood is almost sufficient to make a diagnosis. Visual inspection of the anus by gentle separation of the buttocks will reveal the fissure – together with a sentinel tag in the more chronic fissure. Digital examination or proctoscopy should *not* be done until the child is anaesthetized. Most fissures lie in the midline (at 12 or 6 o'clock) and, as in adults, posterior fissures are more usual in boys.

Anorectal abuse must always be borne in mind when examining even the very young child (of either sex) who presents with an anal problem[2]. Local features of buggery include fissures, very wide dilatation of the inspected anus, venous engorgement, perianal haematomata and oedema.

Such a child usually exhibits other physical signs of abuse, and also behavioural abnormalities. The very early involvement of a paediatrician experienced in the diagnosis and management of child abuse is essential if the child is to be protected from further injury. Cessation of abuse usually allows healing of the anal pathology without the need for local therapy.

### Differential diagnosis

Pruritis ani and inflammatory conditions of the perianal skin may lead to the formation of multiple, radial superficial cracks that do not extend into the anal canal.

Multiple fissures, or those lying laterally or extending above the dentate line should raise the suspicion of Crohn's disease, ulcerative colitis or tuberculosis.

# Management

### MEDICAL

The majority of acute fissures heal in a few weeks if regular defaecation can be established and maintained. A mild stool softener and aperient (e.g. lactulose) should be prescribed, and a diet adequate in vegetable and cereal fibre is encouraged. It is a self-defeating exercise to put the toddler alone 'on a diet'. The whole family should use wholemeal bread rather than white, and join in other dietary adjustments that will also be to their advantage! Local anaesthetic cream is not recommended, since sensitization is common, it is painful to put it into the anal canal where it will be effective, and useful timing of its application demands unusual clairvoyant skills in the mother.

### ANAL DILATATION

The reason for the effectiveness of this procedure is not certain, but it is assumed that it relieves the spasm of the internal sphincter and allows drainage of infected material from the base of the fissure. The lack of spasm permits the resumption of painless defaecation and the re-establishment of normal bowel habits. The existence and cause of this spasm is not proven in adults and has not been tested in children[3, 4].

## Preoperative preparation

Digital examinations, enemas and suppositories are all forbidden. The child is admitted as a day case, starved, and premedicated appropriately for its age.

## The procedure

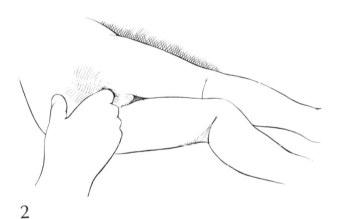

### 2

Under general anaesthesia (deep enough to prevent laryngeal spasm) digital examination is carried out with the child in the left lateral position, (although supine with a nurse flexing the hips is equally suitable for small children). The position, extent and degree of induration round the fissure are noted. A biopsy should always be taken from fissures that appear atypical. The constricting ring described in adults with anal fissures is not so evident in children.

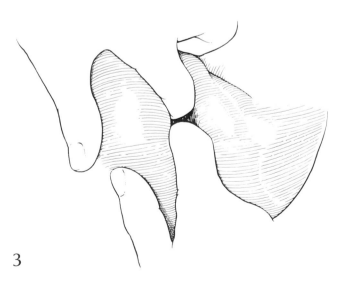

### 3

Dilatation is begun by gentle massage with the right index finger pushing mainly backwards; this hand is then pronated to pull anteriorly and the left index finger is inserted, and gentle but firm stretching carried out anteroposteriorly.

## 4

The hands are rotated and the anal canal is stretched laterally. At this stage it is particularly easy to increase the depth and extent of a posterior fissure, and the amount of force used should be limited in strength and direction to avoid this. Three or four fingers may be used in older children. Hard faeces should be evacuated digitally from the rectum. Adequate dilatation should leave the anal canal lax, but without mucosal tears.

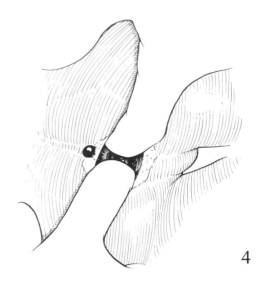

4

### Postoperative care and complications

Regular dilatation of the anal canal is ensured by regular passage of a normal stool. This requires:

1. an aperient such as lactulose;
2. a diet with adequate fibre; and
3. parental support and encouragement.

At an outpatient review 3–4 weeks after dilatation, the dietary and bowel history is checked. The abdomen should be palpated to search for loading of the pelvic colon. The anus can be inspected, but digital internal examination should be avoided. Aperients are gradually withdrawn, and the child should be able to be discharged after a further visit a month or two later.

A little bleeding may be noticed after dilatation and manual evacuation. The short period of incontinence and the bruising secondary to submucosal haemorrhages reported in adults have not been described in children.

### Results

No large series have been reported recently in children, but the great majority seem to experience prompt pain relief. The skin tags usually shrink to insignificance with the passing years. Perhaps 5–10 per cent have recurrence or persistence of symptoms and a further dilatation or sphincterotomy is indicated.

## LATERAL SPHINCTEROTOMY

### Indications

Persistence of a symptomatic fissure after adequate dilatation, which may perhaps have been repeated once or twice, is an indication for lateral sphincterotomy. Such a fissure is usually accompanied by an inflamed or oedematous sentinel skin tag, and is deep enough for the transverse fibres of the lower third of the internal sphincter to be seen. The edges will be undermined and indurated. Simple excision and midline sphincterotomy is not recommended because of the risk of 'keyhole' deformity of the anus with leakage and pruritus.

### Preoperative preparation

No special preparation is necessary. Enemas, suppositories or washouts will be painful and will delay the early and useful postoperative bowel actions.

### The procedure

Under general anaesthesia, a digital examination is performed to confirm the diagnosis; sigmoidoscopy is also necessary. The patient is placed in the lithotomy position and the perineum and anal canal are cleaned and draped. A well-lubricated Parks' retractor of suitable size is inserted and opened to put the anal canal on a slight stretch.

A fine needle is inserted in the 3 o'clock position through the palpable groove between the internal sphincter's inferior border and the external sphincter and 1:250 000 adrenaline (with lignocaine if desired) is injected firstly deep to the anal skin up to the dentate line, and secondly outside the internal sphincter through the intersphincteric space.

# 5

A 2 cm circumferential skin incision is made just outside the anal verge.

A flap of anal skin is raised off the internal sphincter as far as the dentate line. Care must be taken not to button-hole the skin.

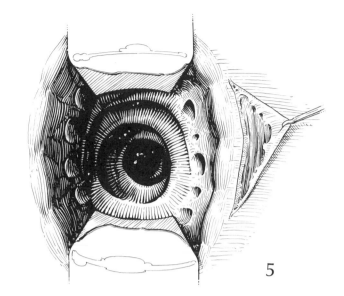

5

# 6

The intersphincteric space is opened for a similar distance on the other side of the internal sphincter, and the lower one-third or one-quarter of the sphincter is divided with scissors or knife to the dentate line. The perianal skin is closed with two or three fine catgut sutures, and if a prominent skin tag is present, it is excised with sharp pointed scissors after the speculum has been removed. Sufficient tissue is removed to prevent any overhang remaining at the external end of the fissure, but damage to the external sphincter or excessive skin removal should be avoided.

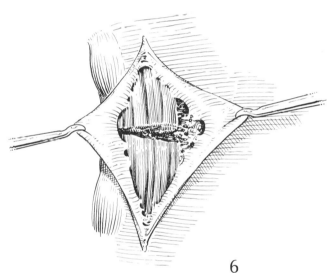

6

## Postoperative care and complications

Mild analgesia may be required, and should be given to ensure comfortable defaecation. Attention to the diet, and the administration of a mild aperient should continue. Cleansing after defaecation is the rule.

Local infection is rare. Haematoma formation has been described, and some surgeons recommend the insertion of a Vaseline gauze pack at the end of the operation to provide local compression. It is not usually necessary, and adds to postoperative discomfort.

## Results

No large series involving children have been described, but it is generally considered a useful procedure. Careful follow-up is necessary for some months to ensure that good habits of regular defaecation are maintained, and that the bowel negativism that so easily develops in children who experience painful defaecation does not occur.

## References

1. Parks, A. G. (1967) The management of fissure-in-ano. Hospital Medicine, 1, 737–738

2. Hobbs, C. J., Wynne, J. M. (1986) Buggery in childhood – a common syndrome of child abuse. Lancet, 2, 792–796

3. Abcarian, H., Lakshmanan, S., Read, D. R., Roccaforte, P. (1982) The role of internal sphincter in chronic anal fissures. Diseases of the Colon and Rectum, 25, 525–528

4. Kuypers, H. C. (1983) Is there really sphincter spasm in anal fissure? Diseases of the Colon and Rectum, 26, 493–494

Illustrations by Gillian Oliver

# Colonoscopy

**Christopher B. Williams**  BM, BCh, FRCP
Consultant Physician, St. Mark's Hospital for Diseases of the Rectum and Colon, St Bartholomew's Hospital;
Honorary Consultant Physician, The Hospital for Sick Children, Great Ormond Street; Queen Elizabeth Hospital for
Children, Hackney, London, UK

## Preoperative

### Indications

Limited colonoscopy is extremely well tolerated by children of any age, paediatric colonoscopes being thinner than an examining little finger. Without either sedation or bowel preparation it is possible to inspect, photograph, and obtain biopsy or other specimens from the rectosigmoid as part of initial assessment of symptomatic patients. Since more extensive or total colonoscopy requires both full bowel preparation and usually some form of sedation, it is reserved for selected patients, usually those with failure to thrive or weight loss, chronic diarrhoea, anaemia, bleeding, and when there is radiological abnormality (e.g. narrowed terminal ileal abnormality on small-bowel follow-through) or a need for therapy (e.g. Peutz–Jeghers polyposis).

Colonoscopy, where it is readily available, is starting to supplant barium enema as the colonic investigation of first choice in children, not only because it can usually be performed without involving irradiation, but because high-quality double-contrast films are not often obtained by paediatric radiologists and X-ray is, therefore, less accurate. When indicated, it is feasible to perform both colonoscopy to the terminal ileum and gastroscopy to the duodenum at a single examination, most of the intestinal tract thus being accessible to inspection, biopsy or instrumentation in one procedure.

### Contraindications and complications

There are few contraindications to colonoscopy in sensitive hands and with appropriate instrumentation. Examination is likely to be difficult and unrewarding in simple constipation or megacolon, where X-ray is preferred, and the diagnostic yield is extremely low in abdominal pain unaccompanied by features to suggest systemic illness. There is a risk of septicaemia in marasmic, immuno-depressed or immuno-suppressed subjects, who should be covered by appropriate antibiotics; prophylactic antibiotics should also be given in the presence of any cardiac lesion. The danger of septic peritonitis contraindicates colonoscopy in the presence of ascites. The availability of immersible instruments and appropriate solutions (glutaraldehyde 2 per cent) means that full sterilization is possible between examinations, preferably with the appropriate automated washing-machine, and there should therefore be no possibility of transmission of infective agents.

In normal subjects the elasticity of the childhood colon means that the theoretical risk of bowel perforation during insertion of the instrument has not been observed in paediatric practice (in contradistinction to adult colonoscopy). The presence of severe acute inflammatory bowel disease with peritonism or deep ulceration, however, contraindicates examination because of the increased possibility of perforation; if unexpectedly severe ulceration is seen during colonoscopy it is wise to terminate the procedure as early as possible and to avoid excessive air insufflation. Even in a normal colon if the procedure proves technically difficult, common-sense and humanity may nonetheless recommend abandonment of an examination; the percentage of failures to reach the caecum varies according to the skill and motivation of the examiner at between 5 and 50 per cent of all colonoscopies. Neonatal examination proves to be the most difficult. The highest percentage of complications, not surprisingly, occurs following therapeutic manoeuvres such as snare polypectomy, when both perforation and bleeding have been reported.

## Bowel preparation

Half a phosphate enema may clear most of the colon of a baby, or clear fluids can be given for 24 hours as complete preparation. For older children oral bowel preparation (without enemas) is generally effective and better tolerated than older purge/enema regimens. Senna syrup and magnesium citrate are pleasant-tasting and, accompanied by 24 hours of fluid diet, give an adequately clean colon except in a few patients – paradoxically often those with colitis whose colon may not empty normally. The alternative is to drink balanced electrolyte solution, or isotonic (5 per cent) mannitol – the latter being contraindicated before polypectomy because of the risk of forming explosive concentrations of hydrogen. Some children become nauseated and vomit before an adequate 1–3 litre volume has been ingested, resulting in failed preparation unless resort is made to large-volume cleansing enemas.

## Sedation or anaesthesia?

Premedication can be useful for apprehensive children in the 5–10-year-old group, in whom reassurance and explanation are often ineffective (antihistamine syrup orally, diazepam rectally, chlorpromazine or pethidine intramuscularly). In babies or older subjects premedication should be unnecessary, assuming a friendly atmosphere and secure parents. Babies can be managed with little or no medication, even during the examination, and older children are frequently more interested and less embarrassed by the prospect of internal examination than adult patients.

Colonoscopic examination is, however, frequently uncomfortable or painful for a short period as the instrument stretches the sigmoid colon mesentery or the visceral peritoneum, and adequate analgesia is, therefore, usually advisable to avoid traumatizing child or parents. There is no contraindication to the use of light general anaesthesia, but this is usually unnecessary and tends to make colonoscopy a 'heavy' procedure, more difficult to organize and less used; it also encourages heavy-handed instrumental technique. With appropriate intravenous medication colonoscopy can be a routine day-case or side-room investigation. A combination of benzodiazepine (for amnesia) and opiate (for sedation and analgesia) is titrated by slow intravenous injection until the child is drowsy enough to accept per-rectal introduction of the instrument without protest. To avoid pain at the injection site, lipid-suspension of diazepam (Diazemuls) or water-soluble midazolam are preferred, and pethidine is diluted 1:5 with water. Initial dosage is based on diazepam 0.1 mg/kg and pethidine 0.5 mg/kg but, according to results, considerably larger amounts may be needed and 50–100 mg intravenous pethidine is not unusual without over-sedating the child. Pethidine is favoured for any incremental doses, since it is more effective in children and reversible by naloxone.

## Choice of instrument

Colonoscopes are more flexible than gastroscopes and it is, therefore, preferable to use an adult colonoscope rather than a paediatric gastroscope if a purpose-built paediatric instrument is unavailable. With lubrication and slow dilatation the anus of even a baby will accept an instrument of 14–15 mm diameter. In small children it is clearly much preferable to have a suitable floppy 10–11 mm diameter instrument, so as to pass small sphincters and variable colonic loops without undue stretching. In well-grown older children an adult colonoscope may sometimes be more appropriate. The length of the instrument is not usually a limiting factor, paediatric colonoscopes being at least 130 cm long, whereas the caecum of a baby may be reached using only 50 cm of instrument and shortened back to 25–30 cm as the colon straightens.

## Is X-ray control needed?

Many examinations do not require X-ray screening control and most colonoscopists never use it. In the learning phase and for the less experienced, however, the extra information given can be invaluable. If X-ray facilities are available difficult procedures can be made quicker, safer and less traumatic. X-ray will also help in the localization of biopsy sites or lesions found unexpectedly at colonoscopy. Irradiation should be kept to a minimum, an occasional brief image being sufficient to demonstrate the position of the instrument and to explain and resolve any looping of its shaft. The best compromise is to avoid use of X-ray in the majority of patients, but to have it available in case of need; if necessary the patient can be transferred to an X-ray table with the colonoscope *in situ*.

# Technique

## 1

### Position of patient

Babies are examined on their backs and this position is also appropriate if general anaesthesia is used. Otherwise most endoscopists start with the patient in the left lateral position, and it is often possible to complete the examination without a change. If there are mechanical difficulties at any stage of the procedure a change of position may alter the configuration of the bowel and make examination easier. Changing to the right lateral position will make the splenic flexure less acute and can also help to drain fluid from the descending colon and facilitate air distension within it if the view is poor.

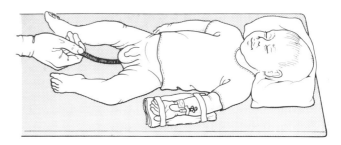

1

### Insertion and passage through rectosigmoid

The colonoscope tip and perianal region are lubricated with jelly, the anus being dilated if necessary with tubes of increasing diameter until digital examination is possible. On insertion initially there may be no view because the tip is against the wall of the rectum. The instrument must be withdrawn slightly and air insufflated before a view is obtained, the tip then being angled and the instrument shaft rotated as necessary to follow along the lumen of the rectosigmoid.

In passing the many bends of the rectosigmoid, the object is to avoid distending or stretching the bowel so as to keep it short and pass almost straight to the descending colon. This is easier to suggest than to achieve but is made more likely by observing the following points.

## 2a, b & c

Only as much air as is necessary to see should be insufflated, and any excess aspirated from time to time. The bowel lumen should be followed accurately. If the view is lost, even for a few seconds, releasing the control knobs and pulling back will cause the lumen to reappear automatically.

Blind pushing should be avoided, but on acute bends this may be necessary for a few seconds providing the muscosa continues to move and the general direction is known. If the tip of the colonoscope will not angle round a bend, pulling the shaft back straight and twisting it one way or the other should be successful. A straight colonoscope and a shortened colon will be achieved by pulling back repeatedly after passing each bend, and before starting each inward push.

The instrument shaft should be held in the fingertips – a clenched fist leads to clumsiness.

### Sigmoid 'N' loop – hook and twist manoeuvre

The commonest situation on reaching the junction of the sigmoid and descending colon, in spite of all care, is for there to be an 'N' loop forming an acute tip angle which makes direct passage difficult or impossible. If the tip can be passed a short way around the bend, looking into the retroperitoneal part of the descending colon, it can be held there without consciously hooking while the instrument is withdrawn 10–40 cm to reduce and straighten out the loop. Putting a clockwise twisting force or torque on to the shaft of the colonoscope while it is withdrawn will help to straighten out this loop and keep the tip in the descending colon.

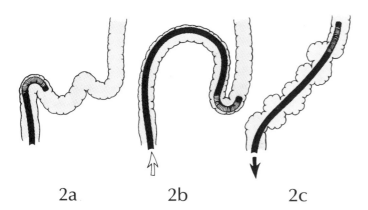

2a        2b        2c

## 3

### Sigmoid 'alpha' loop

Sometimes, especially if there is a redundant colon, a loop is obviously forming but the tip runs in easily without discomfort to the patient. This suggests that a spiral 'alpha' loop is forming (which can be confirmed if fluoroscopy is being used). The correct thing to do is to continue pushing in as far as is comfortable for the patient, at least to the proximal descending colon and preferably to the splenic flexure. If there is little or no discomfort it may be best to push round into the transverse colon before attempting to withdraw and straighten out the instrument.

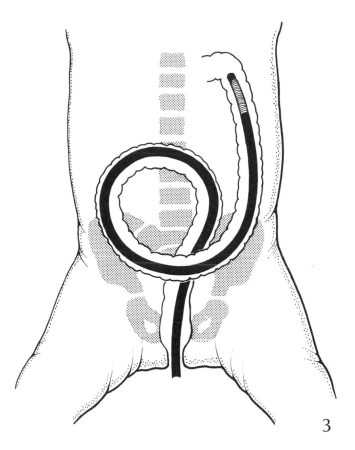

3

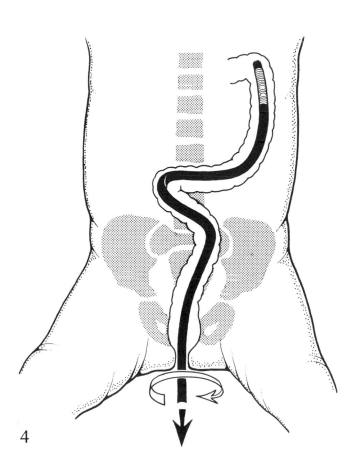

4

## 4

### Straightening out loops

Having reached the upper descending or the transverse colon, the sigmoid colon loop should normally be removed, since loops create friction in the control wires and stress the instrument just as much as they stress the patient. To remove a loop, the instrument shaft is withdrawn until the tip begins to slide or resistance to withdrawal is felt. Whilst pulling back, the application of twist, usually in a clockwise direction, will be found to stop the tip slipping back excessively and facilitate the straightening of the instrument.

The younger the child, the more likely it is that the colon will prove to be hypermobile, without conventional retroperitoneal fixation of the descending colon and splenic flexure. In the 20–30 per cent of patients having a mobile colon, unpredictable and sometimes uncontrollable loops may form which make it difficult or impossible to reach the proximal colon or terminal ileum. Such atypical loops (reversed 'alpha' loop, reversed splenic flexure) can sometimes be successfully removed by first pulling back to reduce their size and then twisting *counter*clockwise as the shaft is further straightened back.

# 5

## Splenic flexure – keeping the sigmoid colon straight

With the colonoscope straightened in the proximal descending colon or splenic flexure, some care may be needed to prevent the sigmoid loop reforming. Continued clockwise (or sometimes anticlockwise) twist on the shaft during reinsertion is often enough to keep it straight. Shaft insertion without tip movement, or losing the 1:1 relationship between shaft and tip, indicates looping. The instrument is immediately pulled back again and the assistant pushes into the left iliac fossa to resist the tendency for the sigmoid loop to rise up from the pelvis. In the splenic flexure this tendency to reloop in the sigmoid colon results because the hooked instrument tip impacts in the splenic flexure. A combination of small corrective measures will usually overcome this.

The instrument shaft should be pulled back straight.

The assistant applies hand/finger pressure over the left iliac fossa.

The instrument shaft is twisted clockwise and re-aimed if necessary toward the lumen, avoiding over-angulation.

The inward push is continued slowly, keeping on the clockwise twist.

Sometimes it is simply easier to reposition the child in the right lateral position to cause the splenic flexure to drop down and flatten out.

## Redundant transverse colon

The transverse colon may sometimes be pushed down by the instrument into a deep loop which makes it difficult and painful to reach the hepatic flexure. Once again the correct procedure is to withdraw the instrument to shorten up this loop. If necessary withdrawal may need to be repeated several times, the instrument advancing a few centimetres on each withdrawal ('paradoxical movement') until the loop is straightened. Keeping the colon deflated also helps to shorten the hepatic flexure region, making it easier both to reach and to pass.

Frequently, difficulty in the transverse colon is actually due to recurrent looping in the sigmoid colon, and the best corrective measures are abdominal pressure in the left iliac fossa and gentle clockwise twisting during reinsertion.

## Passing the hepatic flexure

Having reached and deflated the hepatic flexure, and angled acutely around it into the ascending colon, the transverse loop may remain and make it difficult to pass the rest of the instrument into the ascending colon. By once again withdrawing the colonoscope and straightening out this loop it becomes easier to pass. Deflating the ascending colon by aspiration and simultaneously steering carefully to avoid haustral folds will often cause the colonoscope to descend spontaneously towards the caecum.

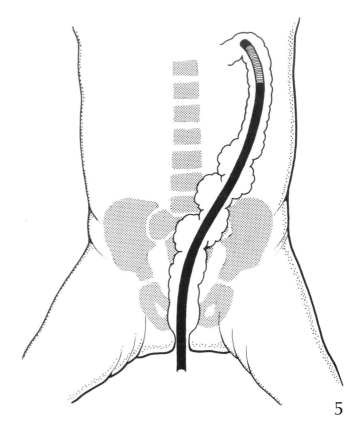

5

## Reaching the caecum

Reaching the caecal pole can be facilitated by change of position (supine or prone), deflation, abdominal pressure, and clockwise twist on the straightened instrument; aggressive pushing usually only results in looping. The colonoscope is seen to have reached the caecum when the bulge of the ileocaecal valve is seen or, 2–5 cm beyond it, the appendix orifice is identified. Brilliant transillumination of the right iliac fossa is usually apparent at this point. The depth of insertion of the straightened instrument is variable according to the age of the patient: 70–80 cm in a teenager down to 25 cm in a small baby. During withdrawal the splenic flexure or descending colon are found at appropriately shorter distances. During insertion, in mobile colons, and if any loops have formed, these distance rules may not apply, but if the room is darkened transillumination will show the position of the instrument tip.

To enter the terminal ileum it is necessary first to identify the bulge of the ileocaecal valve, which may bubble or gush on deflation. The instrument tip is then pushed in just proximal to the bulge, angled in towards it and slowly withdrawn until a 'red-out' indicates embedding into the valve region, at which point air is insufflated to attempt to distend the ileum. Ileal mucosa is characteristically granular or nodulated by lymphoid hyperplasia, in contrast to the shiny surface and vascular pattern of the colon.

In babies under one year of age, entry into the ileum may be impossible, either because the orifice is too narrow or because the dimensions of the caecum are too small to allow the instrument to make the necessary right-angle turn.

## Examination

The colon is visualized to some extent during insertion of the instrument but active examination, biopsy taking, or polypectomies are normally undertaken during withdrawal because the instrument is then straight and easy to manoeuvre, the view is better and the patient is comfortable. At all stages during the examination, but particularly during withdrawal, it is best for the endoscopist to control the instrument himself, using a one-handed technique. Very active manoeuvring of the controls, with rotation and to-and-fro movements of the shaft, allows a good view to be obtained of nearly all areas, although around acute bends and convoluted folds there may be some blind spots.

## COLONOSCOPIC POLYPECTOMY

The principles of colonoscopic polypectomy are identical to those for proctosigmoidoscopic polypectomy, but it is particularly important that full coagulation of polyp stalk vessels is achieved before transection, since any haemorrhage is difficult to control endoscopically. Most polyps in paediatric practice are hamartomatous, thin-stalked, and easy to coagulate. If a thick stalk (1 cm or more) is to be snared it may be wise to inject it with adrenaline (1 ml of 1:100 000 solution), using a long Teflon sclerotherapy needle before applying the polypectomy snare.

Endoscopic snare wires are characteristically thick to guard against too fast cutting, but care should be taken not to apply excessive mechanical pressure before adequate electrocoagulation has occurred. A low power coagulating current (15–25 watts) is employed until local whitening or swelling of the stalk indicates adequate coagulation, at which point tight strangulation should result in severance of the head. If bleeding does occur the stalk remnant can be quickly regrasped with the loop and strangulated for 15 minutes, after which bleeding will not normally recur.

Small polyps up to 6–7 mm size can be destroyed using plastic-insulated 'hot-biopsy' forceps which simultaneously obtain a small biopsy specimen. The smallest hamartomatous polyps (1–3 mm diameter) can be numerous and frequently disappear spontaneously, so that it may be safer to ignore them. Larger polyps can be retrieved by grasping them with the polypectomy snare or alternatively by aspirating on to the tip of the instrument – which risks missing any other polyps during withdrawal unless the instrument is reinserted. Small polyps may be retrieved by aspirating them through the suction channel into a bronchial mucus trap placed in the suction line. Large numbers of polyps in polyposis subjects can be washed out after suction by passing the colonoscope proximal to them and infusing 500 ml saline into the colon through the suction channel, followed by a phosphate enema or stimulant suppository after the instrument has been withdrawn.

Follow-up is probably unnecessary if only one to three juvenile polyps are present in the colon; larger numbers may suggest the possibility of juvenile polyposis which mandates follow-up because of the rare association with dysplastic foci. For Peutz–Jeghers subjects colonoscopy is normally repeated every two years, often combined with gastroscopy as 'top and tail' endoscopy.

## OTHER THERAPEUTIC MANOEUVRES

Electrocoagulation of telangiectases or cavernous haemangiomas (blue rubber-bleb naevus syndrome) is easy through the colonoscope. The use of laser photocoagulation for this purpose has been described but is probably unnecessary, since careful local electrocoagulation with hot-biopsy forceps or judicious sclerotherapy of raised lesions, repeated as necessary, gives excellent results. Strictures, particularly anastomotic strictures after resection of Crohn's disease, can be successfully dilated with transendoscopic balloon dilators. The colonoscope can be used to introduce guide wires, tubes and other devices to any point in the colon, although this is rarely indicated in paediatric practice. The use of submucosally injected indian ink can be useful as a long-lasting marker. Surface irrigation with colorant (1:4 dilution of washable blue fountain-pen ink is convenient) can be helpful in demonstrating the smallest lesions in conditions such as familial adenomatous polyposis.

# Postoperative care

In most cases no special care is needed after colonoscopy, apart from a short period of rest until the after-effects of sedation or anaesthesia wear off. Food and drink can be taken immediately. When the patient appears and feels well, normal activities can be resumed, many examinations being performed on a day-case basis.

# Rectal prolapse in childhood

**R. C. M. Cook**  MA, BM, FRCS
Consultant Paediatric Surgeon, Alder Hey Children's Hospital, Liverpool, UK

## Introduction

Children are said to be more susceptible than adults to rectal prolapse because of the vertical configuration of the pelvis and sacrum, but it remains a rare condition in the otherwise healthy child. Pelvic-floor weakness due to neurogenic disorders leads to prolapse in many children with myelomeningocele or sacral agenesis. It is sometimes precipitated by straining at stool due to diarrhoea, constipation, worms, rectal polyps, or too early and over-zealous 'potty training'. Loss of weight (specifically perirectal fat loss) is blamed for prolapse in children with cystic fibrosis and other malabsorption syndromes, though the voluminous stools, and the chronic cough of the former must also play a part. Pertussis and pulmonary tuberculosis are not uncommonly complicated by prolapse for similar reasons. Assessment of the child presenting with a prolapse must always include a general history and physical examination to exclude these aetiological factors. A sweat test is strongly advised since rectal prolapse may be the presenting symptom of cystic fibrosis[1].

Rectal prolapse in the absence of systemic illness or specific abnormality has a peak incidence in the second and third years of life. Boys and girls are equally affected. The prolapse occurs only on defaecation at first, but may descend at other times later. The mother can usually reduce it easily, though this often happens spontaneously soon after defaecation. If it remains outside it becomes oedematous and there may be a discharge of blood and mucus.

## Appearance

### 1

It is most commonly an incomplete, mucosal prolapse protruding 2–3 cm from the anus and displaying radial folds.

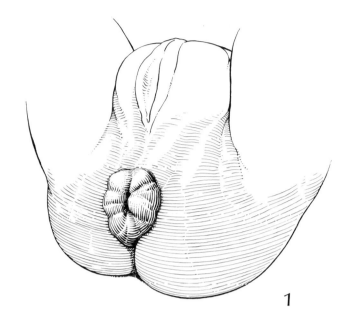

### 2

A complete prolapse of all the layers is rare. The mucosal folds in this are said to be circumferential, but this distinction is lost in both types of prolapse after an hour, when the mucosa becomes oedematous, smooth and featureless. The size and palpable thickness of the wall of the prolapse will differentiate the two. The distinction is, however, not necessarily important in planning treatment. After reduction of a prolapse, digital rectal examination usually reveals no abnormality, but polyps should be felt for (even if not obvious on the prolapsed portion), and the sacrum checked for any deformity or agenesis.

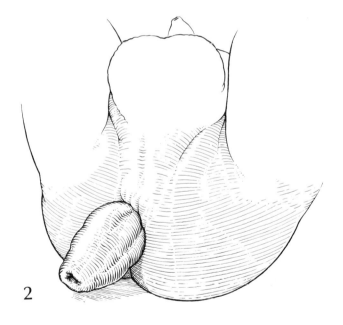

# Management

### CONSERVATIVE TREATMENT

In the absence of generalized disease that predisposes to prolapse, treatment should be supportive, optimistic, and minimal. Efforts are directed at correcting bowel habits in three ways:

1. prescribing an aperient (e.g. lactulose);
2. encouraging a diet containing more vegetable and cereal fibre; and
3. ensuring that defaecation is prompt, quick and performed in a sitting position. Prolonged straining and squatting must be avoided.

   If this fails, support to the perianal region during defaecation should be added to the above regimen. Most simply this consists of the mother holding the child out with her hands under the buttocks, fingers just inside the ischial tuberosities beside the anus.

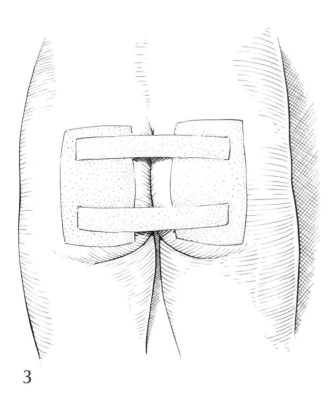

## 3

More prolonged support can be given by strapping the buttocks together. A wide piece of strapping is stuck to each buttock and left for as long as possible. Two narrower strips are put across, stuck to the permanent pieces. They are left in position during defaecation, but removed after to cleanse the perianal region before being replaced with new lengths.

**3**

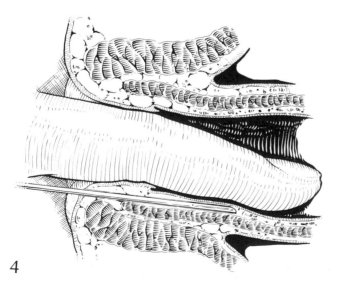

### INJECTION OF MUCOSAL PROLAPSE

## 4

With one index finger in the anal canal, a long 23 gauge needle is guided in the submucosal plane to the lower rectum 4–5 cm from the anal verge. One to two millilitres of 5 per cent phenol in almond oil is injected in each of the four quadrants.

Postoperatively the child can usually be allowed home on the same day, and early resumption of normal bowel habits is encouraged as in the conservative management.

**4**

## THIERSCH OPERATION (MODIFIED)

The rectum and lower colon must be cleared before operation by the use of suppositories and/or washouts. After induction of anaesthesia, sigmoidoscopy is performed to rule out the presence of rectal polyps. The child is placed in the lithotomy position, and the perianal region and the anal canal are cleansed.

## 5

Two small radial incisions are made, each 2 cm from the anal verge, at 12 and 6 o'clock. Using a fully curved aneurysm needle, a length of No. 1 catgut is threaded from posterior to anterior incisions around the anus just deep to the external sphincter muscle. The needle is rethreaded and the catgut pulled from anterior to posterior round the other side of the anal canal.

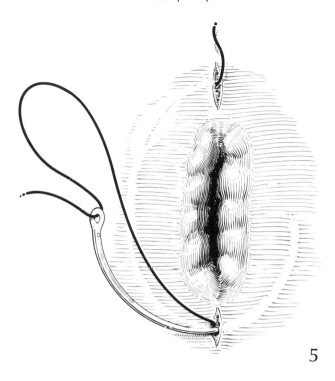

5

## 6

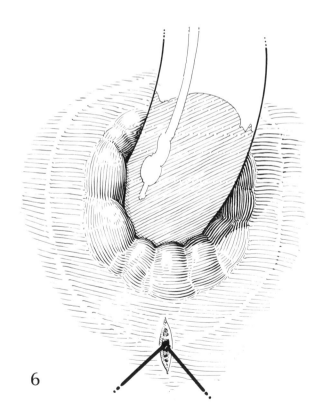

6

With an assistant's finger, or a No. 10 or 11 Hegar's dilator held in the anal canal, the catgut is pulled and tied inside the posterior incision. Fine catgut or other absorbable sutures are used to close the two incisions.

Postoperatively, mild aperients and appropriate dietary measures are used to ensure easy passage of a soft stool. Faecal impaction must be avoided. The catgut will be absorbed within a few weeks but would seem to leave sufficient reaction to support the bowel.

## Results

Recurrence is unusual, although about 5–10 per cent of children will have further prolapse after injection therapy. The injection may be repeated 4–6 weeks later. Cauterization, rectosigmoidectomy, and fixation of the rectum in the presacral space have all been advocated for persistent or severe prolapse in childhood, but in the author's experience have never proved necessary. They are well described in textbooks of adult surgery[2].

### References

1. Stern, R. C., Izant, R.J., Boat, T. F., Wood, R. E., Matthews, L. W., Doershuk, C. F. (1982) Treatment and prognosis of rectal prolapse in cystic fibrosis. Gastroenterology, 82, 707–710

2. Rob, C., Smith R. (1977) Operative Surgery, 3rd ed.: Colon, Rectum and Anus. I. P. Todd (ed). London: Butterworths

# Portal hypertension

**E. Thomas Boles Jr.** MD
Chief, Department of Pediatric Surgery, Children's Hospital, Columbus, Ohio; Professor and Director, Division of
Pediatric Surgery, Department of Surgery, Ohio State University College of Medicine, Columbus, Ohio, USA

**Scott J. Boley** MD, FAAP, FACS
Professor of Surgery and Pediatrics, and Chief of Pediatric Surgical Services, Albert Einstein College of Medicine,
New York, USA

# CENTRAL SPLENORENAL SHUNT

## Preoperative

### Indications

During the past 30 years the centrally placed modification of the standard splenorenal shunt has been found to be of particular value in children with extrahepatic portal hypertension[1]. Such a shunt lowers the portal pressure, decreases the size of or eliminates oesophageal varices, and thus prevents further episodes of variceal bleeding. The operation is not done as an emergency, since bleeding from varices in a child with extrahepatic portal hypertension will invariably stop with non-operative treatment. A less common indication is prevention of further bleeding in children with cirrhosis of some type and intrahepatic portal hypertension.

### Contraindications

As indicated above, the procedure should not be performed in children as an emergency to control acute variceal bleeding. Generally speaking, the operation should not be done unless the splenic vein is large enough to permit a shunt that is at least 10 mm in diameter. Hence, contrast radiographic studies of the portal venous system are essential preoperatively. Microvascular techniques may well permit the operation to be done successfully in younger children with smaller veins, but as a rule the outlook for long-term success increases with the age of the child and the size of the splenic vein[2].

### Position of the patient

The patient is first placed supine. The left side of the trunk is then elevated 10–20° by pads placed under the left shoulder and buttock. The left arm is extended, and the forearm is attached to the horizontal bar of the anaesthetic screen, using sheet wadding and adhesive tape.

# The operation

## 1

### The incision

A transverse upper abdominal incision is made, carrying the incision to the left into the interspace between the eleventh and twelfth or tenth and eleventh ribs. Both rectus muscles as well as the left lateral abdominal muscles are divided in the direction of the incision.

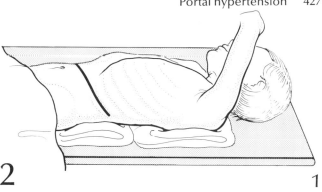

2                                                                       1

## Splenectomy

The splenic flexure of the colon is retracted downward using a pad and appropriate retractor. This manoeuvre brings the spleen downward as well as improving exposure. The spleen is then displaced medially and anteriorly with the surgeon's left hand, exposing and putting tension on the lateral peritoneal reflection of the spleen. This peritoneal reflection is then divided about 1 cm away from its reflection onto the spleen, and the division is carried around the superior portion of the spleen to the highest short gastric vessel. Because this peritoneal reflection usually contains numerous collateral veins, the division must most often be done by sequential division between curved haemostats. These haemostats are controlled with suture ligatures of fine silk as the division proceeds.

After complete division of the peritoneal reflection the spleen can be lifted totally outside the wound, giving excellent exposure to the short gastric vessels, the hilar vessels, and the tail of the pancreas. The short gastric vessels are next individually divided between clamps and secured with suture ligatures. If necessary the tail of the pancreas is carefully displaced downward to expose the vessels in the hilus of the spleen posteriorly. If the tail of the pancreas extends up to the spleen it is absolutely essential that the pancreas be properly displaced. After this manoeuvre, the splenic artery and vein can be visualized and individually divided between clamps and tied. The spleen is then removed.

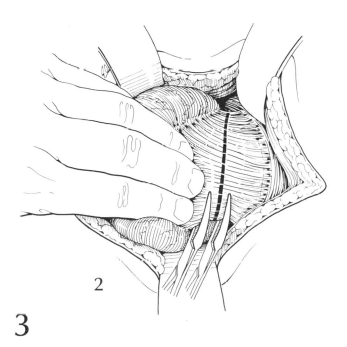

2

## 3

### Exposure of splenic and left renal veins

The tail of the pancreas is held anteriorly and medially by the suture ligatures left long on the splenic vein. The plane between the pancreas and left kidney is bloodless and easily developed, retracting the stomach superiorly and the transverse colon and mesocolon inferiorly during this dissection. The anterior surface of the left renal vein comes into view and is cleared medially from the hilus to the midline. The kidney itself is not mobilized. The gonadal vein inferiorly and the adrenal vein superiorly join the renal vein close to the hilus, but these veins do not ordinarily require division. The renal vein is completely mobilized medial to these tributaries, and tapes are passed around it.

With the pancreas held upward as shown and reflected medially, the splenic vein is exposed and the length of vein medially necessary for the shunt is estimated. The medial segment of the vein is then carefully mobilized from the pancreas, dividing the small pancreatic veins individually between suture ligatures of fine silk. The distal portion of the splenic vein which is not necessary for construction of the shunt is left in place. The splenic vein is then divided between a suitable vascular clamp medially, and a suture ligature of silk distally at a point which will ensure an adequate length of medial or central splenic vein for the shunt.

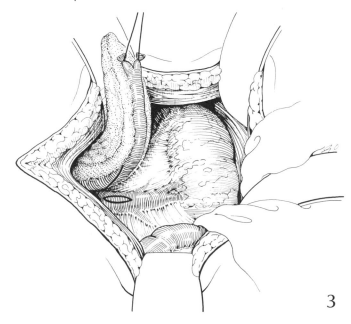

3

# 4 & 5

### Construction of shunt

The anastomosis is planned for that part of the left renal vein immediately anterior to the aorta, and as short as possible a length of the medial or central portion of splenic vein is used. The divided end of the splenic vein is cut obliquely to permit a smooth approximation to the renal vein and to increase the diameter of the shunt. A small haemostat is used to hold the anterior wall of the renal vein upward at the location for the shunt as a Satinsky clamp is applied across it. Alternatively, the medial segment of renal vein to be used for the shunt can be isolated between two tapes. Significant venous congestion of the left kidney will not occur if this latter technique is used, as long as the adrenal and gonadal veins are not disturbed.

A longitudinal ellipse of the renal vein on its anterior aspect is then excised. The medial and lateral angles of the two veins are then approximated with stay sutures of 6/0 non-absorbable material (silk or polypropylene). The superior half of the anastomosis is then made with a running suture. The shunt is completed with a similar running suture to close the inferior half of the anastomosis. Both are technically easier if the sutures start medially and progress laterally. Periodically during the anastomosis the open veins are gently irrigated with heparinized saline. When the shunt has been completed the Satinsky clamp or the tapes are first loosened. After a few moments the vascular clamp on the splenic vein is released. In a properly constructed shunt the splenic vein will curve smoothly without angulation. Frequently blood can be observed rushing through the shunt.

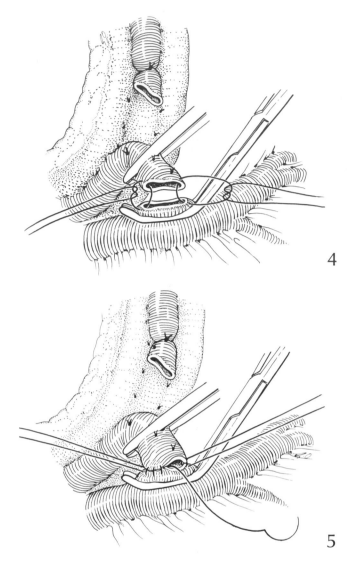

4

5

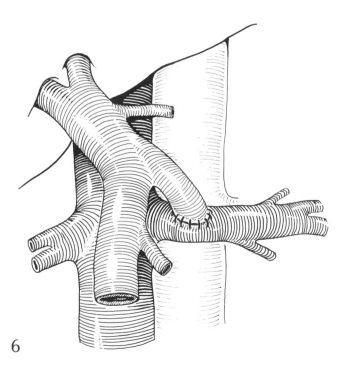

6

# 6

### Completed anastomosis

The shunt uses a short, central segment of splenic vein approximated to the left renal vein at its location over the aorta. Pressures in the portal venous system are measured before and following construction of the shunt.

# Postoperative care

Postoperative morbidity should be minimal. If the left pleural cavity has been entered, a plastic chest tube is placed through a stab incision just above the diaphragm, and left in place for 24 hours. The nasogastric tube is left in place until normal peristalsis returns. No drains are left in the operative field.

# MESOCAVAL SHUNT

## Preoperative

### Indications

These are identical to those for a central splenorenal shunt. Preference for one or the other of these shunts is an individual matter. The procedure is technically easier to perform than a splenorenal shunt. It can also be used if a splenectomy has previously been performed or if a splenorenal shunt has failed.

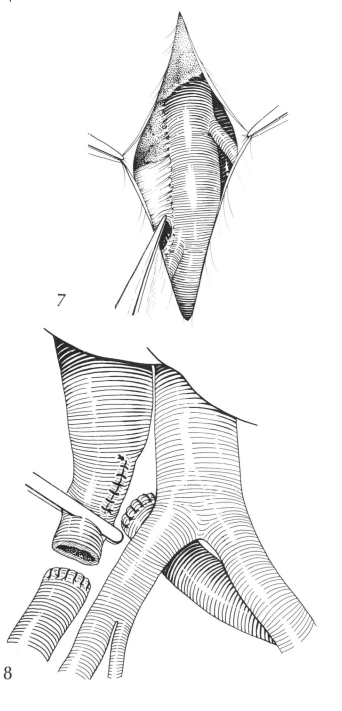

### Contraindications

The procedure is not recommended as an emergency to control bleeding from varices in children with extrahepatic portal hypertension. It should not be done if the superior mesenteric vein is less than 10 mm in diameter or shows evidence on venography of having been involved in a thrombotic process. It should not be done in patients with venous disorders of the lower extremities, a very rare circumstance in childhood.

### Position of patient

The patient is placed supine.

## The operation

### Incision and exposure

The abdomen is entered through a long vertical midline incision or a right paramedian incision. A transverse incision should be avoided because of subsequent interference with venous collaterals from the lower extremities.

An intravenous plastic cannula is introduced into a peripheral mesenteric vein for pressure measurements and, when indicated, venographic studies.

## 7

### Dissection of superior mesenteric vein

The transverse colon and mesentery are lifted upwards, and the small intestinal mesentery is retracted inferiorly. A vertical incision is made through the peritoneum overlying the superior mesenteric vessels. The superior mesenteric artery can be identified by palpation, and the vein lies just to the right of the artery. The vein is dissected free for a distance of about 4 cm inferiorly from the inferior border of the pancreas.

## 8

### Dissection of inferior vena cava

The right colon is mobilized by dividing the lateral peritoneal reflection and is reflected to the left. The duodenum is mobilized by the Kocher manoeuvre and is also reflected to the left. The inferior vena cava is then mobilized from the renal veins to its bifurcation, dividing the lumbar veins between ligatures of fine silk.

If the length of mobilized vena cava is sufficient to permit its approximation to the superior mesenteric vein, it is divided at the bifurcation between vascular clamps, and the distal end oversewn with a running suture of fine arterial silk or polypropylene. If its length is inadequate, the left common iliac vein is divided between vascular clamps at its junction with the vena cava and both openings closed with running sutures. The right common iliac vein is then mobilized to the internal iliac vein, divided, and its distal end closed.

# 9 & 10

### The anastomosis

By blunt dissection a wide opening is made in the posterior mesentery adjacent to the cleared superior mesenteric vein, and the divided end of the vena cava or right common iliac vein is drawn through this tunnel. The vena cava must make a smooth curve around the duodenum, with no angulation. Two straight vascular clamps are applied to the superior mesenteric vein and the clamps rotated to expose the right posterior aspect of the vein. The end of the vena cava or iliac vein is trimmed to approximate the superior mesenteric vein. The latter vein is then opened with vascular scissors at the site for the anastomosis, and a thin ellipse of vein wall of the proper length is excised. Stay sutures of 6/0 arterial silk or polypropylene are placed and tied at the angles, and the posterior anastomosis made with a running suture. The anterior anastomosis is done in a similar fashion. The shunt is irrigated with heparinized saline periodically during the anastomosis. The clamps are removed, and a good flow of blood through the anastomosis should be observed. A few sutures are used to reapproximate the mesenteric peritoneum, and the portal pressure is again measured. The abdomen is closed in anatomical fashion.

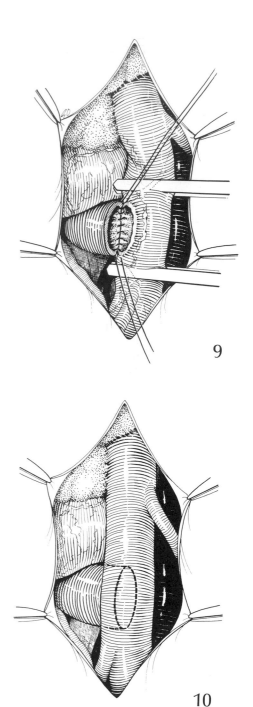

9

10

## Postoperative care

No special care is ordinarily required. The nasogastric tube is left in place until normal intestinal activity returns. The patient should be ambulant on the following day. Elastic stockings and early active exercises of the extremities are advisable.

## Results and complications

The long-term results with both splenorenal and mesocaval shunts have been good in our experience. Eight of ten of the former and six of seven of the latter have been free of further bleeding over follow-up periods averaging approximately 15 years[3]. Similar results have been reported by others, although most authors indicate long-term prevention of bleeding in closer to 50 per cent of patients[2,4-6]. There are disadvantages and possible long-term complications to both shunts. With the central splenorenal technique splenectomy is performed, and the child therefore becomes at risk of post-splenectomy sepsis[7]. This is a small but significant risk which should be lessened by active immunization using polyvalent pneumococcal vaccine. Venous stasis in the lower extremities occurred as a late complication of the mesocaval shunt in five of 12 patients in our series, although the generally reported incidence is less[3,4,8].

# END-TO-SIDE PORTACAVAL SHUNT

## Preoperative

### Indications

The ideal patient for this operation is one with extrahepatic portal hypertension causing bleeding episodes from varices, who has a sufficient length of uninvolved portal vein for the anastomosis, but such patients are exceedingly rare. The operation is well suited for children with congenital hepatic fibrosis, an intrahepatic, presinusoidal form of portal hypertension. The most common indication has been cirrhosis, and it is very effective in preventing further bleeding. The long-term effects of this shunt with regard to encephalopathy have not been well documented in children.

A second more recently developed indication is in the management of glycogen storage disease[9]. Such patients have large livers, prolonged bleeding times, hypoglycaemia, and metabolic acidosis.

### Contraindications

These are largely concerned with the status of the liver functions and the estimated risk of post-shunt encephalopathy in children with cirrhosis. As with adults, ascites, a rising bilirubin level, and a serum albumin level below 3 g/dl indicate a high risk.

### Preoperative preparation

No special preparation is ordinarily required if the procedure is performed electively for portal hypertension. In the unusual situation of an emergency shunt to control bleeding, temporary control by gastro-oesophageal tamponade should be gained if at all possible.

When done for glycogen storage disease, a period of intravenous hyperalimentation for 2–3 weeks before operation is quite helpful in reducing the size of the liver and correcting the bleeding and metabolic abnormalities.

# The operation

### Position of patient and incision

The patient is placed supine with the right side slightly elevated by pads under the right shoulder and hip. The right arm is extended with the elbow flexed at a right angle and suspended to the cross-bar of the anaesthesia screen. This is the mirror image of the position used for the central splenorenal shunt.

A long, upper-abdominal, transverse incision is extended to the posterior axillary line on the right, dividing the interspace between the tenth and eleventh or eleventh and twelfth ribs. The muscles are divided in the direction of the incision, including both rectus muscles.

### Exposure of inferior veva cava

The hepatic flexure of the colon is freed and retracted downward and medially. A wide Kocher manoeuvre allows the duodenum to be mobilized and displaced to the left. Division of the lateral peritoneal reflection of the duodenum may have to be done sequentially between haemostats because of the venous collateral circulation. This dissection exposes the inferior vena cava, and the adventitia over the anterior portion of this vessel is removed from the level of the renal veins to the liver.

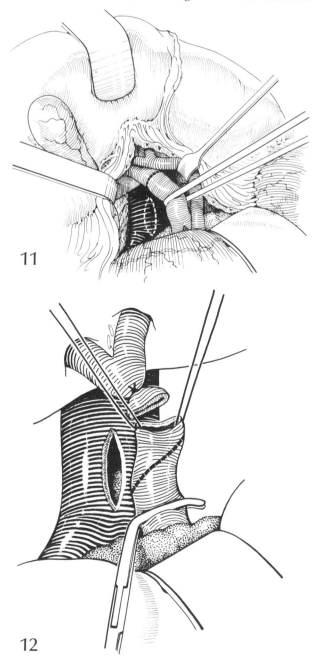

## 11

### Exposure of portal vein

Rather large lymph nodes are found along the lateral edge of the hepatoduodenal ligament, and these are best removed at this stage. The portal vein is approached most easily by dividing the peritoneum over its posterolateral aspect. The superior edge of this peritoneum together with the common bile duct are retracted to the left. Once exposed the vein is freed around its circumference by careful blunt dissection, and an umbilical tape passed around it for traction and exposure. Inferiorly the vein is freed to the pancreas. The coronary vein is often encountered medially, and is divided between silk ligatures. Superiorly the vein is freed to its bifurcation and is divided just proximal to this bifurcation between a right-angled vascular clamp proximally and a ligature plus a suture-ligature of silk distally.

## 12

### Preparation for shunt

The proximal divided end of the portal vein is trimmed obliquely as shown so that the end fits appropriately to the vena cava. The vena cava at the point selected for the anastomosis is grasped with a fine haemostat and tented anteriorly, and a Satinsky vascular clamp is applied to isolate this segment. An ellipse of the anterior wall, of suitable size, is excised with scissors. This is usually about 15 mm in length.

# 13 & 14

### Construction of shunt

The shunt is aligned with interrupted sutures of 6/0 silk or polypropylene, placed and tied at the superior and inferior angles of the shunt. The knots are on the outside. The needle on the superior suture is then passed inward between the left cut edges of the veins. This suture then takes a stitch of the superior portion of the posterior edge of the vena cava close to the angle suture, and is then continued as an over-and-over continuous suture approximating the left edges of the anastomosis. At the inferior angle it is passed from within outwards through the portal vein adjacent to the angle suture, and is then tied to that suture.

During the placement of the posterior suture the anterior or free edge of the portal vein is held upwards with a traction suture. The right suture line is also a simple continuous over-and-over suture approximating the free edges with closely placed stitches, beginning superiorly and finishing at the inferior angle. During the anastomosis the insides of the veins are irrigated with heparinized saline at frequent intervals. On completion of the shunt the Satinsky clamp is loosened from the vena cava, followed by unclamping of the portal vein. Bleeding from the anastomosis is usually minimal, and stops spontaneously with a little patience. The clamps are then removed. Portal venous pressures are taken prior to the shunt through a mesenteric vein and again after the shunt has been completed. The abdomen is closed in anatomical fashion. If the pleural cavity has been entered, a chest tube connected to a water-seal bottle is left in place for 24 hours.

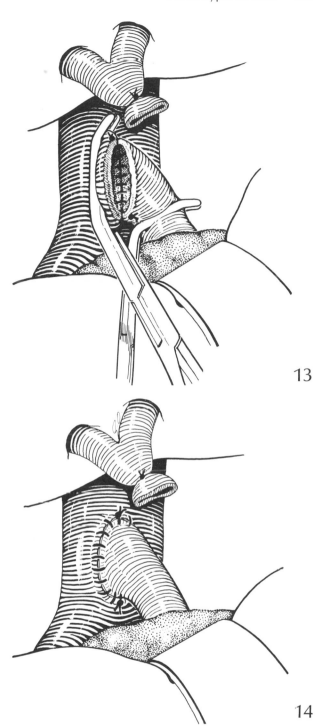

13

14

## Postoperative care and complications

Postoperatively the care is routine for a major laparotomy, with nasogastric suction until the ileus resolves, and appropriate intravenous replacement fluids. Measures to prevent atelectasis are important. Post-shunt encephalopathy is possible in patients with cirrhosis, but has not been a major problem in children.

## Results

The procedure has been very effective in lowering portal pressure and preventing further haemorrhage from varices. The reported experience of the procedure with glycogen storage diseases (types I, II and VI) has shown marked improvement in these children, with decrease in liver size, increased rate of growth, and marked improvement in the hypoglycaemia, acidosis, and hyperlipidaemia[9].

# TRANSOESOPHAGEAL LIGATION OF VARICES

## Preoperative

### Indications

The operation is useful in the control of acute bleeding from varices in children with either the extrahepatic or intrahepatic form of portal hypertension when non-operative techniques (oesophageal tamponade or vasopressin) fail. This is a relatively uncommon indication.

A second and more common indication is to prevent further episodes of bleeding in children whose veins in the portal system are too small to permit a high success rate with a shunt. The operation has been as successful for this purpose as have more complex direct procedures such as oesophageal division or gastric division with lower oesophageal disconnection. Transoesophageal ligation often prevents further haemorrhage for several years. This is particularly true in those with extrahepatic portal hypertension.

### Preoperative preparation

A nasogastric tube should be in place preoperatively. A gastric-oesophageal tamponade tube may be quite useful if the indication is control of acute haemorrhage.

### Anaesthesia

Gas inhalation via an endotracheal tube with ventilatory control is used.

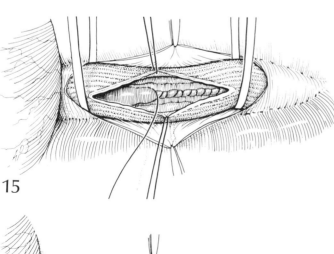

15

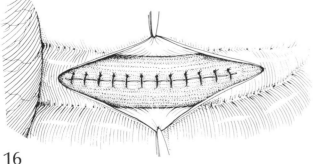

16

## The operation

### Position of patient and incision

The patient is placed in the straight lateral position with the left side up. A standard transverse thoracotomy incision is made just inferior to the tip of the scapula. The left chest is entered through the sixth or seventh interspace.

### Exposure

The inferior pulmonary ligament is divided and the lung retracted superiorly. The lower mediastinal pleura is divided over and parallel to the oesophagus for a distance of 6–7 cm above the hiatus. The lower oesophagus is mobilized by blunt dissection. This is ordinarily easily accomplished, since the para-oesophageal veins are not usually troublesome. The vagus nerves are freed from the oesophagus and not damaged.

## 15

### Ligation of varices

The oesophagus is temporarily encircled by umbilical tapes or unloaded Penrose drains at the superior and inferior limits of the mobilization. The nasogastric tube is withdrawn. The oesophagus is entered longitudinally on its left or uppermost aspect, and the incision is extended for a distance of 5–6 cm. Distally the incision should extend close to the oesophagogastric junction but not into the stomach. There are usually three enlarged tortuous submucosal venous channels. Each is oversewn with a running lock suture of 3/0 or 4/0 chromic catgut. This is started as far proximally as is convenient and is then extended downward. By maintaining upward traction on the suture as the suturing progresses downward, each vein can be obliterated down to and including the level of the oesophagogastric junction.

## 16

### Closure

The oesophageal incision is closed in two layers with interrupted sutures of fine silk. The tapes are removed, and the mediastinal pleura closed loosely with a few interrupted sutures of fine silk.

The chest is closed in anatomical fashion. A plastic chest tube is placed through a stab incision in an interspace just above the diaphragm in the midaxillary line. It is connected to an underwater seal chest bottle or to a three-bottle set with 10 cm of water negative pressure.

## Postoperative care

This procedure is usually well tolerated and no special care is required. The patient is, of course, carefully watched for evidence of bleeding. The chest tube is removed the following day after a chest X-ray has been obtained, and normal ambulation and diet are encouraged.

# TRANSECTION AND REANASTOMOSIS OF THE OESOPHAGUS

## Preoperative

### Indications

Interruption of the submucosal oesophageal veins may be accomplished by transection of the lower oesophagus and reanastomosis. Alone, this procedure is comparable to transoesophageal ligation of varices and has the same indications; it may be expected to produce similar results in terms of controlling acute variceal bleeding. It may also be used as part of a more extensive procedure in which the blood vessels supplying the upper half of the stomach are interrupted.

The procedure using the EEA stapling device (Auto Suture Disposable EEA. Manufactured by United States Surgical Corporation, Norwalk, Conn., USA.) has the advantages of simplicity and speed as compared to either transoesophageal ligation of varices or division of the lower oesophagus and reanastomosis using conventional surgical instruments and techniques[10]. This device divides and creates an anastomosis simultaneously, forming an inverted anastomosis held in approximation by a circular double staggered row of stainless steel sutures.

### Preoperative preparation

When this technique is used to control active bleeding, temporary control using gastro-oesophageal tamponade (with a Sengstaken tube) may be very helpful, and of course adequate restoration of blood volume is essential. When used as an elective procedure, usually in conjunction with some type of further portoazygous disconnection operation, no special preparation is required.

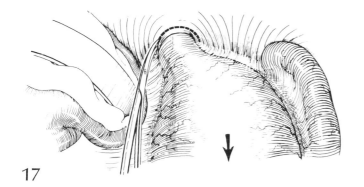

17

# The operation

## 17

With the patient in the supine position under general anaesthesia with endotracheal technique, the abdomen is opened through a vertical midline incision from xiphoid to umbilicus. With appropriate exposure the peritoneal reflection of the lateral segment of the left lobe of the liver to the diaphragm is divided. This segment is retracted to the right. Downward traction on the stomach exposes the gastro-oesophageal hiatus, and the peritoneum over the anterior aspect of the hiatus is divided using scissor dissection.

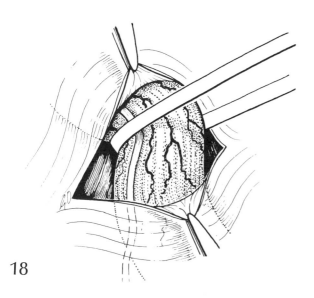

18

## 18

The lower portion of the oesophagus is encircled by blunt dissection and an unloaded Penrose drain passed around it for control and traction. By further blunt dissection the lower 5–7 cm of oesophagus is freed from the mediastinum.

## 19

An opening is made in the anterior gastric wall. The disposable EEA stapling instrument with a cartridge of appropriate size (usually 25 mm) is selected. The anvil at the tip must be securely fixed to the spindle, but the anvil and the adjacent cartridge are slightly separated. This instrument is then passed into the stomach and guided into the lower oesophagus. A heavy suture (1/0 monofilament polypropylene) is then placed encircling the lower oesophagus and is tied tightly down to the spindle of the instrument between the anvil and the cartridge. This suture should be positioned just above the oesophagogastric junction. The cartridge and anvil are then snugged firmly together by tightening the wing nut on the handle. The instrument is then activated by closing the handle at the other end of the instrument, simultaneously transecting the oesophagus and forming the anastomosis. The anvil is again unscrewed from the cartridge and the instrument carefully withdrawn. The gastrostomy is closed in two layers with interrupted silk sutures, and the abdomen closed.

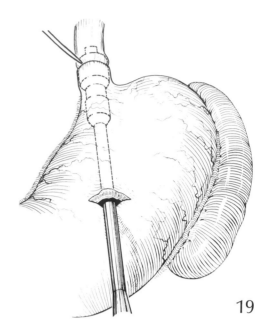

19

## Postoperative care

The stomach is kept decompressed using a nasogastric tube and suction. The child is monitored closely in an intensive care unit. The procedure has been quite successful in controlling acute bleeding, and complications have been few in a small experience. Neither anastomotic leaks nor strictures have thus far been observed[11-13]. Long-term results are not presently available.

# SCLEROTHERAPY

## Preoperative

### Indications

The injection of oesophageal varices with sclerosing fluid to obliterate the dilated venous channels and to prevent further bleeding is not a new technique. It was introduced over 45 years ago, but achieved little popularity because of technical problems and the emergence of shunting operations. In the last decade there has been a remarkable re-emergence of interest in and practice of the technique, to a considerable extent attributable to the studies of Terblanche and his colleagues[14]. The presently available oesophagoscopes with superb fibreoptic lighting and excellent lens systems contribute greatly to the ease and success of the method.

Generally this technique has been used on an elective basis to prevent further episodes of bleeding, although it has also been used successfully to control bleeding during an acute haemorrhage[15–17]. It may be used for children with varices secondary to extrahepatic or intrahepatic portal hypertension. Many children have been successfully managed by this method after failing one or more shunting operations or some form of direct operation. For the child with episodes of bleeding varices whose portal venous branches are thought to be too small for a shunt, the procedure may be ideal.

### Preoperative preparation

In the setting of an elective procedure, no special preparation is required.

### Anaesthesia

General endotracheal anaesthesia has been the rule, with the endotracheal tube being fixed to the left corner of the mouth. An intravenous cannula is of course in place, and the vital signs and ECG are monitored. The procedure is routinely done in adults without general anaesthesia, but our experience to date has been entirely with general anaesthesia.

## The operation

### Position of patient

The patient is placed in the supine position.

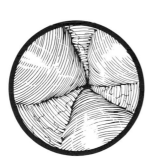

20

# 20

Either rigid or flexible scopes have been employed with success, but we have preferred flexible fibreoptic gastro-oesophagoscopes for several years. The four-way instrument provides excellent visualization and manipulative ease. After induction of anaesthesia the blade of a laryngoscope is introduced down the pharynx and lifted upwards. The entrance to the oesophagus can then be seen, and the oesophagoscope introduced without trauma. The entire oesophagus and stomach are then systematically viewed. The scope is then withdrawn into the oesophagus just above the gastroesophageal junction. In a patient with varices who has not previously undergone sclerotherapy there are usually three good-sized varices in this location.

## 21

The flexible injecting needle is then passed down the appropriate channel until it is seen emerging at the distal end. It is helpful to have measured the distance on the flexible needle required for this passage prior to oesopha-goscopy. The needle can be directed most easily if the end of the scope is positioned 1–2 cm above the unsuspecting varix. The needle is then unsheathed and pushed directly into the varix. One to 1.5 ml of the sclerosing fluid is injected. Sodium morrhuate (5 per cent) or sodium tetradecyl sulphate (1.5 per cent) are satisfactory sclerosing solutions. The varix blanches with the injection, confirming correct placement of the needle. The needle is then withdrawn and sheathed. Often there is some bleeding from the needle wound, and occasionally this is impressive. The scope is advanced into the stomach, and a few minutes allowed to elapse. The scope is then withdrawn back into the oesophagus, and most often irrigation and suction clear the field. Three varices are ordinarily injected at one session, using a total volume of 3–4.5 ml of sclerosing fluid. With completion of the injections the scope is again passed into the stomach, the air in the stomach removed, and then the scope removed.

Repeated sessions of sclerotherapy are necessary to completely obliterate all varices. The interval between sessions in our experience has been 2–4 weeks in most instances, although others have used shorter intervals. Varices do in some cases recur after obliteration has been accomplished so that follow-up endoscopy at six-monthly intervals is advisable[18].

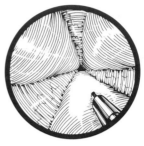

21

## Postoperative care and complications

Careful monitoring of the patient immediately after the procedure is obviously essential, although significant bleeding caused by the technique is rare. The procedures are relatively brief, and recovery from anaesthesia is ordinarily prompt. With increasing experience, competence and confidence on the part of the operator, most of these procedures can safely be done on an ambulatory basis.

A low-grade fever and some retrosternal discomfort are fairly common. Ulceration at the site of an injection may occur, and strictures have been reported. Haemorrhage can of course occur, but fortunately is uncommon. Overall morbidity has been low both in our own experience and in that reported by others.

## Results

In terms of preventing further haemorrhage our results to date have been excellent, although the follow-up periods are still relatively short[18]. Similar results have been reported by other workers[14–16]. The procedure has become very popular, and consequently the number of major operations, including both shunts and extensive direct procedures, now being performed has decreased substantially.

# SUGIURA PROCEDURE

## Preoperative

### Principles and indications

The various types of portal to venous shunting operations are limited to some extent by the small size of the veins in small children, by involvement of major branches of the portal venous system by the thrombotic process, and by failure of the procedure from thrombotic shunt occlusion in a variable proportion of the patients. Furthermore, there is concern as to the possibility of post-shunt encephalopathy, particularly in patients with hepatic disease. A number of techniques have been developed in an effort to obliterate the varices directly. These have often been initially successful, but the long-term results are disappointing.

In 1973 Sugiura published his results with a more extensive direct operation with excellent results in a considerable number of patients[19]. The procedure includes lower oesophageal transection and anastomosis, devascularization of the lower oesophagus and upper stomach, and splenectomy. The para-oesophageal veins, which are naturally occurring shunts, are not interrupted. These results have been confirmed by later publications from Sugiura and his co-workers and by others[20, 21].

The operation may be used for children with either extrahepatic or intrahepatic portal hypertension. It can be used as an initial elective operation in a child with oesophageal varices who has had bleeding, or as a secondary procedure after failure of a previously performed shunt.

## The operation

The operation is performed under general endotracheal anaesthesia with the patient in a straight lateral position, the left side uppermost. The left chest is entered through a long incision either through the seventh interspace or through the bed of the resected seventh rib. The eighth and ninth ribs may be divided posteriorly for greater exposure.

## 22

### Oesophageal devascularization

The oesophagus is exposed by dividing the mediastinal pleura anterior to the aorta from the hiatus to above the inferior pulmonary vein. The oesophagus is then carefully encircled and held outward. The vagus nerves are freed but not divided. All veins from the para-oesophageal veins to the oesophagus are divided and ligated, and all arterial and vagus branches are similarly interrupted. The para-oesophageal veins are not divided. Fine silk sutures are used on the oesophageal side, clips away from the oesophagus. This mobilization and devascularization extends from the hiatus to the inferior pulmonary vein. Ordinarily 40–50 such branches require ligation.

This dissection proceeds downwards from above as far as possible, extending through the hiatus, with preservation of the para-oesophageal veins and the vagus nerves.

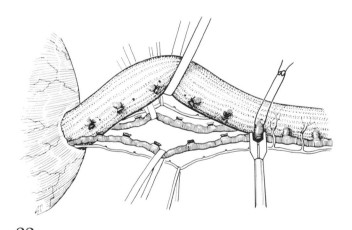

22

## 23

### Opening of diaphragm

The diaphragm is opened radially, beginning at a point 2–3 cm posterior to the phrenic nerve. Multiple suture ligatures are placed along the edges of the diaphragmatic incision for both haemostasis and exposure.

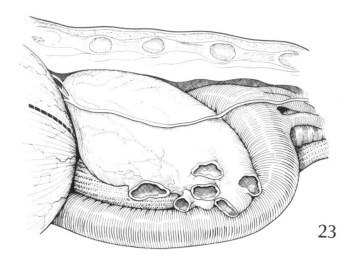

23

### Splenectomy and gastric devascularization

On opening into the abdomen, the peritoneal reflection of the lateral segment of the left lobe is divided. The spleen is next mobilized, securing the collateral vessels in the peritoneal reflection posteriorly and superiorly with ligatures as the mobilization proceeds. The short gastric vessels are then divided, and the hilar vessels are also divided with careful avoidance of the tail of the pancreas.

## 24

After removal of the spleen, all paragastric vessels to the greater curvature of the proximal stomach are interrupted to the left gastro-epiploic vessels. The dissection from the abdomen superiorly joins that from the chest. Next the lesser curvature of the stomach is devascularized by interrupting the branches from the left gastric (coronary) vein and the para-oesophageal veins to the stomach. In essence, a highly selective vagotomy is performed, as this process of devascularization extends downward from the gastro-oesophageal junction, a distance of 6–7 cm.

24

## 25

### Division and anastomosis of oesophagus

Non-crushing clamps are applied across the oesophagus about 3 cm proximal to the cardio-oesophageal junction. These are stronger than vascular clamps and are modified so that they can be screwed together to fix the oesophagus. An incision is made through the presenting half of the oesophageal muscular coat. The submucosa and mucosal sleeve is then mobilized from the muscular coat posteriorly, but without dividing this portion of the muscular coat.

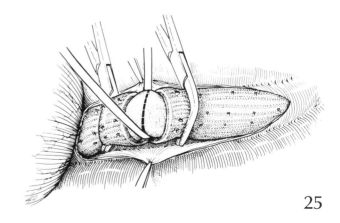

25

## 26

The submucosa and mucosal sleeve is then divided completely. Anastomosis of the mucosa–submucosa is done in a very meticulous fashion, first placing triangulating sutures. Closely placed sutures of 5/0 polyglycolic acid are used to complete the anastomosis, some 100–150 sutures being used. These ligatures occlude the transected varices.

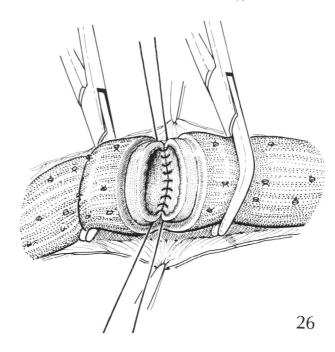

26

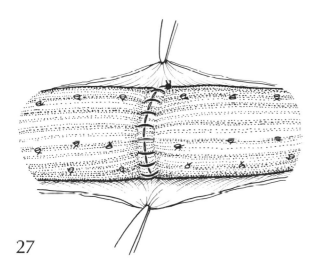

27

## 27

The final step in the anastomosis is suturing of the anterior muscular coat. The clamps, which have been left in place for the entire anastomosis, are then removed.

### Closure

The mediastinal pleura is closed in as watertight fashion as possible. Jackson–Pratt flat suction Silastic drains (manufactured by American V. Mueller.) are placed adjacent to the oesophageal anastomosis and are brought out in the flank under the diaphragm. The diaphragmatic incision is approximated with interrupted silk sutures reinforced with a running polyglycolic acid suture for a wateright closure, to prevent ascitic fluid passing from abdomen to chest. The chest is closed in standard fashion, and a chest tube is left in place.

## References

1. Clatworthy, H. W. Jr., Boles, E. T. Jr. (1959) Extrahepatic portal bed block in children: pathogenesis and treatment. Annals of Surgery, 150, 371–383

2. Bismuth, H., Franco, D., Alagille, D. (1980) Portal diversion for portal hypertension in children. Annals of Surgery, 192, 18–24

3. Boles, E. T. Jr., Wise, W. E. Jr., Birken, G. (1986) Extrahepatic portal hypertension in children: long-term evaluation. American Journal of Surgery, 151, 734–739

4. Auvert, J., Weisgerber, G. (1975) Immediate and long-term results of superior mesenteric vein–inferior vena cava shunt for portal hypertension in children. Journal of Pediatric Surgery, 10, 901–908

5. Fonkalsrud, E. W., Myers, N. A., Robinson, M. J. (1974) Management of extra-hepatic portal hypertension in children. Annals of Surgery, 180, 487–493

6. Cohen, D., Mansour, A. (1977) Extrahepatic portal hypertension. Long-term results. Progress in Pediatric Surgery, 10, 129–140

7. Singer, D. B. (1973) Postsplenectomy sepsis. In H. S. Rosenberg, R. P. Bolande (eds). Perspectives in Pediatric Pathology, 1, 285–311. Chicago: Year Book Medical Publishers

8. Lambert, M. J. III, Tank, E. S., Turcotte, J. G. (1974) Late sequelae of mesocaval shunts in children. American Journal of Surgery, 127, 19–24

9. Starzl, T. E., Putnam, C. W., Porter, K. A. Halgrimson, C. G., Corman, J., Brown, B. I. et al. (1973) Portal diversion for the treatment of glycogen storage disease in humans. Annals of Surgery, 178, 525–539

10. Boerema, I., Klopper, P. J., Holscher, A. A. (1970) Transabdominal ligation–resection of the esophagus in cases of bleeding esophageal varices. Surgery, 67, 409–413

11. Cooperman, M., Fabri, P. J., Martin, E. W. Jr., Carey, L. C. (1980) EEA Esophageal stapling for control of bleeding esophageal varices. American Journal of Surgery, 140, 821–824

12. Wexler, M. J. (1980) Treatment of bleeding esophageal varices by transabdominal esophageal transection with the EEA stapling instrument. Surgery, 88, 406–416

13. Steichen, F. M., Ravitch, M. M. (1980) Mechanical sutures in esophageal surgery. Annals of Surgery, 191, 373–381

14. Terblanche, J., Northover, J. M. A., Bornman, P. Kahn, D., Barbezat, G. O., Sellars, S. L. et al. (1979) A prospective evaluation of injection sclerotherapy in the treatment of acute bleeding from esophageal varices. Surgery, 85, 239–245

15. Lilly, J. R., Van Stiegmann, G., Stellin, G. (1982) Esophageal endosclerosis in children with portal vein thrombosis. Journal of Pediatric Surgery, 17, 571–575

16. Howard, E. R., Stamatakis, J. D., Mowat, A. P. (1984) Management of esophageal varices in children by injection sclerotherapy. Journal of Pediatric Surgery, 19, 2–5

17. Terblanche, J. (1984) Sclerotherapy for emergency variceal hemorrhage. World Journal of Surgery, 8, 653–659

18. Vane, D. W., Boles, E. T. Jr., Clatworthy, H. W. Jr. (1985) Esophageal sclerotherapy: an effective modality in children. Journal of Pediatric Surgery, 20, 703–707

19. Sugiura, M., Futagawa, S. (1973) A new technique for treating esophageal varices. Journal of Thoracic and Cardiovascular Surgery, 66, 677–685

20. Sugiura, M., Futagawa, S. (1984) Results of six hundred and thirty-six esophageal transections with paraesophagogastric devascularization in the treatment of esophageal varices. Journal of Vascular Surgery, 1, 254–260

21. Superina, R., Weber, J. L., Shandling, B. (1983) A modified Sugiura operation for bleeding varices in children. Journal of Pediatric Surgery, 18, 794–799

Illustrations by Gillian Oliver

# Surgery for biliary atresia

**Edward R. Howard**  MS, FRCS
Consultant Surgeon, King's College Hospital, London, UK

## History

Atresia of the extrahepatic biliary system is the end result of a variable inflammatory process of unknown aetiology which affects the lumen of the bile ducts in the perinatal period and which leads to death from cirrhotic liver failure. The incidence is between 0.8 and 1.0 per 10 000 births.

The patency of the hepatic and common hepatic ducts is preserved in a minority of patients (approximately 15 per cent) and bile may be aspirated from the ducts at surgery. These cases were originally called 'correctable' as they may be managed with conventional biliary-enteric anastomosis, e.g. hepaticojejunostomy. A majority of cases, however, suffer obliteration of the hepatic ducts up to the capsule of the liver in the porta hepatis, although in some of these the distal common bile duct may remain patent with free drainage from gall bladder to duodenum. Occlusion of the hepatic and common hepatic bile ducts was previously believed to be 'non-correctable'. The severity of biliary atresia is reflected in the finding of only 52 reported successes after operations performed between 1927 and 1970[1].

A new approach to the condition was suggested by Kasai[2], who observed that excision of all remnants of the extrahepatic bile ducts could allow drainage of bile from the porta hepatis in some 'non-correctable' cases.

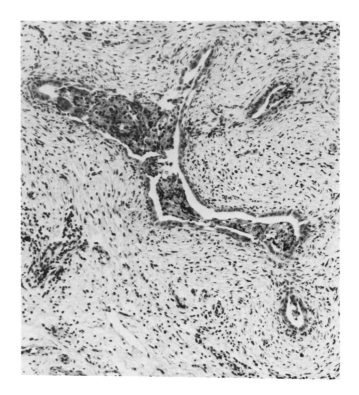

## 1

Microscope studies of the excised tissue reveal, within the area of fibrous tissue, epithelium-lined channels measuring up to 300 μm in diameter. There is destruction and desquamation of epithelium, and inflammation in the surrounding stroma.

Haematoxylin and eosin, × 13. Courtesy of Dr M. Driver    1

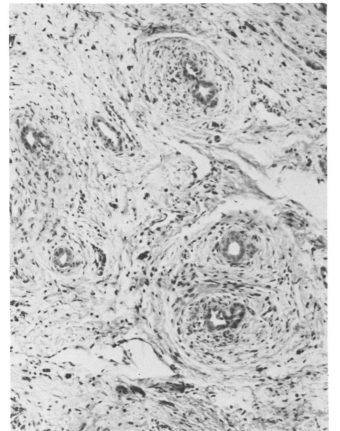

2    Haematoxylin and eosin, × 16. Courtesy of Dr M. Driver

## 2

Large ducts are sometimes absent from the porta hepatis, and 'ductules' are seen surrounded by fibrous tissue.

Serial section techniques showed communications with intrahepatic ducts, but these appeared to be destroyed progressively with age. Kasai devised the operation of portoenterostomy in which a Roux-en-Y loop of jejunum is anastomosed to the edges of the area left after excision of all bile duct remnants in the porta hepatis, and he showed that this procedure is most effective when performed before the patient reaches 60 days of age[3].

# 3

## Classification

The traditional division of biliary atresia into 'correctable' and 'non-correctable' types which depends on the presence or absence of a segment of bile-containing proximal duct has now been replaced by the classification which includes three major categories. The Japanese Society of Paediatric Surgeons has subdivided these main groups to include details of the structure of the distal bile ducts and the macroscopic appearances of the tissues in the porta hepatis[4]. These subdivisions have been omitted from the illustration as they have little influence on surgical treatment.

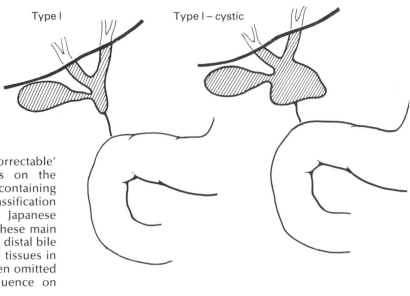

Type I        Type I – cystic

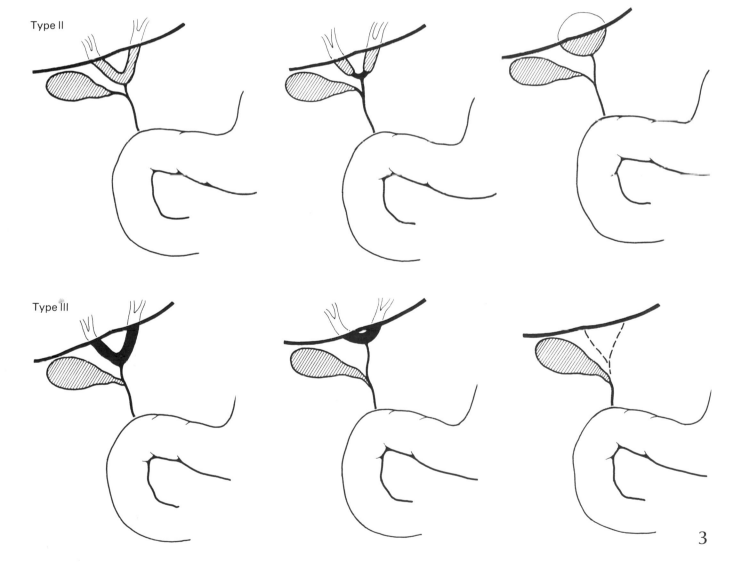

Type II

Type III

# Diagnosis

The differential diagnosis of prolonged jaundice in infancy includes neonatal hepatitis syndrome, intrahepatic biliary hypoplasia, choledochal cyst, spontaneous perforation of the bile ducts, inspissated bile syndrome and biliary atresia. Infection, metabolic abnormalities and alpha-l-antitrypsin deficiency can be detected as causes of neonatal hepatitis by appropriate screening tests, but the aetiology remains unknown in nearly 70 per cent of infants with intrahepatic cholestasis, and this group must be separated rapidly from the 'surgical' causes of jaundice.

Choledochal cyst, bile duct perforation and inspissated bile syndrome may be confidently diagnosed with ultrasonography and hepatobiliary scintigraphy. Definitive investigations of biliary atresia include both percutaneous liver biopsy and [131]I rose bengal faecal excretion[5]. Gamma glutamyl transpeptidase estimation and hepatobiliary scintigraphy are also useful, but infants with severe intrahepatic disease will often show a range of results compatible with a diagnosis of biliary atresia.

Alpha-l-antitrypsin deficient patients pose a particular problem, as features of bile duct obstruction are present on liver biopsy and it is essential to rule out this condition with alpha-l-antitrypsin phenotyping.

Other investigations of biliary tract patency include duodenal intubation for the identification of bile in duodenal aspirate, percutaneous transhepatic cholangiography and laparoscopy combined with gall bladder cholangiography. Unfortunately no single test is diagnostic in all cases, but two or more tests in combination usually differentiate biliary atresia from other causes of prolonged jaundice. Accurate preoperative diagnosis is imperative, as laparotomy findings may be difficult to interpret and may be misleading in up to 20 per cent of patients. It may be particularly difficult, for example, to identify the small bile ducts in cases of biliary hypoplasia and the patency of proximal bile ducts may not be obvious even with intraoperative cholangiography[6].

# Preoperative

Vitamin K (phytomenadione, 1.0 mg per day) is administered intramuscularly for at least four days. Blood is crossmatched, and oral neomycin (50 mg/kg per day) given in six divided doses for 24 hours preoperatively. An adequate intravenous line is set up and a nasogastric tube passed. The patient is placed supine on a thermostatically controlled heated surface. The operating table must have facilities for intraoperative cholangiography.

Intravenous antibiotics (a cephalosporin) are given after the induction of anaesthesia and are continued for five days. An oral cephalosporin is then substituted for a further three weeks as a prophylactic measure against ascending bacterial cholangitis.

# The operation

The traditional management of suspected cases of biliary atresia was separated into two stages, and this is still advised in some centres. The first stage, performed through a short, transverse right incision, consists of operative cholangiography via the gall bladder and a liver biopsy. Confirmation of the diagnosis is followed by definitive surgery a few days later. However, cholangiography is only possible in approximately 25 per cent of cases of atresia, as the gall bladder and distal common bile duct are frequently involved with the atretic process. We therefore prefer to make a preoperative diagnosis with percutaneous liver biopsy, radionuclide studies, etc. and restrict surgery to only one operative procedure.

## PORTOENTEROSTOMY (ORIGINAL KASAI PROCEDURE)

## 4

### The incision

A right subcostal incision is made extending across the right rectus muscle to expose the inferior surface of the right lobe of the liver. A note is made of the macroscopic appearance of the liver, and the presence or absence of ascites and portal hypertension.

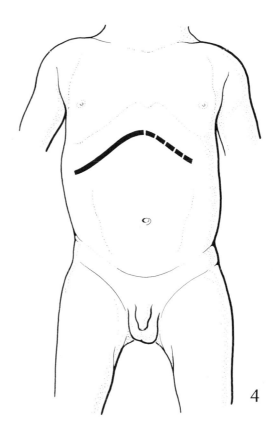

## 5

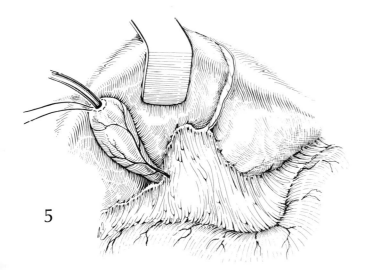

Associated anomalies, which may be found in up to 10 per cent of cases, include intestinal malrotation, situs inversus, polysplenia and preduodenal portal vein[7]. The diagnosis is confirmed in most cases by the observation of a thick-walled, contracted gall bladder containing clear mucus and which may be hidden within a cleft in the liver; cholangiography is often not possible.

## 6

### Cholangiogram

Operative cholangiography is usually performed when the gall bladder is of normal size. *The presence of bile within the gall bladder is an absolute indication for X-ray studies* and the visualization of a patent biliary tract terminates the operation.

In a proportion of cases the cystic and distal common bile ducts are patent, and contrast material will therefore flow into the duodenum but fail to outline the atretic proximal ducts, even after occlusion of the supraduodenal duct with a soft clamp.

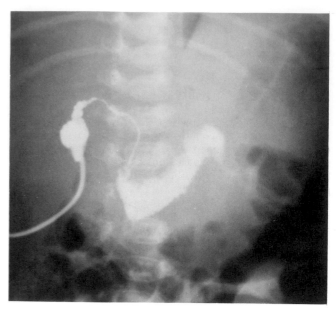

6

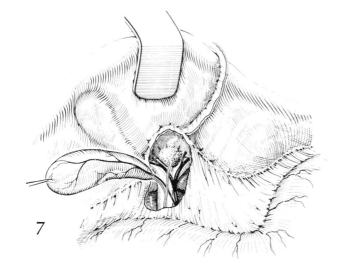

7

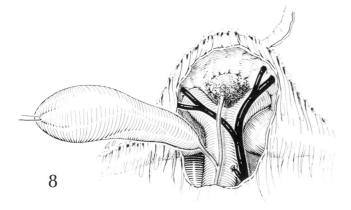

8

### Mobilization of gall bladder and bile ducts

## 7 & 8

Confirmation of the diagnosis of biliary atresia is followed by a lengthening of the incision across the left rectus muscle. The liver is retracted and the gall bladder mobilized from its bed. The cystic artery is often enlarged and is divided between ligatures at this stage. The mobilized gall bladder is used as a guide to the fibrous remnant of the extrahepatic bile ducts, which may be obscured by thickened peritoneum and enlarged lymph nodes. The branches and main trunk of the hepatic artery and the portal vein are dissected at this stage.

The distal portion of the common bile duct is divided between ligatures at the upper border of the duodenum.

# 9

## Dissection and exposure of porta hepatis

The gall bladder and attached remnants of the proximal bile ducts are dissected towards the porta hepatis, exposing the hepatic arteries and portal vein along their whole course. Small vascular branches and enlarged lymphatics are tied meticulously, as this helps to prevent postoperative ascites from lymphatic leakage. A small segment of patent proximal hepatic duct containing bile may be found at this stage in a small percentage of cases, and may be used for a conventional hepaticojejunostomy anastomosis.

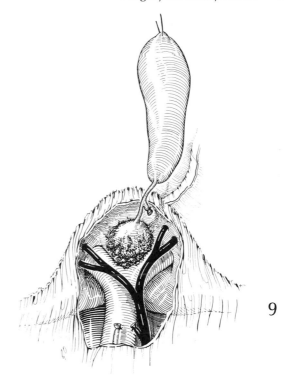

9

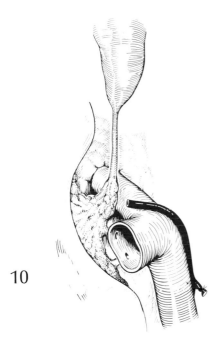

10

# 10

The proximal bile ducts are affected by the atretic process in the majority of cases and the dissection continues to the bifurcation of the portal vein. All the tissue bounded by the right and left branches of the vein is dissected free, and it is usually necessary to divide two or three short tributaries of the portal vein which enter directly into the bile duct remnants.

# 11

## Excision of bile duct remnants

The bile duct remnant and gall bladder are removed after transection of the tissue of the porta hepatis. The plane of transection is made flush with the liver capsule, and as wide as possible within the area bounded by the right and left branches of the portal vein.

This transection extends behind the posterior surface of the portal vein. Bleeding points in the porta hepatis are controlled with direct pressure.

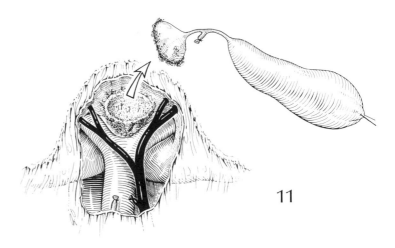

11

## Preparation and anastomosis of Roux loop

# 12

A 40 cm Roux-en-Y loop is prepared by transecting the jejunum just distal to the duodenojejunal flexure. The distal end is oversewn and passed in a retrocolic manner to the hilum of the liver. Small-bowel continuity is re-established with an end-to-side anastomosis in the usual manner.

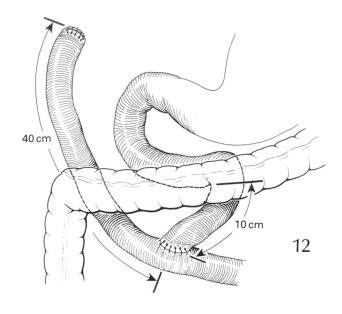

# 13 & 14

An anastomosis is fashioned between the transected tissue in the porta hepatis and the side of the Roux loop, using interrupted sutures of 4/0 catgut. The anastomosis is achieved by positioning all of the posterior sutures before they are tied. The jejunal loop is 'railroaded' into position and the sutures tied serially. Placement of the anterior row of sutures completes the anastomosis. A small drain is placed down to the porta hepatis before closure of the abdomen.

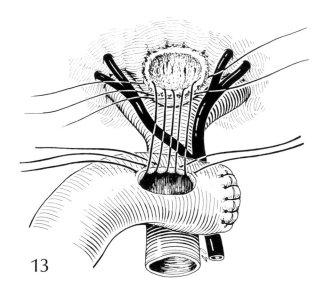

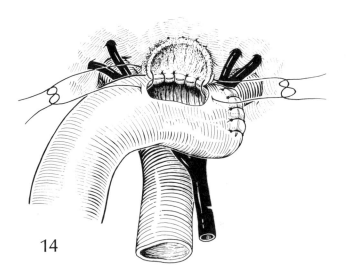

# 15

## CUTANEOUS ENTEROSTOMY

Surgical attempts to prevent ascending bacterial cholangitis after portoenterostomy have often included a cutaneous enterostomy in the bile conduit. The technique illustrated was devised by Kasai so that the cutaneous stoma could act as a vent to prevent any high intraluminal pressure at the portoenterostomy. Numerous types of enterostomy have been described[8], but their beneficial effect on the overall incidence of cholangitis remains in doubt[9]. There was no reduction of cholangitis in a personal series of cases treated with enterostomies and we have now returned to the original Kasai operation.

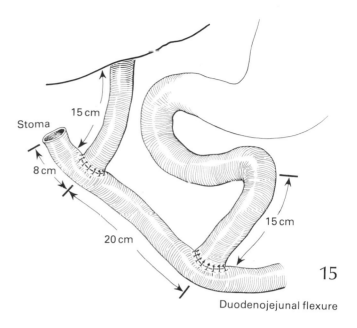

15

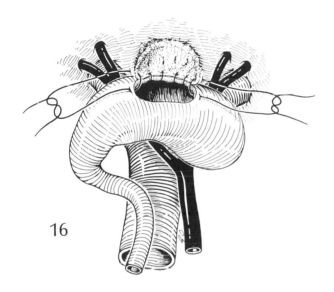

16

## CHOLECYSTPORTOENTEROSTOMY

# 16

Patency of the gall bladder and distal common bile duct demonstrated by operative cholangiography may allow the construction of a more natural conduit for bile drainage after anastomosis of the gall bladder to the transected tissue of the porta hepatis[10].

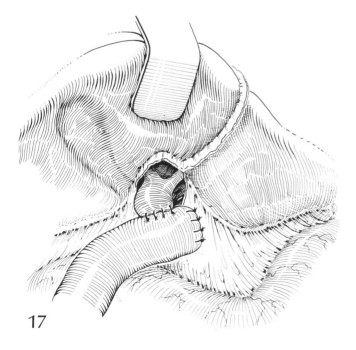

17

# 17

## HEPATICOJEJUNOSTOMY

The presence of a patent common hepatic duct allows the construction of a hepaticojejunostomy as an end-to-side anastomosis between the bulbous end of the common hepatic duct and the side of the Roux loop.

# Postoperative care

Nasogastric drainage is continued until bowel activity returns, and intravenous antibiotics are administered for five days. The onset of any unexplained pyrexia, particularly if accompanied by increased serum bilirubin levels, suggests an ascending bacterial cholangitis, which must be identified with blood and liver biopsy cultures. Possible organisms include *E. coli*, *Proteus* and *Klebsiella*.

The onset of effective bile drainage and an improvement in liver function tests are difficult to predict after operation for biliary atresia and may not occur until several weeks later. Histological analysis of tissue excised from the porta hepatis may help with prognosis and satisfactory bile flow may be anticipated with the identification of duct-like structures with diameters greater than 150 μm.

Any bile draining from cutaneous enterostomies is refed, and the serum electrolytes are checked regularly. Phenobarbitone, cholestyramine and vitamins D and K are prescribed for all cases.

At the time of discharge the parents and the referring hospital are given full information on the signs and hazards of possible attacks of cholangitis, together with instructions on the administration of intravenous antibiotics.

Cutaneous enterostomies are closed at approximately one year after operation.

## RESULTS

Since the introduction of the portoenterostomy operation 25 years ago the achievement of postoperative bile drainage has improved. The results are related to the ages of patients at the time of operation, and this was illustrated in the series from King's College Hospital which showed extended bile drainage in 55 per cent of patients under 12 weeks of age but only 27 per cent of older children[11]. Altman has recently reported similar results with 42 per cent of children under 12 weeks becoming jaundice-free compared with only 20 per cent of those over 12 weeks[9].

The oldest survivors after portoenterostomy are now over 20 years of age, but most continue to show abnormalities of hepatic histology and function. Postoperative complications include recurrent cholangitis, hepatic fibrosis and consequent portal hypertension, which becomes evident with the appearance of oesophageal varices in approximately 30 per cent of long-term survivors. Recent reports suggest that injection sclerotherapy is the treatment of choice for this complication[12].

Current surgical techniques and postoperative care has increased the 4-year survival of patients with extrahepatic biliary atresia from 2 per cent to over 40 per cent.

## References

1. Bill, A. H. (1978) Biliary atresia introduction. World Journal of Surgery, 2, 557–559

2. Kasai, M., Kimura, S., Asakura, Y., Suzuki, H., Taira, Y., Ohashi, E. (1968) Surgical treatment of biliary atresia. Journal of Pediatric Surgery, 3, 665–675

3. Kasai, M. (1983) Hepatic portoenterostomy for the so-called 'non-correctable' type of biliary atresia. In Extrahepatic Biliary Atresia, F. Daum (ed.), p. 85. New York and Basel: Marcel Dekker

4. Hays, D. M., Kimura, K. (1980) Biliary atresia: the Japanese experience. Cambridge, Mass: Harvard University Press

5. Manolaki, A. G., Larcher, V. F., Mowat, A., Barrett, J. J., Portman, B., Howard, E. R. (1983) The prelaparotomy diagnosis of extrahepatic biliary atresia. Archives of Disease in Childhood, 58, 591–594

6. Kahn, E. I., Daum, F. (1983) Arteriohepatic dysplasia: evaluation of the extrahepatic biliary tract, porta hepatis, and hepatic parenchyma. In Extrahepatic Biliary Atresia, F. Daum (ed.), p. 194. New York and Basel: Marcel Dekker

7. Lilly, J. R., Chandra, R. S. (1974) Surgical hazards of co-existing anomalies in biliary atresia. Surgery, Gynecology and Obstetrics, 139, 49–54

8. Howard, E. R. (1980) Extrahepatic biliary atresia. In Maingot, R., ed. Abdominal Operations, R. Maingot (ed.), 7th ed., p. 1176–1185. New York: Appleton-Century-Crofts

9. Altman, R. P. (1983) Long-term results after the Kasai procedure. In Extrahepatic Biliary Atresia, F. Daum (ed.), p. 96. New York and Basel: Marcel Dekker

10. Kasai, M. (1974) Treatment of biliary atresia with special reference to hepatic porto-enterostomy and its modifications. Progress in Pediatric Surgery, 6, 5–52

11. Howard, E. R., Driver, M., McClement, J., Mowat, A. P. (1982) Results of surgery in 88 consecutive cases of extrahepatic biliary atresia. Journal of the Royal Society of Medicine, 75, 408–413

12. Howard, E. R., Stamatakis, J. D., Mowat, A. P. (1984) Management of oesophageal varices in children by injection sclerotherapy. Journal of Pediatric Surgery, 19, 2–5

Illustrations by Kevin Marks

# Choledochal cyst

**R. Peter Altman**  MD
Professor of Surgery and Pediatrics, Columbia University College of Physicians and Surgeons, and Director, Pediatric Surgery, Babies Hospital, Columbia-Presbyterian Medical Center, New York, New York, USA

## 1

Choledochal cyst was initially recognized by Douglas in 1852[1]. The cyst is not an isolated defect restricted to the bile duct but is more appropriately regarded as the sentinel feature of a constellation of anomalies affecting the pancreatobiliary system. This concept has important therapeutic implications[2]. The lesions were first classified in 1959[3]. Several descriptions and classifications of choledochal cyst have since been offered. Among the most useful is that proposed by Todani et al.[4]. The type I choledochal cyst predominates. The cyst is solitary and characterized by fusiform dilatation of the common bile duct. The gallbladder and cystic duct, almost invariably dilated, enter the cyst. Usually, but not always, the pancreatic duct drains into the distal common bile duct, forming a common channel for the transmission of bile and pancreatic exocrine secretions into the duodenum. The common hepatic duct proximal to the cyst is most often normal, although occasionally distortion and dilatation may extend cephalad to involve one or both hepatic ducts in the liver. The hepatic histology also varies from normal in some patients to advanced fibrosis and cirrhosis in others.

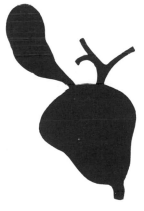

1

## Aetiology

The aetiology of choledochal cyst remains speculative. It has been proposed that the cause is distal narrowing of the bile duct originating *in utero*[5]. A more commonly accepted explanation is that an abnormal junction of the bile duct with the pancreatic duct[6,7] creates an anatomical common channel which allows reflux of pancreatic juice into the bile duct, thereby weakening its wall by enzymatic destruction and resulting in inflammation, dilatation and cyst formation. However, a common channel is also occasionally found in normal individuals and not all patients with choledochal cyst demonstrate this anatomy. Whatever the cause, the result is dilatation of the bile duct, biliary stasis, cholangitis and cirrhosis, unless the process is remedied surgically.

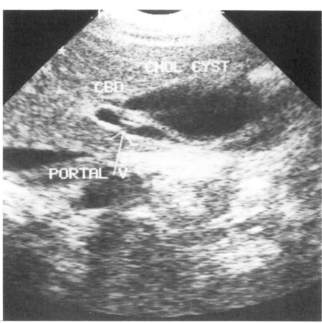

**2**

*Ultrasonogram of 5-year-old with choledochal cyst. Note particularly the relationship of the portal vein to the posterior cyst wall. Also seen is the transition from cystic dilatation to normal-calibre common bile duct (CBD)*

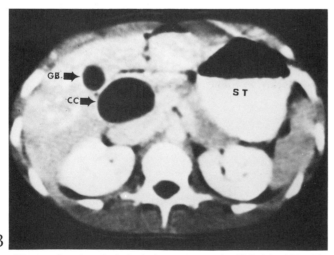

**3**

*CT scan showing choledochal cyst (CC) and gallbladder (GB). The stomach (ST) is filled with contrast.*

## Clinical features

Presentation is variable. Symptoms usually appear in the first decade of life. Females are more often affected than males (ratio 4:1). The classic symptom complex of pain, mass, and jaundice is in fact uncommon. In older patients the usual presentation is vague recurrent abdominal pain associated with minimal jaundice, which may not be readily apparent. In such patients the condition may not be recognized until there are serious hepatic sequelae. In younger patients, and particularly in infants, the obstructive component predominates so that they frequently present with jaundice and an abdominal mass. Infection and pain are not characteristic in this age group, perhaps because of the high-grade ductal obstruction and thus the absence of reflux of intestinal contents into the cyst.

## Diagnosis

# 2 & 3

The diagnosis is readily confirmed by any of several imaging modalities. The most important and reliable confirmatory studies are ultrasonography and CT scanning. The diagnosis can be made antenatally[8,9]. Both these techniques clearly define the dimensions of the cyst and identify the transition to normal ductal calibre. They also provide information about the configuration of the ducts, and particularly the presence of dilatation. If the regional anatomy remains obscure after these non-invasive studies, endoscopic retrograde cholangiopancreatography (ERCP) is a valuable adjunct[10,11,12]; as it defines the distal pancreatobiliary system precisely. However, routine use is not advocated. Because of the risk of inciting cholangitis periendoscopic antibiotic cover is recommended.

## Choice of treatment

Internal drainage of the cyst by cyst enterostomy, while expedient, cannot be recommended. The cyst wall is composed of thick fibrous tissue devoid of mucosal lining, and even after drainage the cyst persists as a receptacle for stagnant bile. Anastomotic stricture and bile stasis result in cholangitis, stone formation and biliary colic so that almost one-half of patients will require subsequent surgery for management of these complications[13,14,15]. Furthermore, it has been shown that cancer develops in the retained cyst in approximately 3 per cent of patients[16,17,18,19]. For these reasons, surgical excision is now the treatment of choice.

# The operations

## 4

An accurate operative cholangiogram is essential. After aspirating the gallbladder and cyst, radio-opaque contrast is instilled through a catheter placed within the gallbladder to outline the gallbladder, choledochal cyst and extrahepatic ductal anatomy. If there is a common channel, it is important to identify the entry of the pancreatic duct into the bile duct in order to protect it when the distal part of the cyst is transected.

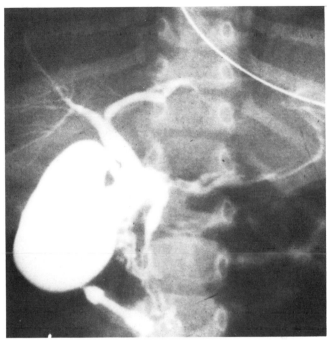

4

*Operative cholangiogram of a 10-month-old infant showing the cyst and normal-calibre common bile and common hepatic ducts. The pancreatic duct is seen entering the common bile duct to form a common channel.*

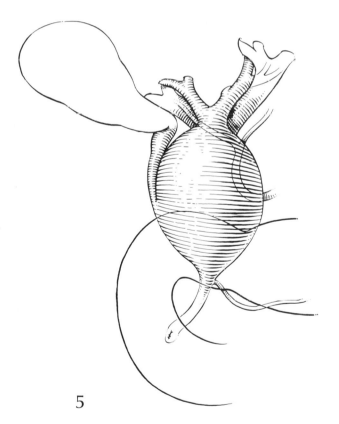

5

## Circumferential dissection

## 5

The choice of procedure depends on the degree of inflammatory reaction encountered in the porta. If the regional anatomy is readily defined, dissection of the gallbladder and choledochal cyst from the intimately associated vascular structures proceeds rather easily. The cystic artery is divided and the gallbladder mobilized from its bed, leaving the cystic duct in continuity with the choledochal cyst from which it invariably arises.

## 6

When it is safe to do so, the cyst is next mobilized by dissection laterally and posteriorly, thereby separating its back wall from the vascular structures in the porta. When scarring and inflammation render dissection behind the cyst hazardous, an alternative technique for resection is proposed (see below).

The transition from cyst to normal calibre hepatic duct is then identified and the duct divided. Once the cyst has been freed superiorly, the posterior and remaining lateral dissection proceeds until the distal limit of the cyst is defined. At this point, the bile duct is transected and secured by suture, taking care to ensure that pancreatic duct drainage is unimpaired should this duct enter the common bile duct to form a common channel (see Illustration 5). The biliary drainage system is reconstructed by a standard retrocolic Roux-en-Y hepatic duct-jejunostomy.

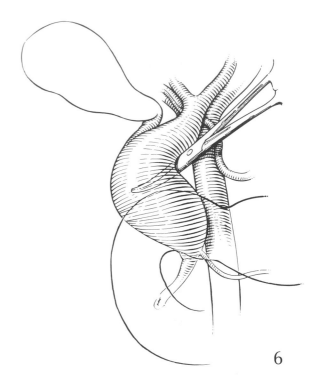

6

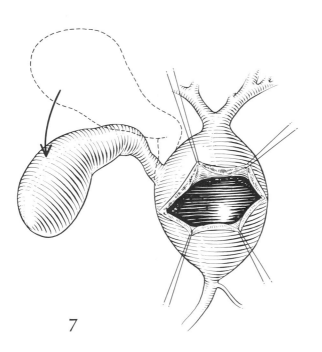

7

## Alternative technique

If pericystic inflammation obscures the anatomy, circumferential dissection of the cyst can be hazardous and may result in unacceptable blood loss, especially if there is already established liver disease and portal hypertension. For such patients, Lilly[20,21] has described a technique of resection in which the plane between the posterior wall of the cyst and the underlying portal vein need not be disturbed.

## 7

The regional anatomy is defined by cholangiograms. The gallbladder and cystic duct are then mobilized as described above. The anterior cyst wall is incised transversely and the cyst contents evacuated.

## 8

An arbitrary plane is then entered by dissecting within the lateral cyst wall in a posterior direction, thereby establishing an intramural separation of the thick inner cyst lining from the thinner outer posterior wall immediately under which lies the portal vein.

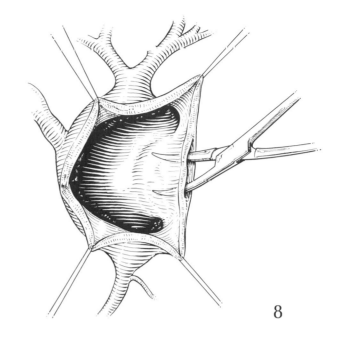

8

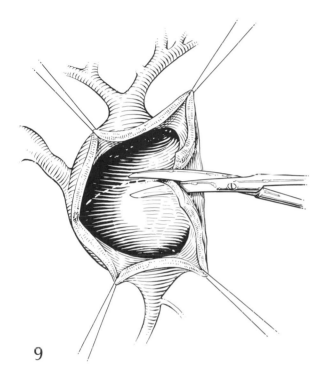

9

## 9

After developing the proper plane within the cyst posteriorly, the cyst lining is divided. Intramural dissection is continued cephalad and caudad as the remainder of the cyst is mobilized anterolaterally to the point at which the hepatic duct and common bile duct assume normal or near-normal dimensions.

## 10

The cyst, with attached gallbladder, is resected and the distal common bile duct closed. By this technique, the cyst and its lining are removed but a portion of the outer posterior wall remains, thereby avoiding the hazardous dissection between the back wall of the cyst and the portal vein. Biliary drainage is re-established by a Roux-en-Y hepatic duct-jejunostomy.

If dilatation of the choledochal cyst extends distally into the duodenum, it is necessary to divide the distal cyst leaving some residual expanded duct (cyst) above the duodenum. The cyst lining is readily stripped and removed before the walls are opposed and secured. Great care should be taken to avoid injury to the pancreatic duct. As mentioned earlier, distortion and dilatation may extend cephalad along the common hepatic duct to involve one or both of the hepatic ducts within the liver. In such patients, the resection is extended as far as feasible, removing as much of the involved ductal structure as possible and filleting the hepatic ducts preparatory to anastomosis with the jejunal conduit.

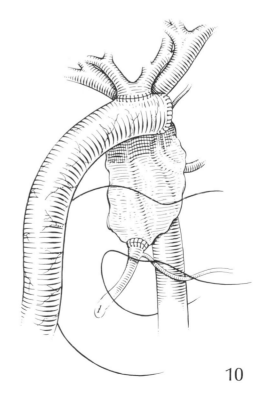

10

# Results

The outlook after cyst resection varies considerably. For some, particularly those coming to surgery later after established liver disease, the outlook is guarded. Furthermore, cyst excision does not completely eliminate the risk of malignancy and biliary cancer has been reported even after resection[18]. Nonetheless, the outcome is generally favourable and for most patients the prognosis is excellent[22,23].

## References

1. Douglas, A. H. (1852) Case of dilatation of the common bile duct. Monthly Journal of Medical Science, 14, 97–101

2. Rattner, D. W., Schapiro, R. H., Warshaw, A. L. (1983) Abnormalities of the pancreatic and biliary ducts in adult patients with choledochal cysts. Archives of Surgery, 118, 1068–1073

3. Alonso-Lej, F., Rever, W. B., Jr, Pessagno, D. J. (1959) Congenital choledochal cysts, with a report of two and an analysis of 94 cases. International Abstracts of Surgery, 108, 1–30

4. Todani, T., Watanabe, Y., Narusue, M., Tabuchi, K., Okajima, K. (1977) Congenital bile duct cysts. Classification, operative procedures, and review of thirty-seven cases including cancer arising from choledochal cyst. American Journal of Surgery, 134, 263–269

5. Ito, T., Ando, H., Nagaya, M., Sugito, T. (1984) Congenital dilatation of the common bile duct in children – the etiologic significance of the narrow segment distal to the dilated common bile duct. Zeitschrift für Kinderchirurgie, 39, 40–45

6. Babbitt, D. P. (1969) Congenital choledochal cysts: new etiological concept based on anomalous relationships of the common bile duct and pancreatic bulb. Annals of Radiology, 12, 231–240

7. Babbitt, D. P., Starshak, R. J., Clemett, A. R. (1973) Choledochal cyst: a concept of etiology. American Journal of Roentgenology, 119, 57–62

8. Dewbury, K. C., Aluwihare, A. P., Birch, S. J., Freeman, N. V. (1980) Prenatal ultrasound demonstration of a choledochal cyst. British Journal of Radiology, 53, 906–907

9. Howell, C. G., Templeton, J. M., Weiner, S., Glassman, M., Betts, J. M., Witzleben, C. L. (1983) Antenatal diagnosis and early surgery for choledochal cyst. Journal of Pediatric Surgery, 18, 387–393

10. Agrawal, R. M., Brodmerkel, G. J., Jr. (1978) Endoscopic retrograde cholangiopancreatography diagnosis of choledochal cyst. American Journal of Gastroenterology, 70, 393–396

11. Altman, M. S., Halls, J. M., Douglas, A. P., Renner, I. G. (1978) Choledochal cyst presenting as acute pancreatitis. Evaluation with endoscopic retrograde cholangiopancreatography. American Journal of Gastroenterology, 70, 514–519

12. Okada, A., Yoshiro, O., Shinkichi, K., Yoshikazu, I., Yashnaru, K., Saito, R. (1983) Common channel syndrome – diagnosis with endoscopic cholangiopancreatography and surgical management. Surgery, 93, 634–642

13. Flanigan, D. P. (1975) Biliary cysts. Annals of Surgery, 182, 635–643

14. Fonkalsrud, E. W., Boles, E. T. (1965) Choledochal cysts in infancy and childhood. Surgery, Gynecology and Obstetrics, 121, 733–742

15. Filler, R. M., Stringel, G. (1980) Treatment of choledochal cyst by excision. Journal of Pediatric Surgery, 15, 437–442

16. Flanigan, D. P. (1977) Biliary carcinoma associated with biliary cysts. Cancer, 40, 880–883

17. Tsuchiya, R., Harada, N., Ito, T., Furukawa, M., Yoshihiro, I., Kusano, T. et al. (1977) Malignant tumors in choledochal cysts. Annals of Surgery, 186, 22–28

18. Nagorney, D. M., McIlrath, D. C., Adson, M. A. (1984) Choledochal cysts in adults: clinical management. Surgery, 96, 656–663

19. Voyles, C. R., Smadja, C., Shands, C., Blumgart, L. H. (1983) Carcinoma in choledochal cysts: age-related incidence. Archives of Surgery, 118, 986–988

20. Lilly, J. R. (1979) The surgical treatment of choledochal cyst. Surgery, Gynecology and Obstetrics, 149, 36–42

21. Lilly, J. R. (1978) Total excision of choledochal cyst. Surgery, Gynecology and Obstetrics, 146, 254–256

22. Saito, S., Tsuchida, Y., Hashizume, K., Makino, S. (1976) Congenital cystic dilatation of the biliary ducts: surgical procedures and long-term results. Zeitschrift für Kinderchirurgie, 19, 49–59

23. Yamaguchi, M. (1980) Congenital choledochal cyst. Analysis of 1433 patients in the Japanese literature. American Journal of Surgery, 140, 653–657

Illustrations by Gillian Oliver

# Splenectomy in childhood

**J. D. Atwell** FRCS
Consultant Paediatric Surgeon, Wessex Regional Centre for Paediatric Surgery, The General Hospital, Southampton, UK

## Indications

In childhood there are three main groups of conditions which require splenectomy[1]: haematological disease, trauma, and a miscellaneous group of conditions.

### Haematological disease

The two main indications for splenectomy in childhood in this group are congenital haemolytic anaemia (congenital spherocytosis) and idiopathic thrombocytopenia resistant to steroid management. There are other haematological indications for splenectomy but these are better considered under the miscellaneous heading.

## Trauma

### 1

The spleen is a friable, vascular organ which is relatively immobile except during respiration. The range of splenic injuries includes transverse tears which may include the hilum, longitudinal injuries, subcapsular haematoma, and complete disruption.

In the past, injuries of the spleen usually required a splenectomy, but since the complications of splenectomy in childhood became apparent the policy has changed, and every attempt is now made to preserve splenic tissue. Only if the spleen becomes totally separated from its blood supply is splenectomy now indicated. Non-operative management[2] or repair of the spleen[3] are the current preferred courses.

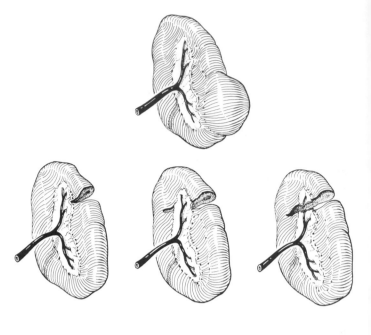

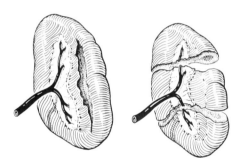

### 1

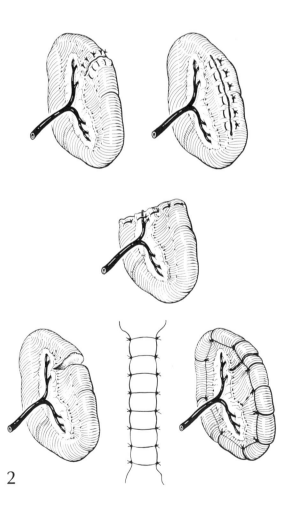

### 2

Repair of the spleen is possible with simple capsular ligatures (with either horizontal or vertical mattress sutures of absorbable material), or partial splenic resection with omental or adhesive support.

The late complications of rupture and traumatic splenic cysts have not been reported following repair of the spleen. In a recent report, splenectomy was performed in only one of 46 patients admitted with traumatic rupture of the spleen[4].

## Miscellaneous group

This group would include splenectomies performed for thalassaemia, relief of hypersplenism associated with portal hypertension or prior to constructing a proximal splenorenal shunt, various tumours, acquired haemolytic and aplastic anaemia, inborn errors of metabolism, histiocytosis, hypersplenism of unspecified types, Hodgkin's disease, and primary splenic diseases such as splenic cyst or torsion of the spleen. In this group should also be included the incidental splenectomy required as a complication of other surgery; in childhood this occurs less frequently than in adult surgical practice.

# Management

## Non-operative management

It should be possible to preserve the spleen without an operation in 70–95 per cent of patients admitted following splenic trauma[2,4,5]. In the majority of patients the critical time is the first 4 hours following the injury, and if surgery has not been indicated by 24 hours it is usually unnecessary.

The diagnosis must be confirmed by ultrasonography and a [99m]Tc scan of the liver and spleen. The progress of the patient will have to be monitored continuously for 48 hours, and at any time an operation may be required. Adequate support from anaesthetic and blood transfusion services is essential. Thus, the conservative approach can be safely implemented only in a well-equipped and fully staffed general or paediatric hospital.

Blood is replaced as required, and nasogastric aspiration is continued for as long as necessary. The patient is kept on strict bed rest for 7 days and can usually be discharged home within 2 weeks. Prior to discharge a [99m]Tc scan of the liver and spleen is repeated to confirm the presence of functioning splenic tissue.

## Operative management

### Preoperative preparation

*Blood transfusion*

In the severely anaemic child a blood transfusion will be required before operation.

*Platelet transfusion*

A platelet transfusion may be required in approximately 20 per cent of patients with idiopathic thrombocytopenia, either preoperatively or at the time of operation.

*Nasogastric intubation*

This is required preoperatively in cases associated with trauma because of the risk of aspiration of gastric contents. In other patients undergoing splenectomy as a routine procedure, the passage of the tube can be carried out at the time of the operation, thus avoiding distress to the child.

### Position of the patient

The patient is placed in the supine position, with a small sandbag under the left chest to raise the left upper quadrant of the abdomen.

### Anaesthesia

General anaesthesia is required, and in cases of traumatic rupture of the spleen, careful assessment and adequate replacement of blood loss is essential.

## Principles of the operation

### The accessory spleen

As haematological conditions are the largest group of indications for splenectomy, in particular with congenital haemolytic diseases and hypersplenism, location and removal of any accessory spleens at the time of splenectomy is of paramount importance. Failure to do this will lead to a failure of the haematological condition to improve, and will necessitate a second exploratory laparotomy. An accessory spleen may be found in approximately 16 per cent of patients. The commonest sites are the splenic hilum, tail of the pancreas, and the greater omentum; other sites are along the gastrosplenic ligament, along the splenic artery and pancreas, splenocolic ligament, and splenorenal ligament.

## Age at operation

Splenectomy for rupture of the spleen may become essential irrespective of the age of the patient, and may even be required in the neonatal period following birth trauma. Other traumatic causes requiring splenectomy are nearly always in the child over 5 years of age.

In congenital haemolytic anaemia and in idiopathic thrombocytopenia, the majority of children will require splenectomy after 3 years of age. Due to the risk of intercurrent infection in childhood following splenectomy, the removal of the spleen should be delayed for as long as possible[6,7].

# The operation

## 3

### The incision

A left upper quadrant transverse muscle-cutting incision is the incision of choice. The transverse incision is particularly useful in traumatic ruptures as it is easily extended and allows careful inspection of the other abdominal viscera. (In the large spleen, rarely found in childhood in this country, the thoracoabdominal approach through the bed of the tenth or eleventh rib should be considered.)

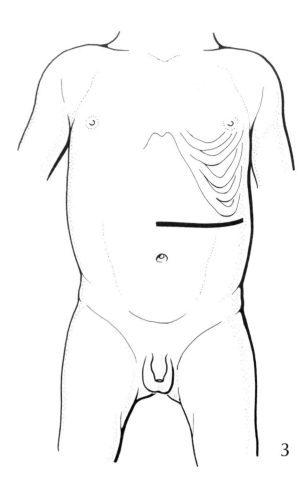

3

## Exploration

Palpation and inspection of the spleen, stomach, duodenum, pancreas, liver and gall-bladder is carried out, looking in particular for splenunculi and for gall-stones in the patients with congenital haemolytic anaemia.

# 4, 5 & 6

## Mobilization of the spleen

A hand is passed over the outer surface of the spleen, between it and the diaphragm, and by gentle traction the spleen may be delivered into the wound. The lienorenal ligament is often divided with the tips of the fingers, but occasionally it may have to be divided under direct vision with a scalpel or the dissecting scissors. At this stage the short gastric vessels are seen in the gastrosplenic ligament. They are divided between ligatures, but difficulty may be experienced here, especially in the very young, due to the extreme shortness of these vessels. The fundus of the stomach is then separated from the spleen.

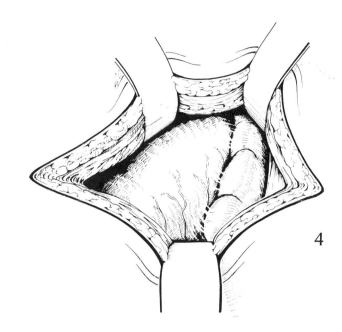

4

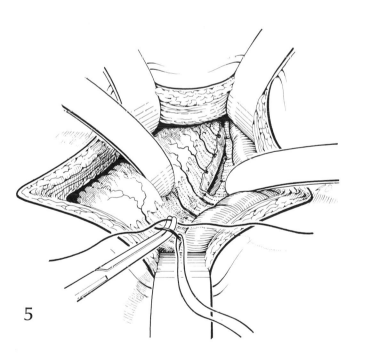

5

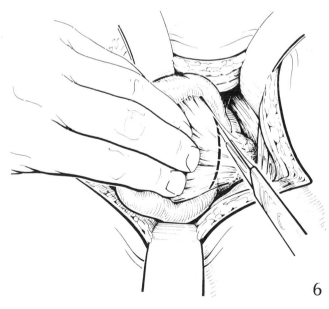

6

# 7

### Ligation of the splenic artery and vein

The spleen and its vascular pedicle are now delivered out of the wound. With a finger behind the vascular pedicle and by gentle gauze dissection, the splenic artery and vein are identified. The artery is then doubly ligated either by using clamps or by using an aneurysm needle to pass the ligatures which are then tied. After an interval of a minute or two the splenic vein is ligated in a similar manner. This pause allows the patient to receive an autotransfusion from the blood trapped in the spleen[8]. Great care must be taken during this stage of the operation to avoid any damage to the tail of the pancreas, which abuts onto the splenic vessels at the hilum. After ligation of the vessels the spleen is removed.

### Inspection of the splenic bed

Careful inspection of the splenic bed is made and any bleeding points are either diathermied or ligated. Usually there is only a gentle ooze, which may be controlled by a hot pack left for a few minutes. A *second careful search* of the abdominal cavity is made for any accessory spleens which may have been missed at the initial exploration.

The wound is closed in layers with absorbable sutures. Drainage of the subphrenic spaces is not necessary unless there has been damage to the tail of the pancreas; a closed-system drainage (Redivac) is then advisable.

# Complications

### Complications of non-operative management

Conservative treatment of injury may have to be abandoned because of continued bleeding. Intermittent bleeding causing a haematoma under the diaphragm may result in a pleural effusion. The pleural effusion usually settles, but occasionally aspiration is required.

### Complications of operative management

### Thromboembolic disease

Following splenectomy there is a rise in the platelet count, which is maximal by the tenth postoperative day. In a review, only 14 of 1413 children undergoing splenectomy were treated with heparin postoperatively, and there was no report of thromboembolic disease in any patient[1].

### Pancreatitis

This is extremely rare (5 out of 1413 children[1]) and should be avoided by careful dissection of the tail of the pancreas from the hilum of the spleen.

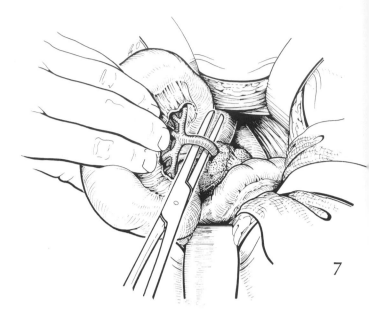

7

### Infection

The late mortality from overwhelming infection following splenectomy has caused considerable discussion among paediatricians, who will often advise postponement of splenectomy until later in childhood, or even avoidance of the operation entirely. In the combined review of 1413 children splenectomized in the USA between 1956 and 1965[1], only two patients of 394 with congenital haemolytic anaemia died (0.5 per cent), and of 34 deaths from sepsis, 16 were in children of less than 2 years of age. The highest death rate was 6 per cent and was found in the group of children with more serious primary disease, where even the value of splenectomy was debatable.

Postoperative infections follow a characteristic pattern. The course is fulminating and the mortality high, the infecting organism is often the pneumococcus, and the patient is liable to recurrent attacks[6,7].

Immunization with a polyvalent pneumococcal vaccine is started shortly after surgery. Prophylactic antibiotics may be used and include penicillin, ampicillin and co-trimoxazole. The duration of prophylaxis required is debatable, but it should probably continue until adult life. The threat of postsplenectomy sepsis is lifelong.

### Haemorrhage

This should be avoidable by careful ligation of the main vessels and inspection of the splenic bed before closure.

### Pulmonary complications

These are rare in childhood following surgical operations, but postoperative physiotherapy is recommended in this group of patients.

# References

1. Eraklis, A. J., Filler, R. M. (1972) Splenectomy in childhood: a review of 1413 cases. Journal of Pediatric Surgery, 7, 383–388

2. Wesson, D. E., Filler, R. M., Ein, S. H., Shandling, B., Simpson, J. S., Stephens, C. A. (1981) Ruptured spleen – When to operate? Journal of Pediatric Surgery, 16, 324–326

3. Buntain, W. L., Lynn, H. B. (1979) Splenorrhaphy: changing concepts for the traumatized spleen. Surgery, 86, 748–760

4. Linne, T., Eriksson, M., Lannergren, K., Tordai, P., Czar-Weidhagen, B., Swedberg, K. (1984) Splenic function after non surgical management of splenic rupture. Journal of Pediatrics, 105, 263–265

5. Filler, R. M. (1984) Experience with the management of splenic injuries. Australia and New Zealand Journal of Surgery, 54, 443–445

6. Horan, M., Colebatch, J. H. (1962) Relation between splenectomy and subsequent infections: a clinical study. Archives of Disease in Childhood, 37, 398–414

7. Ein, S. H., Shandling, B., Simpson, J. S., Stephens, C. A., Bandi, S. K., Biggar, W. D. et al. (1977) The morbidity and mortality of splenectomy in childhood. Annals of Surgery, 185, 307–310

8. Macpherson, A. I. S., Richmond, J., Donaldson, G. W. K., Muir, A. R. (1971) Role of the spleen in congenital spherocytosis. American Journal of Medicine, 50, 35–41

Illustrations by Gillian Oliver

# Liver resections in children

**John R. Lilly** MD
Professor and Chief of Pediatric Surgery, University of Colorado School of Medicine, Denver, Colorado, USA

**Gianna P. Stellin** MD
Assistant Professor, Department of Surgery, University of California at Irvine, Orange, California, USA

The first comprehensive description of liver tumours in children was by Yamagiwa in 1911, but series of hepatic resections in children were not reported until the 1950s. In these early publications about half of the children with malignancy were thought to be unresectable. Of those that were resected, 25 per cent died, almost always as a consequence of overwhelming blood loss. Even resections for benign lesions carried a 10 per cent mortality. The recent appreciation of the liver's segmental anatomy has diminished this heavy operative loss. There were no deaths, for example, in the last 10 major hepatic resections carried out at our institution.

About 80 per cent of liver resections in children are performed for tumours, the majority of which are malignant. Hepatoblastoma is the most frequent malignant hepatic tumour under two years of age. Hepatocellular carcinoma has a peak incidence at about 10 years of age. In contrast to the adults, in whom hepatocellular carcinoma and cirrhosis are associated, the non-tumorous liver in children is usually normal. Metastatic tumours, generally from Wilms' tumour and neuroblastoma, account for less than 10 per cent of paediatric liver resections. The most commonly encountered benign tumours are haemangioma, haemangio-endothelioma and hamartoma.

# 1

## Surgical anatomy

The major hepatic veins divide the liver into three relatively bloodless surgical 'corridors'. A right or left hepatic lobectomy is perfomed by following the right or left side of the middle hepatic vein. The right and left hepatic lobes are divided by the right and left hepatic veins, respectively, again providing relatively bloodless segmental corridors. The right hepatic vein divides the right lobe into anterior and posterior segments. The left lobe, however, is anatomically divided by the umbilical fissure into a medial and lateral segment. The left hepatic vein divides the left lateral segment into two subsegments, superior and inferior. Branches of the major hepatic veins further divide the parenchyma into eight subsegments, each of which can theoretically be removed whilst leaving the others intact. Each anatomical segment and subsegment is supplied by its own trinity structures (artery, portal vein and bile duct). There is no collateral circulation between trinity structures.

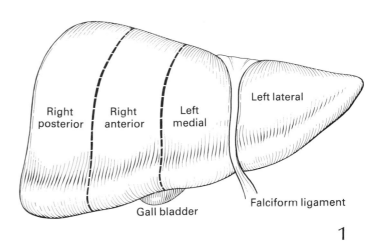

1

## Preoperative evaluation and preparation

Diagnostic evaluation should define tumour resectability and, in the case of malignancy, should exclude non-hepatic metastases. Computerized axial tomography is the most accurate non-invasive diagnostic technique. The hepatic vascular structures, however, can only be delineated by selective arteriography, which will also define the vascular characteristics of the tumour. Arteriography carries the risk of damage to the hepatic artery and is often not done. Ultrasonography is useful in evaluating vena caval integrity.

The most important preoperative serological test is the clotting profile (partial thromboplastin time, prothrombin time, bleeding time). Alphafetoprotein serological determinations in tumour patients are helpful in evaluating residual tumour activity after resection.

Perioperative broad-spectrum antibiotics are administered. A central venous and two large-bore peripheral intravenous catheters are placed in the upper extremities. An arterial catheter may also be useful, particularly in the case of trisegmentectomy. A urinary catheter is left indwelling.

## General principles of intraoperative management

Because of the wide costal angle, shallow abdominal cavity, and relative elasticity of the thoracic wall, a wide bilateral subcostal (chevron) incision of the upper abdomen is usually sufficient in children. In all major resections the xiphoid is excised. Extensions into the chest are optional but rarely necessary. Unless the thorax is open, deep anaesthesia to avoid spontaneous respiratory efforts is mandatory during the cleavage phase of hepatic resection to prevent air embolism. During operation, adequate blood flow to the part of the liver to be retained must be assured. Otherwise, activation and release of fibrinolysins occurs, resulting in a haemorrhagic diathesis. Haemodynamic monitoring must be frequent; twisting of the inferior vena cava and impairment of blood return to the heart often occurs during hepatic mobilization. Blood loss should be replaced immediately, and since banked blood does not contain several clotting factors (V and VIII) fresh frozen plasma should be given periodically if blood loss is heavy.

Except for wedge resection, the first step of liver resection is division of the suspensory ligaments to the lobe or segment to be resected, and identification of the hepatic vein. The second step is the isolation and division of the portal hilar structures, first the hepatic artery, next the portal vein and third the bile duct. An ischaemic (cyanotic) line of demarcation appears along the parenchyma, which is followed during the subsequent hepatic cleavage. The hepatic vein is isolated, clamped, divided, and the venous stumps oversewn using vascular suture. In some cases the hepatic veins cannot be safely dissected, either because of tumour proximity or because of diaphragmatic involvement (which will require resection in continuity). In this situation, extrahepatic division of the hepatic vein should be abandoned and the vein ligated during the cleavage phase of the resection.

The major intersegmental venous drainage is used as a guide during the hepatic cleavage, and is spared. No devitalized tissue is left with the residual liver nor is the raw area covered with omentum or other tissue. Meticulous haemostasis of residual small vessels and ducts is accomplished with fine suture ligature. Adequate drainage of the residual dead space is essential.

# The operations

### RIGHT HEPATIC LOBECTOMY

The right triangular and coronary ligaments are taken down, the bare area is entered and the right hepatic vein identified. The right lobe may be elevated into the wound and retracted towards the left to determine resectability. The falciform ligament is preserved. A cholecystectomy is performed. The right hepatic artery is sacrificed. The right branch of the portal vein is divided either from an anterior approach or, if tumour interferes, by retracting the right lobe of the liver and dividing the right portal vein posteriorly. After dividing the artery and the portal vein, a line of demarcation occurs between the true right and left lobes, extending from the gall-bladder to the vena cava. The right hepatic duct is ligated and divided.

After division of the portal structures the right hepatic vein is dissected. Exposure is improved by retracting the right lobe into the wound. The vein is clamped with paediatric vascular clamps, divided, and closed with a vascular suture. Several small hepatic veins entering the retrohepatic inferior vena cava are ligated.

The liver is divided along the line of colour demarcation. We prefer division by the finger-fracture method, individually ligating major structures as they are encountered. Much of the middle hepatic vein can be preserved and used as a guide during cleavage. Haemorrhage is controlled by compression of the hepatic lobes by the surgeon's and assistant's hands.

After removal of the specimen residual bleeding vessels and duct structures are identified and oversewn. Large intersegmental veins are preserved. The right subphrenic dead space is drained by leaving the mid-portion of the wound open. Five or six soft rubber drains are brought out through the wound.

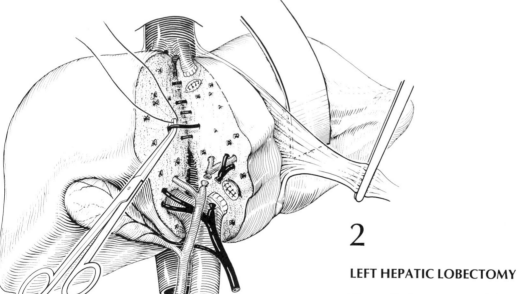

2

2

### LEFT HEPATIC LOBECTOMY

The preliminary steps in left lobectomy are a mirror image of those described for right lobectomy. That is, division of the left triangular ligament and exposure of the left hepatic vein. Unlike right lobectomy, however, the falciform ligament is taken down (to aid in the exposure of the hepatic vein). Cholecystectomy is performed and the left lobe is devascularized by division of the left hepatic artery, left portal vein, and left hepatic duct. The left hepatic vein is divided and oversewn. If all the caudate lobe is to be removed a number of small venous tributaries draining into the retrohepatic vena cava must be individually ligated and divided. Exposure of this rather difficult phase of the resection is helped by retracting the left lobe out of the wound and to the right. Hepatic cleavage is to the left of the middle hepatic vein. Again, meticulous haemostasis of the raw surface and adequate drainage are essential.

## 3

### RIGHT TRISEGMENTECTOMY

The early steps in right trisegmentectomy are identical to those of right lobectomy. After completing the hilar division of the right vascular and duct structures, dissection of the trinity structures to the medial segment of the left lobe is begun. The left portal vein, left hepatic artery and left hepatic duct are dissected from the medial segment by following their course along the segment's undersurface. Individual branches to the liver substance are ligated and divided. Usually one or two fair-sized posteriorly directed vessels enter the caudate lobe and are spared (unless the caudate lobe is also to be removed). The mobilization is stopped just short of the umbilical fissure.

The majority of the vascular and duct structures to the medial segment originate in the umbilical fissure. Dissection is done just to the right of the fissure, however, in order to protect the residual trinity structures to the left lateral segment. Again, we prefer splitting the liver by finger fracture and individually ligating the vascular and duct structures running into the medial segment. Quite early in this cleavage phase the medial segment becomes ischaemic and provides an excellent guide to follow as the liver is split towards the diaphragm. Later, the middle hepatic vein is encountered and ligated. Haemorrhage is controlled during the resection by hepatic compression with the surgeon's and assistant's hands. The entire right lobe and left medial segment are removed in continuity and the massive dead space is completely drained.

Division of the main right hilar and triad structures to the medial segment of the left lobe is completed. The right and middle hepatic veins have been divided and oversewn. The resection line followed the right side of the falciform ligament to the vena cava. In this case the caudate segment was removed.

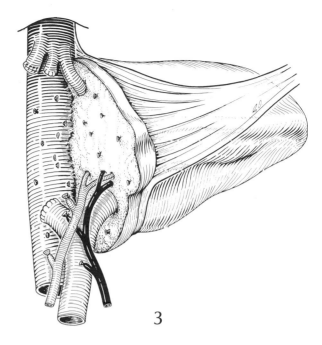

3

## 4

### LEFT TRISEGMENTECTOMY

The falciform ligament is divided and the suprahepatic bare area is entered to expose the main hepatic veins and suprahepatic inferior vena cava. The left triangular ligament is incised, thus fully exposing the left hepatic vein. The left hepatic artery, left portal vein, and left hepatic duct are divided, but the first posteriorly directed branches are spared unless the caudate lobe is to be taken. The left hepatic vein is transected and closed with a vascular suture. If accessible, the middle hepatic vein is also divided. If not, the middle hepatic vein is divided during hepatic cleavage.

Cleavage of the hepatic parenchyma is started along a plane which runs roughly along a line beginning at the left hepatic vein and continuing to the obliterated ductus venosus, the liver hilus, the base of the gall-bladder and the midpoint between the gallbladder and the right lateral extremity of the liver. Often in children a natural groove in this area identifies the separation of the anterior and posterior segments. Superiorly, the dissection is begun at the coronary ligament, just in front of the right hepatic vein. These two planes of dissection are deepened and brought towards each other, ligating all anteriorly directed structures and preserving those running posteriorly. If properly developed, the plane separates the anterior and posterior segments of the right lobe. The entire left lobe and anterior segment of the right lobe are removed in continuity.

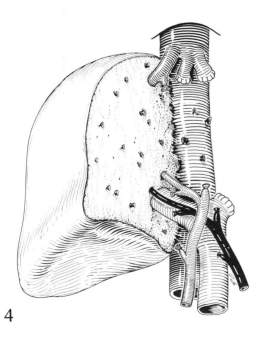

4

## LEFT LATERAL SEGMENTECTOMY

The left triangular ligament is divided, exposing the left hepatic vein. The liver is split just to the left of the umbilical fissure. Again, early in the resection the lateral segment becomes cyanotic, permitting a clear guide to the subsequent excision. The left hepatic vein is identified during hepatic cleavage and divided. Frequently the middle hepatic vein joins the left vein and should be spared by ligation of the left hepatic vein proximal to its junction with the middle hepatic vein.

The left lateral segment may receive its entire arterial supply from an aberrant branch of the left gastric artery. This malformation simplifies the operation as the artery can be sacrificed (after temporary occlusion) early in the operation.

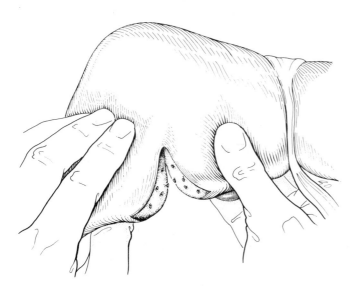

# 5

## WEDGE EXCISION

This operation is reserved for lesions less than 3 cm in diameter which are located near the periphery of the organ. We prefer not to use mattress sutures or other types of infarcting sutures. The liver on either side of the lesion is compressed by the surgeon's and assistant's hands and the lesion sharply excised. Haemorrhage is brisk afterwards and is controlled by individual suture ligation of major arterial, venous, and duct structures. Minor residual bleeding is dealt with by electrocoagulation. The margins of the defect are not reapproximated. Employment of the ultrasonic scalpel for wedge excision reduces blood loss strikingly.

# Postoperative care

Parenteral antibiotics (begun immediately preoperatively) are discontinued after 5 days unless a specific infection exists. Drains are advanced after their effluent ceases. Further advancement is postponed if drainage resumes. In cases of trisegmentectomy the residual dead space may be irrigated with topical antibiotic solutions after drain removal. Serum glucose levels are monitored frequently during the first 24 hours and 10 per cent glucose intravenous solutions are given if levels are low. Albumin and clotting factor synthesis may be diminished during the first 10 postoperative days, and require supplementation. Diet by mouth can usually be started 2–3 days after operation. In the case of malignancy, chemotherapy is initiated as soon as recovery from operation is assured.

# Complications

Subphrenic abscess is not an unusual complication after major liver resection, and particularly after right hepatectomies, unless perfect drainage is provided. Fever is frequently the first indication of the complication. Treatment is best provided by reopening a portion of the wound.

Biliary fistula occurs in many patients but is generally self-limited. Most fistulae close within 10 days, although in one of our patients having trisegmentectomy bile drainage persisted for 52 days before ceasing spontaneously.

After trisegmentectomy most patients become mildly jaundiced for 5 to 10 days. Serum hepatic enzyme levels may be transiently elevated. These biochemical aberrations are a consequence of the massive resection and the small volume of remaining liver. Fortunately, the residual hepatic segment has commonly already undergone hypertrophy due to the slow tumour growth and this,

taken in conjunction with its rapid growth after resection (complete liver regeneration occurs in 2–3 months), accounts for the limited duration of these biochemical aberrations.

Delayed haemorrhage is an unusual complication after liver resection. Mechanical factors may, of course, be responsible, but often haemorrhage is a consequence of intraoperative ischaemia of the residual liver and subsequent fibrinolytic activation.

Prolonged fever, especially in younger children, may occur. The aetiology of this complication is not clear but may be related to transient impairment of the reticuloendothelial function of the residual liver. Coincidentally, increased splenic activity is often noticed in early post-resection radioisotope imaging.

# Results

Contemporary operative mortality for major liver resection should be 5 per cent or less. Morbidity is still significant, approaching 30 per cent in most series. In children with hepatic malignancy and tumour-free resection margins, recent postoperative chemotherapy protocols have more than doubled the short-term survival (25 per cent, historical; 55–70 per cent, current). Since hepatic malignant recurrence may occur 5–10 years after resection, these survival figures must be considered tentative. Chemotherapy also appears to improve the otherwise hopeless prognosis in children with microscopic tumours at the resection margins. Currently, gross residual tumour is incompatible with survival.

The role of preoperative chemotherapy is controversial. A number of publications have noted shrinkage of otherwise 'inoperable' tumours to a point permitting subsequent curative resection. We have observed one patient, in whom extrahepatic metastases became evident during 'preoperative' chemotherapy.

Illustrations by Philip Wilson

# Wilms' tumour – Nephrectomy for renal tumours in children

**Patrick G. Duffy** FRCS(I)
Consultant Urological Surgeon, Hospital for Sick Children, Great Ormond Street;
Senior Lecturer in Paediatric Urology, Institute of Urology, University of London, London, UK

**Philip G. Ransley** FRCS
Consultant Urological Surgeon, Hospital for Sick Children, Great Ormond Street;
Senior Lecturer in Paediatric Urology, Institute of Urology and Institute of Child Health, University of London, London, UK

## Introduction

Nephroblastoma (Wilms' tumour) is the commonest solid malignancy arising in the urinary tract in children. It is an embryonal tumour presenting most usually between the ages of 6 months and 5 years, with a peak at 3 years. Approximately 6 per cent of cases have bilateral tumours. The most common presentation is a painless abdominal mass in an otherwise well child.

## Investigations

Initial investigations include a plain X-ray of the abdomen, ultrasound examination, and intravenous pyelography. An intravenous urogram will show the classical appearances of a space-occupying lesion within the kidney. However, 10 per cent of Wilms' tumours are associated with non-functional kidneys on urography. Ultrasound has the advantage of determining the presence of a solid tumour, and of any extension into the inferior vena cava.

Initial imaging must include demonstration of the contralateral kidney. A chest X-ray is necessary to demonstrate metastases. CT scanning is now widely used for the more sensitive detection of lung secondaries, and may be helpful in assessment of the abdominal tumour or liver metastases.

The principal differential diagnoses to be considered are neuroblastoma, hepatoblastoma, soft-tissue sarcomas, and retroperitoneal teratoma.

Radical nephrectomy is the primary treatment for unilateral Wilms' tumour. The presence of secondary deposits, caval tumour, bilateral disease, or a tumour in a solitary kidney are indications for initial biopsy and chemotherapy, followed by delayed nephrectomy. Bilateral tumours will require open surgical biopsy and complete assessment by full laparotomy.

## The operation

### 1

A generous transverse upper abdominal incision is required to facilitate complete exposure of both kidneys.

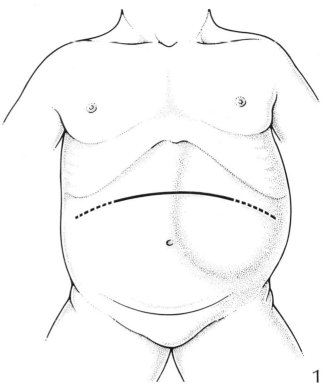

1

### 2

The anterior rectus sheath is incised with diathermy.

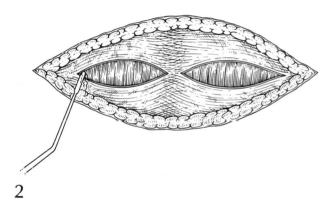

2

### 3a, b

Both rectus muscles are completely divided. The falciform ligament is divided between ligatures.

The peritoneum is entered with care to avoid breaching the anterior surface of the tumour, and the incision is extended laterally under direct vision.

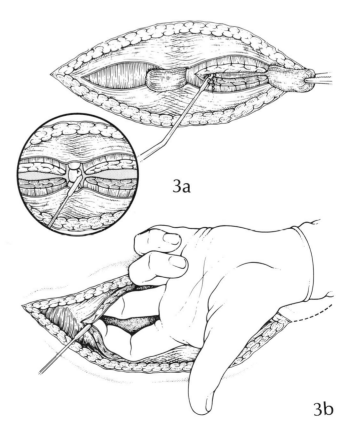

3a

3b

## 4

The abdominal contents are carefully examined for liver and peritoneal secondaries.

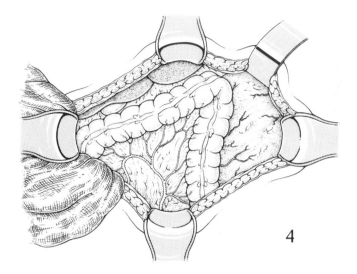

4

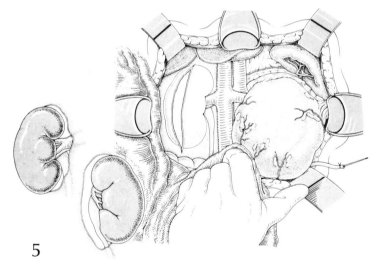

5

## 5

The contralateral kidney is fully mobilized and examined on both anterior and posterior surfaces in order to detect previously unsuspected bilateral disease. Biopsy only from the main tumour and the contralateral lesion is performed under these circumstances.

## 6

The mesocolon is dissected from the anterior surface of the tumour. The ureter and gonadal vessels are ligated at this stage.

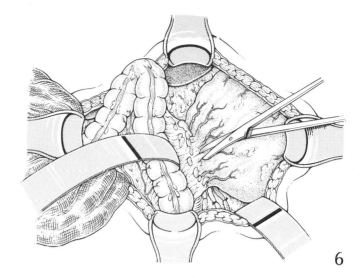

**6**

## 7

A plane is developed posteriorly adjacent to the great vessels by gently inserting a finger into the paravertebral space. The tumour itself is not mobilized at this stage.

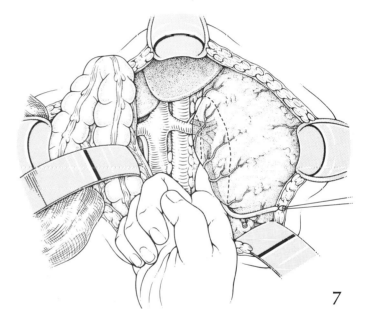

**7**

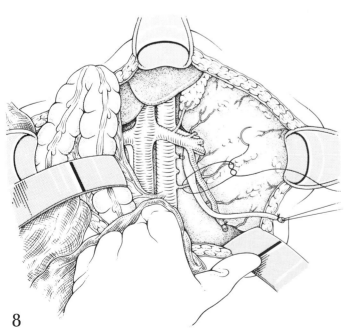

**8**

## 8

Dissection begins caudally, sweeping adventitial tissue and lymph nodes laterally off the great vessels. The renal vein and its branches are gently exposed. Careful palpation of the vein is performed to detect a venous extension of tumour, which demands early ligation of the renal vein. On the right side the second part of the duodenum is encountered during this dissection.

## 9

The renal vein is gently mobilized and elevated by a vascular sling to expose the renal artery. Both vessels are ligated and divided.

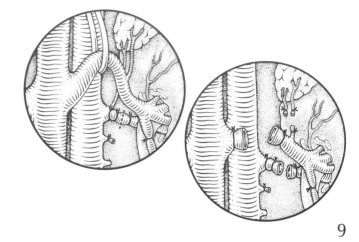

9

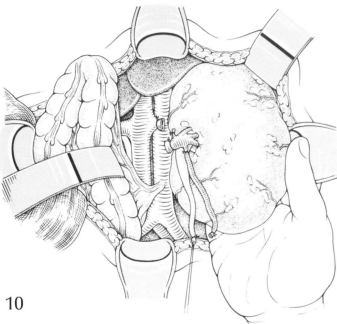

10

## 10

The kidney is partially mobilized by blunt dissection posteriorly.

## 11

Superior dissection is hazardous on the left side, and damage to the spleen and tail of the pancreas must be avoided. The adrenal gland is removed if the tumour is in the upper pole of the kidney.

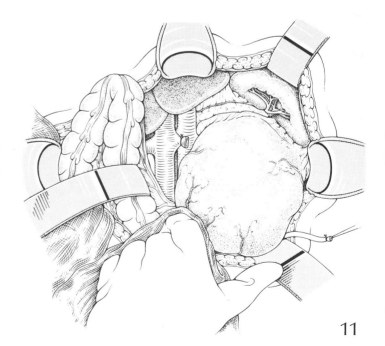

11

# 12

The kidney within Gerota's fascia is lifted out of the abdomen and the posterior dissection is completed under direct vision.

Following removal of the tumour, the renal bed is inspected. Any remaining lymph nodes on the great vessels are removed.

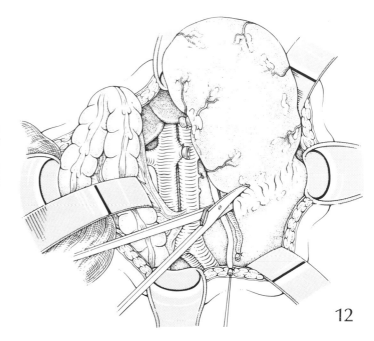

12

# Postoperative management

## UNILATERAL DISEASE

Following nephrectomy, chemotherapy plays an integral part in the management of unilateral Wilms' tumour. Intravenous chemotherapy is commenced within 24 hours of operation. Subsequent adjuvant therapy in the form of radiotherapy and/or chemotherapy will be determined by the pathological stage and tumour type (favourable or unfavourable histology).

## BILATERAL DISEASE

The finding of bilateral disease usually dictates biopsy only and closure of the abdomen. Subsequent surgical management following chemotherapy requires repeat detailed imaging and may include consideration of partial nephrectomy, or bilateral nephrectomy with dialysis and subsequent renal transplantation. Such decisions are complex and require a team approach.

## CONCLUSION

The management of Wilms' tumour consists of surgery with chemotherapy. Chemotherapy has played a major role in decreasing mortality and morbidity in these children. The surgeon should not embark on the management of Wilms' tumour without the aid of a paediatric oncology service.

## Further reading

D'Angio, G. J., Beckwith, J. B., Breslow, N. E., Bishop, H. C., Evans, A. E., Farewell, V. et al (1980) Wilm's tumour: an update. Cancer, 45, 1791–1798

D'Angio, G. J., Evans, A. E., Breslow, N. E., Baum, E., Beckwith, J. B., de Lorimer, A. et al (1982) Management of children with Wilm's Tumour: defining the risk-benefit ratio. Frontiers of Radiation Therapy and Oncology, 16, 30–39 Karger, Basel

Illustrations by John E. Nixon

# Operations for neuroblastoma

**Jay L. Grosfeld** MD
Professor and Chairman, Department of Surgery, Indiana University School of Medicine; Surgeon-in-Chief, James Whitcomb Riley Hospital for Children, Indianapolis, Indiana, USA

Neuroblastoma is the commonest solid tumour of infancy and childhood. This neoplasm is of neural crest origin and can arise from anywhere along the sympathetic nervous chain as well as the adrenal medulla. The vast majority (more than 50 per cent) of tumours arise in the retroperitoneum as a primary adrenal lesion or from paraspinal ganglia. The posterior mediastinum is the site of origin in 20 per cent of cases, while cervical and pelvic tumours are less common.

The best chance for cure in patients with localized neuroblastoma is complete surgical excision of the primary tumour. Unlike other embryonal neoplasms, such as Wilms' tumour, neuroblastoma is not cured by chemotherapy so that expeditious and appropriately performed surgery is critical for a successful outcome.

## Preoperative

The patient should be adequately monitored by electrocardiography, Doppler pulse recording, and measurements of pH, blood gases and blood pressure via an arterial line. Blood pressure must also be carefully monitored during operation to detect any excessive catecholamine release from the tumour. Appropriate large-bore intravenous catheters are placed in the upper extremities. Adequate intravenous support is important, as these neurogenic tumours are quite vascular and blood loss can be excessive. As the neuroblastoma often surrounds the great vessels, an adequate supply of cross-matched blood should be available for the procedure.

# The operations

## MEDIASTINAL NEUROBLASTOMA

Neuroblastoma may arise as a posterior mediastinal tumour and is then best approached by a thoracotomy. Following endotracheal intubation, general anaesthesia is administered. The chest is prepared with iodophor skin solution and draped for a standard posterolateral thoracotomy incision.

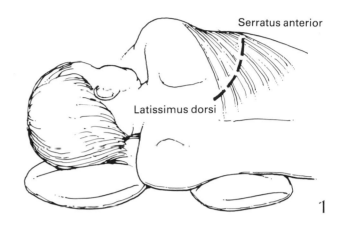

## The incision

# 1 & 2

The patient is placed on his side, affected side uppermost, with a towel under the opposite axilla to allow some expansion of the lowermost lung during the operation. The incision is made below the tip of the scapula. Bleeding points are coagulated. The latissimus dorsi muscle is identified and divided with cautery. The auscultatory space is noted and the fourth interspace identified. The serratus anterior muscle is divided over this interspace and the interspace is entered just above the fifth rib by dividing the external and internal intercostal muscles. An appropriately sized chest spreader (Finochietto) is inserted over chest pads placed on the rib edge.

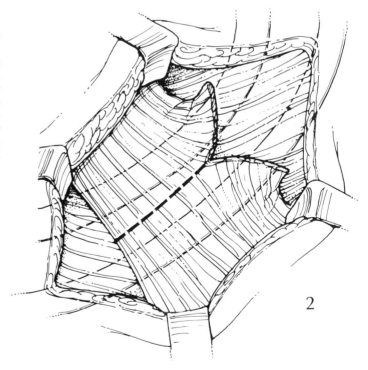

# 3

The lung is retracted medially to reveal the tumour (in this case a large retropleural neuroblastoma). The posterior pleura and the endothoracic fascia around the tumour are opened to allow the surgeon to enter an appropriate dissection plane. The azygos vein is seen coursing over the tumour, which arises from the sympathetic chain.

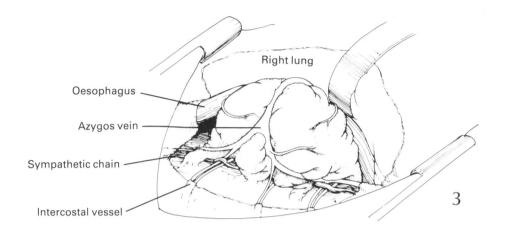

# 4

The azygos vein is divided between 3/0 silk ties. The medial aspect of the tumour is carefully dissected free from the oesophagus, taking care to preserve the vagus nerve. The tumour is mobilized from the paraspinal structures and the rib edges by both sharp and blunt dissection. Great care is exercised to identify and ligate or clip specific intercostal vessels feeding and draining the tumour. The tumour may be attached to a number of sympathetic ganglia and intercostal nerves, and often extends into one or more intervertebral foramina. These extensions are divided between titanium clips which can later be used as markers for possible radiation therapy.

Following excision, the chest is closed in the usual manner. A 24–26 Fr Silastic chest tube is inserted through a stab wound below the incision and placed in the posterior sulcus. We use interrupted 0 Vicryl paracostal sutures to approximate the ribs and running 3/0 Prolene to approximate the divided serratus anterior muscle. It is helpful to have the anaesthetist push the right arm and shoulder caudad to relieve any tension during closure. The latissimus dorsi muscle is reapproximated with a running 3/0 Prolene suture. The subcutaneous fascia is closed with a running 4/0 white Vicryl suture and the skin with a running subcuticular suture of 4/0 white Vicryl. The skin edges are reinforced with Steri-Strips over Mastisol adhesive. Dry sterile dressings are applied. The chest tube is attached to an underwater drainage system with 15 cmH$_2$0 of negative pressure.

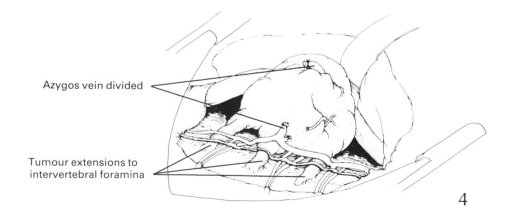

## ABDOMINAL NEUROBLASTOMA

### The incisions

# 5a, b & c

Preoperative preparation of the patient is similar to that for mediastinal tumour excision. The chest and abdomen should be prepared and draped. A variety of abdominal incisions may be used for adrenal neuroblastoma, including a generous chevron-type incision with bilateral subcostal extensions (a) and a supraumbilical transverse incision (b). For extremely large adrenal tumours that significantly elevate the diaphragm or extend into the mediastinum, a thoracoabdominal incision may be useful. (c).

A rolled sheet under the upper lumbar spine pushes up the retroperitoneal structures anteriorly.

A generous transperitoneal incision should be made extending from the midaxillary line on the side of the tumour to the contralateral anterior axillary line. The subcutaneous tissue and Scarpa's fascia are divided with fine-tip electrocautery. The rectus abdominis muscle is divided on both sides of the midline. Bleeding points are controlled with electrocautery. The umbilical vein and epigastric vessels are identified, doubly ligated with 3/0 silk ties and divided. The external and internal oblique fascia and muscles are divided and bleeding points controlled with the electrocoagulator. The transversus abdominis muscle and peritoneum are opened in continuity with the posterior rectus sheath medially on both sides. Once the peritoneum is entered, the liver is examined for possible metastases.

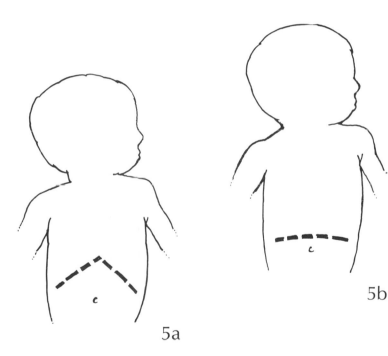

5a

5b

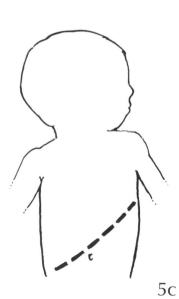

5c

## Neuroblastoma of right adrenal gland

# 6

A large neuroblastoma involving the right adrenal gland is shown. The left adrenal gland is normal. Note the relationship to the aorta, vena cava and adrenal vessels.

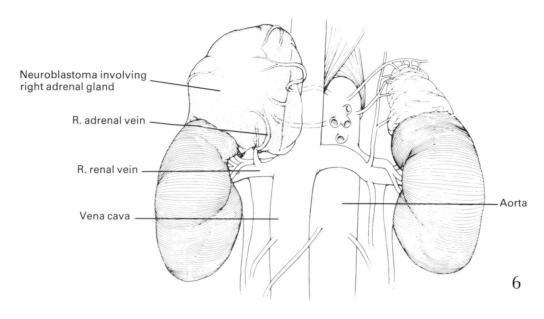

Neuroblastoma involving right adrenal gland

R. adrenal vein

R. renal vein

Vena cava

Aorta

6

# 7

Exposure of the right adrenal is more difficult than that on the left. The hepatic flexure of the colon is retracted medially and inferiorly and the colonic attachments are divided by sharp dissection. A Kocher manoeuvre is performed to elevate the duodenum and mobilize it medially. The liver is retracted superiorly and anteriorly. Division of the lateral hepatic ligaments may improve exposure. Care should be taken to preserve the small hepatic veins that directly enter the vena cava.

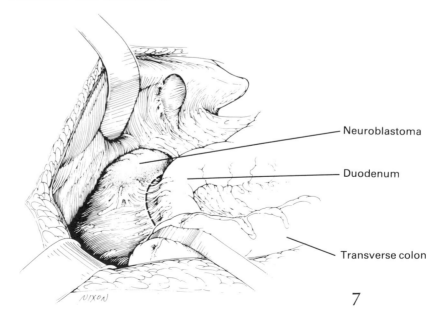

Neuroblastoma

Duodenum

Transverse colon

7

# 8

Once the inferior vena cava has been visualized and the adrenal neuroblastoma identified above the upper pole of the right kidney, Gerota's fascia is opened. Although this illustration shows the right adrenal artery and vein arising from and draining into the right renal vessels, this is frequently not the case. More often the right adrenal vein is a short, stubby vessel that enters the inferior vena cava directly. Care should be taken to isolate this vessel, which is then doubly ligated with 3/0 silk ties and divided.

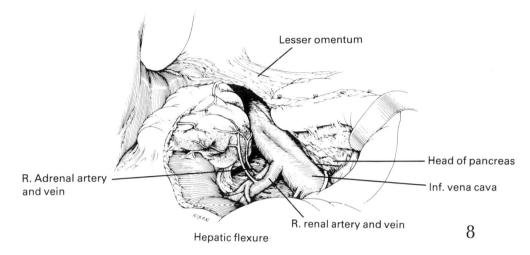

Lesser omentum

R. Adrenal artery and vein

Head of pancreas

Inf. vena cava

R. renal artery and vein

Hepatic flexure

8

# 9

Gerota's fascia completely envelopes the adrenal gland and separates the adrenal from the kidney. This often allows preservation of the ipsilateral kidney. In some cases, however, the tumour invades the kidney and concomitant nephrectomy is then required to ensure adequate tumour removal. The adrenal gland may be nourished by many small arteries, which usually divide before entering the gland. The inferior, middle and superior adrenal arteries should be carefully identified, doubly ligated with 3/0 silk and divided. The right superior adrenal vein and artery are branches of the inferior phrenic artery and vein. Once these vessels have been ligated, the tumour can be mobilized laterally. The crus of the diaphragm is the upper extent of the dissection. Resection of the tumour is completed by carefully dissecting the lesion off the renal capsule. Lymphatic drainage of the right adrenal gland is to the lymph nodes in the right renal hilum and to right para-aortic lymph nodes.

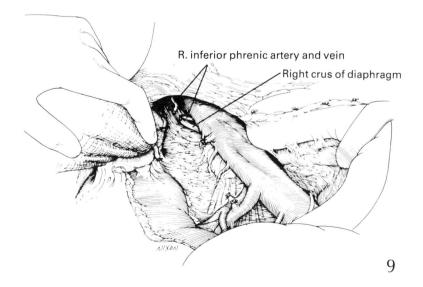

R. inferior phrenic artery and vein

Right crus of diaphragm

9

## Neuroblastoma of left adrenal gland

# 10

A large tumour involving the left adrenal gland is shown.
The right adrenal gland is normal.

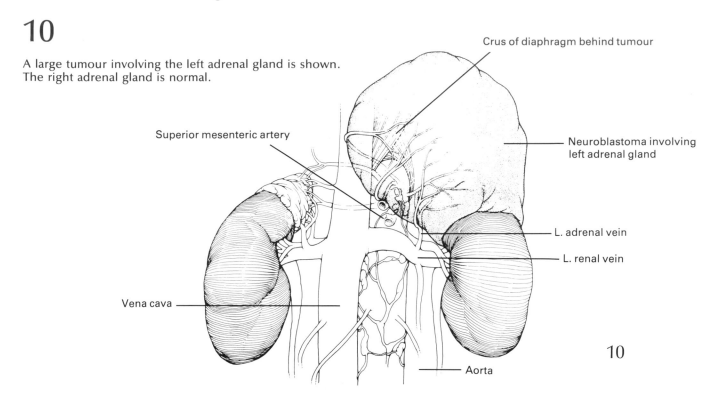

Crus of diaphragm behind tumour

Superior mesenteric artery

Neuroblastoma involving
left adrenal gland

L. adrenal vein

L. renal vein

Vena cava

Aorta

10

# 11

Exposure of the left adrenal gland is facilitated by division
of the splenocolic and splenorenal attachments, thus
allowing entry into the retroperitoneal space.

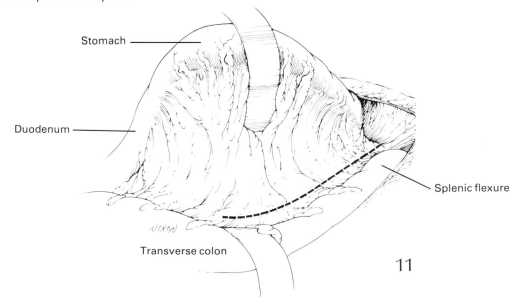

Stomach

Duodenum

Splenic flexure

Transverse colon

11

# 12

The pancreas and spleen are carefully mobilized by dividing the peritoneal attachments, and then elevated upwards and medially. Gentle retraction is important to prevent trauma to these organs. The splenic flexure of the colon is then retracted inferiorly, exposing the kidney and left adrenal tumour. The left renal vein is identified and traced medially to the entry of the left adrenal vein. Gentle downward traction on the kidney improves exposure. The left adrenal vein is doubly ligated in continuity with 3/0 silk

ties and divided. Attention is then turned to the multiple adrenal arteries that are often present. The inferior adrenal artery arises from the left renal artery, the middle adrenal artery arises directly from the aorta, while the superior adrenal artery is a branch of the inferior phrenic artery or occasionally a direct branch from the aorta. These vessels should be carefully doubly ligated or occluded with titanium clips and then divided.

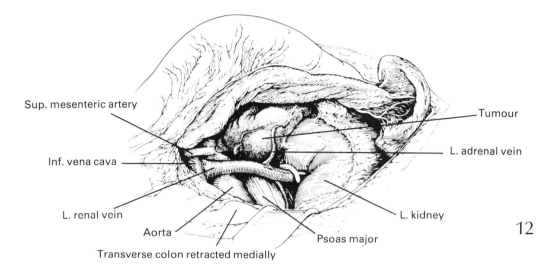

**12**

# 13

Careful dissection of the superior adrenal attachments should continue on the undersurface of the diaphragm near the oesophageal hiatus. An accessory adrenal vein draining into the inferior phrenic vein is sometimes encountered. With most of the vessels ligated, the tumour can now be retracted laterally. During the medial portion of the dissection, care must be taken to expose the

superior mesenteric artery and coeliac axis and to avoid injury to these vital structures. Although not shown in these illustrations, neuroblastoma frequently envelopes the aorta and vena cava, and meticulous dissection is required to avoid accidental entry into these vessels, with consequent life-threatening haemorrhage.

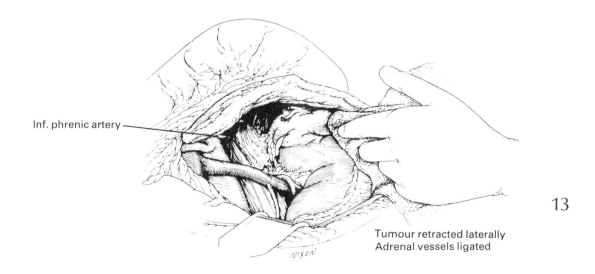

Tumour retracted laterally
Adrenal vessels ligated

**13**

## 14

Once the tumour has been completely removed, the close proximity of the diaphragmatic crura, coeliac axis and superior mesenteric artery becomes apparent.

Lymphatic drainage of the left adrenal gland is to the left renal hilar lymph nodes, para-aortic lymph nodes and through the hiatus of the oesophagus into the inferior mediastinal area. Any suspicious lymph nodes should be excised as lymph node involvement may adversely affect prognosis.

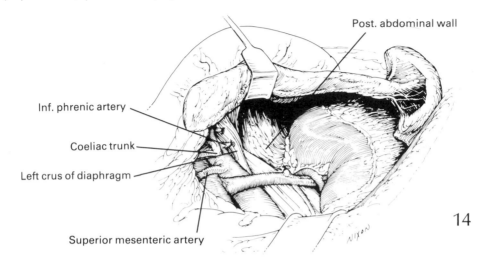

Post. abdominal wall

Inf. phrenic artery

Coeliac trunk

Left crus of diaphragm

Superior mesenteric artery

14

## Paraspinal neuroblastoma

## 15

Paraspinal neuroblastoma may extend into the pelvis, as in this illustration of a left paraspinal neuroblastoma arising from para-aortic sympathetic nervous tissue. Both left and right adrenal glands are normal. The lesion is inferior to the lower pole of the kidney and envelopes the distal aorta and iliac vessels. The ureter passes over the tumour.

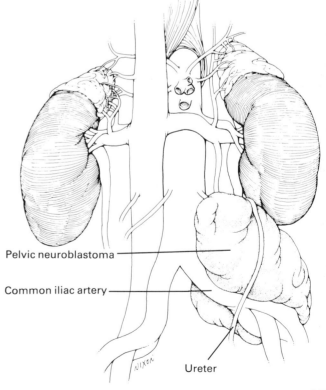

Pelvic neuroblastoma

Common iliac artery

Ureter

15

# 16

The tumour is carefully mobilized and the aorta retracted medially. The ureter is identified and lifted off the lesion. Lumbar vessels must be identified and occluded with ligatures or titanium clips (not shown here). Tumour extending into intervertebral foramina may signify a 'dumb-bell' extension into the extradural space. Careful neurological assessment by CT scanning with myelographic contrast may be useful. Such extensions frequently cannot be excised. Residual tumour and the margins of the resection should be marked with titanium clips to guide radiotherapy. Titanium clips do not result in a scatter effect on subsequent CT scans, as happens with stainless steel or other silver clips.

In some cases resection of the neuroblastoma is not possible and biopsy alone may then be performed to ascertain the diagnosis. This is followed by multimodal chemotherapy, which often shrinks the tumour and allows a later attempt at resection at 'second look' laparotomy. The patient's condition should not be jeopardized by an overzealous surgical approach. *En bloc* contiguous resection of surrounding structures such as spleen, stomach, pancreas, colon, etc. is not recommended.

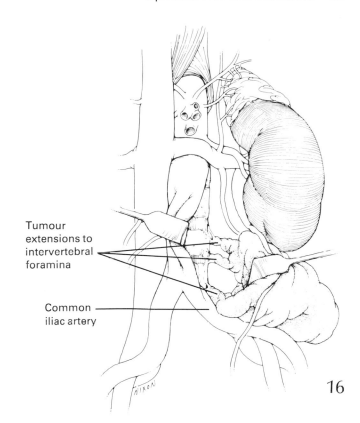

Tumour extensions to intervertebral foramina

Common iliac artery

16

## Abdominal closure

Following tumour resection, the bowel is replaced within the peritoneal cavity in gentle folds and the abdomen closed in layers. The peritoneum, transversus abdominis and posterior rectus sheath are closed together, using a continuous suture of 3/0 polypropylene (2/0 in older children). The oblique fascias (internal and external) are also closed independently by a continuous suture of 3/0 polypropylene. The anterior rectus sheath on both sides is closed with interrupted 3/0 polypropylene sutures, inverting the knot beneath the fascia. Scarpa's fascia is approximated with a running 4/0 white Vicryl suture and the skin with a running subcuticular suture of 4/0 white Vicryl. The skin edges are secured with Steri-Strips over Mastisol adhesive. A dry sterile dressing is applied.

A nasogastric tube is left in place until bowel function resumes. Parenteral nutrition is instituted by a peripheral route if no other therapy is planned. If multimodal treatment with irradiation and chemotherapy is required, a centrally placed Hickman or Broviac catheter is inserted for total parenteral nutrition during the intensive induction phase of anticancer treatment. The patient may also try feeding by mouth but, as cancer treatment frequently causes loss of appetite, protein calorie malnutrition will result if parenteral support is not given.

## Further reading

Grosfeld, J. L. (1986) Neuroblastoma. In: Pediatric Surgery, 4th edn, K. J. Welch, J. G. Randolph, M. M. Ravich, J. A. O'Neill and M. I. Rowe (eds.), pp. 283–293. Chicago: Year Book Medical Publishers

Grosfeld, J. L., West, K. W., Weber, T. R. (1984) The role of second-look procedures in the management of retroperitoneal tumors in children. American Journal of Pediatric Hematology and Oncology, 6, 441–447

McGuire, W. A., Simmons, D., Grosfeld, J. L., Baehner, R. L. (1985) Stage II neuroblastoma – does adjuvant irradiation contribute to cure? Medical and Pediatric Oncology, 13, 117–121

Grosfeld, J. L. (1986) Neuroblastoma in infancy and childhood. In: Pediatric Surgical Oncology, D. M. Hays (ed.), pp. 63–85. Orlando, Florida: Grune and Stratton

Nickerson, H. J. Nesbit, M. E., Grosfeld, J. L., Baehner, R. L., Sather, H., Hammond, N. (1985) Comparison of stage IV and IVDS neuroblastoma in the first year of life. Medical and Pediatric Oncology, 13, 261–268

Rickard, K., Loghmani, E., Grosfeld, J. L., Lingard, C. D., White, N. M., Foland, B. B. et al. (1985) Short and long term effectiveness of enteral and parenteral nutrition in reversing or preventing protein-energy malnutrition in advanced neuroblastoma. A prospective randomised study. Cancer, 56, 2881–2897

Illustrations by Gillian Oliver

# Operation for hyperinsulinism in infancy

**M. Carcassonne**
Professor of Paediatric Surgery; Surgeon-in-Chief, Department of Paediatric Surgery, School of Medicine of Marseille, Marseille, France
**A. Delarue**
Senior Registrar, Department of Paediatric Surgery, School of Medicine of Marseille, Marseille, France

## Description and indications

A wide range of pancreatic organic lesions (diffuse nesidioblastosis, focal adenomatosis, adenoma) are likely to produce hyperinsulinism in infancy. They are collectively known as the islet-cell dysmaturation syndrome. An elevated blood insulin:glucose ratio is generally diagnostic. No current investigation is capable of differentiating diffuse from localized lesions. In infants over 3 months lesions are always diffuse; earlier than 3 months they are diffuse in 70 per cent of cases, but associated or isolated adenomas may be encountered.

Both preoperative arteriography and transhepatic portal catheterization are much too hazardous to be considered in infancy.

As soon as the diagnosis of hyperinsulinism is established, medical treatment should be started to control the hypoglycaemia and prevent permanent brain damage. This treatment consists of hypertonic glucose infusion, and diazoxide to a maximum of 20 mg/kg body-weight per day. If intensive medical treatment fails to correct the hypoglycaemia, or complications of the therapy arise, surgery is indicated.

Before performing any type of pancreatic resection, an extensive exploration of the pancreas is recommended, including macroscopic, microscopic, and biological control.

## Preoperative

### Anaesthesia

A glucose supply through a central venous line is necessary. The use of a computerized extracorporeal monitor (artificial pancreas) can ensure protection against acute hypoglycaemia during the perioperative period.

# The operation

## Position of patient and incision

The infant is placed supine with a roll under his back. A supraumbilical transverse incision provides easy access.

# 1

## Exposure of anterior pancreas

Division of the gastrocolic peritoneum brings into view the body and tail of the pancreas. Gastroepiploic and short gastric vessels are preserved. Ligation of the right colic and gastroepiploic veins allows mobilization of the hepatic flexure of the colon.

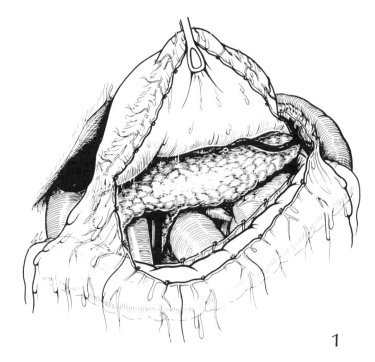

1

# 2

## Exposure of head of pancreas

The peritoneal reflexion is incised along the right side of the duodenum. The Kocher manoeuvre mobilizes both duodenum and the head of the pancreas medially from the vena cava to the right side of the aorta. Gentle blunt dissection is used.

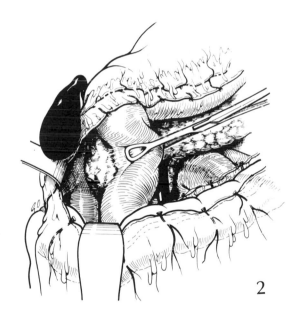

2

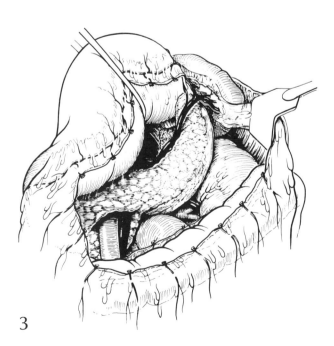

3

## Exposure of tail of pancreas

# 3

Scissor division of the attachments of the spleen to the diaphragm permits medial mobilization of the spleen and tail of the pancreas, separating them from the underlying retroperitoneal structures. This manoeuvre, first described by Allison, mobilizes the pancreas to the right as far as the aorta.

## 4

Once the pancreas is fully exposed it is inspected and palpated. Immediate portal insulin determination is advisable, using radioimmunoassay. In neonates, portal puncture with a fine needle is preferred to extensive catheterization through the splenic vein, in order to avoid portal thrombosis.

Selective resection (adenectomy or distal pancreatectomy) will be undertaken only if a single pure adenoma (nesidioblastoma) has been demonstrated. But after enucleation has been performed, a large biopsy of the tail should be added, in order to eliminate associated nesidioblastosis or multifocal disease, either of which necessitates maximal pancreatectomy.

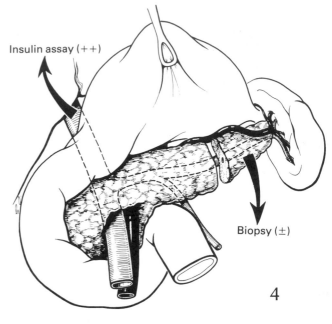

Insulin assay (++)

Biopsy (±)

4

## 5

The majority of infants present with diffuse or multiple microscopic lesions, and palpation of the gland will be negative. Maximal pancreatectomy is the operation of choice when, after a careful exploration of the abdominal cavity, ectopic adenomatous pancreatic tissue is not found.

There is no place for distal blind resection or corporo-caudal pancreatectomy in the surgery of hyperinsulinism in infants; partial resection has shown an unacceptable rate of recurrence, with an overall reoperation rate of 25 per cent.

Maximal pancreatectomy is commenced from the midline and continues to the left and right. The isthmus is first gently separated from the underlying portal vein; the body of the pancreas is then divided. A stapler can be useful.

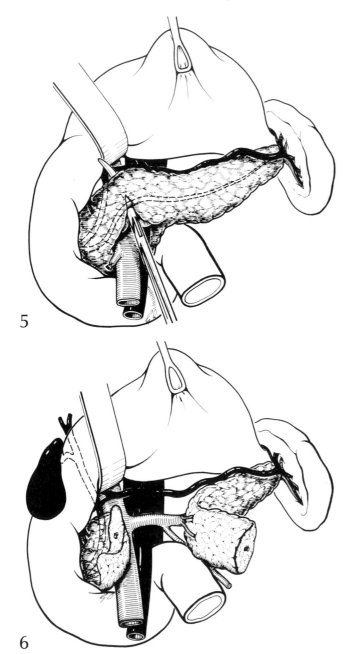

5

6

## 6

Distal pancreatectomy is undertaken from right to left. Short, friable veins joining the splenic vein are ligated and divided. These are more numerous towards the tail of the pancreas than over the body and neck of the organ. The splenic vein is completely separated from the pancreatic tissue. Meticulous dissection is necessary to preserve the vein, but the splenic artery is easily separated.

7

When the left half of the pancreas is resected, it is submitted for frozen section histopathological examination. Resection of the right half of the gland is then undertaken, leaving a small rim of pancreatic tissue between duodenum and common bile duct. Catheterization of the bile duct may be harmful, but patent blue injected into the gall bladder and the use of optical magnification may provide a useful guide.

The blood supply of the duodenum and bile duct is preserved, using cautery on the very distal branches of the right inferior pancreatic artery. Ligature of the left pancreatic vessels, as well as progressive separation of the pancreatic tissue from the border of the duodenum to the ampulla will permit complete separation of the uncinate process. The duct of Wirsung is ligated to the left of the common bile duct, and the rest of the pancreatic tissue is removed.

The portal insulin level at this stage is compared with the initial sample. Although time-consuming, this can detect a missed adenoma in the remaining rim of pancreatic tissue, especially if localized lesions in the resected gland have been identified by the pathologist. At the end of the operation, biochemical as well as microscopical criteria of an effective operation must be satisfied.

A Penrose tube is placed in the pancreatic bed via a separate stab wound.

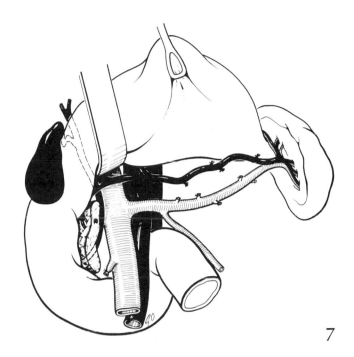

7

# Postoperative care and complications

Total parenteral nutrition using a central venous line and gastric suction are indicated. Hyperglycaemia is often demonstrated in the immediate postoperative period, and may necessitate treatment with insulin. A rise in the blood glucose may be considered valuable proof of an effective resection.

Major operative complications have not been encountered by the authors either during or after extensive primary resections. Serious complications such as biliary and duodenal fistulae have occurred during secondary resections. If an injury of the splenic vessels necessitates ligature, the spleen should be left *in situ*, as it will receive a sufficient blood supply from the left gastric vessels.

A bile-duct injury may be directly repaired using magnification, and a complementary cholecystostomy performed.

A duodenal tear should be recognized and closed.

Long-term endocrine or exocrine pancreatic insufficiencies have not been seen by the authors following primary extensive pancreatectomy, but severe recurrence of hypoglycaemia due to inadequate pancreatectomy has been encountered.

## Further reading

Aynsley-Green, A., Polak, J. M., Bloom, S. R., Gough, M. H., Keeling, J., Ashcroft, S. J. H. *et al.* (1981) Nesidioblastosis of the pancreas: definition of the syndrome and the management of severe neonatal hyperinsulinaemic hypoglycaemia. Archives of Disease of Childhood, 56, 496–508

Carcassonne, M., Delarue, A., Le Tourneau, J. N. (1983) Surgical treatment of organic pancreatic hypoglycaemia in the pediatric age. Journal of Pediatric Surgery, 18, 75–79

Gauderer, M., Stanley, C. A., Baker, L., Bishop, H. C. (1978) Pancreatic adenomas in infants and children: current surgical management. Journal of Pediatric Surgery, 13, 591–596

Illustrations by Kevin Marks

# Sacrococcygeal teratoma

**J. C. Molenaar** MD
Professor of Paediatric Surgery, Erasmus University, Rotterdam; Surgeon-in-Chief, Department of Paediatric Surgery,
University Hospital, Sophia Children's Hospital, Rotterdam, The Netherlands

## Definition[1,2]

A sacrococcygeal teratoma is a monstrous swelling arising
from totipotential cells derived from the primitive knot of
the embryo. It is attached to the coccyx and projects from
the space between the coccyx and the rectum. It contains
a wide variety of tissue derived from ectoderm,
mesoderm, and entoderm. The differentiation of cellular
structure varies from disorganized hamartoma-like tissue
to well-formed organs such as eye, thyroid, intestine, lung
tissue, etc.

Of those operated on neonatally, only about ten per
cent are malignant, but in those operated on later than the
6th month of life, 50 per cent may be so, suggesting
malignant change in a previously benign structure. The
most common types of malignancy are embryonal
carcinoma and yolk-sac carcinoma.

## Diagnosis

Some three-quarters of all sacrococcygeal teratomas occur
in females.

### Prenatal diagnosis

The diagnosis may be made before birth by ultrasound
examination of the gravid uterus. Early prenatal detection
of a sacrococcygeal tumour should not necessarily dictate
abortion as the treatment of choice. The timing of
treatment depends on the health of the child, but should
be within a few weeks of birth. Surgical treatment involves
complete excision of all teratoid tissue and the coccyx;
such complete excision is curative in more than 90 per
cent of cases. Nor is prenatal detection an absolute
indication for caesarean section, although the obstetrician
may prefer this for a large tumour, with the likelihood of
dystocia.

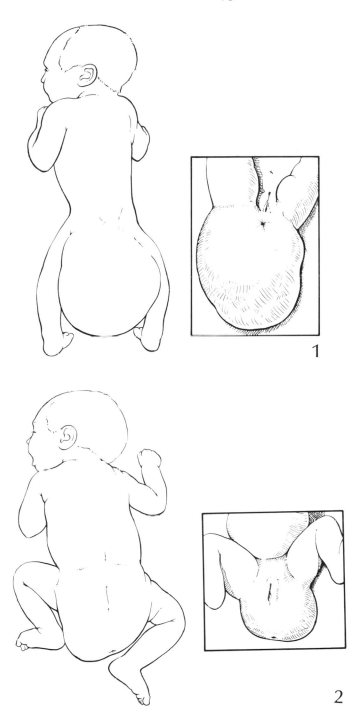

## Postnatal diagnosis

# 1 & 2

The diagnosis of sacrococcygeal teratoma is made immediately after birth from the typical appearance of this anomaly. An important feature is the position of the anus and rectum, which are usually displaced anteriorly by the tumour, but may occasionally be surrounded by it.

Equally important is the upward extension of the tumour into the pelvic space, compressing and elevating the rectum, vagina, bladder, and uterus, which may cause hydronephrosis and bowel obstruction. In such cases a radiographic examination such as a rectogram, IVP, and cystogram may be very helpful. Ultrasound examination is useful in defining the exact location and extent of the tumour. A plain X-ray of the lower abdomen and pelvis may reveal calcification, or the presence of bone or teeth; these findings are pathognomonic. Alphafetoprotein may be elevated in the serum.

## Differential diagnosis

1. Cystic duplication of the rectum. This is a very rare anomaly located in presacral spaces, sometimes extending into the abdominal cavity. Ultrasonography reveals a solitary cystic lesion with no solid components. Complete excision is usually possible, although marsupialization into the rectum may occasionally be a safer course of action.
2. Anterior meningocoele or myelomeningocoele.
3. Chordoma. More than half of all chordomas occur in the sacrococcygeal region.
4. Neuroblastoma.
5. Hamartoma.
6. Lipoma.
7. Haemangioma or lymphangioma.
8. Acute abscess.
9. Presacral teratoma. This is really a variant of presacrococcygeal teratoma without demonstrable external extension.

# Preoperative preparation

1. Blood must be cross-matched and available in the theatre at the time of surgery.
2. A nasogastric tube is passed.
3. Reliable venous access is essential.
4. Central venous monitoring is an advantage.
5. An indwelling bladder catheter is inserted.
6. The rectum is packed with gauze impregnated with Vaseline, liquid paraffin or povidone iodine solution.

# The operation

### Anaesthesia

General endotracheal anaesthesia is mandatory. The anaesthetist should be prepared for possible brisk blood loss during the surgical procedure.

### Position on operating table

The procedure is carried out with the infant in the prone jack-knife position. Rolled towels supporting the pelvis and shoulders achieve this and allow free ventilatory movements of the thoracic and abdominal walls.

# 3 & 4

### Incision

The incision is an inverted V-shape with its apex over the coccyx[3]. It is continued anteriorly across the base of the tumour. This approach facilitates subsequent wound closure and leads to normal appearing buttocks on healing.

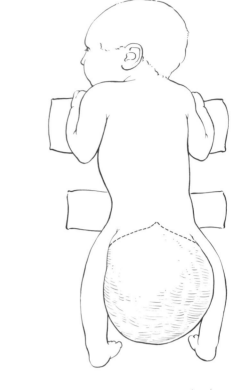

3

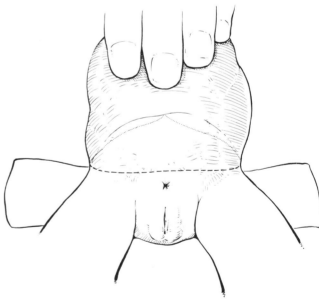

### Dissection

# 5

The tumour is first dissected from the gluteus maximus muscle. The coccyx is then approached and transected from the sacrum by cautery.

The median and lateral sacral vessels should be ligated in continuity and divided. These are the vascular supply to the tumour and early control will allow a more or less bloodless dissection.

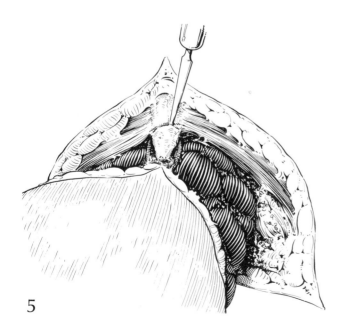

5

## 6

The tumour is gradually freed from the surrounding tissues and the pelvic floor by blunt and sharp dissection.

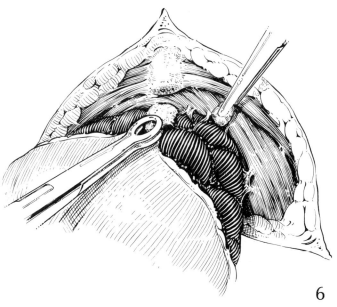

6

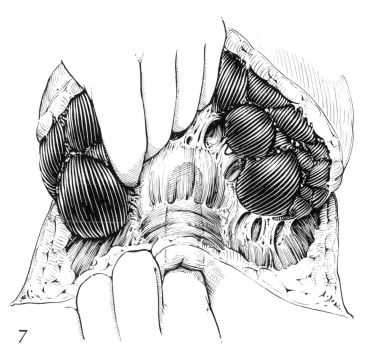

7

## 7

If necessary a finger placed in the rectum will facilitate freeing of the tumour from the rectal wall. Rarely the tumour completely surrounds the rectum, making total excision very difficult.

## 8

After excision, the rectum and the pelvic floor are frequently completely denuded and look rather frightening.

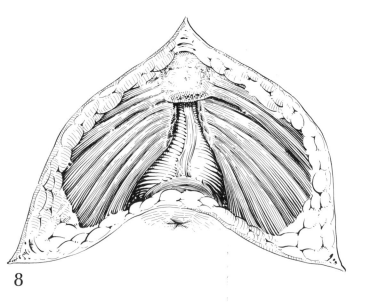

8

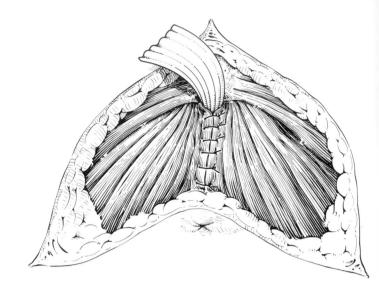

**9**

# 9 & 10

### Reconstruction

It is usually possible to reconstruct the pelvic floor adequately, up to as well as behind the rectum. Good faecal continence is to be expected[4].

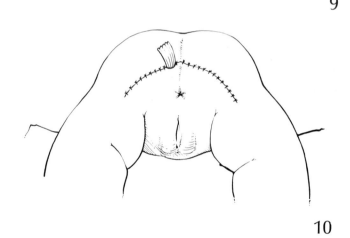

**10**

### Extensive tumour

If clinical and ultrasound examinations raise suspicion of the tumour's extending into the pelvic space above the pelvic floor, then the operation must start with the patient supine. The rolled towels are placed underneath the lumbar region, raising the pelvic floor towards the surgeon. The tumour is then devascularized and dissected through a lower abdominal midline or transverse incision, depending on the extent of the intra-abdominal part of the tumour. Subsequently the abdominal wall is sutured, the patient is turned prone in the jack-knife position, and the operation proceeds as described above.

# Pathology

Thorough histological examination of the tumour is essential to exclude or confirm any malignant element.

# Postoperative management and complications

The nasogastric tube is removed when bowel function is resumed.

The catheter is removed from the bladder on the day after the operation, provided the patient's condition has stabilized. Great care should be taken regarding bladder function. Neurogenic disorders are generally temporary, but may persist[4].

## Follow-up

Regular check-ups are essential. Regular monitoring of serum alphafetoprotein levels are useful for the early detection of recurrent tumour. Ultrasound examinations are also helpful. Recurrent tumours should be excised as soon as possible, except in case of malignancy with deep infiltration. All other patients should be cured by complete excision of all tumour tissue including the coccyx.

## Chemotherapy in malignant cases

Chemotherapy has improved survival in malignant cases. Primarily unresectable malignant sacrococcygeal teratomas or malignant recurrences can now be treated with cisplatin chemotherapy regimens, e.g. BVP (bleomycin, vinblastine and cisplatin) or BEP (bleomycin, VP16-213 and cisplatin). Remarkable shrinkage of the tumour can be achieved, rendering it amenable to secondary resection, and even metastases may be eradicated.

## References

1. Morton, M., Woolley, M. D. (1980) Teratoma. In: Pediatric surgery, T. M. Holder and K. W. Ashcraft (eds.), pp. 960–972. Philadelphia: W. B. Saunders Company

2. Mahour, G. H., Landing, B. H., Woolley, M. M. (1978) Teratomas in children: clinicopathologic studies in 133 patients. Zeitschrift für Kinderchirurgie, 23, 365–380

3. Gross, R. E., Clatworthy, H. W. Jr, Meeker, I. A. Jr. (1951) Sacrococcygeal teratomas in infants and children: a report of 40 cases. Surgery, Gynecology and Obstetrics, 92, 341–354

4. Engelskirchen, R., Holschneider, A. M., Rhein, R., Hecker, W. C., Hopner, F. (1987) Sacrococcygeal teratomas in children: an analysis of long-term results in 87 children, Zeitschrift für Kinderchirurgie, 42, 358–361

## Further reading

Hendren, W. H., Henderson, M. (1970) The surgical management of sacrococcygeal teratomas with intrapelvic extension. Annals of Surgery, 171, 77–84

Raney, R. B. Jr., Chatben, J., Littman, P., Jarrett, P., Schnaufer, L., Bishop, H. et al. (1981) Treatment strategies for infants with malignant sacrococcygeal teratoma. Journal of Pediatric Surgery, 16, 573–577

Illustrations by Kevin Marks

# Hydronephrosis

**John E. S. Scott**   MA, MD, FRCS, FAAP
Senior Lecturer in Paediatric Surgery, University of Newcastle upon Tyne, UK

For the purpose of this discussion the term 'hydronephrosis' is defined as the dilatation of the pelvicalyceal system which occurs as a result of obstruction to the pelviureteric junction or that segment of the ureter immediately beyond it. The condition is common in children and occurs at all ages, the sex incidence being equal. In unilateral cases the left side is more commonly affected than the right but both sides are affected in approximately 15 per cent, with a higher incidence of bilaterality in infancy.

## Diagnosis

### Symptoms and signs

The commonest presenting feature in the newborn is a palpable mass in the flank, often noted during routine physical examination after delivery. In later childhood symptoms are most commonly due to the onset of a urinary infection. Thus, listlessness, anorexia, vomiting, intermittent fever, diarrhoea and malodorous urine may occur. Alternatively, there may be intermittent attacks of abdominal pain, usually central without radiation, lasting at first a few minutes but gradually increasing in duration, severity and frequency. It is only in older children around puberty that the spasmodic flank pain characteristic of adult hydronephrosis appears. A third mode of presentation is haematuria, usually painless and transient. Approximately 25 per cent of obstructed kidneys in children manifest themselves in this way.

## Investigation

### Radiology

# 1

Intravenous urography is the primary diagnostic method and demonstrates the dilatation of the pelvicalyceal system. Initially, the renal pelvis appears fuller than that of the contralateral kidney, and the calyces lose their sharp outline. Later, the renal pyramids disappear so that the calyces become rounded and the renal pelvis enlarges even further. The pelviureteric junction itself cannot be seen: there is a sharp 'cut-off' around the inferior border of the pelvis and a gap of several millimetres between it and the contrast in the upper ureter. Poor concentration of the contrast medium in a dilated kidney may be due to depressed glomerular filtration and/or diminished tubular concentrating capacity, but it may also simply be due to the dilution effect of the increased volume of urine. It is therefore important to take delayed exposures up to four hours or more after the contrast has been injected because only then may the kidney become visible. Delay in renal drainage will also be more apparent on delayed films. In this respect, exposures with the child standing may be informative because, in the vertical position, contrast drains rapidly from a normal kidney but not from an obstructed one. Efforts to demonstrate the lower ureter on at least one of the films should be made so as to exclude ureteric obstruction. A film taken with the child prone will often achieve this.

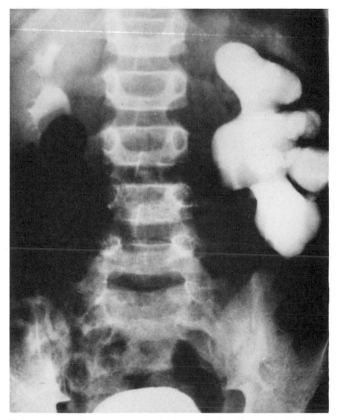

Figure 1    Intravenous urogram showing left pelviureteric junction obstruction.

Micturition cystourethrography should always be performed because pelviureteric junction obstruction is sometimes associated with ureteric reflux. Gross ureteric reflux may produce a degree of pelvicalyceal dilatation which closely resembles pelviureteric junction obstruction.

There are occasions when despite a history highly suggestive of hydronephrosis the intravenous urogram is normal. These are examples of intermittent hydronephrosis, in which dilatation occurs only when there is increased urine flow from the kidney. In ordinary circumstances, intravenous urography is performed after the patient has been deprived of fluid for some hours when urine output is low, but by stimulating a diuresis with increased fluid intake, a higher dose of contrast medium and an injection of the diuretic frusemide (furosemide; Lasix), the kidney may become dilated as a result of the high urine output.

*Ultrasound examination*

# 2 & 3

The introduction of real-time B-mode, linear array ultrasound has provided a major step forward in the diagnosis of renal disease. Because it is non-invasive and possesses no radiation hazard, examinations can safely be repeated. It is particularly useful in the newborn period, when radiology often produces unsatisfactory films. As the dilated kidney may not concentrate the contrast medium, the distinction between hydronephrosis and a tumour may be clinically impossible. The ultrasound scan will not only do this, it will also define the degree of parenchymal atrophy and delineate other abnormalities such as a dilated ureter, duplex renal pelvis or renal cystic disease. The use of ultrasound scanning has virtually eliminated the need for retrograde pyelography in the diagnosis of hydronephrosis.

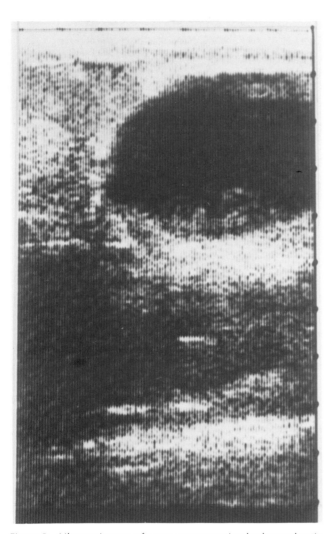

*Figure 2   Ultrasonic scan of a non-concentrating hydronephrotic kidney in a neonate.*

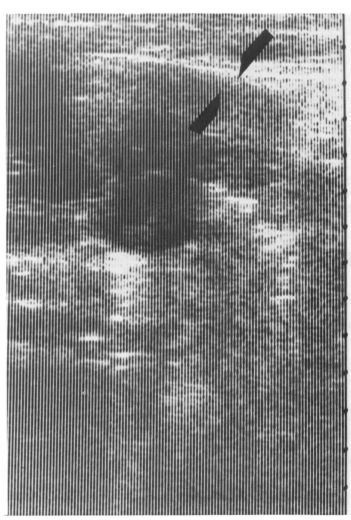

*Figure 3   Ultrasound scan of a hydronephrotic kidney demonstrating thickness of renal parenchyma.*

*Radioisotope renography*

# 4a–e

Renal tubular function and urine transport through the kidney and its drainage system can be measured by using a radioactive labelled substance which is secreted by the renal tubules and excreted from the kidney in the urine. Ortho-iodohippurate (Hippuran) labelled with iodine-123 is suitable for this purpose and radioactivity is recorded with a γ-camera and appropriate computer. The result, however, must be carefully interpreted because it depends on a number of factors. For example, diminished renal tubular secretory activity produces a low, gradually rising time/activity curve (*a*), but a dilated kidney produces a higher level of activity simply because the volume of the renal pelvis is greater (*b*). However, this does not necessarily indicate an obstructed kidney since drainage from the renal pelvis may occur at normal speed if the radioisotope is washed out of the kidney as a result of a diuresis produced by an injection of frusemide (*c*). If, despite administering the diuretic, drainage does not occur (*d*) or occurs more slowly than normal, the kidney is obstructed. This is an important technique for detecting genuine obstruction in a kidney that has a large renal pelvis. Because the radiation dose is small the investigation can safely be repeated at intervals if there is initial doubt about the diagnosis of obstruction. A postoperative renogram will demonstrate whether obstruction has effectively been relieved (*e*).

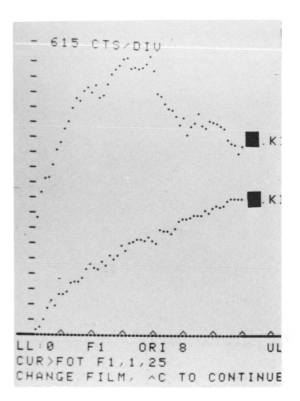

*Figure 4a    Radioisotope renography. Renogram showing diminished tubular function (lower curve)*

# Preoperative

### Preparation of patient

The child is prepared as for any major operation. The only precaution that is particular to the treatment of hydronephrosis is to ensure that the urine is sterile. It is unwise to operate on the kidney if the urine is infected unless an acutely obstructed pyonephrosis is encountered. Even this should be detectable before operation and treated by percutaneous nephrostomy drainage. Emergency surgery is scarely ever necessary and there is time to control bacteriuria with the appropriate antibiotics.

The author favours the dismembered ureteropyelostomy method advocated by Anderson and Hynes[1].

### Position of patient

The child is placed on the operating table in a supine position with the affected side elevated on rolled-up towels (*see Illustration 5*). In neonates and in early infancy it is unnecessary to tilt the child and in bilateral hydronephrosis the child should lie flat if the operator intends to treat both sides at the same session.

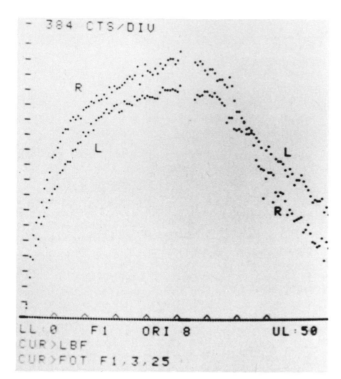

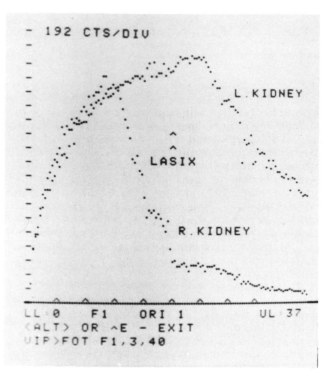

*Figure 4b    Renogram showing high activity in both kidneys of a child who had bilateral renal pelvic dilatation on intravenous urography*

*Figure 4c    Renogram showing a dilated kidney which drained rapidly after administration of frusemide and was therefore not obstructed*

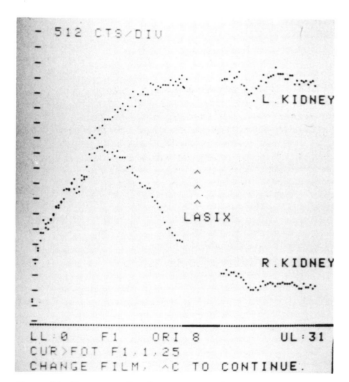

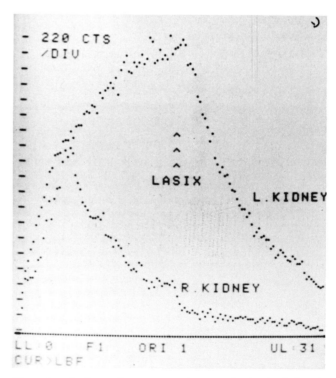

*Figure 4d    Renogram showing retention of radioisotope in the left kidney after administration of a diuretic, indicating obstruction*

*Figure 4e    Postoperative renogram (same patient as in d) showing effective relief of obstruction*

# The operation

## The incision

### 5

The incision is made in the appropriate upper abdominal quadrant from the midline to a point immediately below the costal margin and deepened through the sub-cutaneous fat, dividing the external and internal oblique and rectus muscles. At this point, the operator must decide whether to use a trans- or extraperitoneal approach. Both methods are equally satisfactory and indeed the transperitoneal approach becomes extraperitoneal during the process of exposing the kidney. Moreover, an approach which is commenced extraperitoneally often becomes transperitoneal.

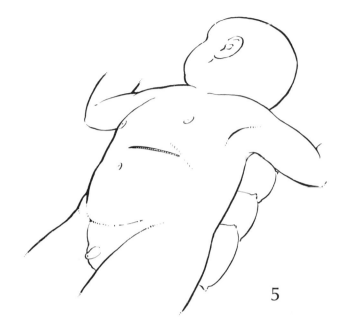

5

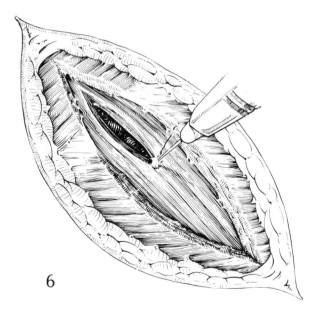

6

### 6

For the extraperitoneal approach, the fibres of the transversus muscle are split at the lateral end of the incision so as to enter the extraperitoneal space, and the peritoneum is stripped off the inner aspect of the lateral and posterior aspects of the abdominal wall. This dissection is commenced laterally where the peritoneum is less adherent and then carried medially to the edge of the posterior rectus sheath which is incised.

# 7

For the transperitoneal approach, the transversus muscle and peritoneum are divided in line with the incision so as to open the peritoneal cavity. The small intestine is displaced medially to expose the colon (ascending or descending), which is lifted out through the incision and drawn medially to display the line of attachment between its mesentery and the peritoneum of the posterior abdominal wall. An incision is made along this line to enter the retroperitoneal space and, when this is widened, the perirenal fascia is exposed.

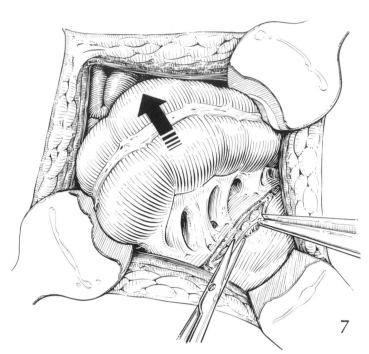

7

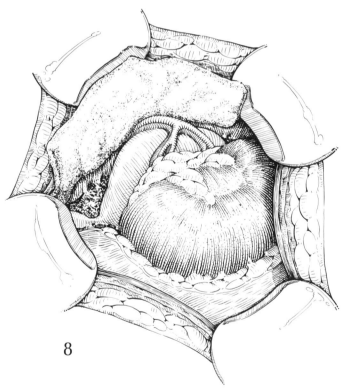

8

# 8

A further incision through this layer reveals the perirenal fat, the renal pelvis and the kidney. Two or three moist packs are inserted to protect the colon, small bowel and liver, which are retracted with the blades of a Denis Browne ring retractor. From this point on, the operation is extraperitoneal.

## 9

The renal pelvis, pelviureteric junction and proximal ureter are now mobilized and cleaned of perirenal fat without lifting the kidney from its bed. The branches and tributaries of the renal artery and vein are carefully lifted off the anterior surface of the renal pelvis so that the pelvis can be drawn downwards. If there is a separate artery crossing the pelviureteric junction to supply the lower pole of the kidney, this should be completely mobilized as well. Three holding sutures are then inserted: (*1*) in the ureter immediately below the pelviureteric junction; (*2*) in the ureter about 5 mm distal to the first; and (*3*) in the inferior border of the renal pelvis 5–10 mm from the kidney. The ureter is divided between sutures 1 and 2 and the medial portion of the renal pelvis is resected with scissors, cutting both anterior and posterior walls simultaneously. This line of resection should be angled to provide a step at the lower border of the renal pelvis.

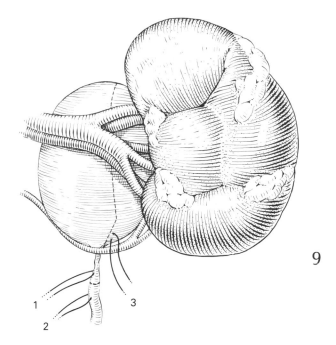

## 10

The advantage of the anterior approach to the kidney will now become apparent because, as the renal pelvis is resected, it will become possible to inspect the interior of the kidney and ascertain the position of entry of the major calyces, particularly the upper one. The direction of the vertical line of resection can be accurately adjusted so that it does not pass too close to the orifice of the upper calyx, thus causing it to become obstructed when the pelvis is repaired. If there are separate vessels supplying the lower pole of the kidney, the ureter is drawn downwards from beneath them and transposed in front.

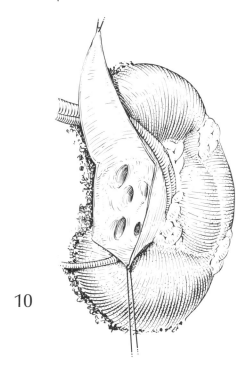

## 11

The reconstruction of the renal pelvis and pelviureteric junction is commenced by repairing the superior two-thirds or three-quarters of the renal pelvis (depending on its size) with a running suture of 4/0 chromic catgut which picks up all the layers. The loops should be placed close together and tightened firmly to produce a suture line which is as watertight as possible.

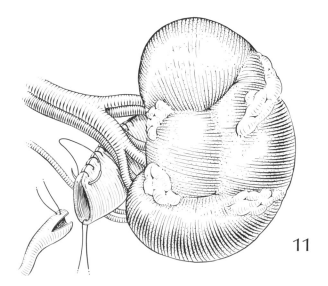

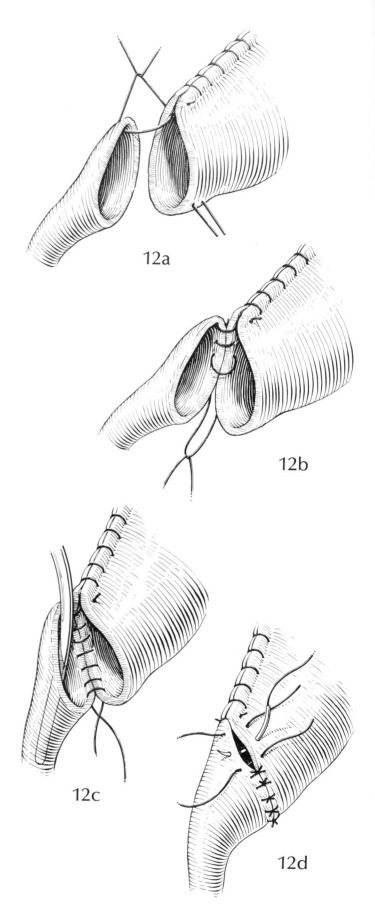

12a

12b

12c

12d

# 12a–d

Before starting the anastomosis between the renal pelvis and ureter, the holding suture in the ureter should be removed so that the ureter can lie in a natural position in its bed. A longitudinal incision is then made through the lateral wall of the ureter for a distance equal to the length of the remaining aperture in the renal pelvis (see *Illustration 11*). It is important to place the ureteric incision correctly or the ureter will become twisted when it is anastomosed to the pelvis. The anastomosis is begun at the superior end with 4/0 chromic catgut sutures placed so that the knots lie on the exterior surface (a and b). When the posterior layer is complete, a probe should be passed into the ureter to ensure that its lumen has not been compromised by one of the sutures (c). The anterior layer of sutures is now inserted but, to ensure that they are accurately located, the final three or four should be placed before being tied (d).

The author does not recommend splinting the anastomosis or draining the kidney with a nephrostomy tube. Careful and accurate suturing should prevent urinary leakage. In babies below the age of 3 months a finer suture material such as 6/0 polydioxanone (Ethicon) should be used because the walls of the ureter and renal pelvis are delicate and the ureteric lumen narrow.

Once the anastomosis is completed, the retractor blades and pads are removed. A narrow length of corrugated polyvinylchloride is led out through a stab incision in the flank to act as a retroperitoneal drain in case the anastomosis does leak. The colon is replaced in its bed and the incision closed in layers. The drain is removed after 48 hours.

## References

1. Anderson, J. C., Hynes, W. (1949) Retrocaval ureter case diagnosed pre-operatively and treated successfully by plastic operations. British Journal of Urology, 21, 209–214

Illustrations by Philip Wilson

# Nephrectomy for non-malignant disease

**Robert H. Whitaker**  MD, MChir, FRCS
Consultant Paediatric Urologist, Addenbrooke's Hospital, Cambridge, and Associate Lecturer,
University of Cambridge, Cambridge, UK

## Principles and indications

### Nephrectomy

The recognition that the infant kidney has a remarkable ability to recover function after relief of obstruction and that a segment of kidney may show localized hypertrophy in reflux nephropathy has led to a more conservative surgical approach and a decrease in the number of nephrectomies performed. Nephrectomy is still appropriate in gross hydronephrosis where there remains only a thin shell of parenchyma; in multicystic kidney; in primary hypoplasia; and in unilateral severe reflux nephropathy, particularly when associated with hypertension. A kidney which has been destroyed by infection (e.g. pyonephrosis, xanthogranulomatous pyelonephritis) may also need to be removed. Similarly, severe trauma may necessitate a nephrectomy.

It is vital when considering such ablative surgery to ensure that the opposite kidney can sustain adequate renal function. In the presence of a normal contralateral organ, a kidney is probably not worth preserving if it contributes less than 10–15 per cent of overall function as assessed by isotope methods after relief of obstruction. If the contralateral kidney is also abnormal, the decision becomes more complex and many other factors have to be taken into consideration.

### Partial nephrectomy

The term heminephrectomy has now been abandoned since, even in the case of a duplex system, it is unusual for precisely half the kidney to be removed. Partial (segmental) nephrectomy implies the removal of an upper or, more usually, a lower pole in an otherwise single kidney. The indications for partial nephrectomy in children are few and are usually stone formation, trauma, or localized anomalies such as caliceal cyst, diverticulum or arteriovenous anomalies. Simple renal cysts can usually be removed with minimal excision of renal tissue. Part of the kidney may need to be removed while separating the two halves of a horseshoe kidney. The vast majority of segmental resections, however, are performed for an abnormality of one moiety of a duplex system. The details of these anomalies are discussed in the chapter on 'Ureteric duplication', pp. 528–533).

## Preoperative

Using X-ray tomography, with or without intravenous contrast, it is usually possible to define accurately the extent of the kidney that needs to be removed, although occasionally it is only when the kidney is exposed that the details of the operation can be planned. Fine sutures and vascular instruments should be available.

# 1

### Position of patient

The kidney is best approached via the loin for partial or complete nephrectomy for benign disease. The full lateral position is used with the 'break' or bridge in line with the lower ribs. In small children it is easier to achieve the correct degree of lateral spinal flexion with a sandbag or foam pillow. The lower leg should be flexed at both the knee and hip and the upper leg should lie straight on top. A pillow between the two legs is optional. The upper arm is supported on an armrest to steady the upper body and the patient is tilted a little head down. Non-stretch strapping is then applied firmly to the table on the abdominal side and, with the body held at the required inclination, the strapping is applied at the level of the hip, across to the other side of the table.

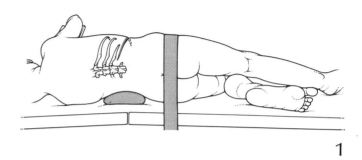

1

## The operations

### The incision

# 2

A subcostal or supra-12th rib incision usually gives adequate access in a child. The muscles are best divided by cutting diathermy. Every effort should be made to avoid damage to the neurovascular bundles although it is difficult to avoid them altogether. The transversus muscle is split along its fibres and the peritoneum swept medially and anteriorly. It also helps to free the peritoneum along the wound edge above and below so that a retractor can be inserted effectively without the risk of tearing the peritoneum.

A Silastic sling is placed around the ureter before the kidney is mobilized, particularly in a child with renal stones. The kidney must then be mobilized completely with blunt and sharp dissection of the perirenal fat. Meticulous haemostasis is essential, particularly in the region of the adrenal vessels. In children the kidney is usually sufficiently mobile that it can almost be delivered from the wound.

The main vessels of the renal pedicle are identified, and it may be an advantage at this stage to put a sling around the main renal artery and to clear it sufficiently for the application of a bulldog clip later.

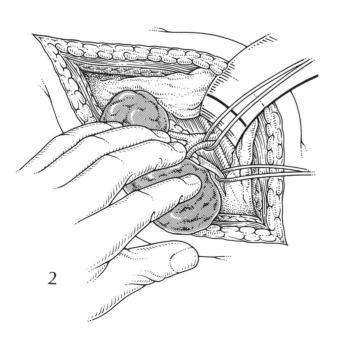

2

## NEPHRECTOMY

If the kidney is to be removed, the main vessels are now ligated in turn, starting with the artery or arteries. It is not always possible to expose the main renal artery and there is no harm with an adherent kidney in dissecting close to the renal hilum and ligating the three to four small arterial divisions separately with linen or black silk ties. It is best to ligate the vessel in continuity using right-angled forceps and to cut the vessel between two such ties. For larger vessels, e.g. the main renal artery and vein, double ligation should always be used on the aortic and inferior vena cava sides. Clamping large vessels is unwise because of the risk of slipping of the clamp and mass ligation of the renal pedicle should be avoided as it may lead to an arteriovenous fistula. After division of the vessels, the kidney is freed from the remaining fat and is held only by the ureter. This is ligated with catgut as low as possible and divided. If the ureter is healthy and there is no reflux, it is not necessary to remove it to the bladder wall. The adrenal should be preserved unless it is part of an inflammatory mass. It is not essential to drain the wound for a simple nephrectomy, but if the dissection has been extensive or the disease process infective, it is wise to use a drain.

## The difficult nephrectomy

After severe or prolonged infection, nephrectomy can be extremely difficult and hazardous, with potential damage to other structures, such as the inferior vena cava, duodenum or spleen, and with a risk of life-threatening haemorrhage. Such accidents can occur even with cautious dissection, usually because other structures have become stuck to or displaced by the kidney. Previous operations on the kidney may have caused severe adhesions, particularly if the perirenal fat has not been replaced.

A subcapsular operation is sometimes useful, approaching the main vessels via an incision through the capsule at the hilum. Alternatively, the vessels can be approached from below by dividing the ureter early and using it as a retractor to displace the kidney so that all structures lateral to the vena cava or aorta can be divided until the renal vessels are reached. It is sometimes impossible to divide the renal artery before the vein from an anterior approach but the artery can sometimes be isolated more easily from behind. The short right renal vein deserves respect and Satinsky clamps should be available to deal with caval tears. In the event of a sudden severe bleed, which is usually venous, packing the wound may be the only solution. This should be followed by a controlled effort to isolate the source: inaccurate clamping in a pool of blood may do more harm than good. Occasionally a large infected pyonephrotic kidney may be impossible to remove safely. It is wiser to drain such a system at the first operation and perform a nephrectomy later.

# 3

## PARTIAL NEPHRECTOMY

Removal of a pole of the kidney, often the lower, is facilitated by dissection of the renal hilum anteriorly to expose the divisions of the renal artery, and posteriorly, in the renal sinus, to expose the appropriate infundibulum. Temporary occlusion of a vessel and injection of a dye such as methylene blue have their place in determining how much tissue is to be removed, but often the decision is based more on arbitrary factors such as the radiographic appearances or distribution of stones.

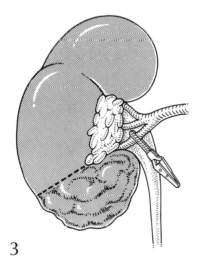

3

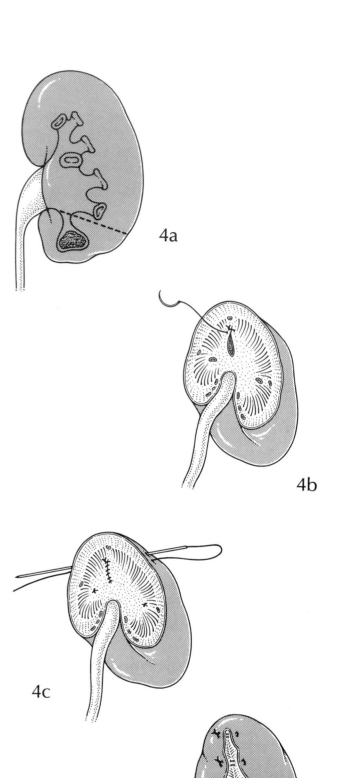

4a

4b

4c

4d

# 4a–d

In a diseased kidney it is not usually possible to strip the capsule off the pole of the kidney and, indeed, it is doubtful if this is of any great benefit. The kidney is cut directly across (and not excised as a V-shaped wedge) while the renal artery is temporarily occluded or the remainder of the kidney gently compressed manually (a). Obvious vessels are doubly underrun with 3/0 or 4/0 chromic catgut (b). The calix is closed with a continuous chromic catgut suture of similar size and the cut surface of the kidney oversewn with horizontal mattress sutures of 2/0 chromic catgut on a straight needle (c and d). If there is still oozing despite this, a piece of haemostatic gauze can be incorporated into the suture line.

If what remains of the kidney is very mobile, it is fixed to the posterior abdominal wall before the perirenal fat is approximated around it. A silicone tube drain should always be used and brought out through a separate stab incision.

# 5

## Partial nephrectomy in duplex kidney

The two moieties of the duplex kidney usually have totally separate blood supplies and caliceal systems, making removal of one part straightforward. Indications for removing the ureter in association with the abnormal moiety of kidney are discussed in the chapter on 'Ureteric duplication', pp. 528–533).

The technique for removal of the upper or lower poles is similar. Access to the lower pole is slightly easier, whereas the plane of dissection is often clearer for an upper pole resection. This demarcation is usually made more obvious by the pathological process that affects the diseased moiety.

The vessels to the affected segment are ligated and divided and the ureter is mobilized to allow a sinus approach (a). In a dysplastic or hydronephrotic upper moiety of a duplex system this sinus extends almost across the full width of the kidney so that the rim of parenchyma can be cut and oversewn progressively around its horseshoe-shaped circumference (b, c and d). Removal of the lower moiety is accomplished in a similar way, although the vascular pedicle is usually more complex. If the cut surface continues to ooze after suture-ligature of obvious vessels, a horizontal mattress suture is used as described for partial nephrectomy.

The remaining moiety is fixed posteriorly to avoid rotation and clothed in perinephric fat. The wound is drained as described earlier and closed in two layers with chromic catgut, polyglycolic acid (Dexon) or Vicryl according to personal preference. The skin is closed with simple nylon sutures or subcuticular polyglycolic acid. Drains are removed 24 hours after drainage has ceased, which is usually after 2–3 days. Limited intravenous urography or radionuclide scintigraphy should be used to check the remaining moiety after 3–4 months, although clinical concern may dictate the need for earlier assessment.

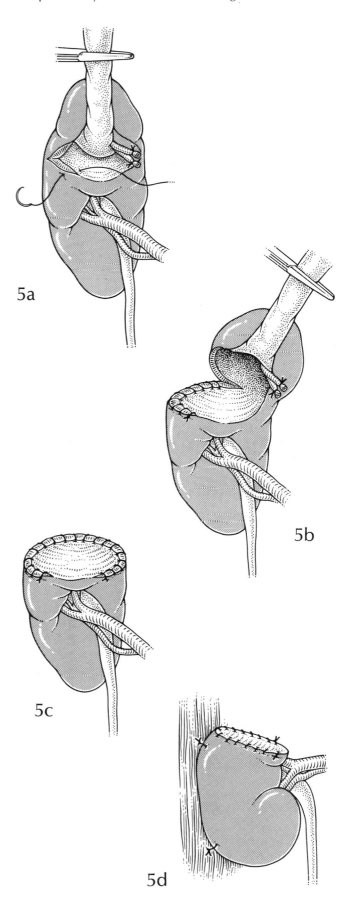

5a

5b

5c

5d

Illustrations by Jean Perry

# Operations for vesicoureteric reflux and obstruction

**S. Joseph Cohen**  MB, BCh, FRCS, MRCP
Consultant Paediatric Surgeon and Urologist, Booth Hall Children's Hospital; Royal Manchester Children's Hospital and St Mary's Hospital; Lecturer in Paediatric Surgery, University of Manchester, Manchester, UK

## Introduction

The vesicoureteric junction is a delicate and effective valve mechanism which opens during ureteric peristalsis, allowing the free flow of urine into the bladder. As the bladder fills its musculature relaxes, allowing further and continuing flow of urine into the bladder with little rise in bladder pressure. When micturition occurs or when pressure within the abdomen rises, intravesical pressure rises sharply, yet the normal functioning ureterovesical valve prevents any retrograde passage of urine into the ureters.

This mechanism may become faulty in one of two ways; (1) by becoming incompetent and allowing vesicoureteric reflux of varying degrees to occur,[1,2] and (2) by being relatively stenosed, causing impedance to the normal peristaltic flow of urine into the bladder.

The results of these conditions have differing effects on the upper urinary tracts.

Vesicoureteric reflux, especially in the presence of urinary infection (and occasionally when there is high pressure, reflux *without* infection) may cause attacks of pyelonephritis which in the long term may result in pyelonephritic scarring or reflux nephropathy[3]. This is one end of a spectrum, the other being reflux of lesser severity which responds well to antibiotic therapy, and routines which ensure effective bladder emptying, for example double micturition.

Vesicoureteric obstruction or stenosed megaureter also has a range of severity, the least being minimal fusiform dilatation of the lower ureter with normal calyces, pelvis and upper ureter. At the other extreme there may be gross dilatation and tortuosity of the whole ureter, with dilatation of the pelvis and calyces and marked thinning of the renal cortex. The more severe lesions are prone to superadded infection which may result in further damage to the renal parenchyma.

## Preoperative investigations

In all cases the patient must be fully investigated to ascertain that the vesicoureteric reflux or the obstruction is primary and not secondary to a neurogenic cause or an obstructed outflow tract, e.g. urethral valves.

1. A straight X-ray of the abdomen and lumbosacral vertebrae is the first investigation. This must be accompanied by an ultrasound examination of the abdomen, which can demonstrate the size, shape and position of the kidneys, and the presence or absence of dilatation of the calyces, pelvis, ureter and bladder.
2. Intravenous urography follows, which will confirm many of the problems already suspected, namely the number, position and size of the kidneys, the presence of renal scarring, the presence or absence of pelvi-calyceal dilatation, and dilatation and tortuosity of the ureters. It will also confirm the size and shape of the bladder.
3. Micturating cystourethrography should outline the whole outflow tract to exclude lesions such as urethral valves, strictures or polyps, as well as demonstrating the degree of reflux when present.
4. Where the investigations suggest an obstructive lesion, diuresis renography can often clarify the position and differentiate between an obstructed and a hypotonic system.
5. Urodynamic studies may be very useful in suspected neurogenic or pseudoneurogenic causes of bladder dysfunction.
6. Cystourethroscopy and vaginoscopy should always precede the operative procedure, firstly to confirm all the findings already demonstrated and also to exclude urethral valves, which may have been missed by the other investigations. In addition the presence of severe or unsuspected cystitis may well cause the postponement of the operation until it is cleared. Vaginoscopy may be important to demonstrate an ectopic opening of a stenosed ureteric orifice.

*In all cases* where the reflux or the obstruction is secondary to other causes, these should be treated first and time allowed for the surgery to take effect. This applies especially in the case of urethral valves where, after successful disruption of the valves, months or even years should elapse before surgery on the ureters is contemplated for either reflux or stenosis.

# Operative techniques

Since the early 1950s many surgical techniques have been devised for the correction of vesicoureteric reflux. The earliest was probably that of Hutch[4], followed by Politano–Leadbetter[5], Paquin[6], Glenn–Anderson[7], Liche–Gregoir[8], and Cohen[9]. The techniques are mainly divisible into two groups: those where the dissection of the ureter is mainly or entirely intravesical (all those mentioned above except the Liche–Gregoir), or entirely extravesical, of which the Liche–Gregoir is the best example.

Recently the endoscopic injection of Teflon submucosally below and behind the ureteric orifice has been introduced by Puri and O'Donnell[10]. The preliminary results are encouraging but time will prove whether this simple and short procedure is as safe and as effective as the operative procedures listed above.

# The operations

A cystoscopy should always precede the opening of the bladder. It often facilitates the dissection if the bladder is left fully distended at the end of the cystoscopy. All intravesical procedures have the following steps in common for the freeing of the ureters from the bladder.

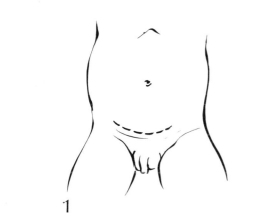

## 1

### The incision

A low transverse suprapubic incision is made. Its position should be such that in later life it will be hidden in the pubic hair, and will not prevent young girls from wearing bikinis.

## 2

### Exposure

The skin and subcutaneous tissues are incised, exposing the rectus sheath. The recti are then separated in the midline, commencing from the pubis and sweeping the peritoneum upwards and off the bladder to prevent its accidental opening. Two stay-sutures are inserted and the bladder opened vertically. The blades of a Denis Browne ring retractor are inserted as illustrated, a Raytec swab under the cranial blade facilitating a wide exposure. A 3/0 or 4/0 Dexon suture is placed at the lowest point of the incision and is held against the edge of the ring retractor by an artery forceps. This is a useful manoeuvre which increases exposure and prevents splitting of the incision downwards into the urethra by the too forceful placement of the retractor blades; later it facilitates bladder closure by marking the lowermost point of the incision. The ureteric orifices are now inspected for number, position, shape and competence, and their tunnels are measured for length. A fine infant-feeding tube, either 3 or 5 Fr, is inserted into the ureter, as shown on the patient's right. A stay-suture is placed around the meatus and loosely tied over the feeding tube. The ureteric meatus is circumcised by an incision around the ureter as indicated by the dotted line on the patient's left.

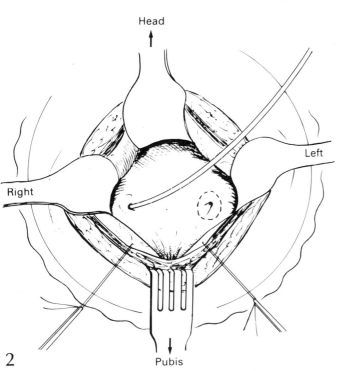

Head

Right

Left

Pubis

# 3

## Dissection

Meticulous dissection of the ureter is performed. The incision is deepened, carefully dividing the muscle fibres that fix the ureter to the bladder musculature. This is done carefully and systematically. It is advisable to commence just below the orifice, and once the plane is entered between the ureter and bladder musculature it is progressively developed circumferentially until the ureter is completely freed. Great care must be taken not to dissect too close to the ureter for fear of damaging its blood supply or its musculature. In addition, the peritoneum, which almost surrounds the ureter, must be carefully teased away from the ureter using a small pledget. In male patients the vas deferens may lie close to this point and care must be taken not to damage it.

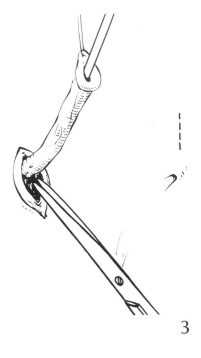

3

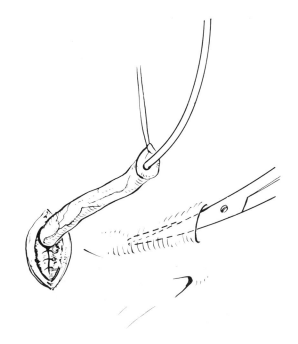

4

## THE COHEN OR TRANSTRIGONAL METHOD OF REIMPLANTATION

# 4

The ureter is now free and ready for reimplantation. In the majority of cases the opposite ureter is freed using the same technique, and reimplantation may commence. The dissection of the ureter may have enlarged its orifice in the bladder wall to such an extent that it should be narrowed with interrupted Dexon sutures. This is done to prevent the formation of a diverticulum. These sutures should narrow the hiatus, but still allow the free movement of the ureter and not restrict or constrict it.

The tunnel is then constructed. A point is selected above and perhaps a little lateral to the opposite ureteric orifice. An incision in the mucosa is made, and after inserting the closed blades of a pair of scissors, it is advanced under the mucosa by an opening and cutting movement. It is prudent to keep advancing the scissors with each cutting of the blades, and not to withdraw them, for this may lead to false passages which could complicate the later stages. Tunnelling is continued until the ureter is reached. The tunnel should be a gentle curve, which is a prolongation of the original entrance of the ureter into the bladder. Care must be taken as the midline is approached, for it is here that the mucosa is most easily button-holed. This can be best avoided by placing a pair of Allis forceps just lateral to the commencement of the tunnel, and by gently retracting this laterally the posterior bladder wall can be straightened and the problem averted. The new tunnel must be wide enough to hold the ureter comfortably, and long enough to prevent reflux. The minimal length is two to three times the ureteric diameter.

# 5

The ureter is now gently threaded through its new tunnel. This is best accomplished by passing a pair of Denis Browne divulsers into the tunnel, grasping the stay suture and drawing the ureter into place, taking care not to twist or kink it in the process.

5

# 6

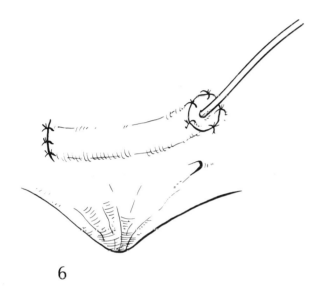

6

The cuff of the ureter is then sutured in position. First a 3/0 Dexon suture is inserted laterally through the full thickness of the ureter and also through the full thickness of bladder muscle. This prevents it from retracting. Next, three or four 5/0 Dexon sutures are inserted, joining the bladder and urethral mucosae. The incision in the mucosa of the original orifice is then similarly closed with fine Dexon sutures. Many surgeons do not believe in retaining this cuff of mucosa, but if it has not been devascularized or traumatized I believe it is worthwhile preserving. If any doubt exists, the terminal part of the ureter should be excised.

# 7

## Obstruction or stenosis

In cases of obstruction or stenosed megaureter, the terminal portion of the ureter must be excised. In the majority of cases this allows the ureter to deflate, and if not too dilated it may be reimplanted as already described. If the ureter is still very dilated, then remodelling may be necessary before reimplantation (see Reimplantation of the grossly dilated ureter, page 520).

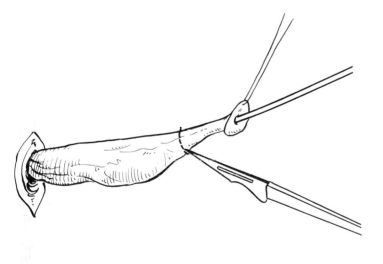

7

# 8

## Bilateral reimplantation

The dissection of both ureters having been carried out as described, the two ureters are held and assessed as to which would sit most comfortably in the upper tunnel. If both seem equally well suited, the author tends to use the upper tunnel for the ureter which has the more severe degree of reflux. The second tunnel is then constructed by the same technique as above. Its position is below the tunnel already made, and goes from the ureteric entrance to the orifice of the opposite side. The second ureter is threaded through its tunnel in the same manner and similarly fixed in its new position. Some surgeons use a single tunnel for both ureters and I believe that there has been no trouble from this, but on the theoretical ground that the two ureters could adhere to one another and cause problems later, I still prefer to use two separate tunnels.

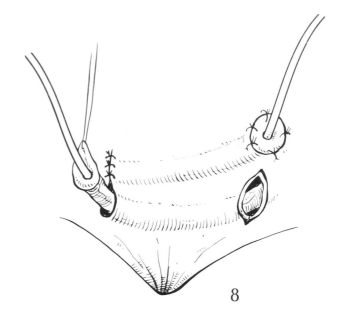

8

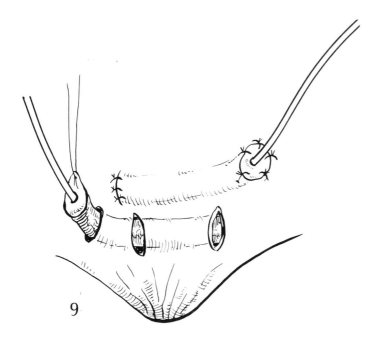

9

# 9

In the very young where the intratrigonal distance is very short, the lower tunnel may be too short for the above procedure. In these cases the tunnel is extended beyond the opposite orifice to a point more lateral.

## Bladder closure

The Raytec swab under the upper retractor blade is removed and the closure commenced. The suture at the lower end of the incision is tied and held up; a pair of Allis forceps applied to the upper end facilitates closure. The mucosa is closed with a continuous 4/0 or 5/0 Dexon suture, and the musculature with 2/0 or 3/0 interrupted Dexon sutures. Fine feeding tubes are left in as ureteric stents, and the bladder drained with a Malecot No. 12 or 14 Fr catheter. The remaining layers are closed with 2/0 or 3/0 Dexon to approximate the recti, 4/0 Dexon to the subcutaneous tissue and a subcuticular Dexon for skin closure. A Jackson Pratt or suction drain is placed retropubically. Some surgeons nowadays dispense with the ureteric splints unless remodelling of the ureters has been carried out.

## THE POLITANO–LEADBETTER TECHNIQUE

### 10

Further dissection is now carried out through the hiatus and the peritoneum is freed from the back of the bladder by blunt dissection. This plane is enlarged upwards towards the dome of the bladder, care being taken not to open the peritoneum (shown by the dotted lines) or to damage any of the intraperitoneal structures. If any difficulties are encountered at this stage it is safer to proceed with an added extravesical dissection of the ureter. A pair of forceps is now inserted through the hiatus into this plane and the tip pressed into the bladder wall as shown. An incision is made at this point, creating the new hiatus of entrance of the ureter.

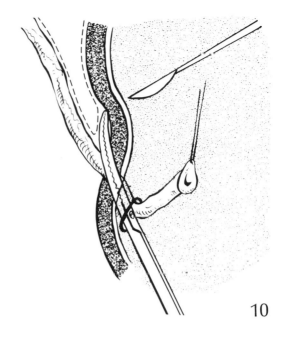

10

### 11

A second pair of forceps is grasped by the first and is led into the lower orifice in the bladder. The ureteric stay-suture is then gently drawn up into the bladder, bringing the ureter into its new entrance.

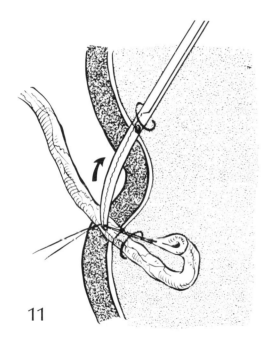

11

### 12

The new submucosal tunnel is fashioned by blunt scissor dissection between the old hiatus and the new. This is similar to the technique already described. Once this has been adequately prepared, the stay-suture on the ureter is grasped and gently threaded through the new tunnel.

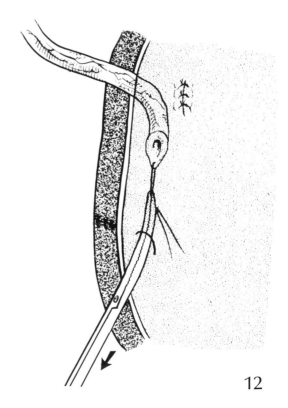

12

# 13

The end of the ureter is excised and is then spatulated. The ureter is now sutured back into the site of the original meatus.

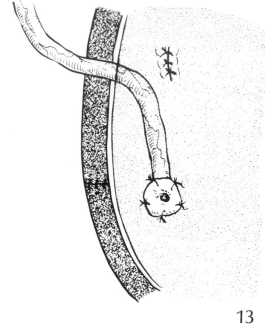

13

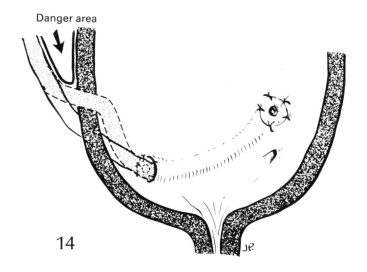

14

# 14

This shows the difference between the two techniques. The stippled ureter indicates the method of Politano–Leadbetter and shows its new hiatus of entrance and new tunnel down to the original meatus; the danger area indicated by the arrow is where the unwary may accidentally and unknowingly open the peritoneum and damage the adjacent organs (bowel, ovary, fallopian tube, etc). In the cross-trigonal method one can see clearly why these problems do not arise and how the new ureteral tunnel is a gentle extension of the curve of the ureter.

## THE LICHE–GREGOIR TECHNIQUE

# 15

This is the only purely extravesical technique still used and it is only applicable in certain conditions; it cannot be used in severely dilated ureters. The Liche–Gregoir technique exposes the bladder in the normal way and then rotates it to the opposite side and slightly forward. The ureter is exposed by dividing the obliterated umbilical artery and the few vessels which cross the ureter at this point. Once the ureter has been exposed, the incision is made as indicated by the dotted line. Note that this is on the back wall of the bladder.

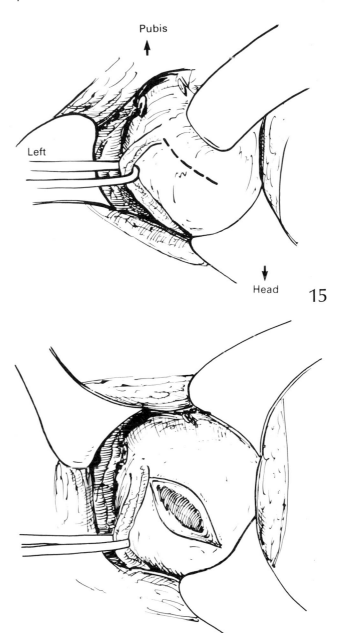

# 16

The incision is carried down to the bladder mucosa, taking care not to injure the mucosa, and freeing the muscle sufficiently to allow the mucosa to fall away; the muscle can then be sutured over the ureter. An important point is that the dissection must be carried out well down to the junctional area between the ureter and the bladder musculature; a shelf must not be left here.

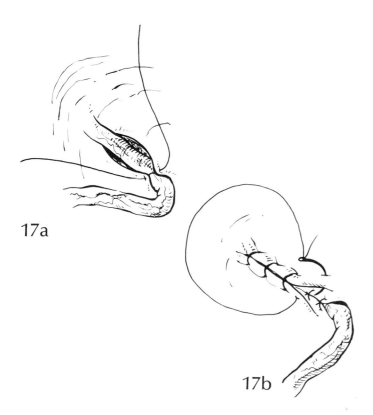

# 17

Once this is carried out, resuturing commences. Interrupted Dexon sutures are inserted, beginning at the proximal end of the tunnel as indicated, and making sure the ureter is not constricted by the sutures. A two-layer closure is recommended and care must be taken to ensure that the ureter is not strangulated anywhere along its reimplanted length. The bladder is then allowed to fall back into its position and the ureter assumes its natural course, but with a longer submucosal segment. The problem with this technique is that it can only be used in moderately dilated ureters.

## REIMPLANTATION OF THE GROSSLY DILATED URETER

# 18

A No. 8 feeding tube is passed up the ureter and sutured in position with Dexon. The ureter may be mobilized sufficiently from within the bladder (see Dissection, page 514) but if any difficulty is encountered a combined intra- and extravesical dissection is carried out[12]. The ureter having been dissected out, is then exposed extravesically and drawn into the extravesical space, but retaining the catheter through the hiatus to facilitate later repositioning. All kinks and bends must be straightened out, taking care not to damage the blood supply, and also keeping as much periureteric alveolar tissue as possible. This dissection often produces an excessive length of dilated ureter, which can be shortened to an adequate length.

Having ascertained exactly where the main blood vessels run, the object is to excise the excess and redundant ureter along the dotted line and also to excise any excess length (this includes the stenosed area in cases of obstruction).

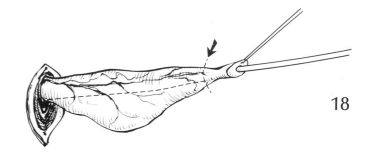

**18**

# 19

Hendren clamps are applied and the incision made as indicated[11].

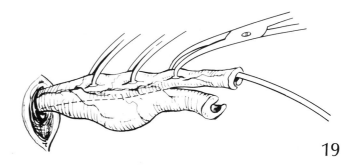

**19**

# 20

The ureter is reconstituted using a continuous Dexon suture, preferably of an inverting or Connel type. In addition the writer usually inserts a few interrupted sutures as well, to make sure that the ureter does not dehisce. The newly remodelled ureter is now ready for reimplantation as in the transtrigonal method, page 514. If the dissection has been carried out extravesically, then traction on the feeding tube will resite the ureter into its old entrance and the transtrigonal procedure can be carried out.

Some surgeons prefer to use the Politano–Leadbetter technique for reimplantation after the above remodelling (see page 517). Bladder closure is as described on page 516, but the use of ureteric stents is obligatory.

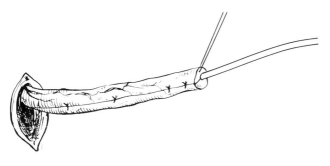

**20**

# Conclusions

Reimplantation of the ureters is recognized as a method of correcting vesicoureteric reflux and obstructed megaureters. Its efficacy has been proven over the last decade and success should be expected in virtually all cases. The complication rate is being reduced steadily, and stands currently at only 1–4 per cent. Unfortunately complications are more common in those cases where there was originally gross dilatation of the ureters, or where the bladder was thickened and trabeculated due to a neurogenic abnormality or to previous outflow obstruction.

## References

1. Dwoskin, J. Y., Perlmutter, A. D. (1973) Vesicoureteral reflux in children: A computerised review. Journal of Urology, 109, 888–890

2. Heikel, P. E., Parkkulainen, K. V. (1966) Vesico-ureteric reflux in children: a classification and results of conservative treatment. Annales de Radiologie (Paris), 9, 37–40

3. Smellie, J., Edwards, D., Hunter, N., Normand, I. C. S. Prescod, N. (1975) Vesicoureteric reflux and renal scarring. Kidney International, 8, Suppl 4, 565–572

4. Hutch, J. A. (1963) Ureteric advancement operation: anatomy, technique and early results. Journal of Urology, 89, 180–184

5. Politano, V. A., Leadbetter, W. F. (1958) An operative technique for the correction of vesicoureteral reflux. Journal of Urology, 79, 932–941

6. Paquin, A. J. Jr. (1959) Ureterovesical anastomosis: the description and evaluation of a technique. Journal of Urology, 82, 573–583

7. Glen, J. F., Anderson, E. E. (1967) Distal tunnel ureteral reimplantation. Journal of Urology, 97, 623–626

8. Gregoir. W., Van Regemorter, G. (1964) Le reflux vésico-urétéral congenital. Urologia Internationalis, 18, 122–136

9. Cohen, S. J. (1975) Ureterozystoneostomie: eine neue antirefluxtechnik. Aktuelle Urologie, 6, 1–6

10. O'Donnell, B., Puri, P. (1986) Endoscopic correction of primary vesicoureteric reflux. British Journal of Urology, 58, 601–604

11. Hendren, W. H. (1969) Operative repair of megaureter in children. Journal of Urology, 101, 491–507

12. Ahmed, S. (1980) Transverse advancement ureteral reimplantation: pull-through alternative in megaloureter. Journal of Urology, 123, 218–221

# Endoscopic correction of vesicoureteric reflux using subureteric teflon injection

**Prem Puri** MS, FACS
Associate Paediatric Surgeon, Our Lady's Hospital for Sick Children, Crumlin, Dublin, Eire;
Consultant Paediatric Surgeon, National Children's Hospital, Dublin, Eire;
Lecturer in Paediatric Research, University College Dublin

**Barry O'Donnell** MCh, FRCS, FAAP(Hon)
Professor of Paediatric Surgery, Royal College of Surgeons in Ireland, Dublin, Eire; Consultant Paediatric Surgeon,
Our Lady's Hospital for Sick Children, Crumlin, Dublin, Eire

## Introduction

Primary vesicoureteric reflux is due to congenital absence or deficiency of the longitudinal muscle of the submucosal ureter. This results in upward and lateral displacement of the ureteric orifice during micturition, thereby reducing length and obliquity of the submucosal ureter. It is generally agreed that vesicoureteric reflux in a dilated system is unlikely to cease spontaneously in most cases, and is therefore a surgical problem. Recently reflux induced in piglets was corrected by subureteric injection of Mentor Polytef paste.[1] Subsequently this technique has been used successfully to treat primary and secondary vesicoureteric reflux in children by endoscopic injection of Polytef paste.[2–6]

The procedure consists of endoscopic injection of the paste into the lamina propria behind the submucosal ureter. The Polytef particles stimulate an ingrowth of fibroblasts at the site of injection, which helps to hold the particles within the tissues.[7] The subureteric Polytef mass is encapsulated by a thin layer of fibrous tissue, which provides a firm anchorage to the submucosal ureter and prevents it from sliding upwards and outwards during micturition, thus preventing reflux. Mentor Polytef paste has been used for 25 years by otolaryngologists to enlarge displaced or deformed vocal cords in patients with dysphonia[8, 9] and by urologists to treat urinary incontinence.[10, 11] No untoward side-effects from these uses of Polytef paste in man have been reported.

# Preoperative

### Indications

The indications for endoscopic correction of vesico-ureteric reflux are the same as for open antireflux operations. It is generally agreed that lesser grades of reflux (grade I or II international classification) can be managed conservatively. Grade III reflux is conservatively managed unless there are 'breakthrough infections' while on antimicrobial therapy, or poor compliance on medical management. Children with grade IV or V vesicoureteric reflux are by general convention considered candidates for surgery.

## EQUIPMENT

# 1

Mentor Polytef paste is a suspension of biologically inert polytetrafluoroethylene particles in glycerin. The glycerin is 50 per cent of the paste by weight. After injection, the glycerin is absorbed into the tissues and the Polytef implant achieves firm consistency, retaining its shape and position at the injection site.

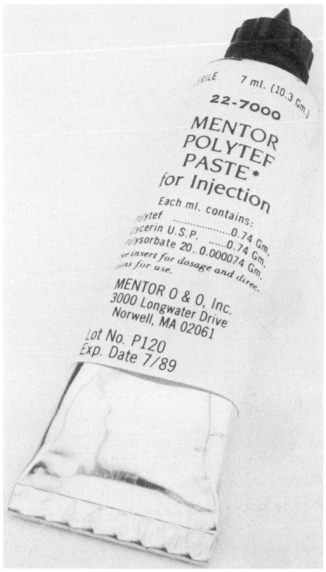

1

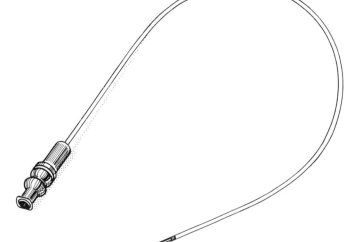

## INSTRUMENTS

# 2

The disposable Puri catheter for teflon injection (Storz) is a 5 Fr nylon catheter onto which is swaged a 21-gauge needle with 1 cm of the needle protruding from the catheter. Alternatively a rigid needle can be used.

2

# 3

A 1 ml tuberculin syringe is filled with Polytef paste, and is then enclosed in the metal syringe holder, which assures a secure connection between syringe and injection catheter. Using the metal piston which comes with the metal syringe holder the injection catheter is filled with Polytef paste.

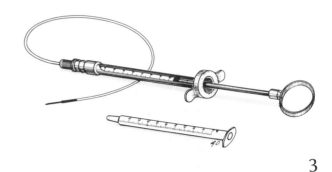

**3**

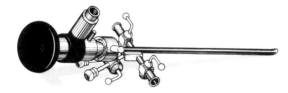

**4a**

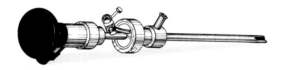

**4b**

# 4a, b & c

All cystoscopes available for infants and children can be used for this procedure. The injection catheter can be introduced through a 14 Fr or 11 Fr Storz cystoscope (a) or 13 Fr Wolf cystoscope (b). There is a specially designed instrument made by Wolf 'The Stinger' (11.5 Fr) (c) through which a rigid needle or injection catheter can be used for injection.

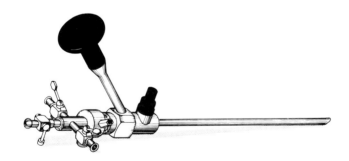

**4c**

## TECHNIQUE

The patient should be placed in a forward lithotomy position with the thighs flexed to 45°. The cystoscope is passed and the bladder wall, the trigone, bladder neck, and both ureteric orifices inspected. The bladder should be almost empty before proceeding with injection, since this helps to keep the ureteric orifice flat rather than away in a lateral part of the field.

# 5

When using Storz or Wolf cystoscopes, it is necessary to pass the injection catheter with the telescope removed.

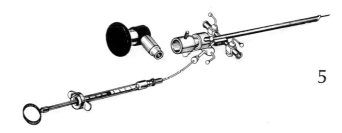

5

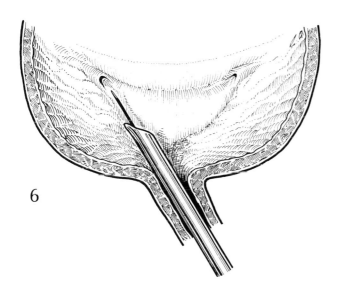

6

# 6

The injection of Polytef paste should not begin until the operator has a clear view all around the ureteric orifice. Under direct vision through the cystoscope the needle is introduced under the bladder mucosa 3–4 mm below the affected ureteric orifice at the 6 o'clock position.

# 7

The needle is advanced about 8 mm into the lamina propria beneath the submucosal ureter and 0.2–0.5 ml of paste is injected. It is important to introduce the needle with pinpoint accuracy. Perforation of the mucosa or the ureter may allow the paste to escape and may result in a failure. As the injection begins, a bulge appears in the floor of the submucosal ureter and gradually increases in size as more paste is injected. Occasionally one may need to inject a little more than 0.5 ml of paste, but the total amount should never exceed 1 ml.

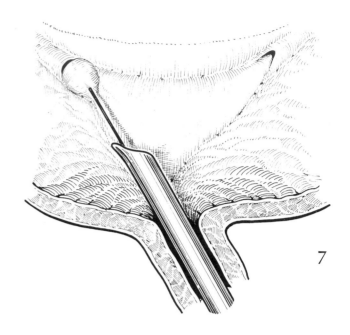

7

# 8

A correctly placed injection creates the appearance of a nipple on the top of which is a slit-like or inverted crescentic orifice. If the bulge appears in an incorrect place, e.g. at the side of the ureter or proximal to it, the needle should not be withdrawn, but should be moved so that the point is in a more favourable position. The non-injected ureteric roof retains its compliance while preventing reflux.

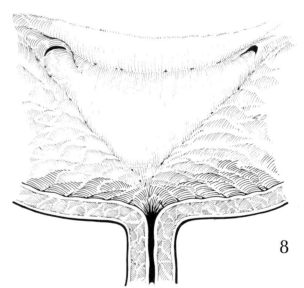

8

## Postoperative care

Postoperative urethral catheterization is not necessary. Loose Polytef paste in the bladder is harmless and is passed out painlessly. The majority of patients are treated as day cases. Co-trimoxazole is prescribed for 2 weeks after the procedure. A micturating cystogram and renal ultrasound are performed 3 months after discharge. A follow-up micturating cystogram and an intravenous urogram are obtained at 12 months following endoscopic correction of reflux.

### COMPLICATIONS

Procedure-related complications are rare. The only complication with this procedure has been failure. This may be initial failure, i.e. the reflux is not abolished by the injection, or recurrence, where initial correction is not maintained. About 20 per cent of refluxing ureters require more than one endoscopic injection of Polytef paste to correct the condition.

## References

1. Puri, P., O'Donnell, B. (1984) Correction of experimentally produced vesicoureteric reflux in the piglet by intravesical injection of Teflon. British Medical Journal, 289, 5–7

2. O'Donnell, R., Puri, P. (1984) Treatment of vesicoureteric reflux by endoscopic injection of Teflon. British Medical Journal, 289, 7–9

3. Puri, P., Guiney, E. J. (1986) Endoscopic correction of vesicoureteric reflux secondary to neuropathic bladder. British Journal of Urology, 58, 504–506

4. O'Donnell, B., Puri, P. (1986) Endoscopic correction of primary vesicoureteric reflux: results in 94 ureters. British Medical Journal, 293, 1404–1406

5. Puri, P., O'Donnell, B. (1986) Endoscopic correction of grades IV and V primary vesicoureteric reflux: Six to 30 month follow-up in 42 ureters. Journal of Pediatric Surgery, 22, 1087–1091

6. Schulman, C. C. (1986) Traitement endoscopique du reflux vésico-urétéral chez l'enfant. Chirurgie Pediatrique, 27, 181–184

7. Stone, J. W., Arnold, G. E. (1967) Human larynx injected with Teflon paste. Histologic study of innervation and tissue reaction. Archives of Otolaryngology, 86, 550–561

8. Arnold, G. E. (1963) Alleviation of aphonia or dysphonia through intrachordal injection of Teflon paste. Annals of Otology, Rhinology and Laryngology, 72, 384–395

9. Lewy, R. B. (1976) Experience with vocal cord injection. Annals of Otology, Rhinology and Laryngology, 85, 440–450

10. Schulman, C. C., Simon, J., Wespes, E., Germeau, F. (1984) Endoscopic injections of Teflon to treat urinary incontinence in women. British Medical Journal, 288, 192

11. Vorstman, B., Lockhart, J., Kaufmann, M., Politano, V. (1985) Polytetrafluoroethylene injection for urinary incontinence in children. Journal of Urology, 133, 248–250

Illustrations by Philip Wilson

# Ureteric duplication

**Robert H. Whitaker**  MD, MChir, FRCS
Consultant Paediatric Urologist, Addenbrooke's Hospital, Cambridge, and Associate Lecturer,
University of Cambridge, Cambridge, UK

Although there are exceptions, most ureteric duplications conform to a definite pattern of anomalies. Many are incidental findings with little or no clinical importance, and symptoms are often too easily attributed to them. A general principle is that the upper ureter drains only the upper pole group of calices, while the lower ureter drains the middle and lower calices. All such anomalies are more common in girls and are frequently bilateral.

A combination of ultrasound, intravenous urography and micturition cystography gives an accurate diagnosis in the vast majority of children with duplications, and cystoscopy is usually superfluous and unwarranted.

# SIMPLE DUPLICATION

## Partial duplication

### 1

The ureters may join anywhere between the renal pelvis and the bladder; it is unusual for such anomalies to have any clinical significance. Occasionally the symptoms or urographic appearances may suggest incoordinate emptying (yo-yo reflux) so that one or other moiety becomes permanently or intermittently dilated, leading to stasis, infection or stone formation. This can be demonstrated by fluoroscopy or radionuclide studies, and in such instances surgery may be needed to avoid further dilatation or infection. The problem is solved by removing the upper pole ureter down to the ureteroureteric junction and anastomosing it at a higher level to the lower pole pelvis as a ureteropelvicostomy or bifid pelvis.

Such a partially duplicated ureter is neither more nor less likely to be affected by vesicoureteric reflux than any other ureter. However, if reflux does occur in a ureter that becomes duplex just outside the bladder, it may be necessary to reimplant the two ureters in their common sheath but as two orifices.

Pelviureteric junction obstruction may occur in the lower half of a duplex system but almost never in the upper moiety. Pyeloplasty can be difficult if the ureters join high up and a lower pole partial nephrectomy may be needed.

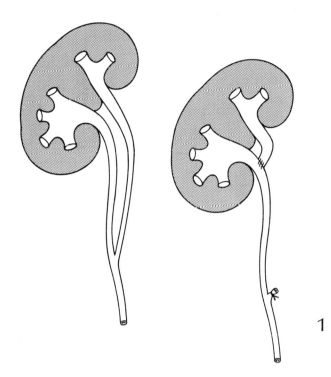

1

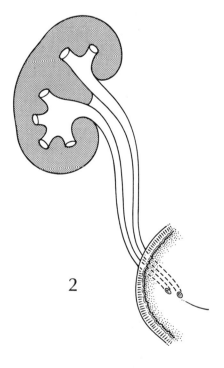

2

## Complete duplication

### 2

When both ureters enter the bladder separately, the duplication is complete and the ureteric orifices are close together on the trigone. If the upper pole ureter opens towards the bladder neck or beyond, it is ectopic (see below). In all cases, however, the upper pole ureteric orifice is situated medially and below the lower pole ureteric orifice. There are adequate embryological explanations for this.

If a child with a simple complete duplication is asymptomatic and free from urinary tract infections, and the urographic appearances are normal (apart from the duplication), there is no indication for further investigation. If reflux is suspected, a micturating cystogram should be obtained. Even with a normal kidney, reflux may occur into the lower pole ureter because of its more direct course through the bladder wall. If reflux occurs into both ureters, it is likely that they join just outside the bladder and that the reflux is into a common stem.

# 3

More commonly, the lower pole of the duplex kidney shows evidence of reflux nephropathy and is small and scarred. If reflux is confirmed by a micturating cystogram, a decision must be made whether an operation is required. The following possibilities exist.

1. *Reimplantation of the two ureters* in their common sheath (*a*). This is appropriate if the lower pole is worth preserving since this type of reflux is less likely to cease spontaneously than reflux into a single ureter. Although theoretically this jeopardizes the non-refluxing upper pole ureter, in practice, with a reliable method such as the Cohen technique, the success rate in preventing reflux should be in excess of 95 per cent.
2. *Partial nephrectomy.* If the lower pole is severely damaged, it is best to perform a lower pole partial nephrectomy with removal of the lower pole ureter as low as possible (*b*). It passes into a common sheath with the upper pole ureter but can be excised below this level by leaving a thin strip of its mucosa attached to the good ureter and carefully using a purse-string suture to close off its lower limit. Even then a small stump of ureter may be left, but this is better than jeopardizing the good upper pole ureter by dissecting any lower.
3. *Ureteroureterostomy.* If the lower pole is worth preserving but a reimplant is contraindicated, then it is best to excise the lower pole ureter and join the two renal pelves or upper ureters together (*c*).

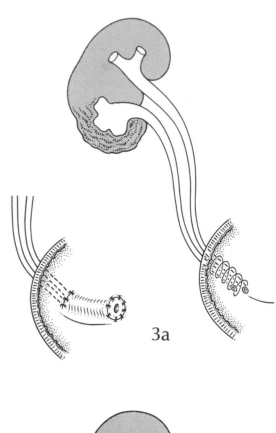

3a

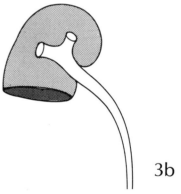

3b

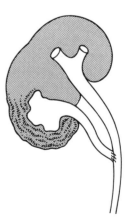

3c

# COMPLETE DUPLICATION WITH ECTOPIC URETER

When the ureteric orifice of the upper pole ureter is situated more ectopically along the trigone towards the bladder neck (*see Illustration 4a*, position A, B or C), the lower pole ureter becomes normal and reflux into it is much less likely. Conversely, the upper pole itself is more likely to be dysplastic or hydronephrotic. Thus the urogram alone showing the typical drooping-flower appearance is a good guide to the likely anatomical arrangement. However, a cystogram is still indicated to exclude reflux into the ectopic ureter, the ipsilateral ureter or the contralateral system. It also determines whether an ectopic ureterocele is present.

## Ectopic ureter at bladder neck

# 4a & b

This anomaly, seen more commonly in girls, is sometimes confirmed when the urethral catheter, passed to perform cystography, inadvertently enters the ectopic ureter. Resiting of the catheter in the bladder and introduction of contrast usually fails to show reflux in these patients. However, reflux into such a ureter low on the trigone or at the bladder neck is not so unusual, but equally the orifice may be narrow and the system obstructed.

The treatment of choice is partial nephroureterectomy, usually starting with an upper pole partial nephrectomy via a loin incision and then a lower ureterectomy via a lower abdominal incision. The ureter is removed as low as possible, but it is unwise to attempt to remove the last few millimetres if it is close to the bladder neck structures. In the acutely ill child with a closed system full of pus it may be necessary to institute urgent, but temporary, drainage by percutaneous puncture.

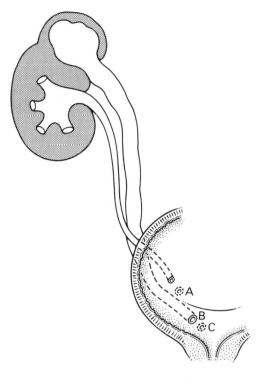

4a

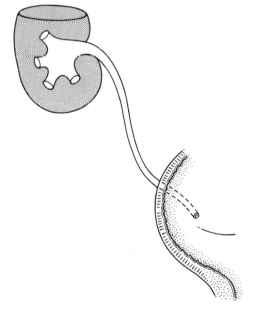

4b

# Ectopic ureterocele

The management of ectopic ureterocele (*see Illustration 5*) is controversial, but some guidelines can be put forward. Single-stage treatment is not necessarily appropriate for all children, since ectopic ureteroceles come in many shapes, sizes and positions. The characteristic features are summarized below.

1. The opening of the ureterocele is at or just beyond the bladder neck.
2. The ureterocele extends into the proximal urethra to a greater or lesser extent.
3. The ureter above it is usually grossly dilated and the upper pole of the kidney poorly functioning, hydronephrotic or dysplastic.
4. The ipsilateral ureteric orifice may be displaced on to the upper surface of the ureterocele and allow reflux.
5. There is frequently a duplex system on the opposite side, with either reflux or other complications and the ureterocele may even displace these ureters.
6. The condition is more common in girls and may be bilateral.

In addition, the ureterocele may cause outflow obstruction by occluding the bladder neck or even by prolapsing through the urethral meatus. Very occasionally, a ureterocele is small and almost orthotopic in situation with a good functioning moiety of kidney above it.

## Emergency treatment

In a severely ill child with an infected system, antibiotics may not produce resolution and it may be necessary to drain the pus. This can be done by percutaneous puncture of a dilated upper pole or by endoscopic resection of the ureterocele. For reasons discussed below, the latter procedure should not be embarked on lightly. After adequate drainage, one of the following operations will be needed. In children who have responded to antibiotics and do not need emergency drainage, either of these may be used as primary treatment.

## Radical operation

# 5a & b

The standard or classical operation for ectopic ureterocele (*a*) is partial nephroureterectomy with excision of the ureterocele and reimplantation of any refluxing ureters or the displaced ipsilateral ureter (*b*). This is a lengthy procedure necessitating two incisions, and the dissection of the distal ureterocele from the proximal urethra is often difficult and carries a risk of leaving a flap which can act as a valve.

This approach, however, is suitable for large or prolapsing ureteroceles and those associated with marked ipsilateral or contralateral reflux. The ipsilateral ureter can be reimplanted into the space left after excision of the ureterocele but it is probably best to take it across the trigone, or above it, by the Cohen technique. The defect left in the muscle after excision of the ureterocele must be closed.

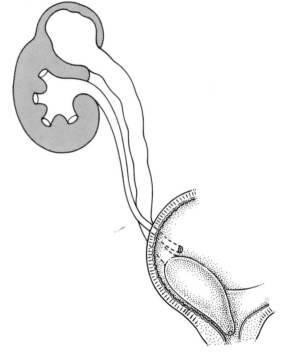

5a

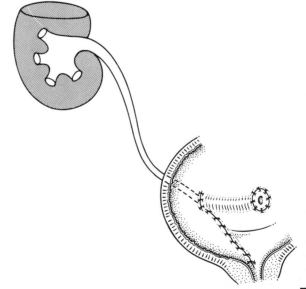

5b

## 6

### Limited operation

Many paediatric urologists now believe that it may only be necessary to perform an upper pole partial nephroureterectomy, leaving a lower portion of the ectopic ureter with its ureterocele *in situ,* and to drain the distal ureteric stump. This view is based on the belief that the ureterocele collapses and that any ill-effects the ureterocele may have had on the other ureters or bladder neck are reversed. Indeed, it is suggested that coincidental or secondary reflux may then cease spontaneously. This method has now been well assessed and 75 per cent of cases treated in this way give no further trouble on short-term follow up. The long-term risks of urinary tract infection or the development of malignancy in these residual ureteric stumps, which cannot be assessed radiologically, are as yet unknown. This method is ideal for cases in which there is no reflux and in which the ureterocele is relatively small, but clearly cannot be used after endoscopic resection of the ureterocele.

An alternative to partial nephrectomy in this situation, when the upper moiety of the kidney is functioning well, is a ureteropelvicostomy (*see Illustration 1*) with appropriate excision of the lower part of the ectopic ureter as outlined above.

## 7a & b

## Ectopic ureter opening outside the bladder

Males and females must be considered separately in this subgroup.

In females, the ectopic ureter can enter the urethra below the sphincter area, the vagina or the vulva; affected girls will be permanently wet between otherwise normal voids, but dryness at night *is* possible because of pooling in the abnormal system. The orifice may be difficult to find but the search is helped by filling the bladder with a dye and then looking for a source of clear urine. Upper pole partial nephrectomy with excision of the ureter as low as possible in the pelvis is curative.

Boys are never continuously wet as a result of an ectopic ureter since the ureter never enters the urethra below the sphincter. However, there may be a spurious wetness due to urine pooling in the urethra from an ectopic ureter entering in the posterior urethra. Alternatively, the ureter may enter the ejaculatory duct, seminal vesicle or vas, resulting in epididymitis or occasionally, in older boys, in haemospermia. Typically, there is a multilocular mass felt rectally. The treatment in all such cases is partial nephroureterectomy. The ureter should be excised as low as possible but extensive dissection should be avoided to minimize damage to the ejaculatory mechanisms. The vas should be ligated on the affected side if the ureter enters the seminal tract.

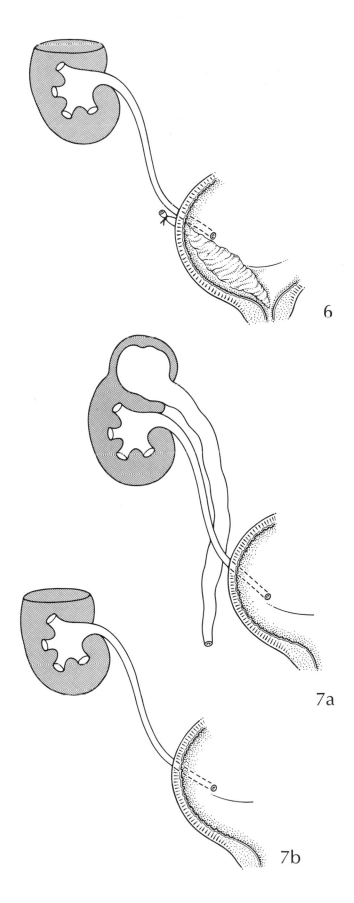

6

7a

7b

# Urinary diversion

**I. S. Kirkland**   FRCS (Ed), FRCS (Glas)
Lately Consultant Paediatric Surgeon, Edinburgh, UK

## Introduction

Urinary diversion may be indicated:

Temporarily for (1) gross vesicoureteric reflux; (2) ureterovesical obstruction; (3) intractable infection; (4) some urethral obstructions.
Permanently for (1) neuropathic bladder; (2) ectopia vesicae; (3) cystectomy.

Diversion can be achieved by constructing an ileal or sigmoid loop conduit to which the ureters are attached by ureteroileal or ureterosigmoid anastomosis, provided that the anal sphincters are intact. There is a growing tendency, when anal continence is assured, to anastomose the ureters directly to the sigmoid, leaving the sigmoid loop in continuity. In these procedures an antireflux type of anastomosis of ureter-to-bowel is made.

Cutaneous ureterostomy should be considered, especially with a unilateral kidney and ureter, but the social implications of bilateral cutaneous ureterostomy must be considered. In the author's experience this procedure appears to offer the best long-term outlook for the preservation of renal function. Temporary urinary diversion by percutaneous pyelostomy under ultrasound control can be undertaken to improve renal function reduced by obstruction or intractable infection.

Permanent nephrostomy and cystostomy are now rarely used.

The author's preference is to construct either an ileal loop conduit or a ureterostomy. The ileal loop is preferred because of its greater intrinsic activity and the relative sterility of its lumen compared with the colon. There is much less risk of reabsorption of urine from the ileal loop.

Long-term follow-up after 10–20 years of patients with an ileal conduit show a significant number (up to 70 per cent) of deteriorating renal units from infection and obstruction. Careful selection and regular long-term follow-up are essential for patients with this type of operation. Diversion should be undertaken before the upper urinary tract is dilated.

The introduction of Silastic balloon catheters which can remain indwelling, or intermittent clean catheterization, may avoid diversion, and the construction of a Silastic urethral 'sphincter' holds promise for the future in patients with complete urinary incontinence.

# ILEAL LOOP CONDUIT DIVERSION

## Preoperative

The most convenient site for the stoma should be determined, taking into account the contour of the abdominal wall, the effect of scoliosis, the degree of lower-limb paralysis which may necessitate the wearing of calipers, and the ability of the patient to look after the stoma. Urostomy bags should be applied to test the suitability of the chosen site for retention of the bag. A stoma therapist is invaluable both at this stage and later to help the family cope with management.

It is convenient that the ileal loop should be free from faecal content. This can be achieved in the ileum by two days' treatment with Senokot syrup and the introduction of an elemental diet with half-strength Vivonex, depending on the age of the patient.

As the operation can take up to 2 hours, and there is a possibility of postoperative intestinal ileus, it is wise to have an intravenous line available to ensure adequate preoperative and postoperative fluid intake.

# The operation

# 1 & 2

### The incision

A transverse skin-crease incision more to the left side than the right is made about midway between the umbilicus and pubic crest. This is deepened by diathermy through rectus sheath and rectus muscles, controlling the inferior epigastric vessels on either side, and dividing the urachus between ligatures. The fascia transversalis is then divided in the line of the incision and the peritoneal cavity entered. (Some surgeons prefer a midline incision, particularly in the younger patient, to be sure of keeping the scar clear of the area to which the adhesive for the bag will be applied.)

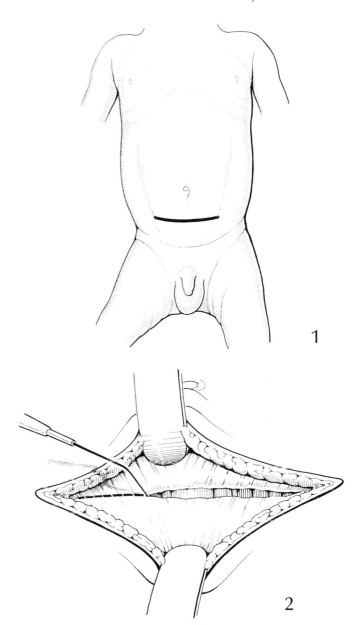

# 3

### Division of ileum

The caecum and terminal ileum are identified and turned upwards to identify the distal ileal branch of the superior mesenteric artery before it divides into upper and lower branches. A suitable length of ileum, as short as is practicable, is selected to form a conduit and double clamps applied before the ileum is divided by diathermy. The upper branch of the ileal artery is divided between ligatures and the distal branch at a suitable point where it anastomoses with the ileal branch of the ileocaecal artery. The mesentery is then divided to the point of origin of the ileal artery. Adequate blood supply to the isolated ileal loop is determined at this time. The venous return follows the arterial supply very closely.

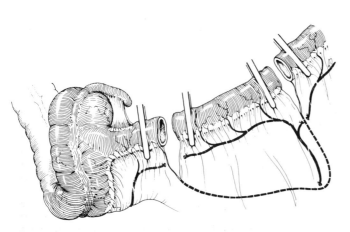

3

## 4

### Ileal reconstitution

The ileal lumen is reconstituted by end-to-end anastomosis with interrupted 3/0 silk sutures in one layer, and the cut ends of the mesentery are also approximated with interrupted silk sutures. Appendicectomy is usually performed.

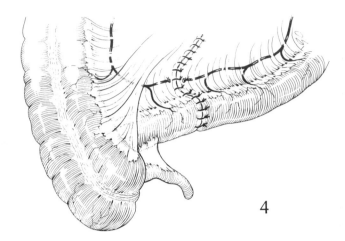

4

## 5

### Division of ureter

The proximal end of the isolated ileal loop is closed with two layers of interrupted silk sutures, using 2/0 silk on an atraumatic needle.

The left ureter is identified through the pelvic mesocolon, exposed and dissected down as near as is possible to its junction with the bladder, making sure that the adventitia on the medial aspect is disturbed as little as necessary to ensure an adequate blood supply. The ureter is divided, its distal stump being closed with a transfixing suture of 2/0 silk. The ureter is dissected proximally to allow sufficient length to reach beyond the promontory of the sacrum. Its free end is 'fish-tailed' for about 0.5 cm. A longitudinal incision 1.5 cm long is made in the seromuscular coat of the ileum at its antimesenteric border. At the distal end a small opening is made in the mucosa to reach the lumen of the ileal loop.

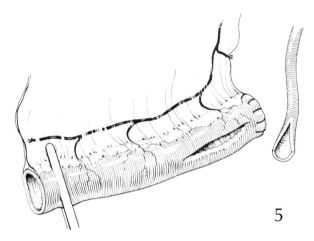

5

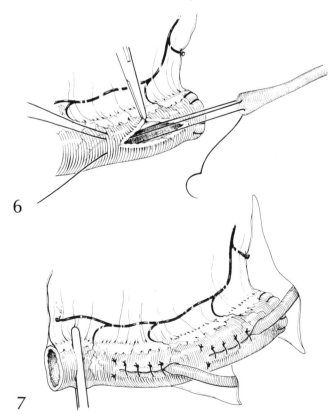

6

## 6 & 7

### Anastomosis of ureters

Anastomosis of the left ureter is then accomplished by a simple two-stitch method as shown in the illustration – again using 2/0 silk sutures. The seromuscular coat is closed with interrupted 2/0 silk sutures over the course of the ureter, creating a tunnel. The right ureter is identified as it passes over the pelvic brim at the division of the right common iliac artery, and is thereafter dealt with similarly to the left ureter.

7

# 8

The uretero-ileal anastomoses are thereafter covered with parietal peritoneum.

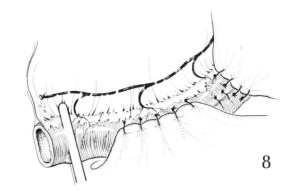

# 9a & b

## Construction of stoma

The distal end of the ileal loop is brought through a separate abdominal incision above and to the right of the original incision (excision of a circle of skin reduces the risk of stenosis). A few interrupted 2/0 silk sutures attach the ileal conduit to the lateral abdominal wall below the caecum.

The free end of the ileal conduit is fixed to the skin with four sutures placed as shown to leave a 'spout'.

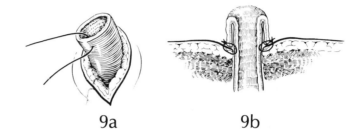

9a                9b

# 10

## Closure of wound

The abdominal wound is closed in layers with continuous 2/0 chromic catgut for the peritoneum, interrupted Dexon sutures for the muscle, sheath and subcutaneous layers, and a subcuticular 4/0 Dexon suture for the skin.

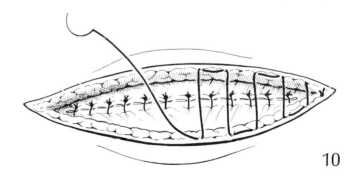

## Postoperative care

It is convenient to have a transparent collecting apparatus so that the state of the stoma can be inspected. Urinary output should be measured carefully and appropriate antibiotics are given if indicated. Although this operation does not cause much discomfort, early postoperative sedation should be considered.

## Potential complications

Early complications include urinary leak from the uretero-ileal anastomosis, arterial or venous infarction of the isolated ileal loop, intestinal obstruction from adhesions, and pyelonephritis. The late complications include uretero-ileal obstruction, stomal obstruction, calculi, intestinal obstruction, excessive length of ileal conduit from growth, and residual cystitis.

# CUTANEOUS URETEROSTOMY

Although various types of cutaneous ureterostomy are described, e.g. T-tube drainage, loop ureterostomy, the author prefers an end-ureterostomy, which affords free drainage.

## 11

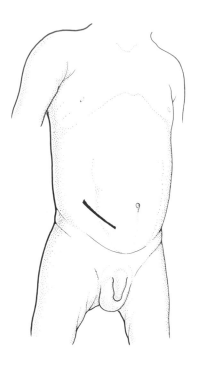

### The incision

A skin-crease incision is made in the right iliac fossa, and deepened through the muscle layers and transversalis fascia down to peritoneum in the same line as the skin wound.

The peritoneum is separated from the lateral and posterior abdominal wall to the point of division of the right common iliac artery. At this point the ureter can be identified closely adherent to the peritoneum. The ureter is dissected distally to as near the bladder as possible.

**11**

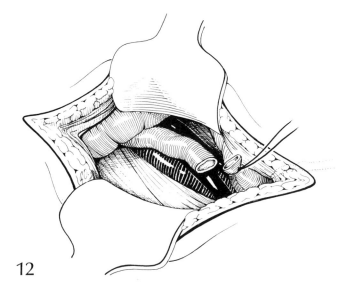

**12**

## 12

The ureter is then transfixed with a 2/0 silk suture, which is tied and the ureter is divided just proximal to the suture.

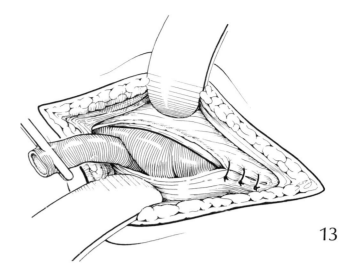

13

# 13 & 14

The ureter is brought to the upper end of the wound, which is closed in layers with interrupted 2/0 silk sutures.

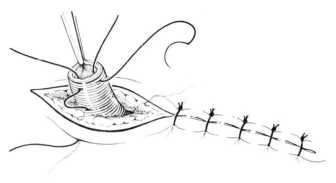

14

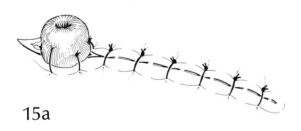

15a

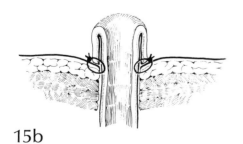

15b

# 15a & b

The ureter is everted to form a spout, using 2/0 silk sutures. A collecting urostomy bag can be applied immediately.

## BILATERAL URETEROSTOMY

When bilateral ureterostomy is indicated this operation can be carried out on each side. This has the disadvantage that two urostomy bags will have to be worn.

If the ureters are long enough and tortuous then both can be brought together at the midline as a double-barrelled ureterostomy.

# Results

Cutaneous ureterostomy can be trouble free for many years, allowing free drainage of the upper urinary tract. In young children, grossly dilated ureters with poor peristaltic activity can improve in size and function, so that urinary tract reconstruction may well be possible at a later date. In the author's experience this was possible after six years of bilateral cutaneous ureterostomy.

# Complications

The commonest complications are arterial infarction of the exteriorized ureter, stenosis of the ureter at the level of the external oblique aponeurosis, and stricture at the mucocutaneous junction, especially if retraction of the ureter occurs.

Illustrations for this chapter by Paul Andriesse

# Urinary diversion and undiversion

**W. Hardy Hendren**  MD, FACS
Chief of Surgery, The Children's Hospital, Boston; Visiting Surgeon, Massachusetts General Hospital; Robert E. Gross
Professor of Surgery, Harvard Medical School, Boston, USA

## Introduction

In the past decade the indications for urinary diversion in children have diminished greatly. For example from 1955 into the early 1970s many children with neuropathic bladders were diverted either to provide a means for getting the incontinent child dry, or to prevent upper urinary tract damage in those with vesicoureteral reflux[1-3]. Today many of these youngsters can be managed by intermittent catheterization to empty the bladder, and reconstructive measures such as ureteral reimplantation, narrowing the bladder neck, augmentation of the small, non-compliant bladder, and the use of artificial sphincters[4]. The author has not used artificial sphincters in young patients because many subsequently need revisional surgery for failure of the device or erosion of the bladder outlet. Similarly, many children with exstrophy of the bladder who were diverted formerly can now be functionally reconstructed. Boys with urethral valves are managed better today than in former years, and therefore fewer are diverted[5-7]. Various other uropathies which were formerly diverted have been amenable to functional repair as surgery has improved for ureteral reimplantation[8-11], repair of megaureters[12-17], bladder outlet reconstruction for continence, etc.

Similarly, techniques have changed considerably for diversion of the urinary tract in those who are presently not well suited for functional reconstruction, such as wheelchair-bound children with myelodysplasia, certain patients with exstrophy not suitable for reconstruction, children requiring removal of the bladder for sarcoma, and a variety of other malformations where normal ureteral drainage and bladder function cannot be achieved.

In 1950 Bricker[18] introduced the ileal-loop urinary diversion for patients undergoing radical pelvic surgery for cancer. Soon after, the ileal loop was being used widely in children with the urological problems described above. Long-term follow-up of ileal loops in young patients, however, showed an unacceptable incidence of recurrent bacilluria, progressive upper-tract deterioration, and stone formation[19-26].

Laboratory studies on dogs showed a high rate of pyelonephritis from reflux in renal segments diverted with an ileal loop (82 per cent) as compared to much better preservation when diversion was performed with a reflux-preventing colon conduit urinary diversion (7 per cent pyelonephritis)[27, 28]. Since 1971 in those relatively few children requiring cutaneous diversion of urine we have carried out the procedure with a colon segment which does not allow reflux[29-34].

# REFLUX-PREVENTING COLON-CONDUIT URINARY DIVERSION

The bowel is thoroughly prepared preoperatively. This can be done using a clear liquid diet for at least three days, cleansing enemas, and antibiotic preparation of the bowel. More recently we have used copious bowel lavage with Go-Lytely*. This is a polyethylene glycol electrolyte gastrointestinal lavage solution which passes quickly through the bowel, cleansing it thoroughly.

## TECHNIQUE FOR COLON CONDUIT

### 1

A segment of colon, usually sigmoid, is selected after carefully assessing the blood supply. The mesentery of the conduit should be maintained as broad as possible, incising the mesentery only enough to give sufficient mobility to anchor the conduit at the desired location. The bowel segment should be of ample length to allow for some shortening from contraction of the taenia, especially when it is contemplated that the conduit may be taken down at a future date, resecting the stoma, and joining the conduit to either the colon or the bladder. If the sigmoid colon is not satisfactory (previous pull-through procedure, malrotation, etc.) a segment from the descending, transverse, or ascending colon can be used.

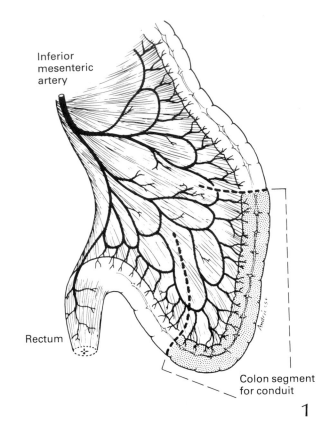

1

### 2

The proximal end of the conduit is closed with two layers of chromic catgut. Permanent, non-absorbable sutures are not used because of the risk of stone formation.

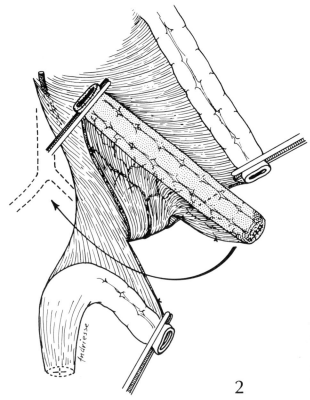

2

* Braintree Laboratories, Braintree, Massachusetts, USA

## 3

The conduit is rotated 180 degrees clockwise and is anchored at the aortic bifurcation above the sacral promontory when both ureters are of normal length. Colon continuity is re-established, generally taking down the splenic flexure to be sure that this anastomosis is without tension. Mesenteric traps should be closed. Note how the ureters lie adjacent to the base of the conduit. When the ureters are mobilized, their adventitia should be preserved to ensure a good blood supply.

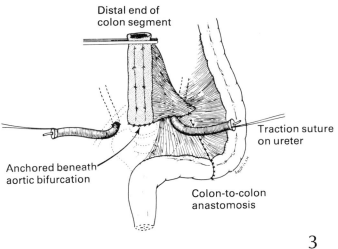

Distal end of colon segment

Anchored beneath aortic bifurcation

Traction suture on ureter

Colon-to-colon anastomosis

3

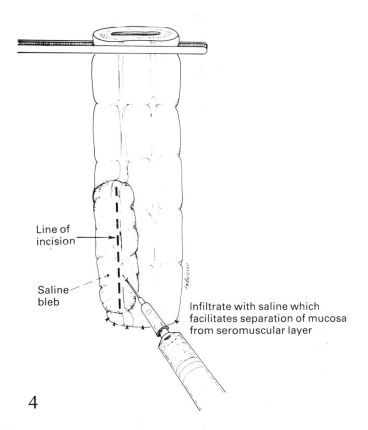

Line of incision

Saline bleb

Infiltrate with saline which facilitates separation of mucosa from seromuscular layer

4

## 4

Saline is injected with a 25 gauge needle to facilitate raising the lateral seromuscular flap from the underlying mucosa.

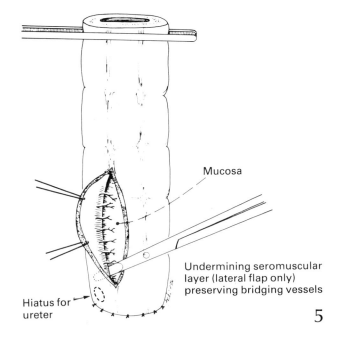

Mucosa

Undermining seromuscular layer (lateral flap only) preserving bridging vessels

Hiatus for ureter

5

## 5

The lateral seromuscular flap is raised, bringing into view the small vessels running from the seromuscular layer to the underlying mucosa. Blunt dissection is performed, which can be facilitated with a peanut gauze held in a curved haemostat. In some cases the seromuscular flap is not easy to raise from the underlying mucosa.

# 6

The ureter is brought through a separate opening of adequate size in the seromuscular layer, or through the end of the opening made when raising the flap. It is placed beneath the bridging vessels; this is a part of the bowel wall that is perhaps a little better supported, for it lies in the mesentery. However, it may be just as satisfactory to lay the ureter on top of those vessels as beneath them. The ureter is cut straight across, not spatulated, and is anastomosed end-to-side with an opening in the colon mucosa. The opening in the colon mucosa should be small, for it tends to enlarge as the anastomosis proceeds. Interrupted 5/0 or 6/0 chromic sutures are used. Forceps handling of the ureter should be minimal.

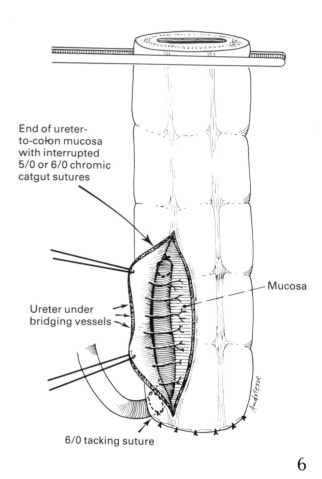

End of ureter-to-colon mucosa with interrupted 5/0 or 6/0 chromic catgut sutures

Mucosa

Ureter under bridging vessels

6/0 tacking suture

6

Stoma

Closure of ureter-to-colon mucosa

Closure of seromuscular layer

Ureter in submucosal tunnel 4–5 cm long

Ureter enters tunnel between seromuscular layer and mucosa

End of loop anchored beneath aortic bifurcation

7

# 7

The completed conduit with submucosal ureteric tunnels 4–5 cm long is shown. The seromuscular flap closure is usually performed using a running, fine non-absorbable suture. The author uses a coloured suture so that the location of the ureterosigmoid tunnel can be seen on the outside of the bowel by external inspection at a later time – for example if the conduit is to be taken down from the abdominal wall and implanted into the colon or bladder. If the two ureters are implanted at the same level in the colon, it is important not to raise the seromuscular flap on both sides of the tunnel, as this could lead to necrosis of that segment of colon wall between the two implants. A drainage stent catheter is not used unless the ureter is dilated and requires tapering. If a drainage stent catheter is passed up to a kidney, it should be fastened to the ostium with a fine catgut suture to hold it in place for a few days. Ureteral peristalsis can dislodge a catheter if it is not secured. Obviously, the anchoring suture should be very fine, so that it will break when the catheter is extracted.

## 8

The completed conduit is shown. No attempt is made to close the space on either side of the conduit, but mesenteric traps are closed. The stoma can be on the left side, the midline, or right side, depending on the location of the laparotomy incision, or whether there was a previous ileal loop, etc. In a previously unoperated case, the author usually makes a right paramedian laparotomy incision and places the stoma on the left, on the belt line, which is satisfactory for an appliance. The bud should be fashioned as a turn-back stoma so that it will protrude slightly. Subcuticular absorbable sutures are used between the bowel edge and skin. Skin sutures should be avoided as they tend to form scar around the stoma, which can cause a poor fit and subsequent leakage from the appliance.

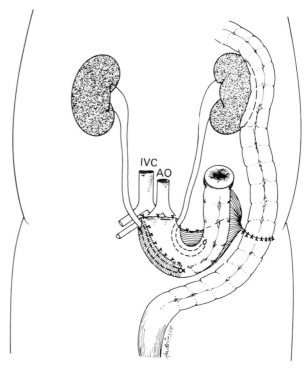

8

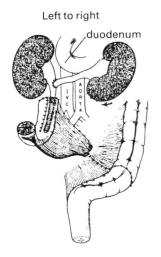

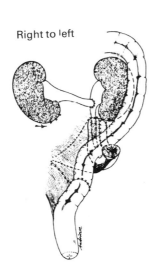

Left to right        Right to left

9

## VARIATIONS FOR SPECIAL CIRCUMSTANCES

## 9

### When one ureter is too short

Sometimes the patient will not have two good ureters to be tunnelled. In that case the better ureter can be used to perform a tunnel, draining the second across the abdomen as a transureteroureterostomy or transuretero-pyelostomy. The conduit is not rotated. The butt end of the conduit is brought high in the right or left gutter, close to the renal pelvis, to attain a tunnel of maximum length.

# 10

## Tapering a dilated ureter

If the ureter is very dilated it can be tapered as shown, taking care not to make it too narrow lest its blood supply be jeopardized. When a ureter is tapered the upper tract should be drained for 10–12 days using a soft plastic catheter.

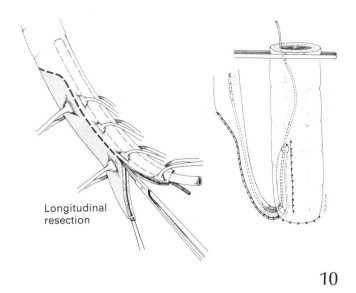

Longitudinal resection

**10**

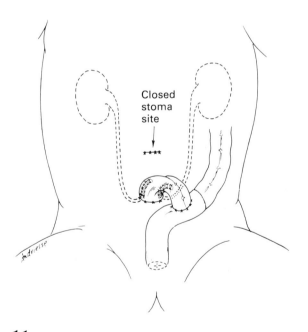

Closed stoma site

**11**

# 11

## Implantation of colon conduit back into the colon

This is suitable in patients who have normal rectal control (e.g. some patients who have undergone anterior pelvic exenteration for malignancy, and bladder exstrophy patients deemed unsuitable for primary bladder reconstruction. It is not suitable for patients with myelodysplasia)[35, 36]. The non-refluxing colon conduit can be used as a temporary diversion, with the intention of subsequently anastomosing the conduit to the rectosigmoid, thereby accomplishing diversion of the urine into the faecal stream in two stages. Primary one-stage ureterosigmoid diversion should not be performed coincidentally with anterior exenteration for cancer, because recurrence in the pelvis could present a serious problem. Furthermore, radiation therapy can cause proctitis, a contraindication to diversion of urine into the faecal stream. In the author's experience, primary ureterosigmoid diversion should be avoided in young infants, because it can lead to several years of malodorous incontinence of combined urine and faeces. Socially it is better to wait until bowel control is well established before diverting urine to the rectosigmoid. This staged approach is a good way to accomplish that. It is well recognized that ureterosigmoidostomy carries a 10 per cent risk of colon carcinoma in the long term[37, 38]. Whether the staged technique will offer protection from this remains to be seen. Routine colonoscopic follow-up of these patients is advisable every two years.

**Ileocaecal conduit**[39-42]

# 12

Alternatively, caecum can be used for cutaneous diversion, creating a non-refluxing nipple by intussuscepting the terminal ileum, which is fastened to the caecal wall, to prevent its prolapse. Ureters can be joined to the ileum in more than one fashion, depending on their size. The

ileocaecal conduit has a tendency to prolapse through its cutaneous stoma unless it is thoroughly anchored by taking sutures at its base and to the peritoneum of the abdominal gutter as well.

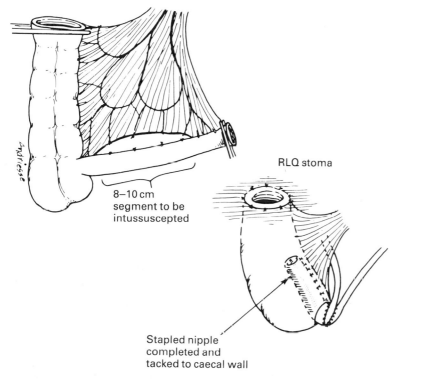

8–10 cm segment to be intussuscepted

RLQ stoma

Stapled nipple completed and tacked to caecal wall

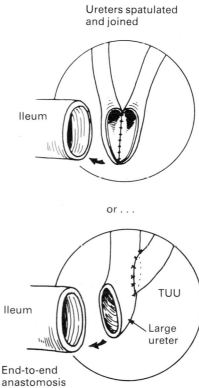

Ureters spatulated and joined

Ileum

or . . .

Ileum

TUU

Large ureter

End-to-end anastomosis

12

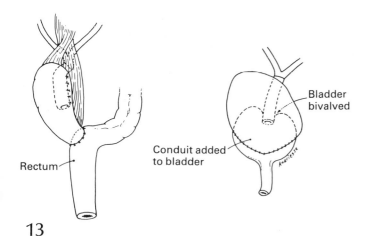

Rectum

Conduit added to bladder

Bladder bivalved

13

# 13

## Implantation of ileocaecal conduit into colon or onto bladder

In some cases the ileocaecal conduit, like the colon conduit, can be rejoined to the colon. In other cases it can be joined to the bladder. The bladder must be bivalved widely, to give a large anastomotic union of the caecum with the bladder, so that it will not behave as a diverticulum.

# CONTINENT URINARY DIVERSION

In the past few years there has been a trend towards creating an intra-abdominal urinary reservoir which can be catheterized through a continent abdominal-wall stoma, thereby avoiding a bag on the abdomen[43-47]. Space precludes illustrating all the various methods which have been used. These methods are much more often performed in adults to provide a catheterizable reservoir following cystectomy for bladder cancer. Fewer children will be considered as candidates for continent diversion, since most problems in children can be solved today without any type of diversion.

# 14

### KOCK POUCH[45, 48-50]

A long segment of ileum is used to create this continent reservoir. The two limbs are sewn together and folded into a reservoir pouch. At each end an intussusception is created to prevent efflux from the pouch. One is brought to the surface as the stoma, which will be catheterized to empty the pouch. The other nipple provides a non-reflux mechanism from the pouch to the upper tracts. The Kock pouch has been used widely to reconstruct patients after cystectomy for cancer. It can be used for children also. There is a 30 per cent incidence of postoperative complications in these patients, including incontinence of the mechanism designed to prevent leaking on the abdominal wall, difficult catheterization, parastoma hernia, stoma complications, and electrolyte disorders. Many of these patients have asymptomatic bacilluria, but pyelonephritis is rare in the absence of reflux.

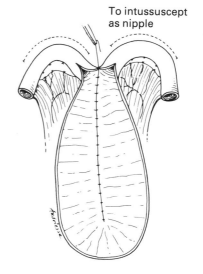

To intussuscept as nipple

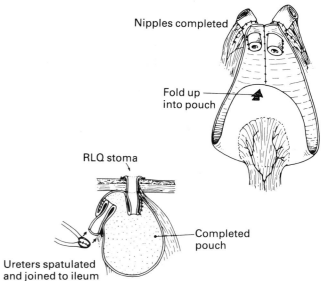

Nipples completed

Fold up into pouch

RLQ stoma

Completed pouch

Ureters spatulated and joined to ileum

14

# 15

## MAINZ POUCH[44]

The ascending colon and terminal ileum can be fashioned
into a reservoir, to which the ureters are joined by
tunnelling them into the colon wall. The terminal ileum
can be intussuscepted as a nipple, which is sewn to the
wall of the reservoir to prevent its unravelling.

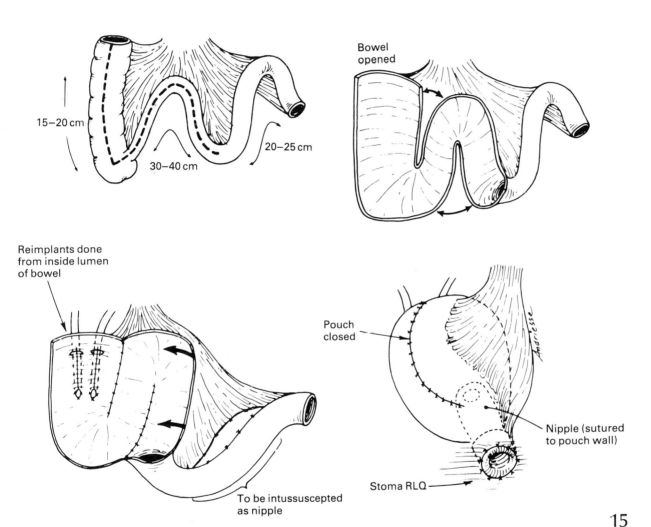

15

# 16

## RIGHT COLON POUCH[51,52]

The colon is opened widely, and laid back on itself to form a reservoir of high capacity but which is incapable of creating peristaltic waves which could give high contractile pressures in the system. A nipple is created to prevent leakage through the stoma, which is emptied by intermittent catheterization.

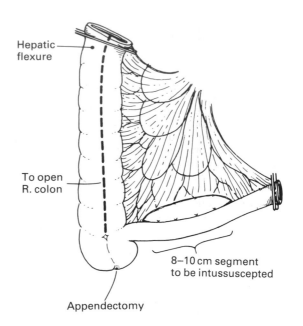

Hepatic flexure

To open R. colon

Appendectomy

8–10 cm segment to be intussuscepted

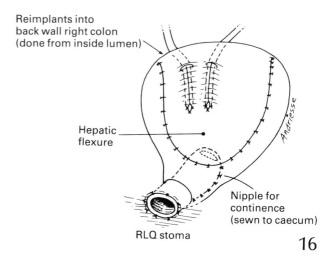

Reimplants into back wall right colon (done from inside lumen)

Hepatic flexure

Nipple for continence (sewn to caecum)

RLQ stoma

16

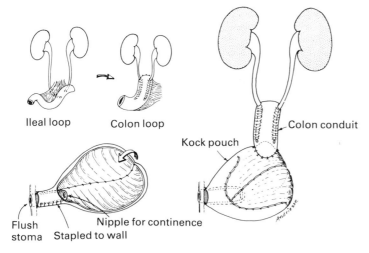

Ileal loop

Colon loop

Kock pouch

Colon conduit

Flush stoma    Nipple for continence    Stapled to wall

17

# 17

## HEMI-KOCK POUCH

There are many different uses for the principles illustrated above. It is generally agreed that the young patient with ileal-loop urinary diversion is at risk of upper-tract deterioration. Such a patient should at least be considered for conversion to a non-refluxing colon conduit. Shown here, is a half-Kock reservoir with its catheterizable limb which can be brought to the abdominal wall (or to the bladder neck or urethra), joining the colon conduit to it as the non-reflux mechanism.

Other types of urinary diversions used widely in past years include: pyelostomy, loop ureterostomy, end ureterostomy, and vesicostomy[53–56]. It is the author's belief that the majority of these can now be avoided by a proper reconstructive operation.

# URINARY UNDIVERSION

The many advances in reconstructive urology which have occurred in the past two decades mandates a reconsideration of patients who underwent various types of urinary diversion in the past. Some could be switched from a refluxing ileal loop to a non-refluxing colon conduit. Others could be changed to a continent-type diversion, and still others could be candidates for refunctionalization of their long-diverted bladders. Since 1969 the author has performed urinary undiversions in 164 patients (Table 1)[57–61]. The bladder in these patients is usually small from long disuse. This precludes complete preoperative urodynamic testing for bladder function. These bladders may be fragile, and during preoperative evaluation, instillation of contrast medium into the bladder using only mild pressure caused rupture and extravasation in three cases. However, this did not present any special problem in a defunctioned bladder.

**Table 1. Urinary Undiversion (1969–1987) (164 Cases)**

| Type of undiversion | Other details |
| --- | --- |
| 62 Ileal loop (14 pyeloileal) | 121 Permanent diversions |
| 12 Colon conduit (three had been ileal loops) | 43 Temporary diversions |
| | 61 Females |
| 38 Loop Ureterostomy or pyelostomy | 103 Males |
| 17 End ureterostomy | 41 Patients had only one kidney (one was a transplant) |
| 27 Cystostomy or vesicostomy | |
| 7 Nephrostomy | 1 Patient was anephric (to be transplanted) |
| 1 Ureterosigmoidostomy | |
| | 11 Personal diversions |
| | 153 Previously diverted elsewhere |

Percutaneous insertion of a small catheter into the bladder during cystoscopy can allow instillation of saline to 'cycle' the bladder[62]. This will give information concerning sensation, continence, and the ability to empty the bladder, and will show whether a small bladder will stretch up to normal capacity. If it does not, augmentation may be necessary. If there is incontinence when the bladder is filled, an operation may be required to correct this.

There are several important technical principles in performing undiversion surgery. First, these are always long, difficult operations, which must be done with patience and meticulous surgical technique to avoid potentially disastrous complications such as urinary leakage, stricture, reflux, or loss of a kidney. Operations of this magnitude should not be attempted unless a high standard of anaesthetic care is available. It has been the author's good fortune to work with superb anaesthetists in the Departments of Anesthesia at the Massachusetts General Hospital and the Children's Hospital, Boston. In ordinary paediatric surgical cases, fluid volume replacement is generally in the range of 5 ml/kg of body weight per hour. In undiversion surgery, where there is mobilization of the bladder, extensive retroperitoneal dissection, and long exposure of the intestines, fluid replacement is often in the range of 20–25 ml/kg per hour. If this fact is not appreciated, fluid replacement can fall behind, leading to hypovolaemia which can produce renal tubular necrosis.

Operative exposure is always a long, vertical midline incision from the symphysis pubis to the xyphoid, using a large, self-retaining ring retractor for global exposure.

When mobilizing the ureter, all periureteral tissue should be maintained with it. This includes the gonadal vessels, which are divided at the internal ring in the male or near the ovary in the female, to keep them with the ureter as collateral blood supply. If the gonad is not disturbed, it will survive with its collateral blood supply.

Transureteroureterostomy[63–65] or transureteropyelostomy are often needed, joining the better ureter to the bladder and draining the contralateral ureter into it. It is important to avoid wedging a ureter beneath the inferior mesenteric artery.

The psoas hitch is another important tool in these reconstructions. After implanting a ureter or a tapered bowel segment, the bladder is hitched to the psoas muscle to fix the point of entry of the ureter so that it will not angulate when the bladder fills.

Bladder augmentation has been used increasingly, not only in cases undergoing undiversion, but in a variety of reconstructive procedures where more volume and better compliance is needed.

Since bowel is often needed in undiversion cases, a thorough bowel preparation is standard. To accomplish this, the patient is instructed to take clear fluids only for two days. Go-Lytely, a proprietary polyethylene glycol electrolyte gastrointestinal tract lavage solution is then used the day before operation. The amount given varies with the patient's size. For a child under 10 kg, 80 ml is given every 10 minutes up to a volume of 1100 ml. In older patients over 50 kg, 240 ml is given every ten minutes up to a volume of 4000 ml.

In performing undiversions it is best to defer a decision on the precise procedure until all anatomy is laid out at the operating table. Then the various options can be considered and the best chosen.

# 18

## ILEAL-LOOP UNDIVERSION

There are several means by which an ileal loop can be taken down to redivert the urine to the bladder. Rarely are two good ureters present. More often the author has found one good ureter which can be hooked to the bladder with the adjunct of a psoas hitch, draining the other by transureteroureterostomy. When necessary the ileal loop can be tapered and implanted into the bladder. This can be done only if it is a good bladder in which a long tunnel can be constructed, together with a psoas hitch. The same thing can be done with a pyeloileal conduit. Bladder augmentation is often necessary. Some of the techniques are illustrated. Rarely, autotransplantation will be feasible[66].

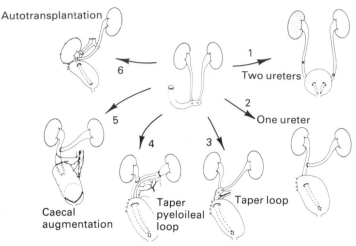

## IMPLANTING ILEAL CONDUIT INTO BLADDER

# 19a & b

The mesentery is incised to straighten the bowel.

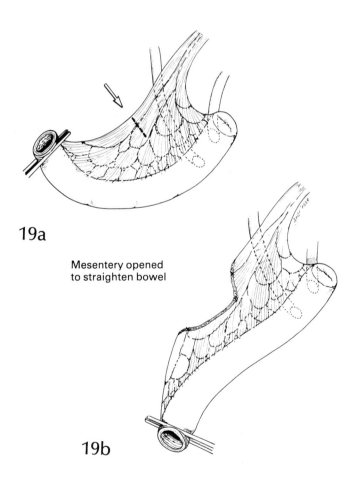

19a

Mesentery opened
to straighten bowel

19b

# 20

Catheters are passed up the ureters to identify their ostia, and the bowel segment is tapered using megaureter clamps. Note that the bowel must not be made too narrow, e.g. sometimes only a very thin strip should be removed, since a two-layer closure will use up more bowel wall. It is important to avoid creating a stenosis.

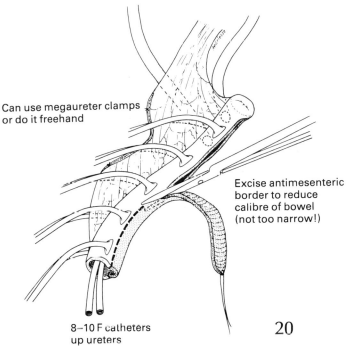

Can use megaureter clamps or do it freehand

Excise antimesenteric border to reduce calibre of bowel (not too narrow!)

8–10 F catheters up ureters

**20**

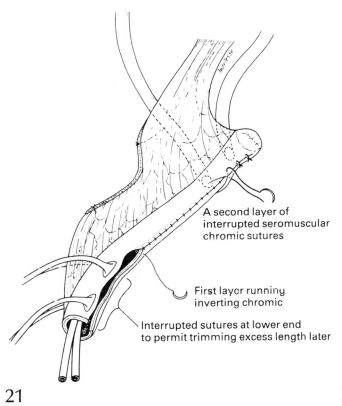

A second layer of interrupted seromuscular chromic sutures

First layer running inverting chromic

Interrupted sutures at lower end to permit trimming excess length later

**21**

# 21

Two-layer closure with chromic catgut is a tedious procedure and must be done with great care to avoid a leak. The lower several centimetres of this closure should be with interrupted sutures, in order to facilitate the trimming of excess length at an appropriate point later in the operation when the conduit is placed in its bed in the bladder.

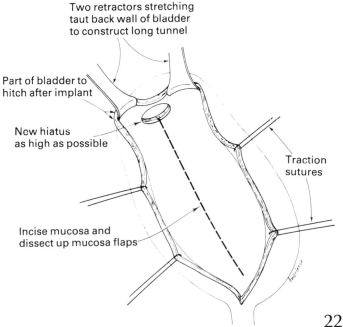

Two retractors stretching taut back wall of bladder to construct long tunnel

Part of bladder to hitch after implant

New hiatus as high as possible

Traction sutures

Incise mucosa and dissect up mucosa flaps

**22**

# 22

A hiatus is created as high as possible on the back wall of the bladder, but not in the side or dome where it may angulate when the bladder fills. An incision is made in the mucosa diagonally across the back wall of the bladder in order to prepare a bed for the 'ureter'. Blunt tunnelling beneath the mucosa of a defunctioned bladder is usually unsatisfactory.

## 23

Mucosal flaps are dissected back widely, usually by knife dissection. Cautery controls the fine bleeding points.

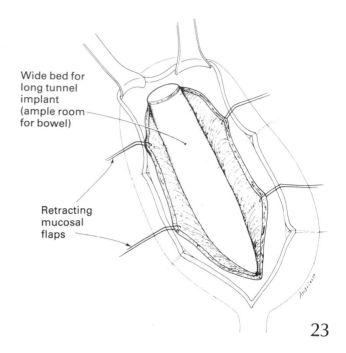

Wide bed for long tunnel implant (ample room for bowel)

Retracting mucosal flaps

23

## 24

The tapered conduit is placed in its bed with the suture line closure posteriorly against bladder muscle to avoid two adjacent suture lines which could result in a fistula. The bowel mesentery lies anteriorly.

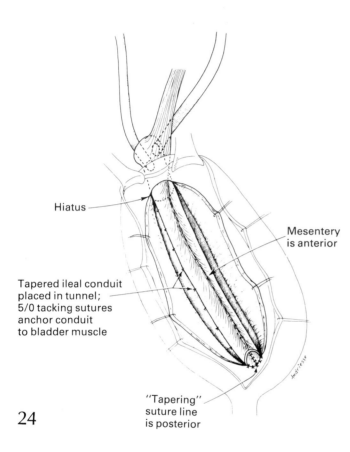

Hiatus

Mesentery is anterior

Tapered ileal conduit placed in tunnel; 5/0 tacking sutures anchor conduit to bladder muscle

"Tapering" suture line is posterior

24

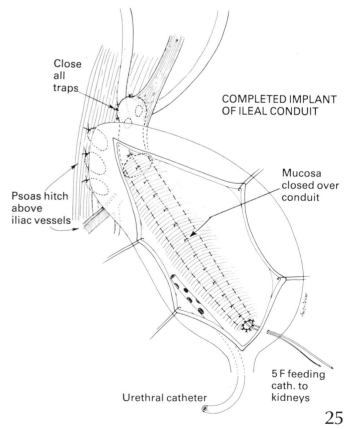

Close all traps

COMPLETED IMPLANT OF ILEAL CONDUIT

Psoas hitch above iliac vessels

Mucosa closed over conduit

Urethral catheter

5 F feeding cath. to kidneys

25

## 25

Completed tunnelling of conduit is shown, obtaining as long a tunnel as possible (5–6 cm). Catheters drain the bladder and each kidney for 10–12 days postoperatively. Note hitch of the bladder to the psoas muscle. This elongates the trigone, giving extra tunnel length. It also prevents angulation of the conduit at the hiatus where it enters the back wall of the bladder, by fixing that part of the bladder wall so that it does not move during filling. This technique for implanting tapered bowel into the bladder is useful only when the tissues are ideal. The bowel must be of good quality, without scar or stricture. The bladder must be large enough to get a good tunnel, and be of soft, resilient tissue. This procedure will not work in a small, contracted, non-compliant bladder.

## ILEOCAECAL CYSTOPLASTY

# 26

The ileocaecal segment is selected, retaining as broad a pedicle as possible for its blood supply.

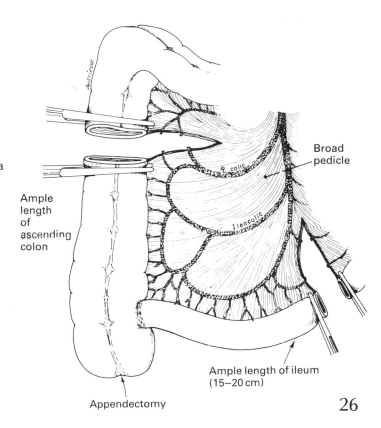

ISOLATED
ILEOCAECAL SEGMENT

Broad pedicle

Ample length of ascending colon

Ample length of ileum (15–20 cm)

Appendectomy

26

# 27

Mesentery is removed from the terminal ileum for 8–10 cm to facilitate intussusception of that bowel segment. A good vascular arcade should be preserved at each end of this bowel segment.

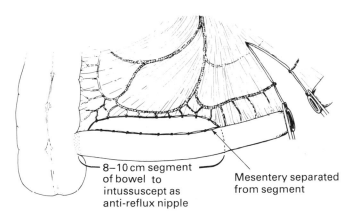

8–10 cm segment of bowel to intussuscept as anti-reflux nipple

Mesentery separated from segment

27

# 28 & 29

The intussusception is created by combined pulling with a Babcock clamp and pushing with blunt forceps. Sutures are placed between the bowel wall and caecum to maintain the intussusception.

# 30

Two or sometimes three rows of staples are placed through the 'nipple' to help hold it. Staples are used only when it will be possible to endoscope the segment postoperatively, because small stones can form on some staples which do not get covered by mucosa. When placed on the bladder, exposed staples and stones can be plucked out endoscopically at a later date, using alligator forceps through a cystoscope. When the nipple cannot be reached endoscopically (as in Illustrations 15 and 16) it is better to use sutures rather than staples.

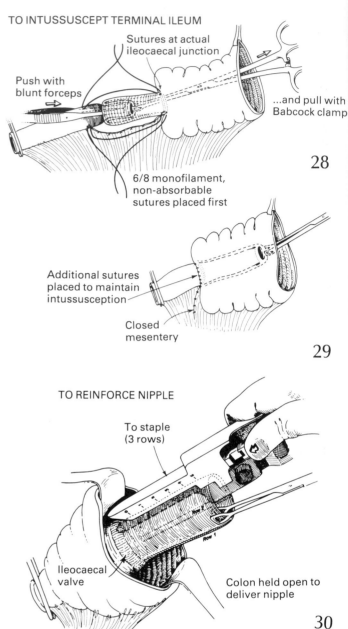

TO INTUSSUSCEPT TERMINAL ILEUM

Sutures at actual ileocaecal junction

Push with blunt forceps

...and pull with Babcock clamp

6/8 monofilament, non-absorbable sutures placed first

**28**

Additional sutures placed to maintain intussusception

Closed mesentery

**29**

TO REINFORCE NIPPLE

To staple (3 rows)

Ileocaecal valve

Colon held open to deliver nipple

**30**

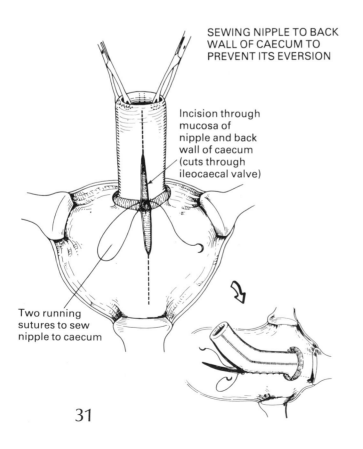

SEWING NIPPLE TO BACK WALL OF CAECUM TO PREVENT ITS EVERSION

Incision through mucosa of nipple and back wall of caecum (cuts through ileocaecal valve)

Two running sutures to sew nipple to caecum

**31**

# 31

Using cautery, an incision is made for the full length of the nipple, through the ileocaecal valve, and along the back wall of the caecum for a corresponding distance. The nipple is then sewn to the adjacent wall of the caecum with two running sutures. If the nipple is not fixed in this manner it can become loose, allowing the intussuscepted bowel to evert and permit reflux.

## 32

The ileocaecal segment is rotated, usually counterclockwise, to be joined to the bladder. Note that the bladder has been opened widely, so that the augmentation will not behave as a diverticulum. Also note the opening of the antimesenteric border of the bowel to match the perimeter of the bladder. A long tubular segment of colon should be avoided to prevent spontaneous contractions which can cause high intravesical pressures and wetting.

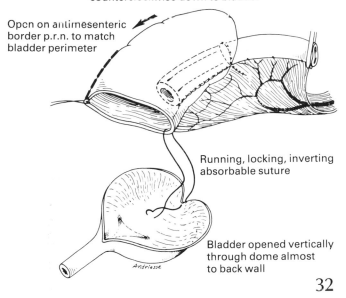

Ileocaecal segment rotated counterclockwise down to bladder

Open on antimesenteric border p.r.n. to match bladder perimeter

Running, locking, inverting absorbable suture

Bladder opened vertically through dome almost to back wall

32

COMPLETED AUGMENTATION

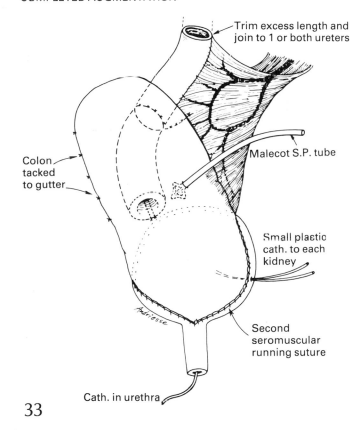

Trim excess length and join to 1 or both ureters

Malecot S.P. tube

Colon tacked to gutter

Small plastic cath. to each kidney

Second seromuscular running suture

Cath. in urethra

33

## 33

The completed augmentation is shown in which the ileocaecal junction is used to prevent reflux. When one or both ureters are of good quality, direct implantation into the back wall of the caecum is used, as shown in Illustration 47a & b.

## 34

### When ileal intussusception is impossible

If there are no ureters, or if an intussuscepted segment cannot be made, another piece of small bowel can be tapered and tunnelled.

CAECAL AUGMENTATION:
Preventing reflux when:
   a. No ureter
   b. Short terminal ileum on caecum
   c. Failed nipple

Opening in back

Bed for "reimplant" bowel muscle

Retracting open caecum (vertical incision)

Mucosal flaps laid back

Transverse closure caecum

Tapered bowel segment to "reimplant"

Gauze to flatten the mucosa

Tapered bowel 8–10 cm tunnel in back caecal wall

34

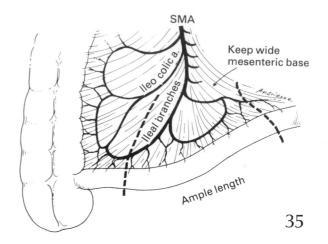

35

# 35, 36 & 37a, b & c

## Small-bowel augmentation

Often small bowel is used to augment the bladder. It should always be detubularized to increase its volume and ablate peristalsis.

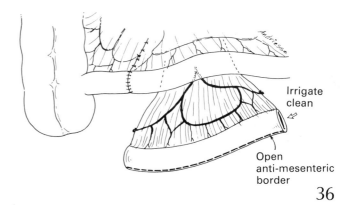

36

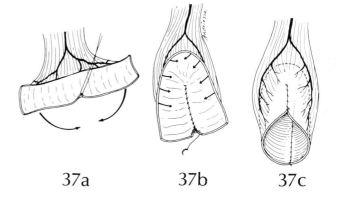

37a        37b        37c

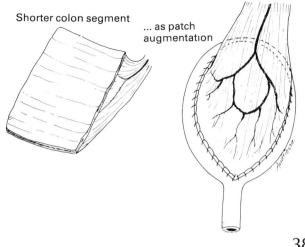

Shorter colon segment

... as patch augmentation

38

# 38

## Colon patch augmentation

A short piece of colon can be used as a patch where only a small increase of bladder volume is needed.

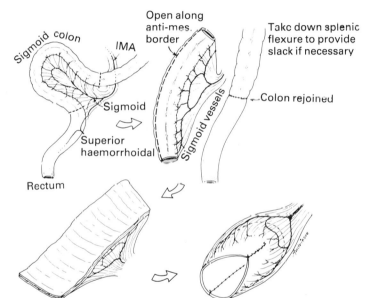

Sigmoid colon    IMA

Open along anti-mes. border

Take down splenic flexure to provide slack if necessary

Sigmoid

Superior haemorrhoidal

Sigmoid vessels

Colon rejoined

Rectum

39

## LARGE AUGMENTATION WITH COLON

# 39

When the native bladder size is very small and a reservoir is needed of a capacity similar to caecum and right colon, sigmoid can be fashioned in the manner shown. The choice of bowel used for augmentation will vary with what is available, the blood supply to the bowel, and what must be accomplished. The caecum is ideal when large ureters must be joined to it, providing a non-refluxing mechanism. The sigmoid is ideal when simple augmentation is needed. Its mesentery lies just next to the bladder on the left side. Small-bowel mesentery may be too short in some cases and it has a pedicle which can serve to trap bowel if not carefully tacked to prevent this.

The sigmoid and left colon may be unavailable in cases where a pull-through operation has been performed for imperforate anus. When caecum is used, loss of the ileocaecal valve can change bowel bacterial flora and interfere with bile-salt resorption in the terminal ileum. However, this is seldom a major problem.

# UNDIVERSION CASES ILLUSTRATED

The following ten cases illustrate the surgical techniques which may be required in refunctionalization of the long-diverted urinary tract. Every case is different and each must be approached with an armamentarium of possible techniques based on sound general surgical principles. The decision regarding specifics of the reconstruction should await a complete laying out of the anatomy at the operating table.

# 40a & b

*Case 1.* Anatomy before and after 'undiversion' in an 11-year-old boy with ileal loop for severe hydronephrosis caused by urethral valves.

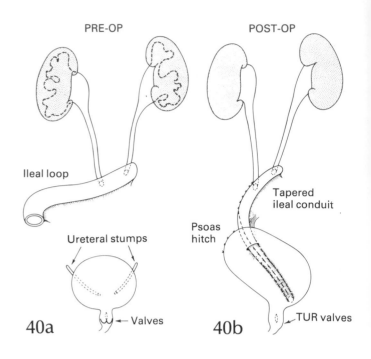

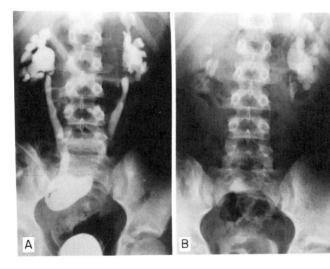

41a                    41b

# 41a & b

(a) Simultaneous loopogram and cystogram preoperatively. Note moderate calycectasis, slightly dilated ureters, small bladder, and short, unusable ureteral stumps.

(b) Intravenous pyelogram 18 months postoperatively. The patient has remained completely well without bacilluria for 14 years. All patients with bowel in the urinary tract, especially as a substitute ureter, require indefinite continuing surveillance, for late stricture can develop in some cases, just as it can when bowel is used for an ileal-loop cutaneous diversion[67,68].

# 42a & b

*Case 2.* (a) A 15-year-old boy with prune belly syndrome. Nephrostomy tubes had been present from 2 weeks of age. An ileal loop had been performed later, but it never drained because both upper ureters were obstructed.

(b) Reconstruction of the urinary tract was performed, discarding the short segment of each ureter and using the bowel to establish upper-tract draining into the bladder.

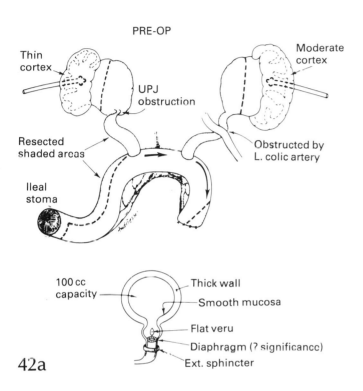

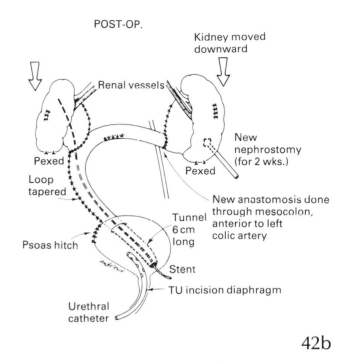

# 43a & b

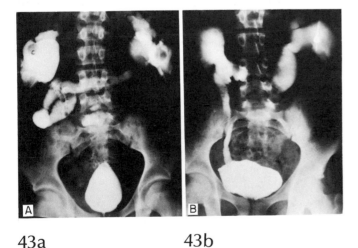

43a                              43b

(a) Preoperative study with simultaneous filling of kidneys through nephrostomy tubes, bowel conduit through a catheter in its stoma, and bladder through a urethral catheter.

(b) Left percutaneous antegrade infusion 18 months postoperatively. Note tapered bowel conduit from left kidney to right and from right kidney into bladder. Bladder capacity and function were satisfactory. There was no reflux. Normal infusion pressures. This patient's life was essentially normal for 10 years after undiversion, with relatively stable renal function of about 30 per cent of normal. At age 25 years his creatinine rose suddenly during treatment of a peptic ulcer with cimetidine, which has been reported to cause acute interstitial nephritis. Renal transplantation was performed; his brother was the organ donor. The patient has done well during the intervening 4 years and he is leading a normal life at age 28 years.

# 44a & b

*Case 3.* (a) A 15-year-old girl with sacral agenesis for whom an ileal loop had been performed 10 years previously for treatment of urinary incontinence. Cycling the bladder by irrigation proved fruitless because the outlet was incontinent.

(b) Reconstruction as shown included narrowing the bladder neck and urethra to provide more outlet resistance, augmenting the bladder with caecum, and preventing reflux with a nipple of terminal ileum.

BEFORE

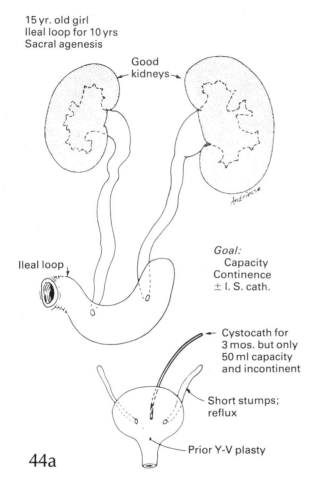

15 yr. old girl
Ileal loop for 10 yrs
Sacral agenesis

Good kidneys →

*Goal:*
Capacity
Continence
± I. S. cath.

Ileal loop

Cystocath for 3 mos. but only 50 ml capacity and incontinent

Short stumps; reflux

Prior Y-V plasty

44a

AFTER

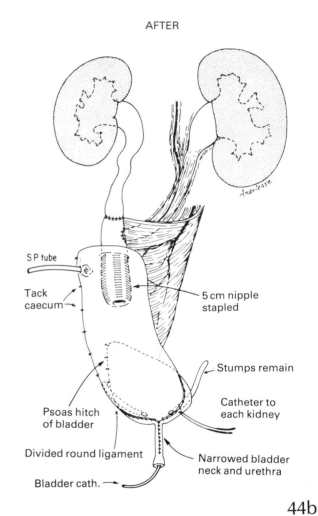

S P tube

Tack caecum

5 cm nipple stapled

Stumps remain

Catheter to each kidney

Psoas hitch of bladder

Divided round ligament

Bladder cath. →

Narrowed bladder neck and urethra

44b

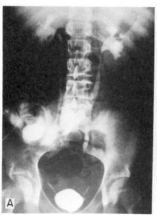

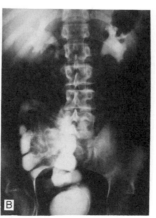

45a          45b

# 45a & b

(a) Preoperative simultaneous loopogram and cystogram. Note small bladder, sacral agenesis, and strictured ileal loop.

(b) Intravenous pyelogram 6 months postoperatively. Nipple with staples can be seen as filling defect in caecal augmentation. No reflux. Patient empties by intermittent self-catheterization using a hollow metal sound. Patient is dry and she is free from urinary infection. Lifestyle is essentially normal now, 5½ years after undiversion.

# 46a & b

*Case 4.*   (a) A 17-year-old girl treated by ileal loop for incontinence at the age of 2 years. Review of subsequent intravenous pyelograms showed progressive deterioration of the upper tracts. Note stricture of the ileal loop.

(b) Reconstruction as shown. The patient is now 5 months postoperative. She is dry. Bladder is emptied by the Credé manoeuver. She catheterizes twice daily to make certain that residuals are low after self-expression of the bladder. This reconstructive operation has not only made her life style more normal, but it will also stop the progressive destruction of her kidneys. Whenever, as in this case, a ureter can be joined to the bladder with a reliable ureteral reimplantation, the author prefers this to joining it to bowel.

BEFORE

AFTER

17-year-old girl
Ileal loop for Myelodysplasia
(at age 2 years)

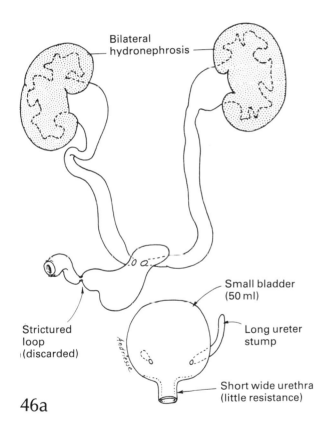

Bilateral hydronephrosis

Small bladder (50 ml)

Long ureter stump

Strictured loop (discarded)

Short wide urethra (little resistance)

46a

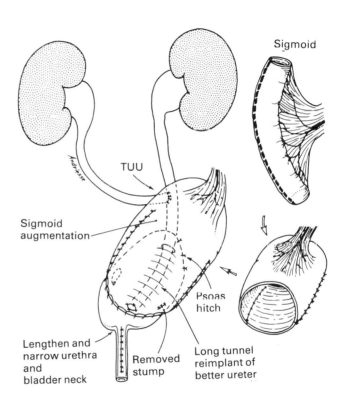

Sigmoid

TUU

Sigmoid augmentation

Lengthen and narrow urethra and bladder neck

Removed stump

Psoas hitch

Long tunnel reimplant of better ureter

46b

# 47a & b

*Case 5.* (a) A 19-year-old male with an ileal loop for 5 years following unsuccessful surgery for vesicoureteral reflux. The problem was complicated by prior partial cystectomy. Neurological evaluation was performed, including magnetic resonance imaging of the lower spinal cord and urodynamic testing, since neurological impairment had been suspected as the cause for failure of surgery when a child. These studies were normal.

(b) One ureter was suitable for tunnelling reimplantation into the back wall of the caecum by Goodwin's technique[69]. The short segment of ileum still attached to the caecum was utilized as a patch to dampen peristaltic activity of the caecum and right colon. The patient is now 18 months postoperative and is well. He has noted failure to ejaculate after undiversion, although nothing was done to the bladder neck at the time of the reconstruction.

BEFORE

AFTER

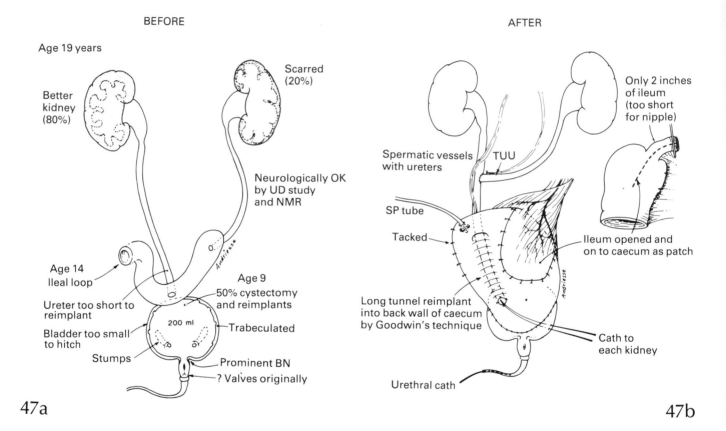

47a

47b

# 48a & b

*Case 6.* (a) A 16-year old boy with an ileal loop for 8 years after failed ureteral implantation surgery. Preliminary cycling of the bladder with saline through a percutaneously placed cystostomy tube demonstrated a good bladder, which increased in size, obviating the need for augmentation. It was felt that it would be best to avoid using bowel if possible, since a stricture had already occurred.

(b) Autotransplantation of the right kidney was used to achieve a good reimplantation on the right, draining the left by transureteropyelostomy. During a 6-year follow up the patient has been well. The intravenous pyelogram remains stable.

BEFORE

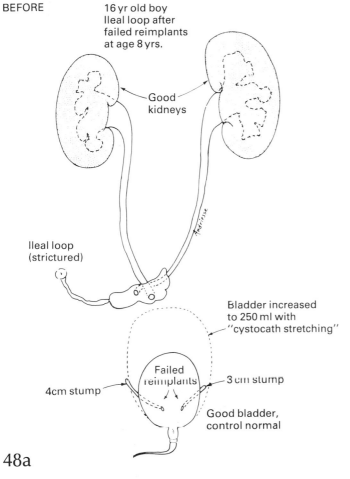

48a

AFTER

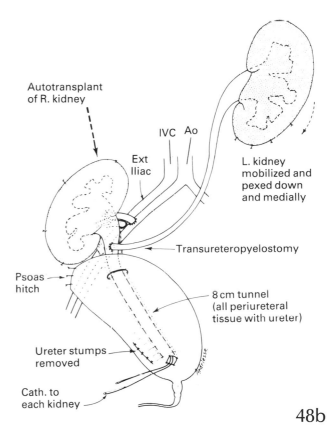

48b

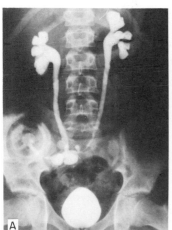

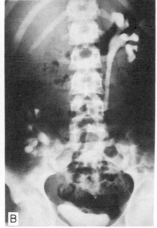

49a

49b

# 49a & b

(a) Preoperative simultaneous cystogram and loopogram. Note strictured ileal loop and moderate bilateral hydronephrosis, with relatively small bladder despite cycling with saline for 2 weeks.

(b) Intravenous pyelogram 1 year after surgery. Autotransplanted kidney is visible in right lower quadrant. There is less hydronephrosis.

# 50a & b

*Case 7.*    Patient had myelodysplasia with urinary incontinence and increasing left hydronephrosis. A non-refluxing colon conduit was constructed at 3 years of age as a temporary measure. This got the patient dry and allowed her upper tracts to return to normal.

Undiversion at age 10 years. Patient is now completely dry. She empties bladder by intermittent self-catheterization. Upper tracts remain stable 3½ years after

undiversion. This child was first treated in 1978. Alternative treatment which would have been considered today would include ureteral reimplantation, bladder-neck narrowing, and possible bladder augmentation depending on the quality of the bladder, avoiding the 7 years with a conduit. None the less, there are patients for whom a temporary conduit can be very useful (see also Case 8).

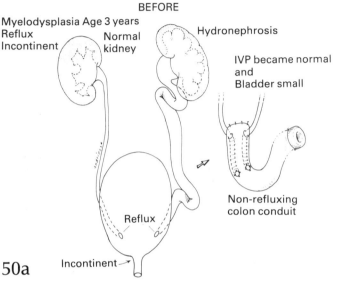

BEFORE

Myelodysplasia Age 3 years
Reflux
Incontinent
Normal kidney
Hydronephrosis
IVP became normal and Bladder small
Non-refluxing colon conduit
Reflux
Incontinent →
50a

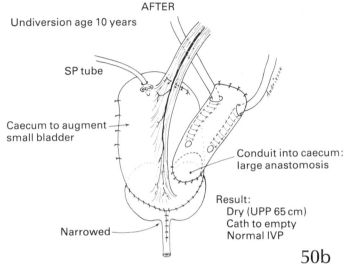

AFTER

Undiversion age 10 years
SP tube
Caecum to augment small bladder
Conduit into caecum: large anastomosis
Narrowed →
Result:
Dry (UPP 65 cm)
Cath to empty
Normal IVP
50b

# 51a & b

*Case 8.*    This patient was seen at 7 years of age in 1978. After multiple previous operations and urinary incontinence, ureterosigmoidostomies had been performed. She was incontinent of stool and urine, and had severe recurrent pyelonephritis.

Non-refluxing ileal caecal conduit was selected as a temporary measure to stabilize the upper tracts and get the patient dry.

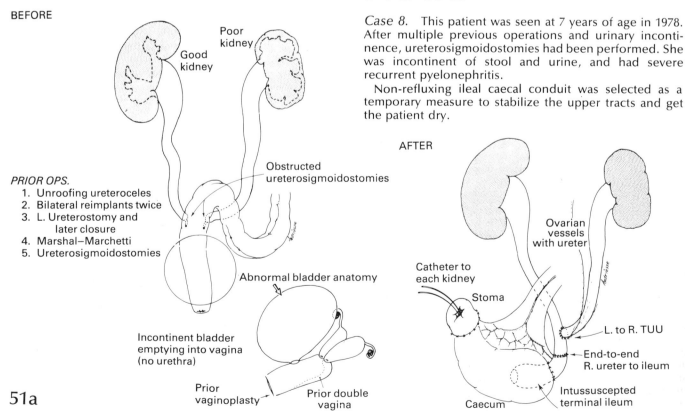

BEFORE

Good kidney
Poor kidney
Obstructed ureterosigmoidostomies

*PRIOR OPS.*
1. Unroofing ureteroceles
2. Bilateral reimplants twice
3. L. Ureterostomy and later closure
4. Marshal–Marchetti
5. Ureterosigmoidostomies

Abnormal bladder anatomy

Incontinent bladder emptying into vagina (no urethra)

Prior vaginoplasty
Prior double vagina
51a

AFTER

Ovarian vessels with ureter
Catheter to each kidney
Stoma
L. to R. TUU
End-to-end R. ureter to ileum
Intussuscepted terminal ileum
Caecum
51b

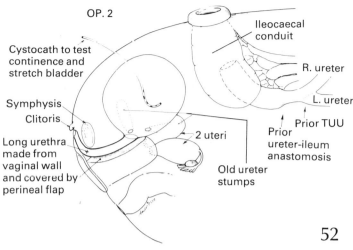

OP. 2

Cystocath to test
continence and
stretch bladder

Symphysis

Clitoris

Long urethra
made from
vaginal wall
and covered by
perineal flap

Ileocaecal
conduit

R. ureter

L. ureter

Prior TUU

Prior
ureter-ileum
anastomosis

2 uteri

Old ureter
stumps

52

# 52

At a second operation 6 months later, a long urethra was constructed by tubularizing the anterior vaginal wall and covering it with a flap from the perineum[70]. Cycling the bladder showed a competent outlet, although the bladder remained small.

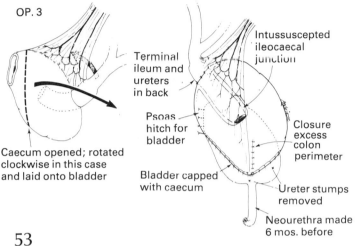

OP. 3

Intussuscepted
ileocaecal
junction

Terminal
ileum and
ureters
in back

Psoas
hitch for
bladder

Bladder capped
with caecum

Closure
excess
colon
perimeter

Ureter stumps
removed

Neourethra made
6 mos. before

Caecum opened; rotated
clockwise in this case
and laid onto bladder

53

# 53

Six months later the caecum was joined to the bladder. Now, 8 years after completion of this staged reconstruction, the patient is dry, voids to completion, has no reflux, and has stable upper tracts. Patients with a neurologically intact bladder outlet can empty an augmented bladder by bearing down with high intra-abdominal pressure, while simultaneously opening the urethral sphincter. In contrast are those patients who cannot open their sphincters, and who must rely on intermittent catheterization to empty the bladder.

# 54a & b

*Case 9.*  (a) This 12-year-old boy with a solitary kidney was referred 8 years after cutaneous pyelostomy. Ureteral reimplantation had been performed at 4 years of age but had been unsuccessful, possibly because Type 1 urethral valves had been overlooked.

(b) Reconstruction was done in a single stage, fulgurating the valves, closing the pyelostomy (dismembered pyeloplasty), and reimplanting the ureter. It is possible to operate on both ends of a ureter simultaneously if the blood supply to the upper ureter is carefully maintained. The ureter should not be mobilized unnecessarily at its upper end. It should never be dissected away from its investing adventitia in which runs the collateral blood supply downward from the renal pelvis. Only that segment to be resected should be disturbed, removing the pyelostomy or ureterostomy, and restoring continuity of the upper tract with a meticulously formed oblique anastomosis without tension, using fine, interrupted sutures. An alternative which might be considered is operating on one end of the ureter, allowing it to heal, and then repairing the other end. However, the author has seen numerous examples where this was impractical, such as where satisfactory reimplantation of the ureter cannot be accomplished because the upper ureter is tethered upward by scar.

Careful complete repair is to be preferred[71].

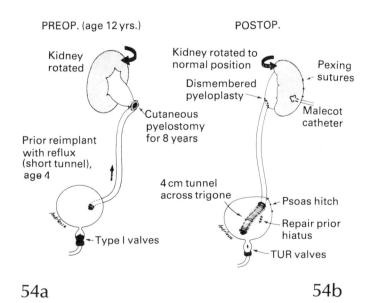

PREOP. (age 12 yrs.)

Kidney
rotated

Prior reimplant
with reflux
(short tunnel),
age 4

Cutaneous
pyelostomy
for 8 years

Type I valves

POSTOP.

Kidney rotated to
normal position

Dismembered
pyeloplasty

Pexing
sutures

Malecot
catheter

4 cm tunnel
across trigone

Psoas hitch

Repair prior
hiatus

TUR valves

54a

54b

# 55a & b

(a) Preoperative filling solitary left system through syringe inserted into cutaneous pyelostomy. Note straight entry of ureter into side wall of bladder, with no ureterovesical tunnel.

(b) Intravenous pyelogram carried out 4 months postoperatively. Note normal size of bladder. Patient is well now, 12 years following this reconstruction. Getting rid of the bag he had worn on his left flank since infancy normalized his life.

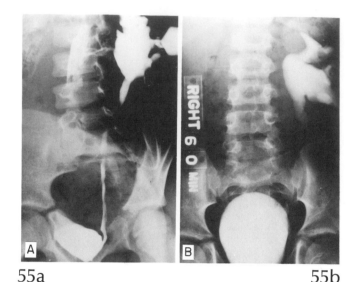

55a                                            55b

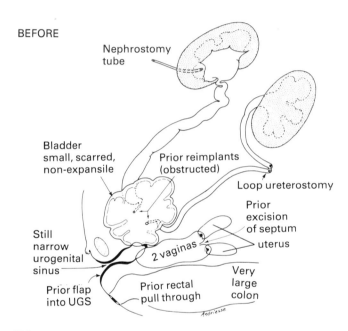

BEFORE

56a

# 56a & b

*Case 10.*   (a) This 5-year-old girl had spent more than half her life in hospitals for treatment of a high cloacal malformation[72]. She had a right nephrostomy tube, a left-loop ureterostomy, and a badly scarred bladder, although it had originally been normal in appearance. A perineal flap had been advanced into the urogenital sinus with the aim of exteriorizing the vagina. This was unfortunate: a vaginal pull-through should have been performed, retaining the urogenital sinus as urethra.

(b) The first procedure was to make a urethra[70] and widen the entry to the vaginas.

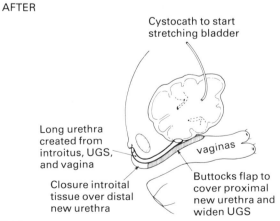

AFTER

56b

AFTER UNDIVERSION (6 mos. later)

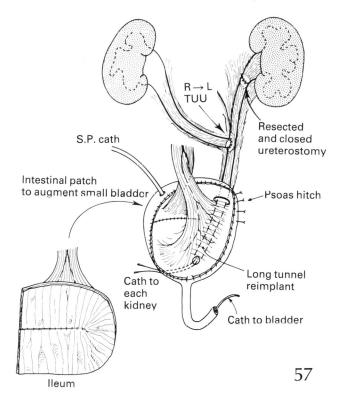

57

## 57

Six months later undiversion was performed, re-establishing urine flow to the bladder which was augmented to give it capacity and compliance. Now, 8 years later, this patient functions well, although intermittent catheterization is needed to assure complete emptying of her bladder. She is dry.

58a        58b

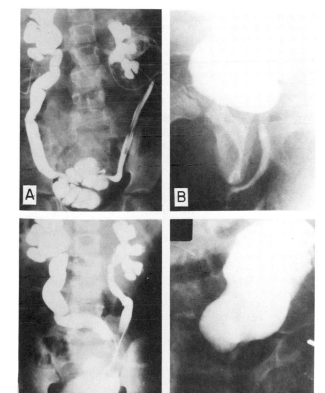

58c        58d

## 58a–d

(a) Shows the badly scarred, contracted bladder and hydronephrotic upper tracts, both requiring external drainage.

(b) Illustrates the reconstructed urethra. As stated, the urogenital sinus should originally have been saved as urethra, disconnecting the vaginas from it and bringing them down to the perineum by a pull-through procedure, or extending their length with a segment of bowel to the perineum.

(c) Postoperative study via drainage catheters 12 days after undiversion to illustrate long-tunnel implantation of the left ureter and right-to-left transureteral ureterostomy.

(d) Cystogram 2 weeks after undiversion via suprapubic tube, illustrating satisfactory bladder volume after augmentation with small bowel.

# Conclusion

Great changes have taken place in diversion and undiversion techniques in recent years. Urinary diversions in children are needed less often than previously because reconstructive surgery has improved, obviating the need for the majority of diversions.

Furthermore, in those children for whom a diversion continues to be needed, it should clearly be by a method which does not allow reflux, which is present with ileal loops and which often leads to deterioration of the kidneys. When there is sufficient bowel and when renal function is sufficient to cope with a certain amount of solute reabsorption which occurs when there is bowel in the urinary tract[73], a so-called continent diversion technique can be considered. Patients are happier with a small stoma which they can empty by intermittent self-catheterization, as compared to a bag worn over a stoma which drains continuously.

Finally, there are many patients with various types of urinary diversion who could be undiverted, refunctionalizing the long-diverted urinary tract, as illustrated in the spectrum of cases shown here.

## References

1. Bill, A. H. Jr, Dillard, D. H., Eggers, H. E., Jensen O. (1954) Urinary and fecal incontinence due to congenital abnormalities in children: Management of implantation of the ureters into an isolated ileostomy. Surgery, Gynecology and Obstetrics, 98, 575–580

2. Bowles, W. T., Tall, B. A. (1967) Urinary diversion in children. Journal of Urology, 98, 597–605

3. Cook, R. C., Lister, J., Zachary, R. B. (1968) Operative management of the neurogenic bladder in children; diversion through intestinal conduits. Surgery, 63, 825–831

4. Light, J. K., Flores, F. N., Scott, F. B. (1983) Use of the AS 792 artificial sphincter following urinary undiversion. Journal of Urology, 129, 548–551

5. Hendren, W. H. (1970) A new approach to infants with severe obstructive uropathy: early complete reconstruction. Journal of Pediatric Surgery, 5, 184–199

6. Hendren, W. H. (1971) Posterior urethral valves in boys: A broad clinical spectrum. Journal of Urology, 106, 298–307

7. Whitaker, R. H. (1973) The ureter in posterior urethral valves. British Journal of Urology, 45, 395–403

8. Cohen, S. J. (1975) Ureterozystoneostomie: eine neue antireflux technik. Aktuelle Urolgie, 6, 1–8

9. Politano, V. A., Leadbetter, W. F. (1958) An operative technique for the correction of vesicoureteral reflux. Journal of Urology, 79, 932–941

10. Hendren, W. H. (1974) Reoperation for the failed ureteral reimplantation. Journal of Urology, 111, 403–411

11. Hendren, W. H. (1980) Reoperative ureteral reimplantation: management of the difficult case. Journal of Pediatric Surgery, 15, 770–786

12. Bischoff, P. (1961) Operative treatment of megaureter. Journal of Urology, 85, 268–274

13. Hendren, W. H. (1979) Megaureter. In Campbell's Urology, 4th edn, J. H. Harrison, R. F. Gittes, A. D. Perlmutter, T. A. Stamey, P. C. Walsh (ed.), pp. 1697–1742. Philadelphia: W. B. Saunders Co

14. Hendren, W. H. (1975) Complications of megaureter repair in children. Journal of Urology, 113, 238–254

15. Hendren, W. H. (1969) Operative repair of megaureter in children. Journal of Urology, 101, 491–507

16. Kalicinski, Z. H., Kansy, J., Kotarbinska, B., Joszt, W. (1977) Surgery of megaureters–modification of Hendren's operation. Journal of Pediatric Surgery, 12, 183–188

17. Paquin, A. J. Jr. (1964) Considerations for the management of some complex problems for ureterovesical anastomosis. Surgery, Gynecology and Obstetrics, 118, 75–92

18. Bricker, E. M. (1950) Bladder substitution after pelvis evisceration. Surgical Clinics of North America, 30, 1511–1521

19. Delgado, G. E., Muecke, E. C. (1973) Evaluation of 80 cases of ileal conduits in children, indication, complication and results. Journal of Urology, 109, 311–314

20. Hendren, W. H., Radopoulos, D. (1983) Complications of ileal loop and colon conduit urinary diversion. Urologic Clinics of North America, 10, 451–471

21. Middletown, A. W. Jr., Hendren, W. H. (1976) Ileal conduits in children at the Massachusetts General Hospital from 1955–1970. Journal of Urology, 115, 591–595

22. Mitchell, M. E., Yoder, I. C., Pfister, R. C., Daly, J., Althausen, A. (1977) Ileal loop stenosis: A late complication of urinary diversion. Journal of Urology, 118, 957–961

23. Ray, P., DeDomenico, I. (1972) Intestinal conduit urinary diversion in children. British Journal of Urology, 44, 345–350

24. Retik, A. B., Perlmutter, A. D., Gross, R. E. (1967) Cutaneous ureteroileostomy in children. New England Journal of Medicine, 277, 217–222

25. Shapiro, S. R., Lebowitz, R., Colodny, A. H. (1975) Fate of 90 children with ileal conduit urinary diversion a decade later: Analysis of complications, pyelography, renal function and bacteriology. Journal of Urology, 114, 289–295

26. Smith, E. D. (1972) Follow-up studies on 150 ileal conduits in children. Journal of Pediatric Surgery, 7, 1–10

27. Richie, J. P., Skinner, D. G., Waisman, J. (1974) The effect of reflux on the development of pyelonephritis in urinary diversion: An experimental study. Journal of Surgical Research, 16, 256–261

28. Richie, J. P., Skinner, D. G. (1975) Urinary diversion: The physiological rationale for non-refluxing colonic conduits. British Journal of Urology, 47, 269–275

29. Althausen, A. F., Hagen-Cook, K., Hendren, W. H. (1978) Non-refluxing colon conduit: Experience with 70 cases. Journal of Urology, 120, 35–39

30. Altwein, J. E., Hohenfellner, R. (1975) Use of the colon as a conduit for urinary diversion. Surgery, Gynecology and Obstetrics, 140, 33–38

31. Hendren, W. H. (1975) Non refluxing colon conduit for temporary or permanent urinary diversion in children. Journal of Pediatric Surgery, 10, 381–398

32. Kelalis, P. P. (1974) Urinary diversion in children by the sigmoid conduit: its advantages and limitations. Journal of Urology, 112, 666–672

33. Mogg, R. A., Syme, R. R. (1965) The treatment of neurogenic urinary incontinence using the colonic conduit. British Journal of Urology, 37, 681–686

34. Skinner, D. G., Gottesman, J. E., Richie, J. P. (1975) The isolated sigmoid segment: Its value in temporary urinary diversion and reconstruction. Journal of Urology, 113, 614–618

35. Hendren, W. H. (1983) Ureterocolic diversion of urine: Management of some difficult problems. Journal of Urology, 129, 719–729

36. Hendren, W. H. (1976) Exstrophy of the bladder–An alternative method of management. Journal of Urology, 115, 195–202

37. Crissy, M. M., Steele, G. D., Gittes, R. F. (1980) Rat model for carcinogenesis in ureterosigmoidostomy. Science, 207, 1079–1080

38. Mueller, C. W., Thornbury, J. R. (1973) Adenocarcinoma of the colon complicating ureterosigmoidostomy: A case report and review of the literature. Journal of Urology, 109, 225–227

39. Gittes, R. F. (1977) Bladder augmentation procedure. In: Reconstructive Urologic Surgery: pediatric and adult, J. Libertino, L. Zinman (ed.), pp 216–226. Philadelphia: W. B. Saunders Co

40. Gil-Vernet, J. M. Jr. (1965) The ileocolic segment in urologic surgery. Journal of Urology, 94, 418–426

41. Skinner, D. G. (1974) Secondary urinary reconstruction: Use of the ileocecal segment. Journal of Urology, 112, 48–51

42. Zinman, L., Libertino, J. A. (1975) Ileocecal conduit for temporary and permanent urinary diversion. Journal of Urology, 113, 317–323

43. Gilchrist, R. K., Merricks, J. W., Hamlin, H. H., Rieger, I. T. (1950) Construction of substitute bladder and urethra. Surgery, Gynecology and Obstetrics, 90, 752–760

44. King, L. R., Stone, A. R., Webster, G. D. (1987) Bladder Reconstruction and Continent Urinary Diversion. Chicago: Year Book Medical Publishers

45. Kock, N. G., Nilson, A. E., Nilsson, L. O., Norlen, L. J., Philipson, B. M. (1982) Urinary diversion via a continent ileal reservoir: Clinical results in 12 patients. Journal of Urology, 128, 469–475

46. Mitchell, M. E., Hensle, T. W. (1987) Total bladder replacement in children. In Bladder Reconstruction and Continent Urinary Diversion, L. R. King, A. R. Stone, G. D. Webster (ed.), pp. 312–320. Chicago: Year Book Medical Publishers

47. Thuroff, J. W., Alken, P., Hohenfellner, R. (1987) The Mainz pouch (mixed augmentation with ileum "N" Zecum) for bladder augmentation and continent diversion. In Bladder Reconstruction and Continent Urinary Diversion, L. R. King, A. R. Stone, G. D. Webster (ed.), pp. 252–268. Chicago: Year Book Medical Publishers

48. Skinner, D. G., Lieskovsky, G., Skinner, E. C., Boyd, S. D. (1987) Urinary diversion. In Current Problems in Surgery 24: pp 407–471. Chicago: Year Book Medical Publishers

49. Skinner, D. G., Boyd, S. D., Lieskowsky, G. (1984) Clinical experience with the Koch continent ileal reservoir for urinary diversion. Journal of Urology, 132, 1101–1107

50. Skinner, D. G., Lieskowsky, G., Boyd, S. D. (1984) Technique of creation of continent internal ileal reservoir (Koch pouch) for urinary diversion. Urologic Clinics of North America, 11, 741–749

51. Goldwasser, B., Barrett, D. M., Benson, R. C. (1987) Complete bladder replacement using the detubularized right colon. In Bladder Reconstruction and Continent Urinary Diversion, L. R. King, A. R. Stone, G. D. Webster (ed.), pp. 360–366. Chicago: Year Book Medical Publishers

52. Goldwasser, B., Barrett, D. M., Benson, R. C. (1986) Bladder replacement with use of a detubularized right colonic segment: A preliminary report on a new technique. Mayo Clinic Proceedings, 61, 615–621

53. Johnston, J. H. (1963) Temporary cutaneous ureterostomy in the managment of advanced congenital urinary obstruction. Archives of Disease in Childhood, 38, 161–166

54. Perlmutter, A. D., Patel, J. (1972) Loop cutaneous ureterostomy in infants and young children: Late results in 32 cases. Journal of Urology, 107, 655–659

55. Perlmutter, A. D., Tank, E. S. (1968) Loop cutaneous ureterostomy in infancy. Journal of Urology, 99, 559–563

56. Williams, D. I., Cromie, W. J. (1975) Ring ureterostomy. British Journal of Urology, 47, 789–792

57. Hendren, W. H. (1985) Urinary undiversion and augmentation cystoplasty. In Clinical Pediatric Urology, 2nd Edn, P. P. Kelalis, L. R. King, A. B. Belman (ed.), pp. 620–642. Philadelphia: W. B. Saunders Co

58. Hendren, W. H. (1978). Some alternatives to urinary diversion in children. Journal of Urology, 119, 652–660

59. Hendren, W. H. (1973) Reconstruction of previously diverted urinary tracts in children. Journal of Pediatric Surgery, 8, 135–150

60. Hendren, W. H. (1976) Urinary diversion and undiversion in children. Surgical Clinics of North America, 56, 425–449

61. Hendren, W. H. (1974) Urinary tract refunctionalization after prior diversion in children. Annals of Surgery, 180, 494–510

62. Kogan, S. J., Kim, K., Levitt, S. B. (1976) Preoperative evaluation of bladder function prior to renal transplantation or urinary tract reconstruction in children: description of a method. Journal of Pediatric Surgery, 11, 1007–1008

63. Hendren, W. H., Hensle, T. W. (1980) Transureteroureterostomy: experience with 75 cases. Journal of Urology, 123, 826–833

64. Hodges, C. V., Moore, R. J., Lehman, T. H., Behnam, A. M. (1963) Clinical experiences with transuretero-ureterostomy. Journal of Urology, 90, 552–562

65. Sharpe, N. W. (1906) Trans-uretero-ureteral anastomosis. Annals of Surgery, 44, 687–707

66. Stewart, B. H., Hewitt, C. B., Banowsky, L. H. W. (1976) Management of extensively destroyed ureter: Special reference to renal autotransplantation. Journal of Urology, 115, 257–261

67. Hendren, W. H., McLorie, G. A. (1983) Late stricture of intestinal ureter. Journal of Urology, 129, 584–590

68. Hendren, W. H. (1978) Tapered bowel segment for ureteral replacement. Urologic Clinics of North America, 5, 607–616

69. Goodwin, W. E., Harris, A. P., Kaufman, J. J., Beal, J. M. (1953) Open, transcolonic ureterointestinal anastomosis: new approach. Surgery, Gynecology and Obstetrics, 97, 295–300

70. Hendren, W. H. (1980) Construction of female urethra from vaginal wall and a perineal flap. Journal of Urology, 123, 657–664

71. Hendren, W. H. (1978) Complications of ureterostomy. Journal of Urology, 120, 269–281

72. Hendren, W. H. (1986) Repair of cloacal anomalies: Current techniques. Journal of Pediatric Surgery, 21, 1159–1176

73. Ferris, D. O., Odel, H. M. (1950) Electrolyte pattern of the blood after bilateral ureterosigmoidostomy. Journal of the American Medical Association, 142, 634–640

# Rhabdomyosarcoma

**J. Siebert** MD
Resident in Surgery, Massachusetts General Hospital, Boston, Massachusetts, USA

**S. Kim** MD
Clinical Associate Professor of Surgery, Harvard Medical School; Visiting Surgeon, Massachusetts General Hospital, Boston, Massachusetts, USA

## INTRODUCTION

Rhabdomyosarcoma is the most common soft-tissue sarcoma and the most common soft-tissue neoplasm of the pelvis in children. It represents 5–15 per cent of all malignant soft-tissue tumours and 5 per cent of all malignant diseases in children under 15 years of age. The overall 2-year survival has improved from less than 20 per cent about twenty years ago to 65–70 per cent currently. There has been an evolution of therapy over the past two decades from radical surgery to a combination of chemotherapy, radiation, and surgery. Due to the improvement in chemotherapeutic agents, chemotherapy now stands as the cornerstone of treatment. This has culminated in better survival, with a gratifying improvement in the quality of life because of less mutilating surgery.

## STAGING

Rhabdomyosarcoma has been broken down into clinical groups by the Intergroup Rhabdomyosarcoma Study:

Group I. Localized disease resected completely, regional nodes are negative, and no *two* organs are involved.
Group II. (A) Grossly resected disease, but with positive microscopic residual.
    (B) Regional disease with involved nodes, completely resected with no microscopic residual.
    (C) Regional disease with involved nodes, grossly resected, but with microscopic residual and/or histological involvement of the most distal regional node in the dissection.
Group III. Incomplete resection with gross residual disease.
Group IV. Distant metastatic disease present at onset. This may represent distant organs or nodes.

## BACKGROUND

In 1972 in the United States, the Intergroup Rhabdomyosarcoma Study–I was instituted. This consisted of 691 patients in a therapeutic trial over a 6 year period. Diagnosis was made by biopsy only. Clinical Group I, treated with vincristine, actinomycin, and cyclophosphamide (VAC), was found to have a relapse-free survival rate at 3 years of 84 per cent, and the overall survival rate was 90 per cent. Radiation therapy did not alter the survival rate. For Clinical Group II disease, double-agent chemotherapy (vincristine and dactinomycin) for one year was as effective as the standard three-drug regimen (VAC). At 3 years, 70 per cent of these patients were relapse free and 75 per cent were still alive. Approximately 90 per cent of the patients in Group III and 75 per cent in Group IV responded favourably to a combination of chemotherapy and radiotherapy, with complete regression of disease in over one-quarter of the patients before the start of radiotherapy, and in approximately 50–65 per cent of patients after the completion of therapy. At 3 years, remission rates were 56 per cent of patients in Group III, and 35 per cent in Group IV. Survival rates were 60 per cent in Group III and 20 per cent in Group IV.

Intergroup Rhabdomyosarcoma Study–II was initiated in 1978 on the basis of findings from IRS–I. This revealed that repetitive courses of intensive pulse chemotherapy for 2 years following diagnosis yielded higher disease-free rates as well as higher survival rates for all patients.

Pelvic rhabdomyosarcoma treated with primary VAC therapy with limited radiotherapy/surgery for tumours arising from bladder, prostate, and vagina, revealed improved bladder salvage rates from 44 per cent in IRS–I to 57 per cent in IRS–II, without jeopardizing survival, which remained at 78 per cent for 3 years. However, only three of 11 patients (27 per cent) treated with chemotherapy alone were relapse free. When radiation was instituted at 16 weeks or later for persistent prostatic disease, repeat biopsies from 2 to 8 months later showed persistent disease in two-thirds of patients. This suggests that radiation should be instituted earlier in the course of pelvic rhabdomyosarcoma, especially where tissue sampling cannot ensure true representation of the disease extent, and where wide local excision means a radical surgical procedure.

The review of IRS–I pathology revealed three cytological patterns with definite prognostic implications. The anaplastic (accounting for 11 per cent) and monomorphous patterns (7.4 per cent) were associated with unfavourable prognoses, whereas the common mixed type was associated with a more favourable outcome. In multivariant analysis of clinical factors, only clinical group and alveolar histology could match the pathological classification. Combining patients in Groups I–III, the survival rate at 3 years was 78 per cent for mixed histology versus 48 per cent for the monomorphous and anaplastic types.

These findings have significant therapeutic implications for pelvic rhabdomyosarcoma. For primary tumours of the bladder, prostate, vagina, and uterus which have a favourable prognosis by clinical stage and pathological pattern, and where organ salvage is an important goal, more intensive primary chemotherapy with or without early radiotherapy may be effective in achieving higher complete and sustained response rates before any major surgery has to be performed.

Today in IRS–III in patients with sarcoma localized to the pelvis, the addition of cisplatinum and adriamycin to pulse VAC will hopefully improve the disease-free survival rate, and also salvage the pelvic organs in an even larger percentage of patients. Radiotherapy is to be instituted at week 6, irrespective of response to chemotherapy for lesions arising from the prostate, bladder neck and/or bladder trigone. The study will limit radiotherapy when possible in the treatment of patients with tumours arising from the vagina, uterus and dome of the bladder. In those patients who fail to respond to more conservative regimens employing chemotherapy alone or chemotherapy/radiotherapy as the initial treatment, pelvic exenteration will continue to be effective salvage therapy.

## CLINICAL PRESENTATION

The genitourinary tract is the third most common site of origin for rhabdomyosarcoma, following the head and neck, and the limbs. Rhabdomyosarcoma arising in the pelvis is an insidious tumour in childhood, but often remains localized for prolonged periods. Vaginal rhabdomyosarcoma presents with vaginal discharge, bleeding, or a mass such as botryoid sarcoma. Bladder and prostate primaries will present with dysuria, haematuria, urinary retention, rectal symptoms such as tenesmus and constipation, or a pelvic or perineal mass.

Pelvic rhabdomyosarcomas are subdivided into three major histological categories. The most common among young children is the embryonal type. The alveolar type is more commonly seen in adolescents. Pleomorphic rhabdomyosarcomas are the least common in children and are typically found in adults. The growth patterns of the various tumours are somewhat predictable. Lesions of the bladder and vagina tend to spread submucosally and present with clusters or masses. Primary prostatic lesions spread directly along fascial planes and disseminate via lymphatic and haematogenous routes.

## TREATMENT

The initial diagnosis is obtained via biopsy which can be obtained endoscopically or by laparotomy. It is essential to obtain an accurate assessment of the extent of the disease in order to stage the patient appropriately and to evaluate the response once therapy is instituted. Extent of the local disease can be assessed by computerized tomography scanning of the pelvis, as well as by intravenous urograms, cystograms, barium-enema studies, cystoscopy, vaginoscopy, and both flexible and rigid proctosigmoidoscopy. Metastatic work-up should include computerized tomography scanning of the chest, bone scan, liver chemistries and scanning, as well as bone-marrow aspiration or biopsy.

Once the patient is assigned to the appropriate clinical stage, chemotherapy can commence according to treatment protocols. If tumour growth occurs after 14 days of chemotherapy, or failure to respond is evident at week 8 of therapy, radiotherapy should commence. If the primary lesion arises from other than the prostate, bladder neck, or bladder trigone, radiotherapy should be instituted as early as week 6, regardless of apparent response to chemotherapy. Failure of both chemotherapy and radiotherapy to control tumour growth prior to week 20 requires surgical intervention. Good salvage, with exenteration if indicated, can still be obtained.

At 20 weeks of therapy, all non-invasive studies described for the initial evaluation are repeated. This is in preparation for evaluation laparotomy and/or endoscopic examinations. At the minimum, this operative procedure should include (1) examination of all intra-abdominal organs; (2) biopsy of pelvic and para-aortic lymph nodes; and (3) cystotomy of bladder or prostate lesions with biopsy of the previously involved site. If the site of the prior tumour mass can be excised without exenteration, this should be carried out at the time of laparotomy. This may include partial cystectomy with or without ureteral reimplantation, ureteroureterostomy, nephrectomy, or other indicated procedures for bladder primaries. In prostatic tumours, it may consist of simple prostatectomy or an excision of prostatic nodules. In vaginal lesions, hysterectomy and partial or total vaginectomy should be performed. If the vaginal lesion is very distal, it may be possible to spare the uterus. Oöphorectomy is not performed unless there is gross ovarian involvement.

In patients with either microscopic residual disease or positive regional lymph nodes, local radiotherapy is instituted for those lesions of the vagina, uterus, and dome of the bladder. In patients with tumours where no limited procedure is feasible but where the patient has had partial response to his chemotherapy, X-ray therapy should be employed at this point if not already instituted.

Patients achieving a clinical response, and with laparotomy biopsies confirming no evidence of disease, are placed on maintenance chemotherapy.

Patients with progressive disease, with no response or with a response less than 50 per cent at the time of laparotomy at 20 weeks, should undergo radiotherapy if feasible. A second evaluation is carried out at 28 weeks with repetition of all studies which were positive at 20 weeks. This evaluation need not include laparotomy if tumours are accessible by endoscopic evaluation and biopsy.

A third evaluation is carried out 6 weeks later at

approximately 34 weeks. If gross residual tumour is present, exenteration now provides the greatest chance for disease-free survival. Primary lesions of the prostate, bladder, and vagina can usually be encompassed by anterior exenteration.

If the patient has residual disease or develops recurrent disease following prior conservative surgery, then he or she should undergo 'curative' resection if this is anatomically feasible and if no distant metastases are evident. Locally recurrent disease can be managed in the same fashion as if only a biopsy had been performed at the initial procedure, provided that no radiotherapy or chemotherapy has been employed. This may occur in circumstances where local surgery was performed initially with an incorrect diagnosis. Treatment of spread of the primary tumour varies. If a patient develops regional lymph-node metastases, a retroperitoneal lymph-node dissection should be considered. If local recurrent disease develops after being treated by chemotherapeutic protocol, then surgical resection should be undertaken. Pulmonary metastases that persist despite radiotherapy and chemotherapy should be resected.

## CONCLUSION

Unlike many benign conditions in paediatric surgery, the treatment of malignant tumours continues to strive for better survival rates and quality of life. The treatment of pelvic rhabdomyosarcoma by anterior, posterior, or total exenteration with double stomas was the only hope for cure until the development of better chemotherapeutic agents. Today's management starts with a surgical biopsy, followed by chemotherapy with or without radiation therapy, and then utilizes surgery for evaluation of therapy or as a final resort on any failure of other modes of treatment. This is typical of the changes in the management of malignant tumours in the paediatric patient. Improvement in disease-free states and survival rates will continue as we employ better and more specific chemotherapeutic agents, coupled with the judicious use of radiotherapy.

## Further Reading

1. Ghavimi, F., Exelby, P., D'Angio, G., Cham, W., Lieberman, P. II., Tan, C., et al. (1975) Multidisciplinary treatment of embryonal rhabdomyosarcoma in children. Cancer, 35, 677–686

2. Maurer, H., Moon, T., Donaldson, M., Fernandez, C., Gehan, E. A., Hammond, D., et al. (1977) The intergroup rhabdomyosarcoma study. Cancer, 40, 2015–2026

3. Neifeld, J. P., Maurer, H. M., Godwin, D., Berg, J. W., Salzberg, A. M. (1979) Prognostic variables in pediatric rhabdomyosarcoma before and after multimodal therapy. Journal of Pediatric Surgery, 14, 699–703

4. Grosfeld, J., Clatworthy, W., Newton, W. A. (1969) Combined therapy in childhood rhabdomyosarcoma: an analysis of 42 cases. Journal of Pediatric Surgery, 4, 637–645

5. Fleming, I. D., Etcubanas, E., Patterson, R., Rao, B., Pratt, C., Hustu, O. et al. (1984) The role of surgical resection when combined with chemotherapy and radiation in the management of pelvic rhabdomyosarcoma. Annals of Surgery, 119, 509–514

6. Hays, D. M. (1980) Pelvic rhabdomyosarcomas in childhood: diagnosis and concepts of management reviewed. Cancer, 45, 1810–1814

7. Tefft, M., Hays, D., Raney, R. B., Lawrence, M., Soule, E., Donaldson, M. H. et al. (1980) Radiation to regional nodes for rhabdomyosarcoma of the genitourinary tract in children: is it necessary? A report from the Intergroup Rhabdomyosarcoma Study No. 1 (IRS-1). Cancer, 45, 3065–3068

8. Hays, D. M., Raney, R. B. Jr., Lawrence, W. Jr., Soule, E. H., Gehan, E. A., Tefft, M. (1982) Bladder and prostatic tumours in the Intergroup Rhabdomyosarcoma study (IRS-1): results of therapy. Cancer, 50, 1472–1482

9. Pedrick, T. J., Donaldson, S. S., Cox, R. S. (1986) Rhabdomyosarcoma: the Stanford experience using a TNM staging system. Journal of Clinical Oncology, 4, 370–378

10. Hays, D. M., Shimada, H., Raney, R. B., Tefft, M., Newton, W., Crist, W. M. et al. (1985) Sarcomas of the vagina and uterus: the Intergroup Rhabdomyosarcoma Study. Journal of Pediatric Surgery, 20, 718–724

11. Ghavimi, F., Herr, H., Jereb, B., Exelby, P. R. (1984) Treatment of genitourinary rhabdomyosarcoma in children. Journal of Urology, 132, 313–319

12. Hilgers, R. D. (1975) Pelvic exenteration for vaginal embryonal rhabdomyosarcoma: a review. Obstetrics and Gynecology, 45, 175–180

13. Kramer, S. A. (1985) Pediatric urologic oncology. Urologic Clinics of North America, 12, 31–42

Illustrations by Philip Wilson and F. Wadsworth

# Surgery of renal calculi

**Patrick G. Duffy** FRCS(I)
Consultant Paediatric Urologist, The Hospital for Sick Children, Great Ormond Street, London;
Senior Lecturer in Paediatric Urology, Institute of Urology, University of London, UK

**Philip G. Ransley** FRCS
Consultant Urological Surgeon, The Hospital for Sick Children, Great Ormond Street, London;
Senior Lecturer in Paediatric Urology, Institute of Urology and Institute of Child, University of London, UK

## Pathophysiology

The majority of renal calculi in children are of infective origin. Boys are more commonly affected than girls and the peak incidence occurs between the ages of 2 and 3 years. The most commonly associated organisms are urea-splitting *Proteus* or *E. coli*. The finding of a *Proteus* organism in urine should raise the index of suspicion. The calculi are soft, containing a large amount of organic matrix, and are often poorly opacified. They contain magnesium ammonium phosphate (struvite) and varying quantities of calcium phosphate (apatite), oxalate, carbonate and urate. They may be discrete or form an extensive cast of the pelvicalyceal system. Soft matrix may be passed per urethram. The kidneys are often normal, but pyonephrosis, perinephric abscess or progressive pyelonephritis may occur.

Metabolic calculi are rare in children. Hypercalcaemia may be idiopathic or due to vitamin D overdosage or hypophosphatasia, and usually results in nephrocalcinosis. Hyperparathyroidism is extremely rare in children.

Hypercalciuria is defined (in the United Kingdom) as greater than 4 mg/kg per 24 hours or as a urinary calcium: creatinine ratio of greater than 0.25. Hypercalciuria also occurs in some children with infective stones, especially following a milk load. Renal tubular acidosis results in an alkaline urine, hypercalciuria, and recurrent urinary calculi in addition to nephrocalcinosis. Hyperoxaluria also produces nephrocalcinosis and recurrent oxalate stones, which may require removal if there is urinary obstruction. Uric acid calculi occur in children with leukaemia and are usually sufficiently calcified to be visible on X-ray film. Cystinuria results in recurrent cystine stones which are radio-opaque but not very dense, and rib shadows are clearly visible through them. Surgical intervention will be required for large calculi or obstructing stones prior to establishing an effective regimen of high fluid intake with or without D-penicillamine. Xanthine and dihydroxyadenine stones are radiolucent.

# Preoperative investigations

## RADIOLOGY

The plain abdominal film must include the whole urinary tract and may need to be repeated following bowel preparation.

The intravenous pyelogram and/or ultrasound scan will reveal urinary obstruction and demonstrate the renal anatomy, including any associated anomaly. A degree of ureteric dilatation is often seen in the ureter draining a kidney containing infected stones, and does not necessarily indicate the presence of obstructing calculi.

A micturating cystogram is essential to detect vesico-ureteric reflux, but may be usefully postponed until the stones have been removed and the urine rendered sterile for some weeks, provided that by doing so it is not overlooked.

## URINALYSIS

Microscopy and culture are performed.

pH determination is carried out on an overnight urine. A pH of less than 5.3 in a sterile urine excludes renal tubular acidosis.

Twenty-four hour urinary calcium and oxalate excretion tests are performed. It is essential that these investigations are carried out preoperatively or very much later when the child is ambulant and eating a normal diet.

A screening test for amino acids is carried out.

## PLASMA

Creatinine, urea, electrolytes, calcium, phosphate, and uric acid tests are performed.

The findings of nephrocalcinosis or recurrent calculi demand more extensive biochemical investigation.

# Management

1. Extracorporeal shock-wave lithotripsy;
2. Percutaneous removal;
3. Open surgery.

The more traditional forms of surgery for renal calculi are being superseded by extracorporeal shock-wave lithotripsy (ESWL), and percutaneous disintegration and removal of the stones. In the adult population routine open renal calculus surgery is being replaced by the lithotripter and the percutaneous approach to the pelvis of the kidney. It is foreseen that as the instruments improve, more children will be treated by these modern techniques.

### EXTRACORPOREAL SHOCK-WAVE LITHOTRIPSY

## 1

The lithotripter, which was introduced into Britain in 1984, has enabled fragmentation of stones without a surgical incision or the insertion of a tube into the kidney. The patient is placed in a water bath. Two X-ray cameras detect the position of the stone and, using a computer, the shock wave from the probe is directed through the water onto the stone.

Second-generation machines do not require the use of a water bath, and the patient does not need general anaesthesia. Smaller and younger patients will eventually be suitable for extracorporeal destruction of calculi.

These machines must be used in major centres, with specialists in percutaneous renal surgery who can overcome the problems of obstruction of the upper and lower ureters by stone fragments.

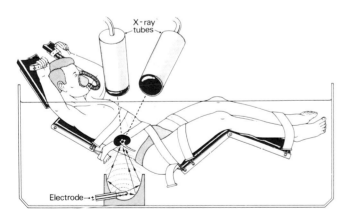

1

## PERCUTANEOUS REMOVAL

### 2

In the adult a percutaneous tract to the kidney is dilated with telescopic steel dilators over a guide-wire. A balloon catheter is placed in the ureter to prevent the stone falling into the lower ureter.

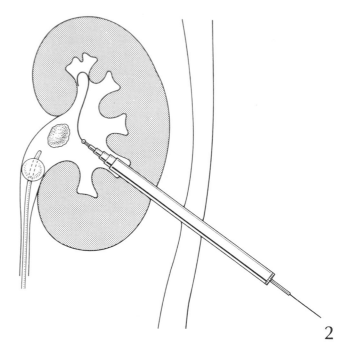

2

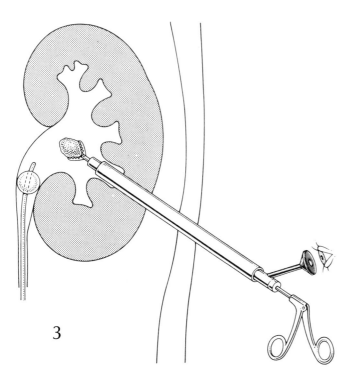

3

### 3

A nephroscope in a sheath with a stone grasper can be used.

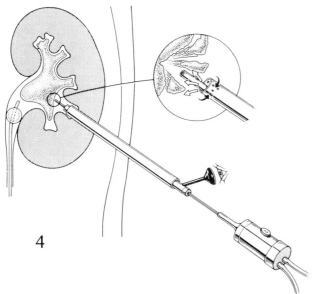

4

### 4

A staghorn calculus can be disintegrated under direct vision using an ultrasound probe.

Suitable endoscopic equipment for approach to the kidney and ureter in the paediatric population has not yet been fully developed.

## OPEN SURGERY

For those centres which do not have this sophisticated equipment, we give the traditional surgical approach to the kidney in children.

## Preparation of patient

The urine should be rendered sterile prior to the operation if possible. Whether or not this is successfully achieved, an appropriate antibiotic should be given with the premedication.

## Anaesthesia

General anaesthesia with an endotracheal tube, relaxation, and artificial ventilation are required. Excessive respiratory movement should be avoided, to reduce the movement of the kidney and the intrusion of the pleura into the operative field.

## Position of the patient

The surgeon should personally supervise the positioning of the patient on the operating table.

The patient is placed in a full lateral position with the lower ribs positioned over the table break or adjustable bridge. The degree of break or bridge elevation will vary with the size of the child. In infants and small children a loosely packed sandbag or foam rubber pad may be more suitable. (Note that if a foil diathermy plate is used the sandbag should go beneath it.) A degree of head-down tilt is convenient and aids venous return. The patient is secured to the table with non-elastic zinc oxide strapping passed over the pelvis and secured to the table on either side. Further strapping of the shoulder may be required in older children, whilst in smaller children a foam pad or sandbag under the dependent side of the chest may aid stability. The child should be held firmly with the back vertical while the strapping is applied, following which a little lateral roll of the table towards the surgeon may be helpful.

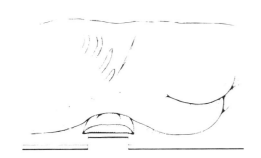

## 5

### The incision

A subcostal incision is suitable in most cases. In older children a supracostal approach (see Urology volume in this series) or via the bed of the twelfth rib may give better access. The incision extends forwards from just below the tip of the twelfth rib and is continued down to the muscle layer. Bleeding is controlled by diathermy.

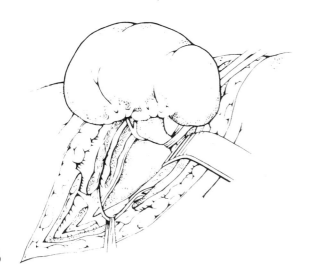

## 6

### Exposure of the kidney

The incision is deepened using cutting diathermy, the peritoneum being pushed forwards with the fingers before completing the anterior portion. The subcostal nerve is identified and preserved. Gerota's fascia is incised longitudinally and a finger swept over the kidney surface to free it from surrounding fat. The ureter is identified and secured with a sling. In most children the kidney may now be delivered into the wound and the posterior surface exposed.

## 7

### Incision into renal pelvis

The surface of the pelvis is freed of fatty tissue and the parenchyma retracted. Formal dissection of the renal sinus is not usually required in children. With a large extrarenal pelvis a vertical incision may be employed. If the pelvis is small, an oblique incision extending up towards the infundibulum of the upper calyx gives better access and may be continued into the lower calyx to raise a triangular flap. Stay sutures are applied to the margins of the incision.

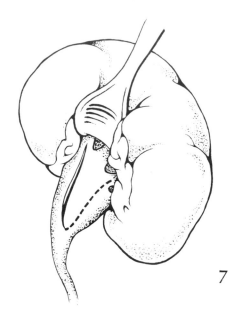

7

## 8

### Removal of stones

A stone in the renal pelvis will now be visible and can be lifted out gently with stone forceps.

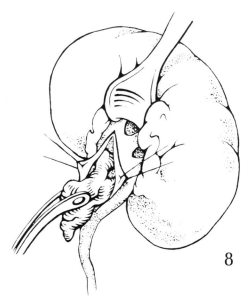

8

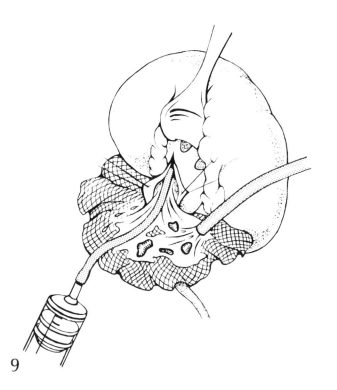

9

### Irrigation of pelvicalyceal system

## 9

Gauze swabs are now placed around the pelvis to catch small stones and debris and to allow suction without fatty tissue occluding the sucker. A soft catheter with an end hole rather than side holes is introduced, and the calyces are irrigated systematically with normal saline. Stones and debris are carefully removed and any lost into the wound must be retrieved to prevent confusion on later X-ray films.

The exposed kidney is then X-rayed to confirm complete clearance. A marker should be included in the film to assist orientation.

## 10

### Removal of calyceal stones

Calyceal stones may be removed via the renal pelvis, using curved stone forceps. If a calyceal stone can be identified using the stone forceps or by palpation, a nephrotomy incision directly onto the stone or the tip of the forceps may be simpler, quicker and less traumatic.

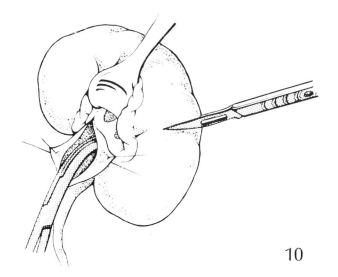

10

## 11

### Exposure of several calyces

Extensive staghorn stones may require the exposure of several calyces. A bulldog clip is applied to the renal artery, or the whole renal pedicle is occluded with a soft intestinal clamp. A longitudinal incision on the posterior surface parallel to the lateral margin of the kidney gives good access. Following removal of the stones the clamps are released intermittently to allow identification and under-running of major vessels. The calyces are approximated with interrupted 3/0 catgut stitches and the kidney parenchyma is apposed with loosely tied horizontal mattress sutures through the capsule. The kidney swells on removal of the clamps, and if these sutures are too tight they will cut out.

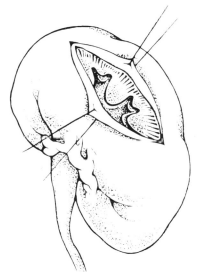

11

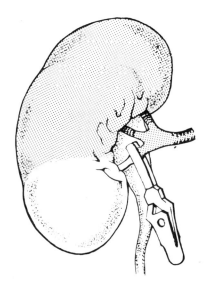

12

## 12

### Lower-pole calculi

The lower branch of the renal artery is readily identifiable and may be occluded with a bulldog clip. Intravenous methylene blue following occlusion may aid demarcation.

# 13

### Incision into lower pole

Simple incision into the lower-pole calyx may then be performed. Lower-pole partial nephrectomy (see pages 507–511) is rarely required in children.

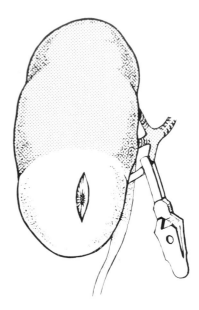

13

### Closure

# 14

Following X-ray confirmation of complete clearance, the incision in the renal pelvis is closed with interrupted 4/0 catgut sutures. A drain is positioned adjacent to the renal pelvis and Gerota's fascia is reconstructed using 3/0 catgut. The wound is closed in layers with catgut and interrupted 3/0 silk for the skin.

The stones should be sent separately for analysis and culture.

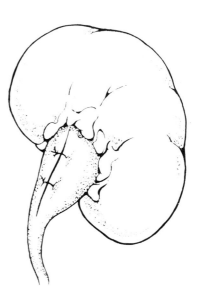

14

# Postoperative care

Intravenous fluids are administered for 24 hours. If the peritoneal cavity has been opened during the course of the operation, they may be required for a longer period.

The drain may be removed after 48 hours if there is no urine leak, or shortened at 5 days if urine leakage has occurred.

Antibiotics are administered throughout the post-operative period and continued prophylactically if vesico-ureteric reflux is present. Where a delayed cystogram is planned reflux must be assumed to be present until the examination has been performed.

### Follow-up

Monthly urine cultures should be carried out and a follow-up pyelogram obtained at 6 months. Further plain films of the urinary tract are taken at 6-monthly intervals for 2 years. Provided the urine remains sterile, recurrences are rare. Further surgery may be required for the correction of vesicoureteric reflux.

### *Further reading*

Barratt, T. M., Williams, D. I. (1974) Urolithiasis. In *Handbuch der Urologie*, Band XV, Supplement, *Urology in Childhood*, D. I. Williams, T. N. Barrett, H. B. Eckstein, S. M. Kohlinsky, G. H. Newns, P. E. Polani, *et al*. (eds) pp. 280–295. Berlin: Springer-Verlag

Illustrations by Kevin Marks

# Posterior urethral valves

**Ian A. Aaronson**   MA, MB, BChir, FRCS
Professor of Urology and Pediatrics, Director of Pediatric Urology, Medical University of South Carolina, Charleston, South Carolina, USA

## Introduction

### Valve anatomy

# 1a, b & c

A posterior urethral valve is a single structure which takes origin from the inferior margin of the verumontanum. Although its embryology is uncertain, it lies in the position of the infracristal ridges which can usually be discerned in the normal posterior urethra (a). When exposed at autopsy through the anterior urethral wall the valve appears as two separate leaflets (b) but endoscopically these are seen to fuse in the midline anteriorly where most of the obstruction occurs (c).

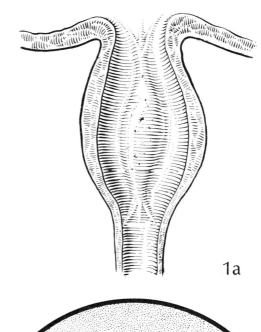

1a

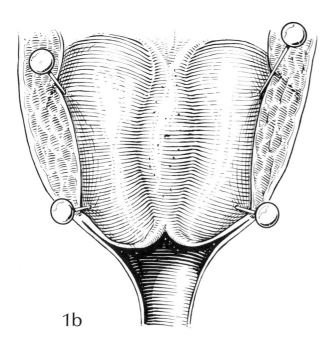

1b

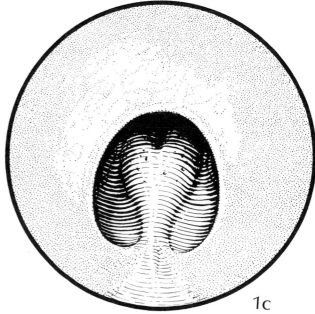

1c

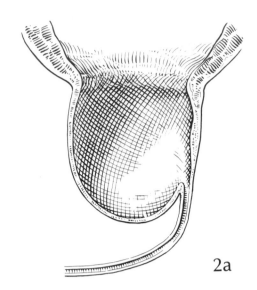

2a

# 2a, b & c

Most valves are thin, filmy structures which balloon downwards during voiding (a). A very lax valve may occasionally prolapse as far as the bulbar urethra (b), whilst one which is rigid forms a transverse diaphragmatic obstruction in the mid-posterior urethra (c). All types, however, take origin from the inferior margin of the verumontanum, and Young's classification, which has been in use for over 50 years, should finally be discarded.

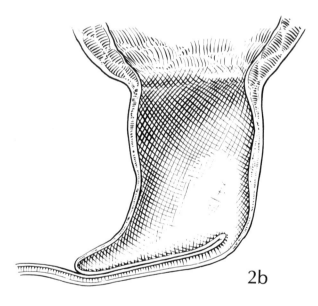

2b

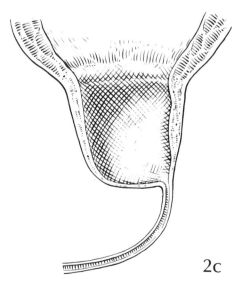

2c

## 3

Minor degrees of valve are sometimes encountered in which the two leaflets blend with the lateral urethral wall. It is highly improbable they ever cause symptoms or require treatment.

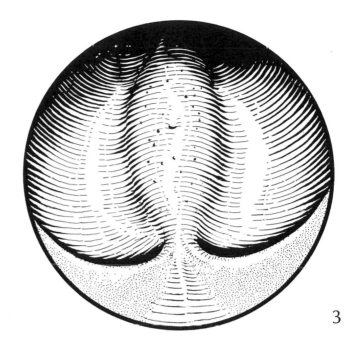

3

## Effect on upper urinary tract

Above the valve, back-pressure effects are nearly always present. These take the form of a widely dilated posterior urethra, a thick-walled and usually trabeculated bladder, widely dilated tortuous ureters and bilateral symmetrical hydronephrosis. Vesicoureteric reflux is common and frequently associated with a varying degree of renal dysplasia.

The bladder neck is always thickened as part of detrusor hypertrophy but hardly ever causes obstruction or requires treatment.

## Presentation

Nowadays the diagnosis is usually made either before birth as a result of antenatal ultrasound, or immediately afterwards because of a persistently palpable bladder. Urinary ascites is an occasional presentation in the first weeks of life.

Infants in whom the diagnosis has been missed usually present with urinary infection and acute-on-chronic renal failure. This is generally accompanied by hyperkalaemia and a severe metabolic acidosis which may lead to respiratory arrest. Water and sodium balance are often also profoundly disturbed. Septicaemia is common and may be complicated by a consumptive coagulopathy.

Older boys may also present with urinary infection but often the main complaint is of a poor stream, straining or urinary incontinence.

The diagnosis will usually be suspected on clinical grounds and supported by the ultrasound findings of a widened posterior urethra, distended bladder, and dilated upper urinary tract.

# Preoperative

### Preparation of infant

On suspicion of the diagnosis a No. 8 Fr plastic infant feeding tube should be passed transurethrally and secured for continuous bladder drainage. Self-retaining catheters should be avoided as the hypertrophied bladder tends to clamp down around the balloon and obstruct the ureters.

It is essential that the bladder drains well and its failure to do so is usually because the catheter has curled up in the posterior urethra. Withdrawing the catheter for a few centimetres and repassing it with a finger in the rectum will usually ensure its passage through the hypertrophied bladder neck. Persistent difficulty can usually be resolved by injecting a few millilitres of contrast medium through the catheter and manipulating it under fluoroscopic control.

When the urine appears to be infected, a blood as well as a urine culture should be taken and intravenous tobramycin or cefotaxime given. Blood coagulation studies are also advisable. Plasma creatinine should be measured and any derangement of acid–base, potassium, sodium, or water balance corrected. In infants with severe metabolic disturbances the aid of a paediatric nephrologist can be invaluable.

In most cases the above actions will result in a rapid improvement in the infant's general condition. If this is not apparent within 24 hours, percutaneous nephrostomy drainage of both kidneys should be considered.

### Confirmation of diagnosis

The presence of a posterior urethral valve is most easily confirmed by a micturating cystourethrogram. However, this should be delayed until urinary infection has been brought completely under control and metabolic disturbances corrected.

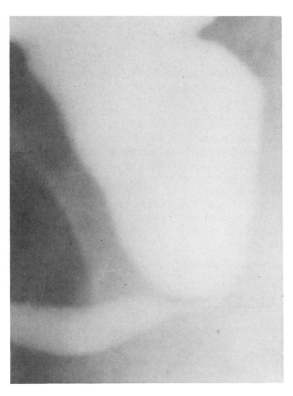

## 4

A voiding film during full micturition is necessary to demonstrate the valve, which appears like a spinnaker sail billowing out before the stream which continues distally from the posterior margin of the obstruction. Dilatation of the urethra proximal to the valve is essential to the diagnosis, and signs of bladder hypertrophy are usually also present.

4

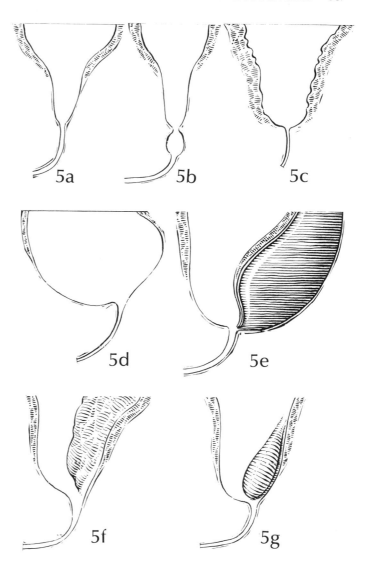

# 5a–g

Normal variants frequently mistaken for a valve include partial hold-up at the level of the external urethral sphincter caused by hesitancy (a) and indentations in the posterior urethral contour produced by the pelvic floor (b). Pathological conditions to be considered in the differential diagnosis are a neuropathic bladder (c), the prune belly syndrome (d), distortion of the posterior urethra caused by an ectopic ureter (e), and urethral filling defects resulting from an ectopic ureterocele (f) or posterior urethral polyp (g).

Endoscopic confirmation of the diagnosis is made immediately prior to valve ablation.

# The operation

### THE FULL-TERM INFANT AND CHILD

Under general anaesthesia the infant is placed in a modified lithotomy position with the buttocks brought well down to the end of the operating table. The legs should be well protected with cotton wool and fixed to the supports with crepe bandage. The skin is prepared and drapes applied, taking care to exclude the anus from the operative field.

The calibre of the penile urethra should first be checked with a well-lubricated No. 10 Fr sound which should only be introduced for about 1–2 cm. If necessary, a meatotomy can be performed, but no attempt should be made to dilate the urethra.

# 6

A No. 10 Fr infant resectoscope with a hooked ball electrode (Storz) is assembled and the alignment of the working parts checked through a 0 degree telescope. The sheath is dried and thoroughly coated with water-soluble lubricant, and with its introducer in place is gently inserted through the meatus. The introducer is now removed and the instrument reassembled and gently advanced under vision into the bladder. The presence of diverticula and the position and shape of the ureteric orifices are noted.

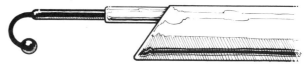

6

## 7

The instrument is now rotated through 180 degrees and, with the irrigation fluid running in under low pressure, gradually withdrawn through the bladder neck. Just beyond the verumontanum the valve will suddenly snap across the field of view like a curtain with a central slit-like aperture. Further withdrawal of the instrument and manipulation of the trigger will cause the ball to engage the valve in the 12 o'clock position. A short burst of cutting current is then applied.

7

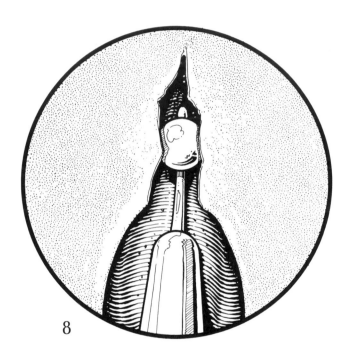

8

## 8

The instrument is turned back to the normal position and re-advanced under vision towards the bladder neck. Withdrawing the instrument will now bring the disrupted valve into view.

## 9

The procedure is repeated, rotating the instrument to engage residual valve tissue in the 10 o'clock, 2 o'clock, 8 o'clock and finally the 4 o'clock positions. Any remaining freely floating tags do not require treatment. The resectoscope is now removed and the presence of an unobstructed urethra confirmed by manual expression of the bladder. Finally, a No. 8 Fr feeding tube is passed to drain the bladder for 48 hours.

If any significant bleeding occurs, attempts at valve ablation should be immediately discontinued and the situation reassessed after two or three days of catheter drainage.

In older children a No. 13 Fr resectoscope may be used, employing a similar technique.

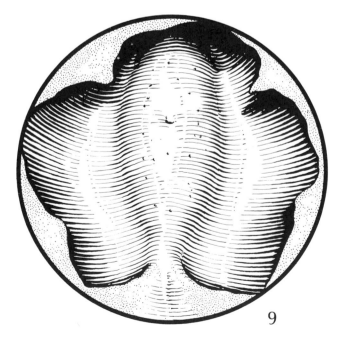

9

## THE PRETERM INFANT

It is inadvisable to attempt to pass a No. 10 Fr resectoscope in infants weighing less than 2.5 kg. Instead, one of the following procedures can be employed:

1. *A No. 8 Fr cystoscope*  The instrument can usually be introduced into the urethra in all but the smallest infants. A modified No. 3 ureteric catheter with a metal stilette may be passed alongside the cystoscope and used to coagulate the valve.

2. *Whitaker hook electrode*  This newly available*,well-insulated and relatively atraumatic instrument can be introduced under fluoroscopic control and withdrawn to engage the valve. A short burst of cutting current in the 9 o'clock and 3 o'clock positions is usually sufficient to relieve obstruction.

3. *Fogarty catheter*  This is passed into the bladder, where the balloon is inflated with 0.1–0.2 ml water. It is then withdrawn until the balloon is felt to engage the valve. Disruption may be achieved by a further short sharp pull on the catheter.

4. *Perineal urethrotomy*  Access to the valve by a No. 10 resectoscope can usually be achieved by a perineal urethrotomy. However, the small calibre of the urethra and the friable nature of urothelium render the operation difficult and postoperative infection, stricture or diverticulum formation are common.

5. *Antegrade endoscopic disruption*  A good view of the valve may be obtained with a No. 10 Fr or 13 Fr resectoscope introduced via the bladder neck through a formal vesicostomy. The valve is then ablated by electrocautery.

6. *Vesicostomy*  This operation is an excellent and safe means of obtaining immediate relief of obstruction in small infants when specialized instruments are not available.

7. *Indwelling urethral catheter*  In very small babies the bladder may be drained by a No. 5 Fr infant feeding tube for several weeks to allow growth to occur. However, frequent monitoring of the urine is necessary to ensure that it remains free of infection.

# Postoperative management

## At 48 hours

The urethral catheter is removed and the bladder checked by clinical examination for adequate emptying. If necessary this can be confirmed by ultrasound. Polyuria, hyponatraemia and metabolic acidosis are commonly present and need to be corrected. Once this is done and infection eradicated the plasma creatinine will usually fall rapidly towards normal.

## At 3 months

The glomerular filtration rate of each kidney is measured by the slope clearance method using $^{99m}$Tc DTPA.

## At 6 months

The MCUG is repeated to confirm adequate resection of the valve, the absence of any stricture of the urethra, and to determine if vesicoureteric reflux is still present. In about one-third of cases it will have disappeared. A renal scan using $^{99m}$Tc DMSA is also carried out to determine the relative renal cortical mass on either side. It is also useful to obtain an IVU to serve as a baseline for any subsequent studies.

### ADDITIONAL SURGERY

This may be indicated in the following situations:

1. *Persistently raised plasma creatinine* Among infants in whom there is little or no improvement in plasma creatinine within 10–14 days of relieving obstruction, the eradication of infection, and the correction of metabolic disturbances, an exploration of the kidney should be considered. This will often reveal bilateral cystic kidneys which on biopsy will be found to be dysplastic. An intraoperative Whitaker test should also be carried out to exclude obstruction at the ureterovesical junction.

2. *Ureterovesical obstruction* Mild hold-up at the ureterovesical junction is common in the first week or two after surgery, but in most cases it is self-limiting and does not require treatment. When significant obstruction is confirmed by a Whitaker test it is most simply relieved by a temporary Sober 'Y' or ring cutaneous ureterostomy. Alternatively the ureters may be remodelled and reimplanted, but this operation is exacting and in inexperienced hands complications are common.

3. *Persistent reflux* When the $^{99m}$Tc DMSA study indicates that the kidney on the refluxing side has negligible function, nephroureterectomy should be carried out. Otherwise the ureter is remodelled and reimplanted.

### LONG-TERM FOLLOW UP

Infants who initially presented with impaired renal function will require supervision until they become adults. A progressive rise in plasma creatinine is often seen throughout childhood, and in the most severe cases renal transplantation may become necessary by puberty.

## *Further reading*

Aaronson, I. A. (1984) Posterior urethral valve: a review of 120 cases. South African Medical Journal, 65, 418–422

Aaronson, I. A., Cremin, B. J. (1984) Lower urinary tract obstruction. In: Clinical Paediatric Uroradiology, I. A. Aaronson and B. J. Cremin, pp. 210–232, Chapter 11. Edinburgh, London and New York: Churchill Livingstone

Illustrations by Philip Wilson

# Hypospadias repair

**John W. Duckett**  MD
Director, Division of Urology, Children's Hospital of Philadelphia, Philadelphia, Pennsylvania, USA

## The operation

## 1a–h

### Anterior hypospadias (subcoronal meatus)

This is the most common lesion: the subcoronal meatus with a blind-ending distal groove accounts for 60–70 per cent of cases. The stream will be deflected ventrally 45–60 degrees. In about 30 per cent the meatus is stenotic, a dorsal preputial hood is present, and the median raphe deviates to one side, creating some torsion.

Repair of this deformity is indicated to correct the direction of voiding. Replacement of thin ventral penile skin by rotated preputial skin may also be required. Reconstruction of an uncircumcised preputial appearance is possible, or the family may choose a circumcised appearance.

## Meatal advancement and glanuloplasty (MAGPI)

Even the very stenotic subcoronal meatus may be repaired with this technique and no prior meatotomy is necessary. The operation is performed at about six months of age. A vertical incision into the glanular groove for a distance of about one centimetre opens the dorsal meatus generously. Transverse closure of the diamond-shaped defect created flattens out the glanular groove and allows a straight stream to emerge.

Sometimes the glanular bridge between meatus and groove is redundant and a wedge is then removed. It is helpful to place 1:100 000 of adrenaline into the glans with a 26-gauge needle, in order to obtain haemostasis and improve visualization of the tissues.

After an adequate meatal advancement has been achieved the ventral lip of the urethra is fixed with a holding stitch and brought forward. This tilts the glans to a more normal conical position and allows the lateral glanular wings to rotate to the ventrum. Holding stitches are frequently placed in the glanular wings to approximate them more normally. The excess ventral epithelium is excised to approximate a nice edge and form a cosmetically normal ventral glans. The glanular tissue beneath the epithelium may be approximated with 6/0 polyglycolic acid sutures, and another layer of chromic catgut used to bring the epithelial edges together. If the newly created urethral meatus has redundant tissue from the lateral glanular grooves this may be excised to improve the appearance.

A sleeve approximation of the penile skin may be done, excising all redundant tissue and leaving a circumcised appearance. Alternatively, the preputial skin may be fashioned so as to recreate the prepuce for the 'European look', but this carries a higher risk of breakdown.

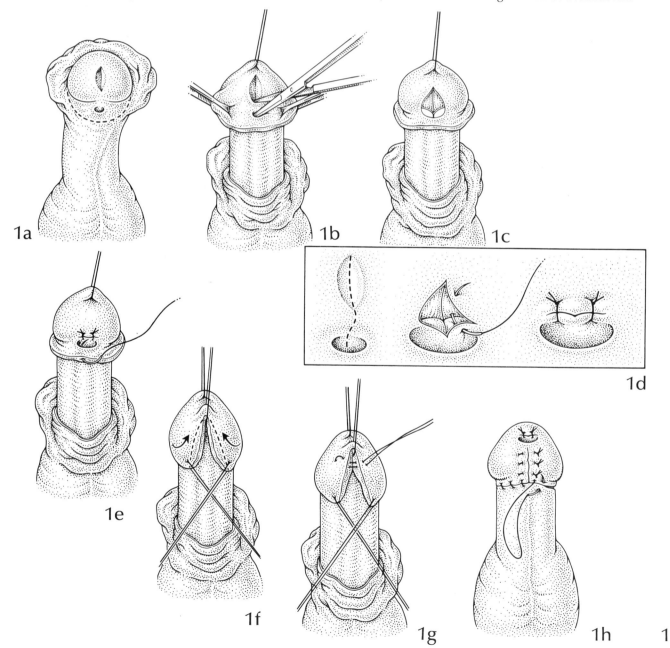

1a

1b

1c

1d

1e

1f

1g

1h

1

# 2a–d

## Perimeatal-based flap (Mathieu procedure)

This technique is utilized for a meatus that is on the distal shaft approximately 1 cm from the corona, but is wide open and fixed, so that it cannot be mobilized and advanced by the MAGPI technique. The ventral skin must be thick, so that a perimeatal-based flap will be adequately vascularized. Subcutaneous tissue should be left attached to this ventral flap to assure this.

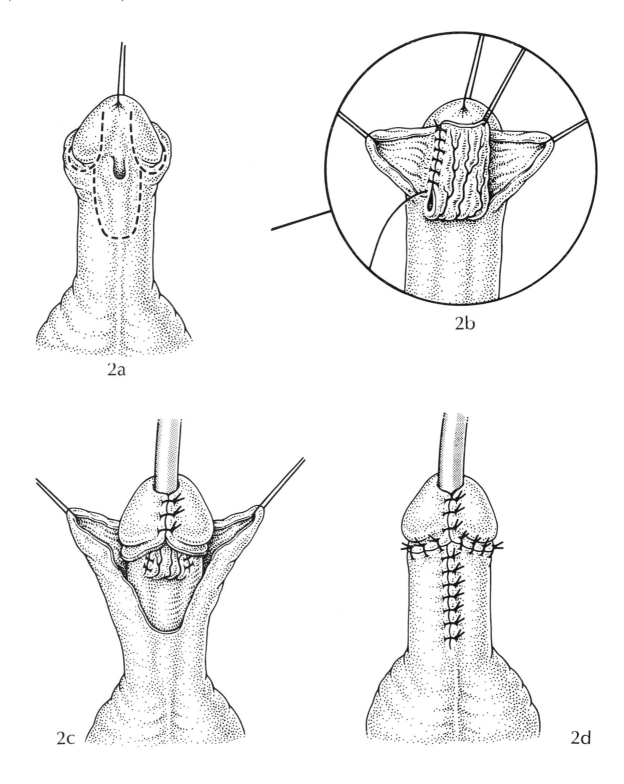

2a

2b

2c

2d

# 3a–j

### Transverse preputial island flap with glans channel

This technique is universally useful for one-stage procedures in which chordee release is done at the same time as urethroplasty. It is reserved for urethral replacement of approximately 2.5–5 cm. The vascularized neourethra heals without the need for revascularization from skin cover. The proximal anastomosis should be fixed to the tunica albuginea, attaching good spongiosal tissue of the proximal urethra so that the anastomosis will not kink. It should calibrate from 10–14 French. The distal glanular groove must be generous in size, 16–20 French, to avoid compromising the vascularized pedicle traversing the glans channel. Compromise of this portion of the neourethra will lead to a long glans stricture which is most difficult to manage whilst maintaining an apical meatus.

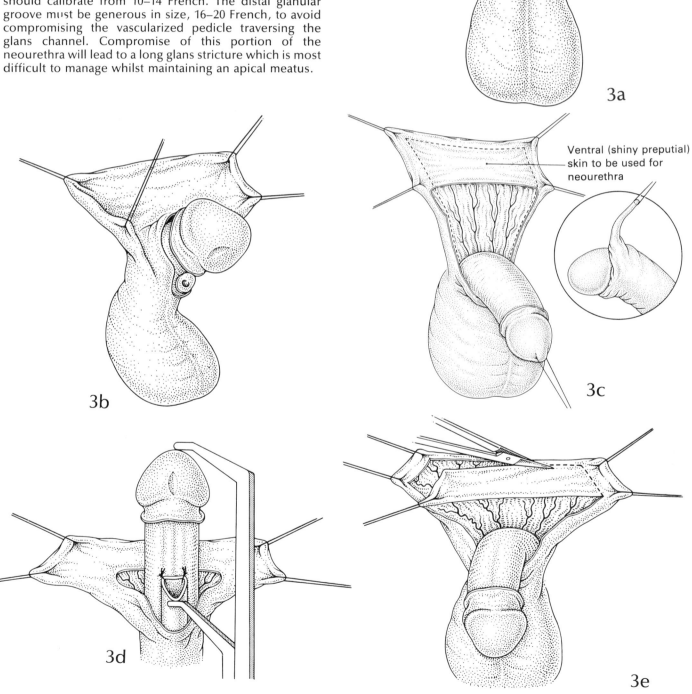

Ventral (shiny preputial) skin to be used for neourethra

3a

3b

3c

3d

3e

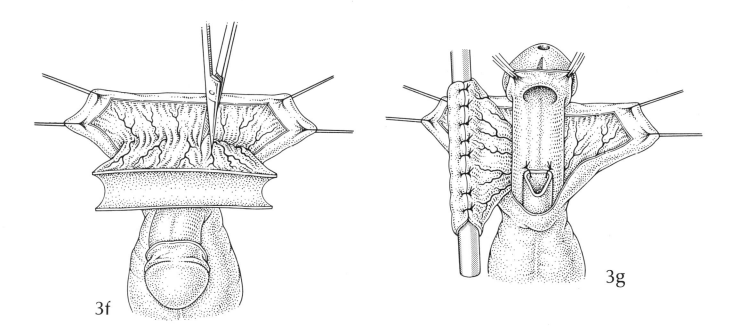

3f

3g

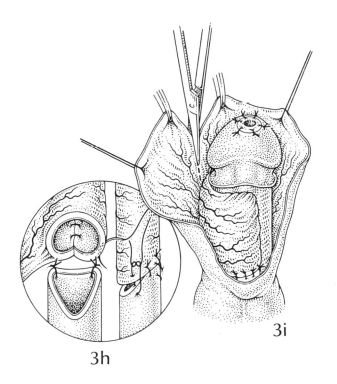

3h

3i

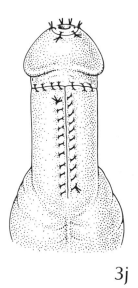

3j

# 4a–d

**Transverse preputial island flap plus perineal
extension for perineal hypospadias with bifid
scrotum**

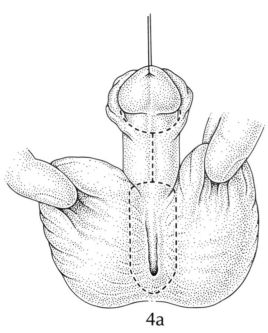

4a

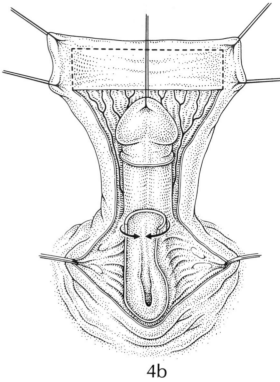

4b

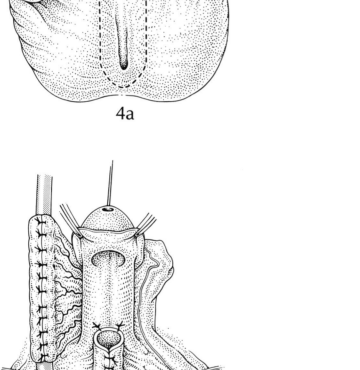

4c

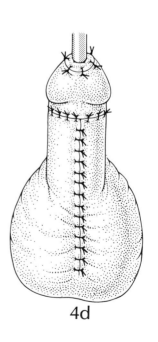

4d

# 5a, b & c

**Transverse preputial island flap variation 'button hole' for transposing wide pedicle to ventrum**

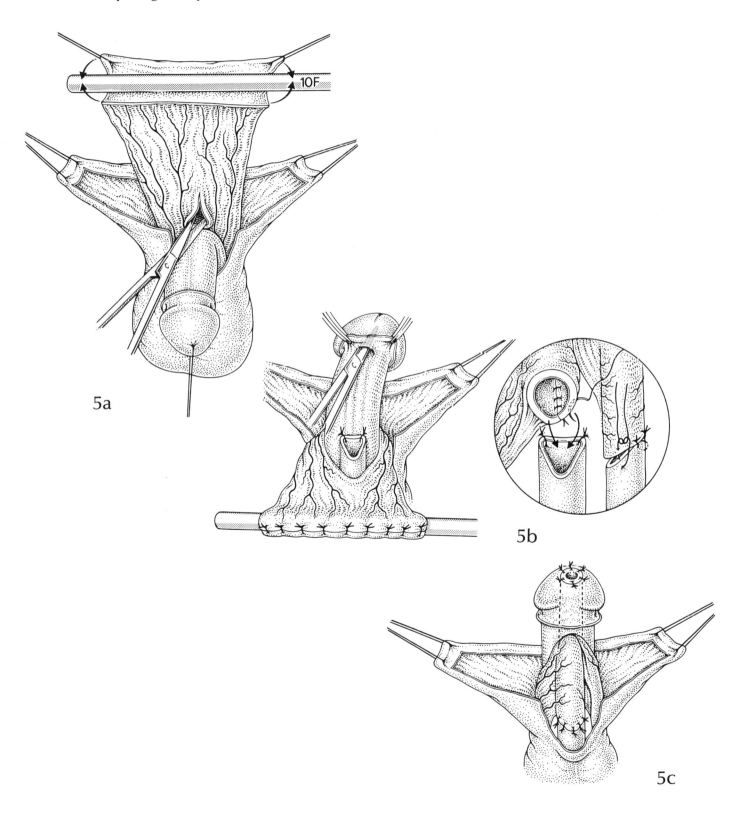

5a

5b

5c

# 6a–g

## Double-faced preputial island flap

This modification of the standard island flap technique allows for a nice ventral skin cover. The dorsal preputial skin is left attached to the island flap and the inner surface rolled into a tube, while the outer surface serves as the ventral skin cover. It takes considerable ingenuity to fashion the skin in order to avoid compromising the neourethra, but will provide a cosmetic skin cover.

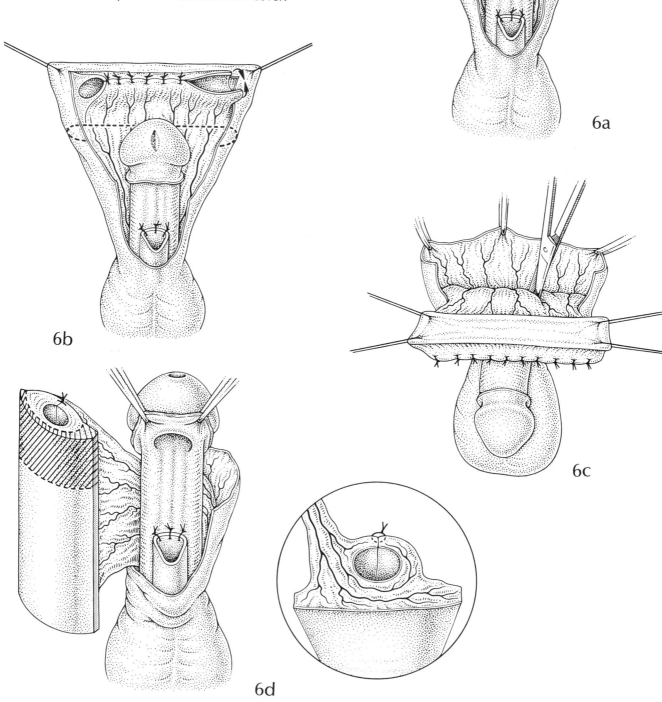

6a

6b

6c

6d

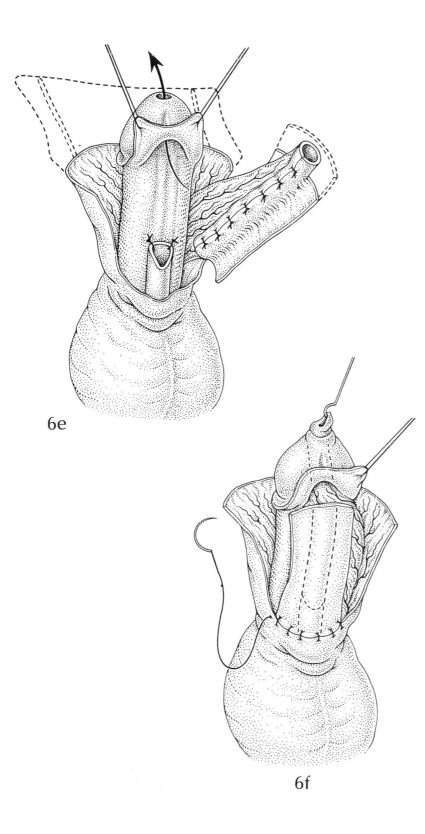

6e

6f

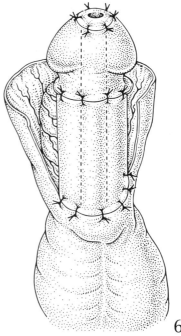

6g

# 7a–h

## Onlay island flap

This is for cases with a proximal meatus without chordee. It is especially appropriate for a meatus that is covered with very thin penile skin which must be cut back to spongiosal tissue. A ventral strip of urethral plate is left intact all the way into the glans. A transverse preputial island flap of approximately 10–12 mm is made and is swung around to the ventrum. It is anastomosed longitudinally on one side with a running suture. Then the flap is turned over as a ventral cover for the urethral plate and a proximal horseshoe closure is made around the proximal meatus with interrupted sutures. The meatus is calibrated to 10–14 French size, and the opposite side is then closed with a running suture up to the glans, making sure that there is not too much redundancy of the onlay flap in case this later forms a diverticulum. The meatus is fashioned by bringing glans wings around the onlay flap, making an apical meatus, and bringing glans around to the ventrum. Skin approximation can be made in a variety of fashions.

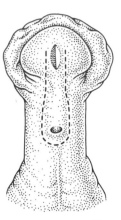

7a

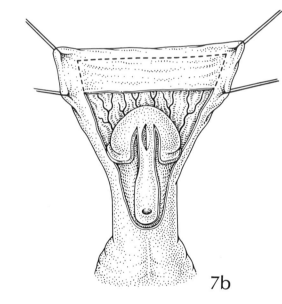

7b

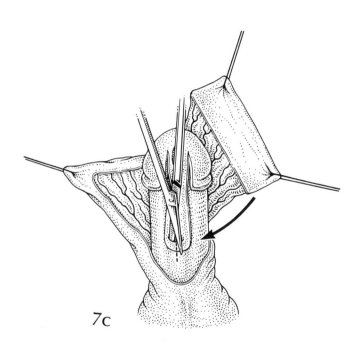

7c

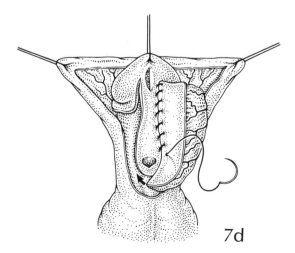

7d

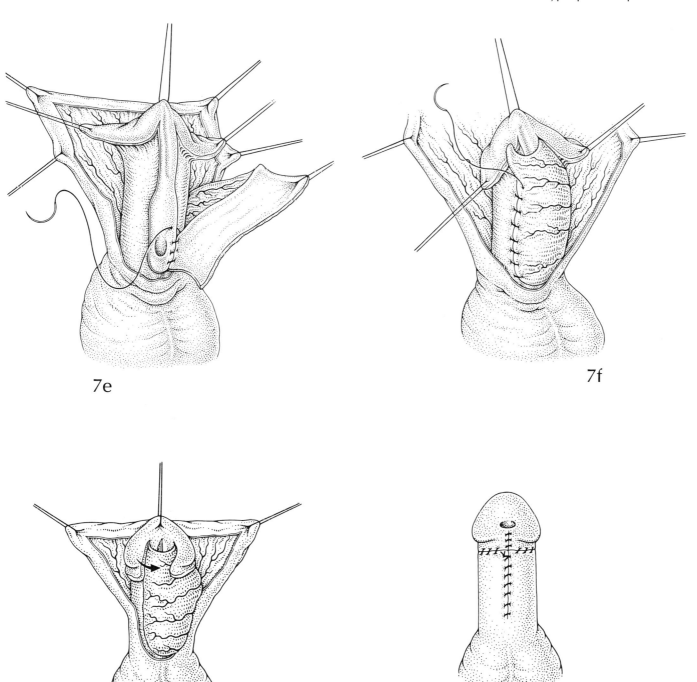

7e

7f

7g

7h

## SUTURES

Polyglycolic or PDS sutures (6/0 or 7/0) are normally used on the internal structures, whereas 7/0 chromic is our preferred suture for the skin and meatus. Unfortunately the 7/0 chromic still leaves some annoying suture tracks. With a cooperative child, those that persist may be opened in the office with local anaesthesia.

## OTHER CONSIDERATIONS

*Age*  We now prefer to operate on children from 6 to 18 months of age, with most between 6 and 12 months.

*Magnification*  We find optical loupes or Optivisor quite satisfactory. The optical microscope has been used, but we have not yet felt the additional magnification to be helpful.

## Diversion

Howard Snyder's contribution of the 6 French Silastic stent sutured to the glans and allowed to drip into the napkin has greatly simplified the management. In older children 4–5 years of age we counsel them in advance and explain that they will go back into napkins, and they have been most cooperative in this regard.

We still prefer to cover the penis with either Xerofoam gauze with an outside gauze wrap and Elastoplast, or a silastic foam dressing. Silastic foam (30 cm$^3$) is mixed with two eye dropper fulls of catalyst. A template of X-ray film or plastic cup is placed around the stretched penis and a cylinder of foam poured into this mould. It forms in 15–60 seconds and the excess is peeled away. Experience is needed to get this foam dressing just right. It will stay on for 7–10 days and the dripping urine on the outside does not soak through.

## OUTPATIENT SURGERY

Almost all of our hypospadias are operated as day surgery cases. The parents of those children from some distance stay nearby and make frequent visits to the hospital. The child is put on suppressive medication while the open tube discharges into the napkin. The parents are instructed to change the napkin frequently, particularly to avoid soiling with stool. The child may take showers with this dressing arrangement, but should not be immersed in a bath.

As Higgins said in 1947, 'Hypospadias is a grievous deformity which must ever move us to the highest surgical endeavor. The re-fashioning of the urethra offers a problem as formidable as any in the wide field of our art.'

Illustrations by Kevin Marks

# Orchidopexy

**Lewis Spitz**   MB, ChB, PhD, FRCS(Ed), FRCS(Eng), FAAP(Hon)
Nuffield Professor of Paediatric Surgery, Institute of Child Health, University of London; Consultant Paediatric Surgeon
Hospital for Sick Children, Great Ormond Street, London, UK

## Introduction

Orchidopexy is one of the commoner surgical procedures performed on the otherwise healthy male child. Maldescent of the testis occurs in 4.3 per cent of male infants at birth (2.7 per cent for full-term and 21 per cent for premature infants). By 6–12 weeks of age two-thirds of these testes will have spontaneously descended into the scrotum. The overall incidence of maldescent at one year is 0.8 per cent. Thereafter the chances of spontaneous descent of the testis are remote.

### EMBRYOLOGY

The gonads develop on the urogenital ridges, which are longitudinal structures on the posterior wall of the coelomic cavity on either side of the root of the mesentery.

Three primordia combine to form the primitive gonad.

1. The primary germ cells, which migrate into the genital ridge.
2. The mesenchyme of the ventromedial aspects of the mesonephros adjacent to the root of the mesentery.
3. The coelomic epithelium overlying the mesenchyme. The latter two components together form the genital ridge.

With the arrival of the primitive germ cells towards the end of the sixth week of intrauterine life, the epithelial cells covering the gonad grow as cords of cells into the mesenchyme. Between the cords lie the germ cells and gonadal mesenchyme.

Early in the eighth week visible sex differentiation commences. The sex cords continue to develop into seminiferous tubules and rete testis. The tubules of the rete testis become secondarily connected with the mesonephric duct which will eventually form the vas deferens.

## DESCENT OF THE TESTIS

The stage of so-called internal descent is the result of elongation and differential growth of the posterior abdominal wall structures. During this process, the mesonephros is carried cranially, leaving the testis behind at the level of the internal inguinal ring, where it remains until the seventh month.

True testicular descent begins at 28 weeks and is usually complete at birth. As the testis enters the internal ring, the gubernaculum emerges from the superficial ring. As soon as the gubernaculum reaches the bottom of the scrotum it contracts, drawing the testis caudally. Descent through the inguinal canal takes only a few days, while complete descent into the scrotum is accomplished within the next four weeks.

Failure of testicular descent is likely to be due to either:

1. a disturbance of the hormonal environment (LHRH, LH, testicular hormone axis); or
2. mechanical failure.

## INDICATIONS FOR ORCHIDOPEXY

1. Spermatogenesis. Degenerative changes commence in the undescended testis during the second or third year of life.
2. Inguinal hernia. Most undescended testes have an associated patent processus vaginalis. A clinical inguinal hernia is rare in childhood but its presence should lead to early surgery to prevent strangulation and/or vascular damage to the testis.
3. Torsion. The undescended testis is more prone to torsion because it lies suspended within the patent processus vaginalis.
4. Trauma. The undescended testis may be more prone to injury because it lacks the normal cushioning effect.
5. Psychological effects. It is generally recommended that for psychological reasons it is beneficial to have both testes in the scrotum by the time the child has to attend school.
6. Malignancy. There is a significantly increased risk of malignancy developing in the undescended testis (40 times that of the normally descended testis). The risk is greatest for the intra-abdominal testis. Although it has been speculated that early orchidopexy may provide some protection against malignant degeneration, placing the undescended testis in the scrotum clearly facilitates early diagnosis of any subsequent malignant swelling. (However, 20 per cent of malignancies occur in the contralateral testes of unilateral maldescents.)

## AGE AT ORCHIDOPEXY

To achieve maximal preservation of spermatogenic function, orchidopexy should be performed around the age of two years.

# Maldescent of the testis

Three types of abnormality of testicular position are recognized.

1. *Retractile testis* is caused by elevation of the testis out of the scrotum and into the superficial inguinal pouch by the action of the cremaster muscle. It is a normal testis and will return spontaneously into the scrotum when the cremaster muscle relaxes, for example in the squatting position, or it can be coaxed back into the scrotum by gentle manipulation from the groin. It may only reach the upper half of the scrotum.
2. *Ectopic testis* is where the testis has emerged through the inguinal canal but has become lodged in an abnormal site, e.g. the superficial inguinal pouch, or the perineal, prepubic, or femoral regions. Strictly, the commonest position (superficial inguinal pouch) is one to which the normally descended testis may retract under stress, and hence is not truly ectopic, although distinct from group 3.
3. *Incompletely descended testis* is caused by an arrest of testicular descent along a normal pathway from the site of development in the urogenital ridges of the retroperitoneum to the scrotum.

# Preoperative preparation

A course of gonadotrophins or luteinizing hormone-releasing hormone is recommended for bilateral impalpable testes as a diagnostic test for the presence of functioning testicular tissue. A rise in serum testosterone level indicates the presence of testes either intra-abdominally or in the inguinal canal. The use of hormones to stimulate testicular descent is still controversial but they may be helpful to differentiate between retractile and maldescended testes.

## Anaesthesia

The operation is performed under general anaesthesia. The side to be operated upon is clearly marked preoperatively. A caudal block will help reduce postoperative discomfort. The child is placed supine on the operating table, with the legs slightly abducted.

## Skin preparation

The operative field, which extends from the umbilicus to the mid-thigh, including both groins and the scrotum, is carefully prepared with an antiseptic solution, e.g. povidone-iodine.

# The operation

The operation consists of two parts:

1. orchiolysis – mobilization of the testis, attention to the associated inguinal hernia, obtaining sufficient length of spermatic cord for the testis to reach the base of the scrotum; and
2. orchidopexy – fixation of the testis in the scrotum.

## ORCHIOLYSIS

### The incision

## 1

A transverse skin incision is made in the lowermost transverse abdominal skin crease. It extends from a point level with the pubic tubercle medially to just above the level of the mid-inguinal point laterally. The incision is deepened through the subcutaneous layers of Camper's fascia (a fatty layer) and Scarpa's fascia (a well-developed fibrous layer) using electrocautery. The superficial inferior epigastric vein is encountered in the subcutaneous tissue on the medial aspect of the incision running obliquely superiorly and laterally. It is coagulated and divided. Immediately deep to the fibrous plane of Scarpa's fascia lies the aponeurotic fibres of the external oblique muscle.

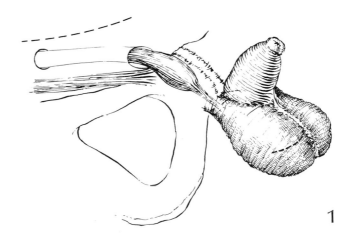

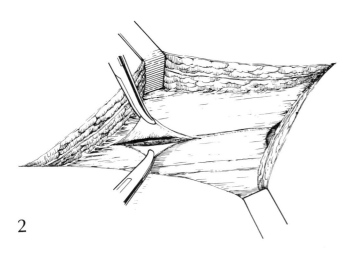

## 2

### Opening the inguinal canal

The lowermost fibres of the external oblique aponeurosis are cleared of overlying fascia, and inferomedially the margins of the external inguinal ring are defined. The spermatic cord will be found passing through the external ring in the case of an ectopic or superficial inguinal pouch testis. A short incision is made in the external oblique aponeurosis above and lateral to the external ring. The edges of the incision in the external oblique are held in artery forceps, exposing the spermatic cord covered by a shiny internal spermatic fascia. The ileoinguinal nerve passes through the inguinal canal on the surface of the spermatic cord. It should be identified and carefully protected. Division of the nerve results in loss of sensation of the upper medial portion of the thigh and the anterior third of the scrotum. The external oblique aponeurosis is carefully mobilized off the surface of the spermatic cord with blunt dissection. The inguinal canal is now opened by extending the incision in the external oblique through the crescentic external ring.

## 3

### Mobilization of the cord structures

The spermatic cord and its coverings are gently lifted out of the inguinal canal using blunt dissection. The testis will usually appear at the medial end of the spermatic cord. As the cord is elevated off the floor of the inguinal canal, the small and fragile cremasteric vessels are encountered. They are secured either by ligation or electrocoagulation and divided. The inferior pole of the testis is attached to the subcutaneous tissues by the gubernaculum, which contains numerous small vessels. The gubernaculum is divided between artery clamps and the ends ligated.

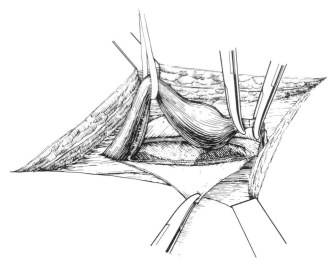

3

## 4

### Dissection of the hernial sac

If a hernial sac is present it is necessary to isolate it from the vas and testicular vessels and to ligate and divide it at the level of the internal inguinal ring. The hernial sac may appear merely as a projection of peritoneum onto the surface of the spermatic cord; this is an incomplete hernia and the sac is easily dissected off the surface of the cord. The complete inguinal hernia appears to surround and envelop the cord structures. It is a thin, friable membrane and is easily torn during rough dissection. To isolate the hernial sac, the cord is drawn upwards over the superolateral part of the incision, to expose its posterior surface. It is here that the two opposing surfaces of the inguinal hernia meet to envelop the vas and vessels. By gently teasing apart the two surfaces, the vas and vessels are exposed.

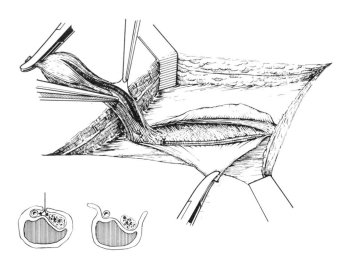

4

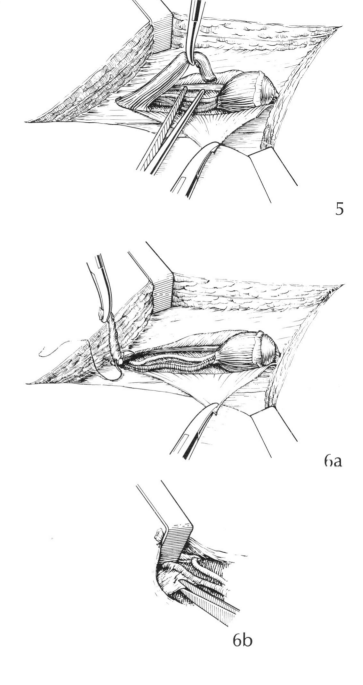

5

6a

6b

# 5, 6a & b

## Isolation of the hernial sac

The vas and vessels are carefully separated from the hernial sac and the distal end divided. The sac is dissected proximally towards the internal ring where it is transfixed with 3/0 Dexon and divided. To obtain an adequate length of the testicular vessels and avoid tension on the testis when it is placed in the scrotum, the lateral spermatic bands from the deep fascia of the abdominal wall are divided. It may be necessary to extend this dissection proximally in the retroperitoneal tissues to the lower pole of the kidney in order to attain sufficient length of the cord.

If, following extensive retroperitoneal dissection, the cord is still too short, an extra few millimetres may be gained by ligating and dividing the epigastric vessels at the medial border of the internal ring. In the case of an impalpable testis, consideration should be given to the higher properitoneal approach[1], or the internal oblique and transversus muscles may be divided laterally to extend the orthodox incision, or high division of the testicular vessels[2] performed.

## ORCHIDOPEXY

A tunnel into the scrotum is made by finger dissection from the medial end of the groin incision. Fibrous tissue barriers are broken down until the tip of the index finger reaches the base of the scrotum.

# 7a & b

### Incision in the scrotum

A shallow skin incision is made through the skin and underlying dartos muscle at the base of the scrotum (*Illustration 7a*).

Using blunt dissection, a pouch large enough to accommodate the testis comfortably is fashioned between the dartos muscle and the underlying loose fascia within the scrotum (*Illustration 7b*).

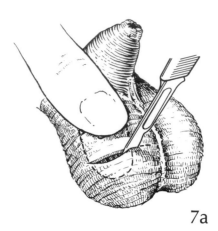

7a

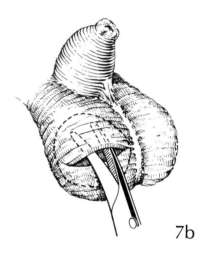

7b

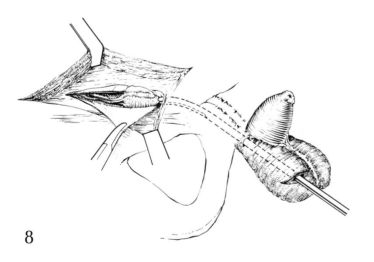

8

# 8

### Bring the testis down into the scrotum

A long, narrow artery forceps is pushed up into the groin through the incision in the scrotum. The opening in the scrotal fascia should be large enough to allow passage of the testis, but small enough to prevent retraction of the testis back into the groin.

The lower pole of the testis is grasped in the jaws of the artery forceps and the testis is drawn into the scrotum, ensuring that torsion of the vas and vessels does not occur.

# 9

## Securing the testis in the dartos pouch

The testis is pulled out through the scrotal incision. If the hole in the scrotal fascia appears too large, it can be narrowed with one or two interrupted Dexon sutures.

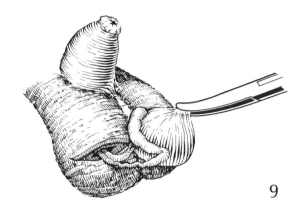

9

# 10

The testis is gently manipulated back into the subdartos pouch. Skin hooks applied to the edges of the scrotal incision facilitate this manoeuvre. The testis is secured in the scrotum with the first skin closure suture and the rest of the scrotal incision is closed with interrupted sutures of 5/0 or 4/0 Dexon or chromic catgut. Tying the sutures on the inside of the scrotum prevents the irritation of sutures on the surface.

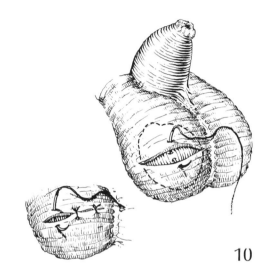

10

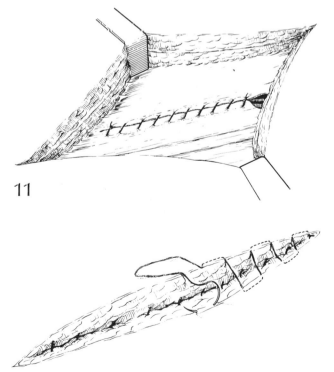

11

12

# 11 & 12

## Closure of the inguinal incision

The cut edges of the external oblique aponeurosis are approximated with a continuous suture of 3/0 or 4/0 Dexon, leaving a snug opening at the external ring for the vas and vessels.

The wound is closed with a continuous suture to the subcutaneous tissues and a subcuticular suture to the skin.

# Postoperative care

The patient may either be discharged from hospital on the evening after the orchidopexy (day-case) or on the first postoperative day. Prolonged hospitalization and bed-rest are unnecessary. During the first few days after surgery the child will crouch forwards while walking, but full recovery is remarkably rapid.

The position of the testis should be checked at 2 weeks and again at 6 months postoperatively.

Full activity and sport may be resumed within 3–4 weeks of the orchidopexy. Complications are rare but may include the following:

1. *Early:*  wound haematoma;
wound sepsis;
testicular necrosis.
2. *Late:*  testicular retraction into the groin;
testicular atrophy;
malignancy.

## References

1. Jones, P. F., Bagley, F. H. An abdominal extraperitoneal approach for the difficult orchidopexy. British Journal of Surgery, 1979; 66: 14–18.

2. Fowler, R., Stephens, F. D. The role of testicular vascular anatomy in the salvage of the high undescended testis. Australian and New Zealand Journal of Surgery, 1959; 29: 92–106.

## Further Reading

Fonkalsrud, E. W., Mengel, W. (eds) The undescended testis. Chicago, London: Year Book Medical Publishers Inc., 1981.

Rajfer, J. Symposium of cryptorchidism. Urologic Clinics of North America, 1982; 9 (3)

Scholtmeijer, R. J., Molenaar, J. C., Chadha, Dev, R. (eds) Symposium on undescended testes, European Journal of Pediatrics, 1982; 139: 247–294.

Scorer, C. G., Farrington, G. H. Congenital deformities of the testis and epididymis. London: Butterworths, 1971.

Illustrations by Kevin Marks

# Torsion of the testis

**John E. S. Scott** MA, MD, FRCS, FAAP
Senior Lecturer in Paediatric Surgery, University of Newcastle upon Tyne, UK

The first report of testicular torsion appeared in 1840 when Delasiauve[1] described a 15-year-old boy who developed sudden severe pain in a pre-existing swelling in the left groin; exploration demonstrated a testis which had twisted on its attachments. This description is particularly significant because the patient was in the paediatric age group and had a pre-existing condition of paediatric surgical interest, namely, cryptorchidism.

## Aetiology

Testicular torsion may be extravaginal or intravaginal. Muschat[2], who carefully studied the mechanics of the condition, doubted whether the former was actually possible. In fact, extravaginal torsion can occur before the testicular coverings are fixed to the walls of the scrotum, as during or immediately after testicular descent. Thus this type of torsion is seen only in the newborn and probably occurs antenatally.

Intravaginal torsion is normally prevented by the attachment of the posterior surface of the epididymis to the wall of the scrotum but if the tunica vaginalis invests the whole of the epididymis and the lower part of the cord with a visceral layer, the testis dangles in the scrotal cavity like a bell clapper, and intravaginal torsion is possible. Another anomaly which may be a predisposing factor is an elongated mesorchium, where the epididymis and testis are separated from each other by a mesentery which may be of sufficient length to permit the body of the testis to twist independently of the epididymis. The spiral cremaster fibres may actually initiate the rotation of the testis when they contract.

The direction of rotation is usually from without inwards, the right rotating in a clockwise direction and the left counter-clockwise from the examiner's viewpoint.

Approximately 50 per cent of cases of torsion affect cryptorchids, including the abdominal testis.

## Diagnosis

Testicular torsion is one of the causes of the 'acute scrotum', the others being acute epididymitis, mumps orchitis, incarcerated inguinal hernia, torsion of a testicular appendage, neoplasm, and acute idiopathic scrotal oedema.

Torsion occurs most commonly between the ages of 10 and 25 years, but many instances of its occurrence in younger or older patients are described. It is probably the commonest acute scrotal disorder in children.

There are two modes of presentation, the *acute* type and the *recurrent* type. The acute type is characterized by sudden severe pain in the testis, frequently following some minor physical exertion, though often occurring during sleep. The pain rapidly increases in intensity, spreads to the groin and lower abdomen, and may be accompanied by vomiting. Shortly afterwards the testis swells and the overlying scrotal skin becomes red and oedematous. On examination, the testis is enlarged, hard and excruciatingly tender. Because of this it is often difficult to distinguish the precise position of the epididymis, which will be in an abnormal position, with the body of the testis lying transversely, high in the scrotum. The spermatic cord is thickened. In acute epididymitis it may be possible to detect that only the epididymis is enlarged and that the testis is lying low in the scrotum. Elevation of the testis may ease the pain in epididymitis but aggravates it in torsion[3]. If there are accompanying symptoms of urinary infection together with pyuria and bacteriuria, the diagnosis of epididymitis is easier, but unfortunately acute epididymitis does occur in young boys without apparent evidence of urinary infection.

Attempts to confirm the diagnosis of torsion and simultaneously to relieve the condition by untwisting the testis are worth making, but the testis may be too tender to manipulate and the overlying swelling may obscure the landmarks. Other techniques which detect arterial circulation in the spermatic cord and testis, such as Doppler ultrasonography[4], have been advocated. This instrument is reliable if flow in the testicular artery is definitely heard, but the apparent absence of flow does not confirm the presence of torsion, since the scrotal oedema may obscure the sounds.

Testicular blood flow may also be detected by the intravenous injection of the radioisotope $99^m$ technetium pertechnate followed by gamma camera photographs of the testis[5]. This method, however, requires the immediate availability for 24 hours every day of the radioisotope service. Even though the technique is claimed to produce reliable results, delay of even a short duration in organizing the investigation may prejudice the viability of the testis.

## Torsion of a testicular appendage

Torsion of a testicular appendage produces symptoms often as severe as those of torsion of the whole testis, but it is usually possible to palpate the pea-sized, hard, tender appendage near the upper pole of the testis.

## Scrotal oedema

In acute idiopathic scrotal oedema there is reddening and oedema of the skin of the scrotum, which spreads into the groin and perineum, but scarcely any pain, merely slight discomfort. The skin may be tender but the underlying testis and cord are normal.

## Orchitis

Virus orchitis as a complication of mumps is uncommon in childhood. There is a painful, tender swelling of the body of the testis only, which has a normal position in the scrotum with a normal spermatic cord.

## Neoplasm

A neoplasm of the testis can produce pain if it enlarges rapidly and there is usually a tense, overlying hydrocele. However, the acute tenderness and scrotal skin changes characteristic of torsion are not usually present and the spermatic cord is normal.

## Recurrent torsion

In the recurrent type of torsion there will have been a history of episodes of testicular pain and swelling every few months or years, which have subsided after a short period of bed rest or a hot bath. If examined between attacks, the testis may seem to lie more transversely in the scrotum than normal and be excessively mobile. However, the history alone should alert the examiner to the need for early surgical intervention.

## Incarcerated inguinal hernia

The symptoms and signs of torsion of an undescended testis closely resemble those of incarceration of an inguinal hernia, namely, severe pain and tenderness in a hard, red swelling in the groin. An empty scrotum on the affected side should raise suspicion, but it may be impossible to distinguish between a twisted inguinal testis and one that has been strangulated by the incarceration of a loop of bowel in the neck of an inguinal hernia sac. Since early surgical exploration is indicated for both conditions, differentiation is perhaps unnecessary. Occasionally an abdominal testis may undergo torsion, producing severe abdominal pain; again, the absence of a testis from the scrotum should alert the examiner to the possibility.

# Management and operation

The long-term results of surgery for testicular torsion are poor. In one series[6], reduction in testicular size was noted at follow-up in 68 per cent of testes which were thought to have been 'saved' by operation. There was a direct relationship between the degree of testicular atrophy and the duration of torsion before correction; even correction within 4 hours of torsion did not guarantee a full-sized testis. Thus, every minute counts, and in view of the inevitable delay between the onset of torsion and the commencement of operation it is worth attempting manual untwisting of the testis at the earliest opportunity.

Success with the manoeuvre, however, does not preclude the need for early operation. The affected testis is gently rotated in the opposite direction to the assumed direction of torsion; thus the left is rotated clockwise and the right counterclockwise. Unfortunately, torsion can occur in the reverse direction, in which case this manoeuvre will increase the strangulation. If the attempt does not immediately ease the pain it should be abandoned.

Exploration is performed through a scrotal incision opening the tunica vaginalis. A blood-stained effusion is usually present.

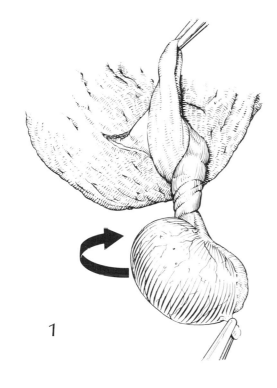

1

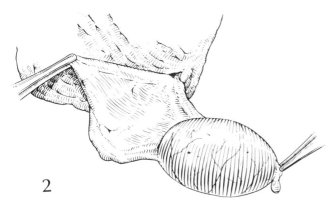

2

# 1 & 2

The testis is delivered through the incision, the direction of the twist is noted, and the testis untwisted. With torsion of the left testis, note that the direction of rotation is counterclockwise. As the spermatic cord is untwisted, redundant tunica vaginalis will be apparent

If the testis is completely infarcted or if its colour does not improve within a few minutes it should be removed.

# 3 & 4

When the testis does appear to be viable the redundant tunica vaginalis should be resected and the testis returned to the scrotal cavity and fixed to scrotal septum and dartos muscle by a row of non-absorbable sutures. The scrotal incision is then closed over a small drain which is removed after 48 hours.

It is important to explore the opposite side of the scrotum at the same operation because the anomaly of testicular fixation which predisposes to torsion will be present in 50–80 per cent of patients, and there is therefore a distinct possibility of torsion affecting the contralateral testis. The testis is similarly anchored.

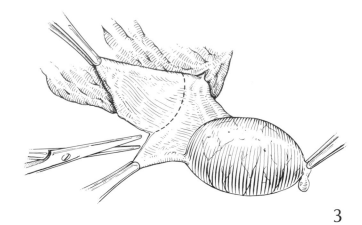

**3**

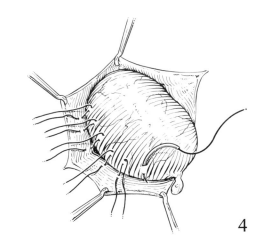

**4**

## Recurrent torsion

When a young boy complains of episodic testicular pain it should be assumed that recurrent torsion is occurring even though the testis may seem to be normal on palpation. The risk of losing the testis as a result of a final unresolved torsion is too great to be ignored. Both testes should be explored through scrotal incisions and anchored in the manner described.

## References

1. Delasiauve Descente tardive du testicule gauche, prise pour une hernie étranglée; opération; gangrène du testicule; extirpation de cet organe; accidents divers; guérison. Revue Médicale Française et Etrangère, 1840; 1:363

2. Muschat, M. Pathological anatomy of testicular torsion; explanation of its mechanism. Surgery, Gynecology and Obstetrics, 1932; 54: 758–763

3. Prehn, D. T. New sign in differential diagnosis between torsion of spermatic cord and epididymitis. Journal of Urology, 1934; 32: 191–200

4. Levy, B. J. The diagnosis of torsion of the testicle using the Doppler ultrasonic stethoscope. Journal of Urology, 1975; 113: 63–65

5. Hitch, D. C., Gilday, D. L., Shandling, B., Savage, J. P. A new approach to the diagnosis of testicular torsion. Journal of Pediatric Surgery, 1976; 11: 537–541

6. Krarup, T. The testes after torsion. British Journal of Urology, 1978; 50: 43–46

# Circumcision, meatotomy and meatoplasty

**J. D. Frank** FRCS
Consultant Paediatric Surgeon and Urologist, Hospital for Sick Children, Bristol, Avon, UK

## CIRCUMCISION

### Indications

### 1

A true phimosis is the *only* medical indication for circumcision. This is usually due to balanitis xerotica obliterans. Circumcision in the neonatal period should be avoided if possible because of the complications of meatal ulceration leading to meatal stenosis. Circumcision for social and religious reasons should therefore preferably be performed when the child is out of nappies.

### Anaesthesia

General anaesthesia is normally employed except in the newborn period, when a penile block may be used. The addition of caudal anaesthesia to a full general anaesthetic ensures a comfortable early postoperative period.

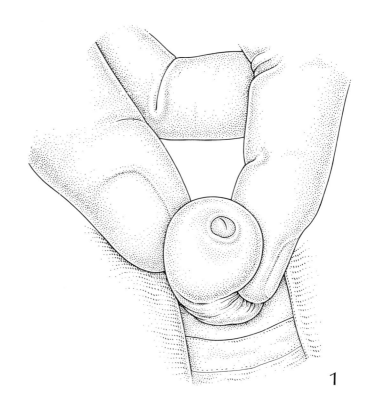

1

## The operation

There are more ways of performing a circumcision than almost any other paediatric surgical operation apart from a hypospadias repair. The two most important considerations in planning the procedure are that it should have minimal complications and give a good cosmetic result. The following method appears to fulfill these criteria.

# 2, 3 & 4

The scarred foreskin is dilated with artery forceps and completely retracted. Preputial adhesions are freed from the glans, and all smegma is removed and the glans cleaned completely.

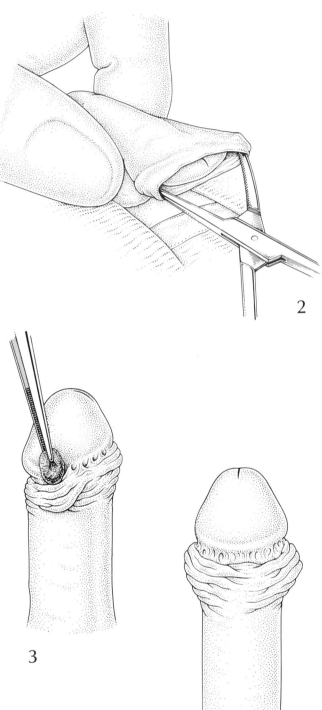

# 5–9

The foreskin is then elevated by placing one artery clip ventrally and one dorsally. A sinus forceps is applied to the skin at the level of the coronal sulcus and closed gently. This movement will make it slide up and over the underlying glans, taking the skin with it. When the glans can be palpated inferior to the forceps, it can be safely closed and held tightly shut. Using long sharp scissors, a clean cut is then made just distal to the sinus forceps to remove the excess foreskin. If sufficient foreskin is not removed with the first cut, the procedure can be repeated and a little more skin excised. It is always better to leave a little too much rather than risk a deficiency of shaft skin.

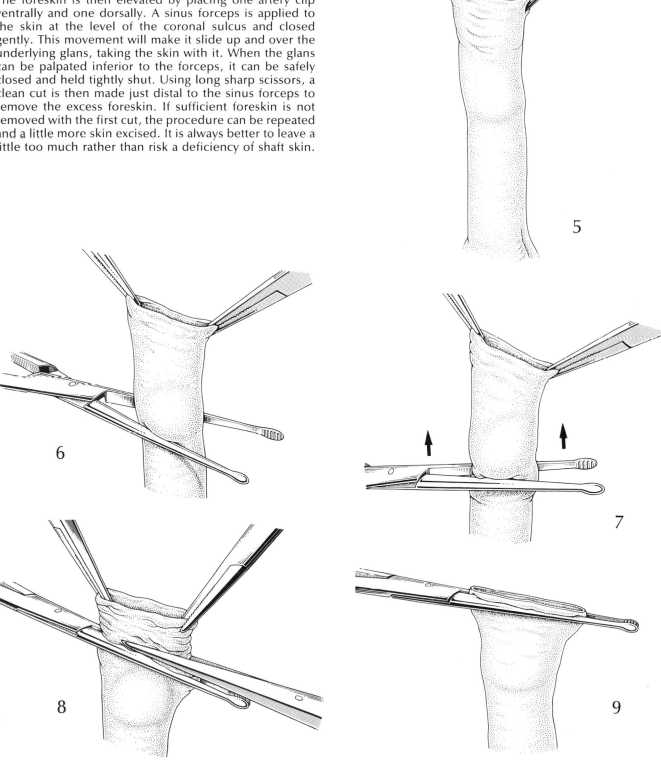

# 10, 11 & 12

The skin is then retracted, and any bleeding points are grasped with artery forceps and ligated with fine catgut. The excess inner layer of the prepuce is trimmed, leaving a margin around the corona of approximately 3 mm. The wound is closed with interrupted 5/0 Dexon or plain catgut sutures.

## Postoperative care

No postoperative dressing is necessary but some liquid paraffin may be poured over the penis to prevent the sheets adhering to it.

The child is allowed home on the same day and may start bathing the next day. No particular postoperative precautions are necessary.

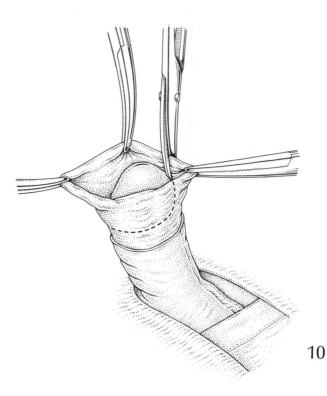

10

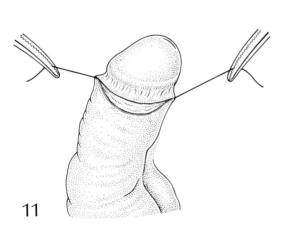

11

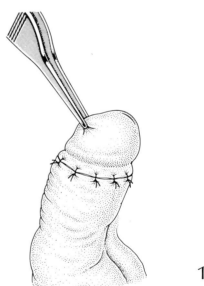

12

# MEATOTOMY AND MEATOPLASTY

The commonest causes of meatal stenosis are ulceration following an ammoniacal dermatitis in the circumcised male and previous hypospadias repair. The majority of these patients can be successfully treated by meatal dilatation, but a meatotomy may be required.

## Meatotomy

## 13a, b & c

Once the meatus has been dilated, a pair of fine scissors is used to make a ventral incision through the meatus. A few fine 6/0 Dexon sutures are used to approximate the urethral mucosa to the skin.

The main complication of this procedure is that it creates a glandular hypospadias. This may affect the direction of the urinary stream but, providing the incision is not carried too far proximally, there should be no major problems.

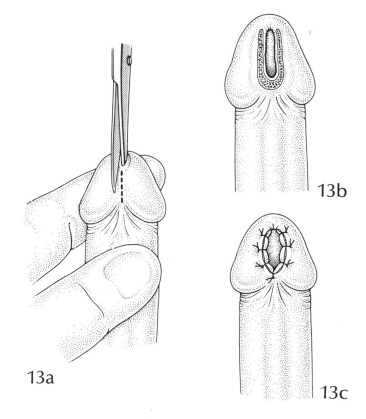

13a

13b

13c

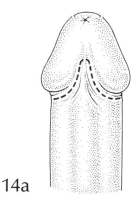

14a

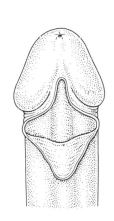

14b

## Meatoplasty

## 14a–f

Occasionally in children stenosis may recur after a meatotomy. Meatoplasty is then required.

A tongue of ventral skin is first mobilized. An incision is then made proximally from the meatus until normal urethra is reached, and the tongue of skin is inlaid into the proximal part of the incision as shown. This repair also creates a glandular hypospadias with occasional spraying. The wound is closed with 6/0 Dexon sutures.

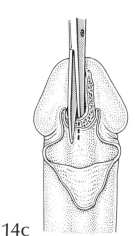

14c

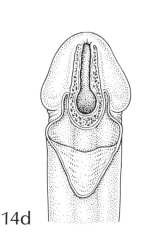

14d

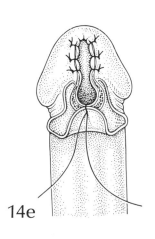

14e

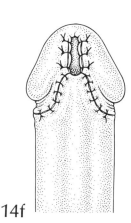

14f

Illustrations by Philip Wilson

# Bladder exstrophy closure and epispadias repair

**P. G. Ransley** FRCS
Consultant Paediatric Urologist, The Hospital for Sick Children, Great Ormond Street, London; and The Institute of Urology, University of London, London, UK

**P. G. Duffy** FRCS
Consultant Paediatric Urologist, The Hospital for Sick Children, Great Ormond Street, London; and The Institute of Urology, University of London, London, UK

**Michael Wollin** MD
Clinical Fellow in Paediatric Urology, The Hospital for Sick Children, Great Ormond Street, London, UK; and Senior Resident in Urology, University of Massachusetts Medical Center, Worcester, Massachusetts, USA

## BLADDER EXSTROPHY CLOSURE

## Introduction

The surgical treatment of the bladder exstrophy complex of anomalies is a highly specialized and difficult area of paediatric urology. Accordingly, it is most appropriate for exstrophy cases to be referred to a specialist centre. The initial closure of the bladder is the beginning of a series of surgical steps aimed at achieving satisfactory cosmesis, urinary continence and a sexually adequate penis.

In the male patient (predominant in a ratio of 3 male to 1 female), the anomaly consists of an exposed everted exstrophic bladder in continuity with an epispadiac penis. The pubic bones are widely separated and the external sphincter complex is represented only by a fibrous interpubic bar and has no recoverable sphincter function. The penis itself is short and with upward chordee. It may be very small and occasionally sex assignment as female may be appropriate.

The umbilicus is low set and there may be an accompanying umbilical hernia. Bilateral inguinal hernias are usual. The perineum is foreshortened with an anteriorly placed anus which may be abnormal.

In the female the anomalies are similar, with a bifid clitoris and a separate vaginal opening. The anus may be vestibular.

When isolated male epispadias occurs, the penile defect ranges from a simple glanular anomaly to symphysial epispadias verging on complete exstrophy. In all but the most distal lesions, the bladder neck and sphincter mechanisms are poorly formed and complete incontinence is usual. Isolated female epispadias is a very rare anomaly in which a bifid clitoris and a patulous urethral opening are obvious in a child with complete urinary incontinence.

The current surgical approach consists of early closure and later surgery for continence, aiming, if possible, to have achieved satisfactory urinary storage, continence and bladder emptying (by voiding or intermittent catheterization) by the time the child enters the junior school. However, some patients will inevitably remain incontinent until later, awaiting either an artificial urinary sphincter or spontaneous improvement at puberty.

The surgical steps may be summarized as follows.

1. In the neonate, closure of the bladder within the first 48 hours of life without osteotomy. (After 48 hours, bilateral osteotomy is required. Osteotomy may be performed with simple gallows traction up to the age of 3 years. After 3 years, external fixation is required or the closure should proceed without osteotomy.)
2. Carefully supervised testosterone therapy at the end of the first year of life. Usually 25 mg intramuscularly monthly for 3 months.
3. Epispadias repair at 12–18 months (single stage).
4. Annual assessment of upper tracts (ultrasound) and bladder capacity (cystogram under anaesthesia).
5. Bladder neck reconstruction with or without enhancement enterocystoplasty.
6. Bladder emptying achieved by voiding or intermittent catheterization.

This chapter describes the basic techniques of bladder closure and epispadias repair and does not attempt to act as a detailed guide to the intricacies of the management of the bladder exstrophy patient.

# Preparation

The newborn infant is transferred to the paediatric urological centre from the maternity unit. It is appropriate that at least one parent should see the anomaly in order to appreciate its gravity and thereby to understand the subsequent surgical procedures. However, neither parent is in a position to accept a detailed discussion at this stage. Surgery may be delayed for up to 48 hours, if necessary, while still avoiding the need for osteotomy. After 48 hours, pelvic ring closure without osteotomy is very difficult and virtually impossible. Cross-matched blood should be available. Before surgical reconstruction, an ultrasound or intravenous pyelogram is recommended to exclude an upper urinary tract abnormality.

General anaesthesia is required with the usual neonatal precautions and an additional caudal anaesthetic is helpful.

The patient is positioned flat and supine. Total lower body preparation with individual wrapping of the legs allows maximum manoeuvrability at the time of pelvic ring closure.

A single intraoperative dose of gentamicin (2 mg/kg), metronidazole (7.5 mg/kg) and ampicillin (6 mg/kg) is administered intravenously as soon as venous access is established.

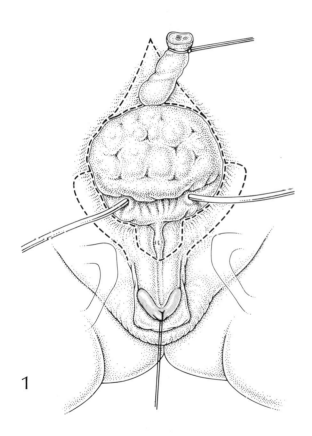

1

# The operation

## 1

### Skin incision

The umbilicus is ligated and trimmed but retained. Incisions are made as shown, beginning in the midline above the umbilicus. The incisions are deepened with diathermy, but the distal incisions outlining the paraexstrophy skin flaps may be left superficial at this stage.

## 2

### Bladder mobilization

The umbilical arteries serve as a guide to the extra-peritoneal plane on each side. Careful blunt dissection opens up a plane behind the rectus muscles on each side, in front of the ureter (stent in position for palpation) down to the pelvic floor at the bladder neck.

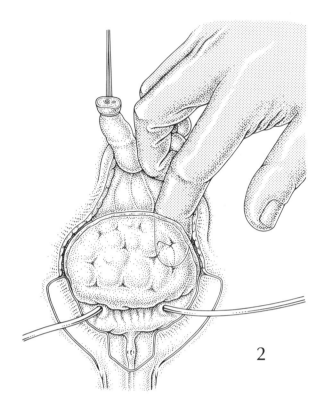

2

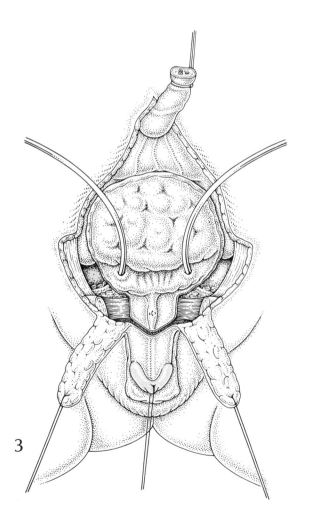

3

## 3

### Mobilization of paraexstrophy flaps

With a finger in position behind the abdominal wall, the distal incisions may be completed with diathermy. Superficial bleeding is encountered from erectile tissue and local infiltration with adrenaline 1:200 000 into the prostate may be helpful. The paraexstrophy skin flaps are preserved. The transverse incision dividing the urethral plate is located distal to the verumontanum. The interpubic bar tissue fusing with the bladder neck is now visible and is an important landmark.

# 4

## Dissection of posterior urethra

The verumontanum and prostate are freed from the underlying corpora cavernosa in order to allow them to recess into the pelvis. No corporal mobilization is performed at this time.

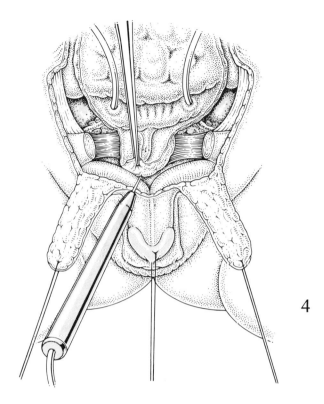

4

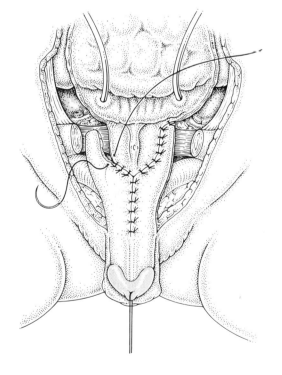

5

# 5

## Formation of urethra

The bladder and prostate drop back into the pelvis and the paraexstrophy skin flaps are used to bridge the gap and create the segment of urethra that will come to lie behind the approximated symphysis, so that the bladder and prostate become totally intrapelvic organs. Interrupted 6/0 polydioxanone or polyglycolic acid suture materials are suitable.

# 6

## Bladder closure

Either a 10FG plastic Jacques or Nélaton catheter with opposed eyes is sutured to the bladder wall with 3/0 chromic catgut. Positioning of the catheter to ensure that all the eyes lie within the closed bladder lumen is important. The bladder margins are trimmed back to fresh muscle tissue and bladder closure begins, using interrupted 3/0 polyglycolic acid sutures.

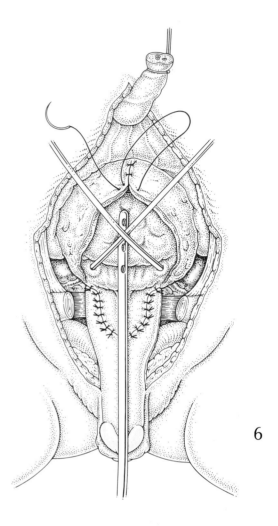

6

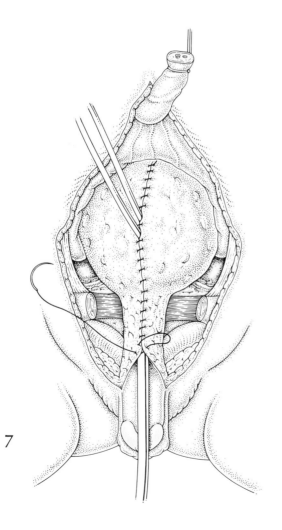

7

# 7

## Closure of urethra

The bladder neck region and the paraexstrophy skin flaps are tubularized. The suture material used for the skin is 5/0 polyglycolic acid.

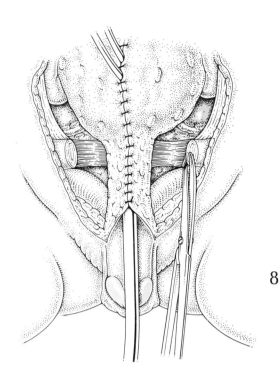

8

# 8 & 9

### Incision of pubic tissue and urethral wrap

The interpubic bar tissue is released from the posterior aspect of the pubic bone. This is an important step to provide support for the paraexstrophy skin flap tube and to define the boundary between the abdominal cavity and perineum. It may not be possible to achieve sufficient mobility for wrapping to be completed at this stage due to the wide separation of the pubic bones. In such circumstances the sutures are laid and closure completed as the pelvic ring is brought together with abdominal closure.

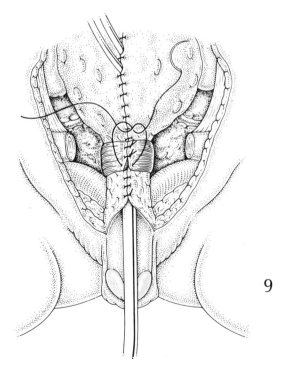

9

## 10

### Approximation of pubic bones

Three heavy sutures are placed in the pubic bones. The precise placement is shown in the small inset diagram and is very important to prevent a bowstring effect cutting back into the urethra if the bones separate a little postoperatively. Heavy (0 or 1) polypropylene sutures have been used, but 1/0 polydioxanone sutures have also proved satisfactory and are currently favoured.

## 11

### Transposition omphaloplasty and wound closure

The umbilicus is displaced to the apex of the abdominal incision.

Closure of the abdominal wound begins by bringing rectus muscles together, starting from above and proceeding downwards. The aim is to even out the tension of closure throughout the whole length of the wound so that the strain of closure is not taken by the symphysial sutures alone. Vertical mattress sutures achieve this, provided that the bights are placed at right-angles to the oblique wound edge and not horizontally, parallel to the transpyloric plane. A 2/0 polydioxanone suture is usually adequate but 0 may be advisable in the lower half of the wound.

Final closure of the pubic bone is completed last. Internal rotation of the hips and compression of the pelvis by an assistant is helpful.

Skin closure is completed in two layers.

# Postoperative management

The patient is placed in a mermaid dressing with adequate cotton wool padding between the knees and ankles. The nursing staff unbandage, massage and rebandage every 4 hours. This dressing is maintained for 3–4 weeks.

During the first few days, immobilization of the child on a crucifix frame prevents hip flexion, which may otherwise occur and which compromises skin healing.

One of the most important factors leading to success in exstrophy closure is the maintenance of good stent and urethral catheter drainage. A high intravenous fluid intake is essential in the first few hours and days postoperatively to prevent crystalline deposits, to which the exstrophy patient seems very prone, blocking these tubes.

Ureteric stents are maintained for 2 weeks provided that wound healing is satisfactory.

At 3–4 weeks, the urethral catheter is removed and the child returns to the theatre for an examination under anaesthesia before going home, in order to check that there is free urethral passage for urinary drainage.

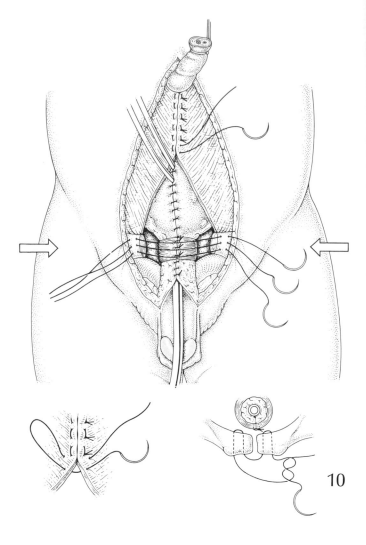

10

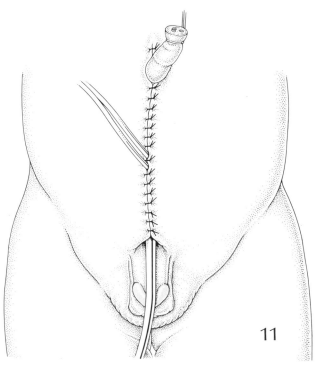

11

# EPISPADIAS REPAIR

## Introduction

Epispadias repair is usually undertaken at 12–18 months of age following a short period of testosterone therapy to enhance the penis. With late presenting exstrophy cases the repair may be performed as a single stage procedure in conjunction with bladder closure, with or without osteotomy.

## Preparation

No special preparation is required. Cross-matched blood should be available.

General anaesthesia is required, with additional caudal anaesthesia.

The patient is again positioned flat and supine.

Antibiotic cover is performed with a single intraoperative dose of gentamicin (2 mg/kg) , metronidazole (7.5 mg/kg) and ampicillin (6 mg/kg).

Preoperative and perioperative infiltration with adrenaline 1:200 000 is helpful, especially around the base of the corpora and into the prostate.

## The operation

## 12

### Preliminary glansplasty

A longitudinal incision is made through the distal fusion of the lateral wings of the glans and distal urethra. This is closed transversely using 6/0 polydioxanone sutures. The manoeuvre makes a great difference to the final cosmetic appearance by displacing the terminal urethral meatus slightly ventrally.

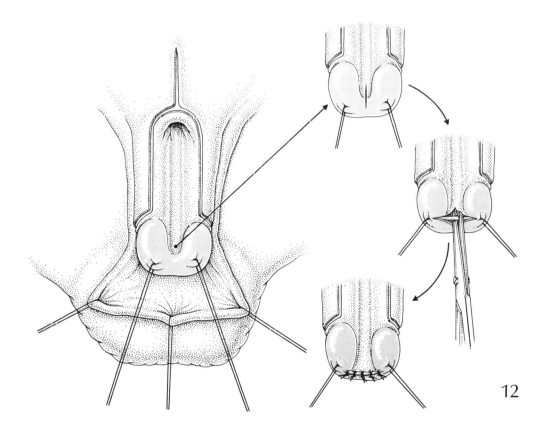

12

## 13

### Skin incision

The incision begins in the midline above the urethral opening and is extended far enough upwards to provide good access to the proximal corpora for mobilization. It continues down on each side of the midline urethral strip (backed by corpus spongiosum) and sweeps ventrally around the coronal sulcus separating the prepuce and ventral skin from the corpora.

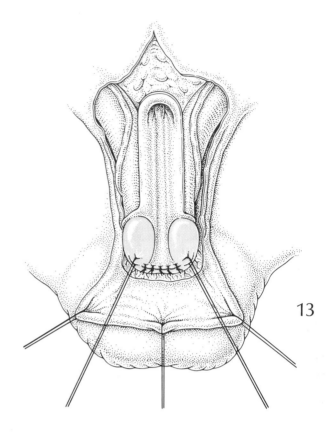

13

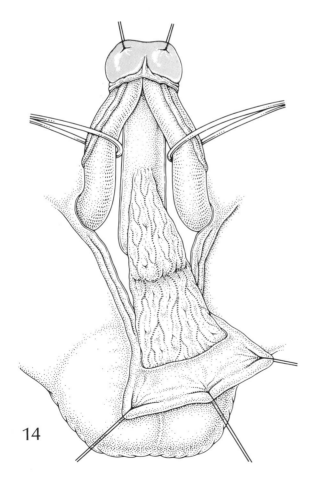

14

## 14

### Mobilization of urethral strip

Dissection of the midline strip commences most easily on the ventral surface, preserving a pedicle to the dartos. Alternate dorsal and ventral dissection is continued until the midline urethral strip is completely free from the corpora. Dissection then continues backwards to separate adhesion of the prostate and interpubic bar from the convex dorsal surface of the corpora. The midline strip from the urethral opening to the glans should be completely free of corporal attachment at completion.

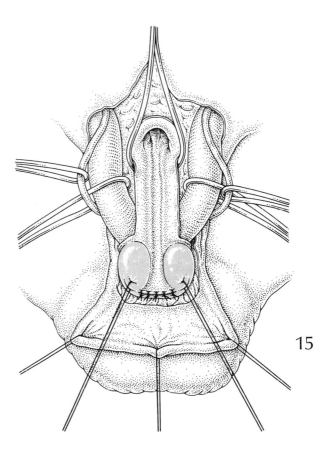

15

# 15 & 16

## Dissection of neurovascular bundles and corporal bodies

The neurovascular bundles are now well seen sweeping laterally and ventrally at the midpoint of the corpora. Artificial erection at this stage will show upward angulation of the corpora at this point.

The corpora are dissected free of adhesion to the pubic rami for 1–2 cm. Further dissection is not advantageous.

The neurovascular bundles are elevated from the bodies of the corpora and retracted.

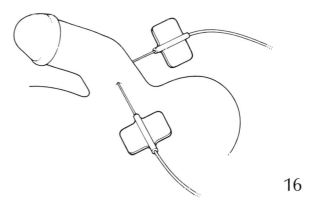

16

## 17

### Tubularization of urethral plate

The urethral plate is now tubularized over a 10FG Silastic (Dow Corning, UK) urethral stent or catheter. It is advisable to place a suprapubic catheter in position by guided puncture before closing the urethra. Urethral closure stops at the proximal end of the glans at this stage.

The urethra and dartos pedicle are displaced onto the ventral aspect of the penis.

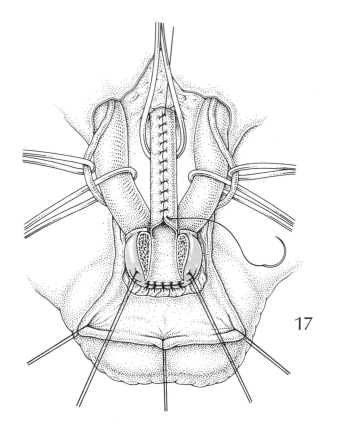

17

## 18

### Cavernocavernostomy and corporal rotation

Cavernocavernostomy and corporal rotation are performed to correct chordee and approximate the corpora on the dorsal aspect of the urethra. An incision is made transversely in the dorsal aspect of the corpora on each side at the site of maximum angulation. This incision opens as a diamond, elongating the dorsal surfaces of the corpora. The adjacent apices of each diamond are sutured together using a double-ended suture of 5/0 polypropylene (knots inside). Using a continuous stitch, the corpora are rotated through 90° as the two diamonds come face-to-face on the medial aspect.

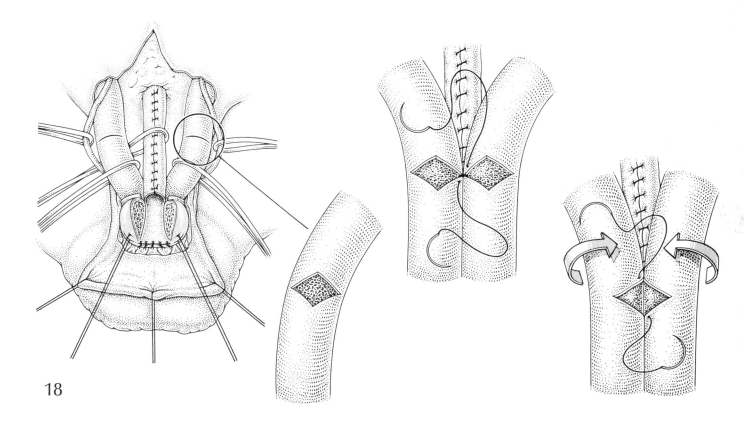

18

# 19

## Closure of glans

A broad strip of glans tissue is excised on each side and the glanular urethra closure completed. The raw surfaces of the glans now come together on the dorsal aspect using vertical mattress sutures of 6/0 polydioxanone. The corporal rotation and approximation is now reinforced with some additional sutures of 5/0 polydioxanone between the site of the cavernocavernostomy and the glans.

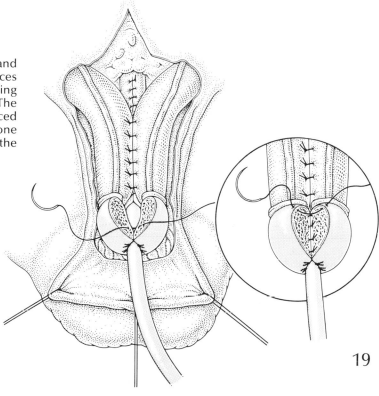

19

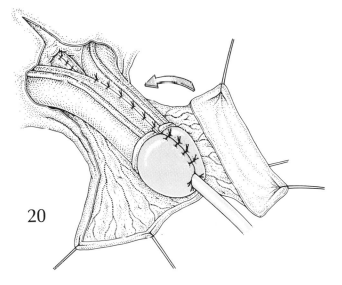

20

# 20

## Mobilization of preputial skin

The inner layer of preputial skin is isolated on a vascular pedicle and brought onto the dorsal surface of the penis for skin cover. The ventral aspect is covered with the outer layer of preputial skin.

# 21

### Skin closure

The base of the dorsum of the penis is covered by employing distally based triangular skin flaps from the margins of the original midline incision to prevent scarring causing bowstringing to the abdominal wall.

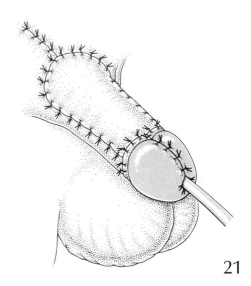

**21**

## Postoperative care

Bedrest for 1 week. The penis is enclosed in a Silastic foam dressing for 1 week. The catheters are maintained for 2 weeks.

Cystoscopy is performed at 3 months.

### *Further reading*

Duckett, J. W. (1977) Use of paraexstrophy skin pedicle grafts for correction of exstrophy and epispadias repair. Birth Defects, 13, 175–179

Lepor, H., Jeffs, R. D. (1983) Primary bladder closure and bladder neck reconstruction in classical bladder exstrophy. Journal of Urology 130, 1142–1145

Lepor, H., Shapiro, E., Jeffs, R. D. (1984) Urethral reconstruction in boys with classical bladder exstrophy. Journal of Urology 131, 512–515

# Intersex abnormalities in the newborn: surgical reconstruction

**Patricia K. Donahoe** MD
Chief of Pediatric Surgery, Massachusetts Hospital; Professor of Surgery, Harvard Medical School, Boston, Massachusetts, USA

A child with ambiguous genitalia must be attended to immediately at birth. The gender which is appropriate to the anatomy of the infant must be assigned as early as possible, since new parents are asked about the sex of the child as soon as the birth is known. They must be able to give an answer that is commensurate with the gender assignment that will eventually provide the most satisfying functional result. Surgical correction must then be done as early as possible so that confusion about sex is not prolonged, and subconscious rejection of the child is less likely to occur.

Four major categories of abnormality can cause gender confusion at birth: female pseudohermaphroditism, male pseudohermaphroditism, true hermaphroditism, and mixed gonadal dysgenesis. The gonads are symmetrical in the first two, but are not if one gonad has differentiated predominantly as a testis and the other as an ovary, as in mixed gonadal dysgenesis or true hermaphroditism.

Genetic females, no matter how severely virilized, should be raised as females. In genetic males the gender assignment must be based on the infant's anatomy, that is, the size of the phallus, and not on the 46XY karyotype. If the phallus is inadequate, one should recommend assignment to the female gender. The average penile length at 30 weeks gestation is $2.5 \pm 0.4$ cm, increasing to $3.5 \pm 0.4$ cm at term, with a width of $1.00–1.5$ cm. A term size below $2 \times 0.9$ cm should cause concern[1]. Exceptions, however, must always be made if the patient presents late and has become fully committed to the male role.

Female pseudohermaphroditism occurs when a genetic female (46XX) is exposed in utero to androgens, either exogenous or endogenous, as in the congenital adrenal hyperplasia syndromes[2,3]. The phenotype can vary from clitoral enlargement alone to complete labioscrotal fusion and formation of an entirely normal male penis with a closed urethra formed to its tip. Cortisol deficiency can lead to salt wasting, which can be life-threatening unless replacement is instituted. All masculinized females have normal child-bearing potential and should be raised as females. The psychologically important clitoral recession should be done as early as possible, particularly if the defect is severe. The timing of the vaginoplasty is determined by the point of entry of the vagina into the urogenital sinus[4–6].

Male pseudohermaphroditism occurs in genetic males 46XY with deficient masculinization of the external genitalia due to insufficient testosterone production, conversion[7,8] or inadequate target organ response[9]. Heritable defects can be detected in only 50 per cent of cases[10]. Many patients with male pseudohermaphroditism have been raised as males. However, if the female gender is chosen, then gonadectomy should be done at the time of perineal reconstruction. In the patient with absent or rudimentary vagina this usually requires only clitoral recession and labioscrotal reduction. The labioscrotal folds should be partially reduced during the first procedure (see Illustration 1) and dilatation and a substitute vaginoplasty planned for the late adolescent or early adult years[11]. Patients with testicular feminization in whom an introitus is often present may have this dilated with bougies at a later age to form a functional vagina.

True hermaphrodites[12] have well-developed, non-dysgenetic male and female gonadal tissue[13] in many combinations, i.e. a testis on one side and an ovary on the other, two ovotestes, or a normal gonad on one side and an ovotestis on the other. Although 80 per cent of these patients have a 46XX karyotype, testicular tissue is present[14]. The patient with a small phallus should be raised as a female; the patient with a large phallus already committed as a male should be raised as a male. Gonads should be bivalved and biopsied longitudinally. The gonadal tissue commensurate with the sex of rearing should be salvaged. Microdissection may be used[15]. Perineal reconstruction should be accompanied by removal of Wolffian structures. If the phallus is adequate for male gender assignment, ovarian and Müllerian structures can be removed, followed by hypospadias repair. Testicular prostheses can be inserted later, should the testicular tissue be inadequate.

Mixed gonadal dysgenesis[16,17] patients have dysgenetic gonads, retained Müllerian structures, internal and external asymmetry and a mosaic karyotype, often 45X/46XY[18]. The dysgenetic gonads can develop neoplasms such as gonadoblastoma[19] or seminoma-dysgerminoma[20]. Children with mixed gonadal dysgenesis should be raised as females with removal of the gonads, perineal reconstruction with flap vaginoplasty, and oestrogen and progesterone replacement at adolescence[18].

If the patient is already committed to the male role, then hypospadias repair will be required[26]. The gonads must be carefully observed for tumour development, which may occur as early as the newborn period. Their removal is advised in the third decade[21].

# 1

Perineal reconstruction[22-25] in infants to be reared as females consists of clitoral recession, vaginoplasty, and labioscrotal reduction. It is similar in all types. Cytoscopic determination of the level of entry of the vagina into the urogenital sinus is crucial. In most it is distal to the external sphincter and the opening can be exteriorized by the simpler flap vaginoplasty (a). The repair can be undertaken at 3–6 months of age, or even in the newborn period if the social circumstances are such that the baby might otherwise be rejected[24]. If the vagina enters the urethra proximal to the external sphincter a more complicated pullthrough vaginoplasty (b) will be required to avoid jeopardizing continence. If no vagina is found (c), then vaginal replacement can be planned for late adolescence. Miniature fibreoptic cystoscopes allow safe assessment in premature newborn or older infants. The bladder must be filled to allow accurate definition of the external urethral sphincter. This manoeuvre accentuates the rounded nature of the structure.

In those to be reared as males the hypospadias repair is the essential and other measures may also be required. If the scrotum drapes around the base of the penis, 'shawl scrotum', it can be corrected by bringing the scrotum caudad by dart flaps, often coordinated with repair of a bifid scrotum. This should be delayed so as not to compromise the Byers flaps[23]. Testicular prostheses may have to be inserted. We suggest the soft Silastic, Heyer–Schulte variety. These must be changed as the male approaches adolescence.

Mastectomy may be necessary if a male develops gynaecomastia on approaching puberty.

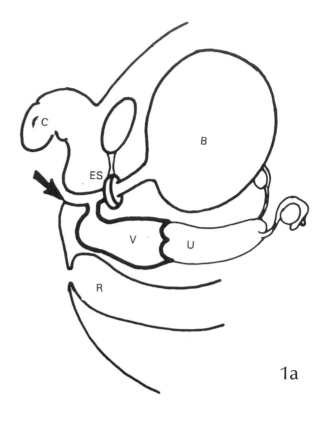

1a

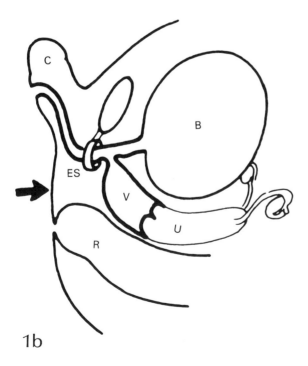

1b

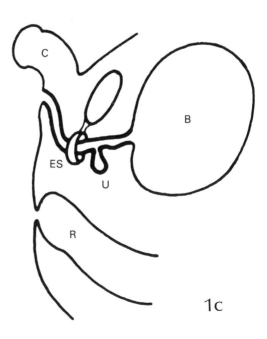

1c

C, clitoris; B, bladder; ES, external sphincter; V, vagina; U, uterus; R, rectum

# Clitoral recession

## 2a

The appearance of the enlarged clitoris is shown. The bifid corpora cavernosa from the pubic rami join, elongate, and form the enlarged glans. The dissection is started by circumscribing 2 mm below the glans. The dorsal flap is usually generous and the ventral flap small.

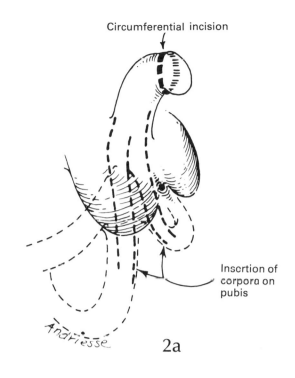

2a

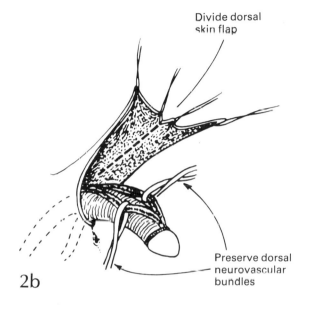

## 2b

The dorsal skin flap is divided cephalad in the midline. On either side of the midline the prominent dorsal neurovascular bundle consisting of two lateral arteries and a central vein is carefully dissected out of Buck's fascia and retracted.

## 2c

Dissection is carried back to the bifurcation of the corpora; the shaft is then divided between that point and the glans, preserving the neurovascular bundles. Haemostasis is secured with gentle diathermy cautery, taking care not to cause undue fibrosis which could prevent later clitoral erection.

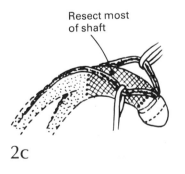

## 2d

The near and far ends of the corpora are approximated with very fine interrupted Vicryl sutures circumferentially. The glans is positioned cephalad between the divided dorsal flaps and is sutured to the mons dorsally and to the ventral mucosa of the urogenital sinus.

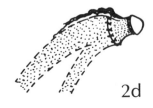

# 2e, f

Excess skin from the clitoral shaft may be placed downward as a shawl to create the labia minora. This technique aims to retain the important sensitivity of the clitoris.

Clitoral recession is commonly combined with low vaginoplasty.

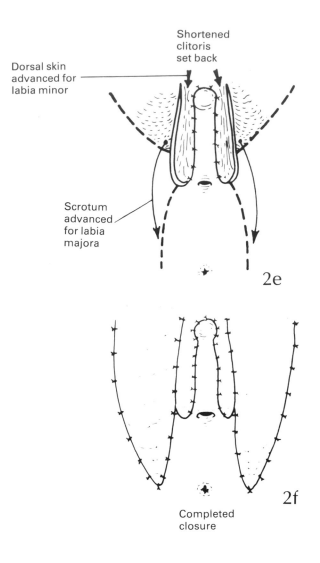

2e

2f

Completed closure

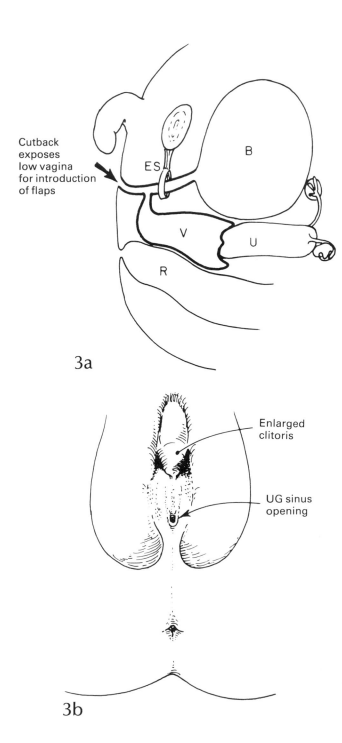

3a

3b

# Low vaginoplasty

# 3a, b

If the vagina enters the urogenital sinus distal to the external urethral sphincter (ES), a low or early vaginoplasty may be performed.

# 3c

After the clitoris has been recessed and the bisected shaft skin rotated around the repositioned glans, U-flaps are outlined on the labioscrotal folds, their extent depending upon the degree of enlargement. An inverted U-flap, outlined on the perineum and broadly based at the level of the anus, is raised. A catheter is placed in the urethra.

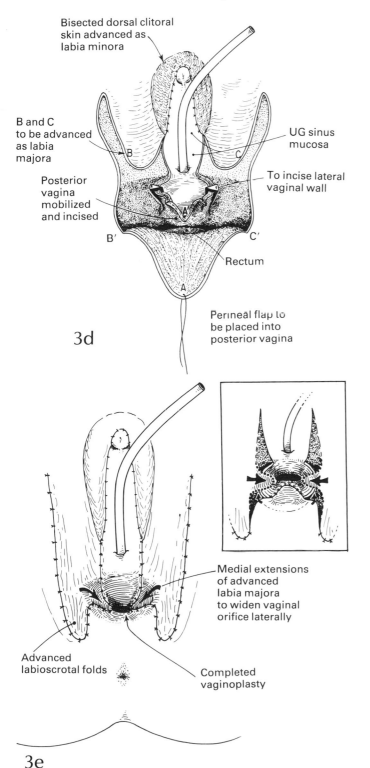

3d

# 3d

The labioscrotal flaps are raised and the shawl of the labia minora sutured medially to the urogenital sinus mucosa. The inverted U-flap based on the rectum is dissected back toward the anus. At this point a finger is placed in the rectum which is dissected away from the back wall of the vagina, often as far back as the peritoneal cul-de-sac. It is more acceptable to err on the side of opening into the vagina rather than the rectum to avoid creating a rectovaginal fistula.

The vagina is opened in the midline posteriorly ('cutback') and flap A laid into A' with interrupted Vycril sutures, which are preferred because they slide so well. Two small incisions are made in the lateral wall of the vagina. The labioscrotal flaps are then advanced into the side-arms of the inverted U-flap created on the perineum (B to B' and C to C').

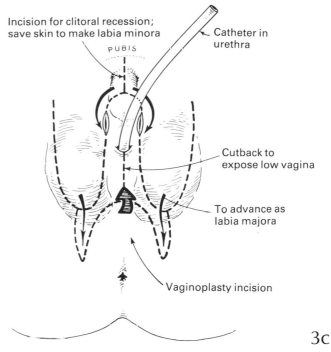

3c

# 3e

This gives an elongated appearance to the refashioned labia majora. The medial portion of the often copious labioscrotal folds is advanced into the lateral incisions on the vaginal wall to enhance the vaginal opening (inset), stenosis of which is one of the commonest long-term complications after these procedures.

If the clitoral skin is particularly long it can be further advanced between the mucosa of the urogenital sinus and the labioscrotal folds to enhance the vaginal orifice. Care must be taken, however, to assess the vascular supply to the distal end of this shaft skin.

# High vaginal pull-through

## 4a

If the vagina enters the urogenital sinus proximal to the external sphincter (ES), exteriorization should be delayed until the child is older and larger, usually at the age of two years, and a high vaginal pull-through performed. The vaginal opening is catheterized with a small Fogarty balloon and a sound passed into the bladder. A cutback of the urogenital sinus is *not* done as in the low vaginoplasty. This manoeuvre would divide the external sphincter and could probably make the child incontinent.

## 4b

A posterior inverted U-flap based on the rectum is raised. Labioscrotal U-flaps are raised, as is an anterior U-flap based on the urogenital sinus mucosa.

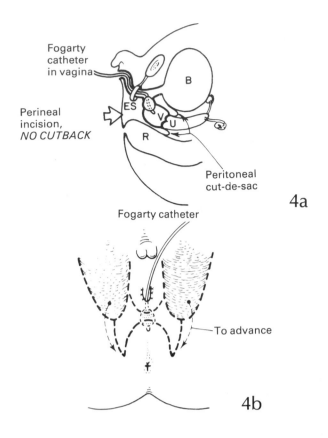

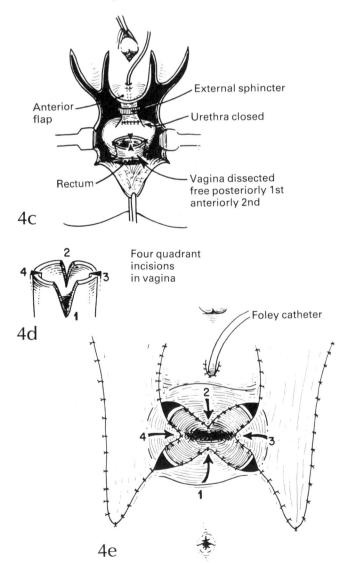

## 4c

Dissection behind the urethra is carried up to the Fogarty balloon with care being taken to avoid the external sphincter, which may be identified by a nerve stimulator. Firm prostatic tissue may be encountered at this point. The vagina is then divided from the urethra which is closed transversely after pulling back the Fogarty balloon. The urethra is closed neither too tightly, to avoid a stricture, not too loosely, to avoid creating a diverticulum.

The urethral sound is then removed and a Foley catheter placed in the bladder. The vagina is mobilized up to the peritoneal cul-de-sac, posteriorly, with a finger placed in the rectum to avoid entering that structure, and anteriorly from the back wall of the bladder.

## 4d, e

The orifice of the vagina is usually exceptionally narrow, so should be opened back to copious tissue. The posterior perineal flap is advanced posteriorly to point 1, the anterior flap of the urogenital sinus (point 2), and the labioscrotal folds into the lateral arms of the perineal flap and into the lateral incisions of the vagina (points 3 and 4).

Even with all these precautions stenosis of the vaginal orifice can be a late complication. We therefore recommend that daily dilatations with a Hegar dilator begin two weeks after high or low vaginoplasty and continue for six months to maintain pliability of the orifice during healing.

# Hypospadias

## 5a

The hypospadias in intersex babies committed to the male gender is often severe.

If the penis is very small and the hooded foreskin is depleted, hypospadias repair may have to be staged. At the first stage the chordee should be straightened and the dorsal flaps rotated to cover the ventral surface. If the dorsal foreskin is ample, hypospadias repair may be accomplished in a single procedure as follows.

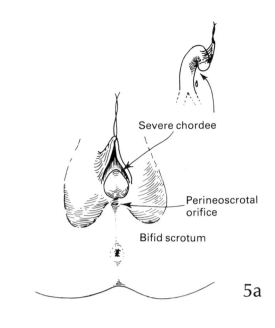

5a

## 5b

The glans is circumscribed. Through a short ventral midline incision the chordee is completely straightened, taking all fibrous tissue (atretic corpus spongiosum) external to Buck's fascia. The shiny skin just adjacent to the perineal meatus is tubularized after a U incision.

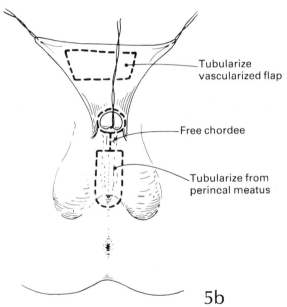

5b

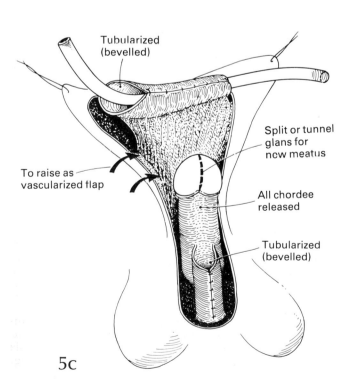

5c

## 5c

After the method of Duckett[26], the folded hooded dorsal foreskin is divided between the mucous membrane and the foreskin. The mucous membrane is outlined to create a patch that can be rolled into a tube. This patch is dissected away from the dorsal foreskin, preserving its vasculature, and rolled into a tube with a running Vicryl suture. The tubularized graft is then rotated ventrally so that its longitudinal suture line faces inward toward the shaft of the penis, and is anastomosed to the urethral tube which has been constructed from the mid-scrotum. The proximal and distal suture lines must be bevelled in order to avoid stricture.

## 5d

The distal end of the vascularized graft may be tunnelled through the glans to the meatus. Alternatively, the glans is opened, the graft laid in, and the glans closed around the distal portion of the graft to create a new meatus.

It is important to close multiple tissue layers over the neourethra. These often consist of the dartos proximally in the area of the scrotum, and shaft subcutaneous tissue distally over the vascularized graft.

The remaining dorsal foreskin, whose blood supply must likewise be secure, is then divided and rotated ventrally over the neourethra which has already been covered with multiple layers of adventitia. The proximal part of the scrotum is brought together in the midline to correct the bifid scrotum and to cover the proximal neourethra.

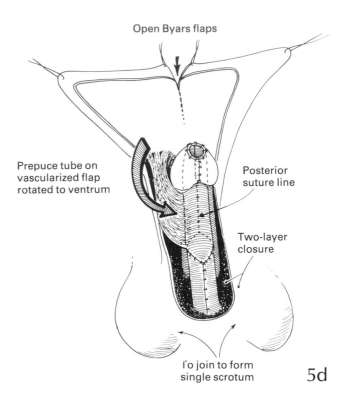

Open Byars flaps

Prepuce tube on vascularized flap rotated to ventrum

Posterior suture line

Two-layer closure

To join to form single scrotum

5d

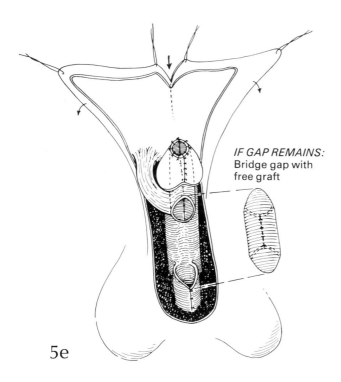

IF GAP REMAINS:
Bridge gap with free graft

5e

## 5e

In the event that the tubularized graft proximally cannot meet the vascularized graft distally, the defect can be bridged with a free skin graft taken with a Reese dermatome from the inside of the upper arm, bevelling the grafts at the points of anastomosis to avoid stricture.

## 5f

The dorsal foreskin is divided as Byars flaps and swung ventrally to cover all defects.

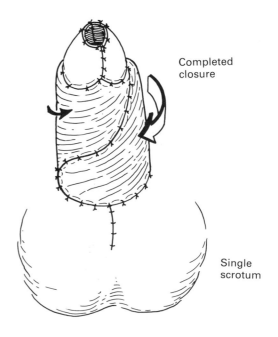

Completed closure

Single scrotum

5f

# References

1. Stephens, F. D. (1983) Congenital Malformations of the Urinary Tract. New York: Praeger

2. Bongiovanni, A. M., Root, A. W. (1963) Adrenogenital syndrome. New England Journal of Medicine, 268, 1283–1289

3. New, M. I., Dupont, B., Pang, S., Pollack, M., Levine, L. S. (1981) An update of congenital adrenal hyperplasia. Recent Progress in Hormone Research, 37, 105–181

4. Hendren, W. H., Crawford, J. D. (1969) Adrenogenital syndrome: the anatomy of the anomaly and its repair. Some new concepts. Journal of Pediatric Surgery, 4, 49–58

5. Hendren, W. H. (1980) Reconstructive problems of the vagina and the female urethra. Clinics in Plastic Surgery, 7, 207–234

6. Hendren, W. H., Donahoe, P. K. (1980) Correction of congenital abnormalities of the vagina and perineum. Journal of Pediatric Surgery, 15, 751–763

7. Opitz, J. M., Simpson, J. L., Sarto, G. E., Summitt, R. L., New, M., German, J. (1972) Pseudovaginal perineoscrotal hypospadias. Clinical Genetics, 3, 1–26

8. Peterson, R. E., Imperato-McGinley, J., Gautier, T., Sturla, E. (1977) Male pseudohermaphroditism due to steroid 5 alpha reductase deficiency. American Journal of Medicine, 62, 170–191

9. Madden, J. D., Walsh, P. C., MacDonald, P. C., Wilson, J. D. (1975) Clinical and endocrinologic characterization of a patient with the syndrome of incomplete testicular feminization. Journal of Clinical Endocrinology and Metabolism, 41, 751–760

10. Eil, E., Crawford, J. D., Donahoe, P. K., Johnsonbaugh, R. E. and Loriaux, D. L. (1984) Fibroblast androgen receptors in patients with genitourinary anomalies. Journal of Andrology, 5, 313–320

11. Donahoe, P. K., Crawford, J. D., Hendren, W. H. (1977) Management of neonates and children with male pseudohermaphroditism. Journal of Pediatric Surgery, 12, 1045–1057

12. Van Nierkerk, W. (1976) True hermaphroditism: an analytic review with a report of 3 new cases. American Journal of Obstetrics and Gynecology, 126, 890–907

13. Donahoe, P. K., Crawford, J. D., Hendren, W. H. (1978) True hermaphroditism: a clinical description and a proposed function for the long arm of the Y chromosome. Journal of Pediatric Surgery, 13, 293–301

14. Ferguson-Smith, M. (1966) X-Y chromosomal interchange in the aetiology of true hermaphroditism and of XX Klinefelter's syndrome. Lancet, 2, 475–476

15. Nihoul-Fékété, C., Lortat-Jacob, S., Cachin, O., Josso, N. (1984) Preservation of gonadal function in true hermaphroditism. Journal of Pediatric Surgery, 19, 50–55

16. Sohval, A. (1964) Hermaphroditism with 'atypical' or 'mixed' gonadal dysgenesis: relationship to gonadal neoplasm. American Journal of Medicine, 36, 281–292

17. Federman, D. D. (1967) Abnormal Sexual Development: a genetic and endocrine approach to differential diagnosis. Philadelphia: W. B. Saunders

18. Donahoe, P. K., Crawford, J. D., Hendren, W. H. (1979) Mixed gonadal dysgenesis, pathogenesis and management. Journal of Pediatric Surgery, 14, 287–300

19. Scully, R. E. (1970) Gonadoblastoma, a review of 74 cases. Cancer, 25, 1340–1356

20. Salle, B., Hedinger, C. (1970) Gonadal histology in children with male pseudohermaphroditism and mixed gonadal dysgenesis. Acta Endocrinologica, 64, 211–227

21. Manuel, M., Katayama, K. P., Jones, H. W. (1976) The age of occurrence of gonadal tumors in intersex patients with a Y chromosome. American Journal of Obstetrics and Gynecology, 124, 293–300

22. Donahoe, P. K., Hendren, W. H. (1980) Intersex abnormalities in the newborn infant. In: Pediatric Surgery, K. W. Holder, T. M. Ashcraft, (eds.), pp. 858–890. Philadelphia: W. B. Saunders

23. Donahoe, P. K., Crawford, J. D. (1986) Ambiguous genitalia in the newborn. In Pediatric Surgery, 4th Ed., J. K. Welch, J. G. Randolph, M. M. Ravitch, J. A. O'Neill, M. I. Rowe (eds.), pp. 1363–1382. Chicago: Year Book Medical Publishers

24. Donahoe, P. K., Hendren, W. H. (1984) Perineal reconstruction in ambiguous genitalia infants raised as females. Annals of Surgery, 200, 363–371

25. Donahoe, P. K., Pena, A. (1986) Abnormalities of the female genital tract. In Pediatric Surgery, 4th Ed., J. K. Welch, J. G. Randolph, M. M. Ravitch, J. A. O'Neill, M. I. Rowe (eds.), pp. 1352–1362. Chicago: Year Book Medical Publishers

26. Duckett, J. W., Hypospadias. Clinics in Plastic Surgery. 1980; 7:149–160

Permission for figures obtained from Annals of Surgery (1984), 200, 363–371, and Yearbook Medical Publishers, Chicago: Pediatric Surgery, 4th edition (1986) P. K. Donahoe and J. D. Crawford.

Illustrations by Gillian Oliver

# Myelomeningocele

The late **H. B. Eckstein**  MA, MD, MChir, FRCS
Consultant Paediatric Surgeon, The Hospital for Sick Children, Great Ormond Street, London and Queen Mary's Hospital for Children, Carshalton, Surrey, UK

**L. Spitz**  MB, ChB, PhD, FRCS(Ed), FRCS(Eng), FAAP(Hon)
Nuffield Professor of Paediatric Surgery, Institute of Child Health; Consultant Paediatric Surgeon, Hospital for Sick Children, Great Ormond Street, London, UK

## Introduction

Myelomeningocele is one of the commoner major congenital abnormalities which may require surgical correction in the neonatal period. There is a failure of fusion of some of the vertebral arches and the spinal cord is either covered by a thin membrane or is exposed on the surface as an open neural plaque. Surprisingly little is known about the aetiology, although it is widely accepted that there are considerable geographical variations in the incidence figures and the abnormality is much more common in social class 4 than in social classes 1 and 2. In the past blighted potatoes and excessive tea-drinking have been implicated as causative factors, while at present attention is focused on a relative folic acid deficiency in the mother at the time of conception and in the first few weeks of pregnancy. There is, however, little doubt that the aetiology is multifactorial.

Myelomeningocele must be distinguished from a meningocele which by definition is covered by an epithelium-lined CSF-containing sac but which does not contain any neural tissue. Meningocele is not associated with neurological deficit, and hydrocephalus is an unusual accompaniment, and seldom requires surgical correction in the first few weeks of life.

# Description

## 1

The lesion is most frequently situated in the lower lumbar spine and upper sacrum, but may occur anywhere along the vertebral column or indeed along the whole of the craniospinal axis. The exposed neural plaque is attached circumferentially by a thin membrane, and this in turn is continuous with the surrounding skin. Encephalocele, which is the related abnormality affecting the cranium, poses totally different problems and will not be discussed.

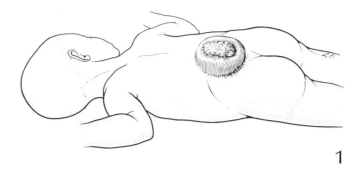

1

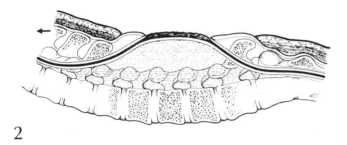

2

## 2

At the time of birth the lesion tends to be flat and the neural plaque is close to the posterior aspect of the vertebral bodies because of the effect of positive intrauterine pressure exerted by the uterus and amniotic fluid on the fetus.

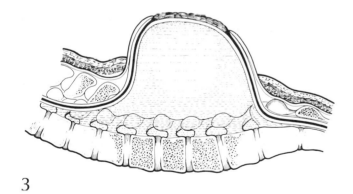

3

## 3

After delivery the pressure of the amniotic fluid disappears, the neonatal cerebrospinal fluid tends to accumulate, and this raises the neural plaque, displacing it posteriorly. This displacement causes increased traction on the nerve roots and results in increasing nerve conduction loss.

## ASSOCIATED PROBLEMS

The vast majority of infants with myelomeningocele have some degree of paralysis of the lower limbs. As a result of the partial denervation, muscle imbalance ensues and this may result in deformities causing flexion of the hips, hyperextension of the knees and calcaneus deformity of the feet. There is always accompanying anaesthesia with loss of cutaneous sensation, and this may lead to problems with pressure sores later in life. Because of the motor and sensory denervation, the majority of infants are incontinent of urine and faeces. A large proportion of children with myelomeningocele develop obstructive uropathy, which may be evident in 10 per cent of patients by the age of 3 months. The obstruction results either from inadequate bladder emptying or from a secondary detrusor hypertrophy which may lead to ureterovesical obstruction.

The problem of obstructive uropathy is greater in patients with sacral myelomeningocele than in those whose lesions are higher up the vertebral column. Patients with sacral lesions tend to have normal lower limb function and a low incidence of hydrocephalus, so that the urinary and faecal incontinence and the obstructive uropathy will become their major problem. Hydrocephalus associated with the Arnold–Chiari malformation is present in the large majority of patients with myelomeningocele, and in at least 70 per cent the hydrocephalus is progressive and will require surgical treatment (see pages 649–658).

## ETHICAL IMPLICATIONS

Before deciding upon surgical closure of the spinal defect, the surgeon must be fully aware of the implications and possible results of surgical treatment. If the spinal lesion is closed and a shunt inserted as necessary, the chances are that the infant will survive. In large published series the mortality of treated patients has been around 30 per cent. The great majority of this 30 per cent will die within one year and late deaths are relatively infrequent. If the spinal defect is not closed, the open lesion is likely to become infected and ascending meningitis tends to supervene. It is likely that 80–90 per cent of untreated children will die, but accurate figures are difficult to obtain. Obviously, if the degree of paralysis and deformity is minimal there will be no question as to whether to perform surgery, but in the infant with complete paraplegia and possible multiple deformities including kyphoscoliosis, it may be very debatable whether surgical closure of the back should be performed. The decision whether to operate or not must be made in relation to each individual patient, and must be discussed fully with senior members of the nursing staff and with the parents.

The concept that all these infants required emergency surgery within 24 hours of birth, as advocated by Sharrard et al. (1963)[1] is no longer valid and 'selection for treatment'[2] has been widely accepted by the profession. The ethical implications have been discussed by the author.[3]

## PRE-OPERATIVE INVESTIGATIONS

Blood should be cross-matched, as bleeding from the vertebral veins may be troublesome and difficult to control. An X-ray of the spine may be helpful to show the presence or absence of hemivertebrae, other malformations, and the degree of kyphosis. A culture swab for microbiology from the myelomeningocele should be taken so that suitable antibiotic therapy can be instituted if required. A pre-operative muscle chart prepared by an experienced physiotherapist is essential to give baseline information regarding the muscle power in the lower limbs. It is important to ensure that the infant is normothermic at the time of muscle charting, since the hypothermic baby, perhaps following ambulance transport from a maternity unit to a neonatal surgical centre, may give the impression of a greater degree of paralysis than is actually the case.

# THE OPERATION

The surgical closure is carried out under general endotracheal anaesthesia in a warm operating theatre. The infant is placed prone on the operating table with the chest and pelvis supported by sponges, rolled towels or sandbags to allow unimpeded ventilation. An intravenous infusion should be established, as blood transfusion may be required for even the smallest lesion. An electric blanket or warm-water mattress should be used to avoid unnecessary cooling of the patient. The infant's temperature should be closely monitored throughout the procedure.

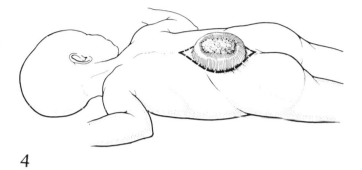

**4**

## 4

An elliptical incision is made into the cerebrospinal-fluid-containing myelomeningocele sac at the junction of the skin and the transparent membrane, i.e. well away from the neural plaque which should at no stage be handled with instruments. Nerve roots will be seen passing from the neural plaque and traversing the myelomeningocele sac. It is important to identify and preserve all these fibres.

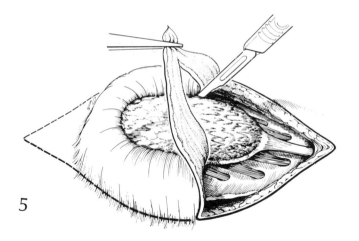

**5**

## 5

The membrane is elevated and mobilized medially, and excised under direct vision up to the edges of the neural plaque. It is important to excise the entire membrane, as there is a distinct risk of dermoid cyst formation should any tissue containing epidermal cells be left *in situ*.

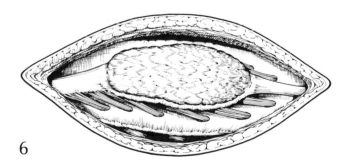

**6**

## 6

The dura mater is now clearly visible lining the base of the myelomengocele cavity. It is a glistening white fibrous layer. A circumferential incision is made through the layer as far laterally as possible, and the dura is carefully dissected off the underlying muscle laterally and the neural arches medially, until the emerging neural roots are encountered. The mobilization is completed superiorly and inferiorly so that the dural layer can be closed as a tube over the neural plaque as a watertight layer.

# 7

The dura is closed with an interrupted or continuous suture of 4/0 silk or polyglycolic acid.

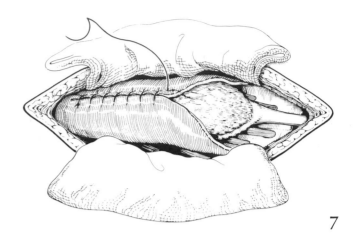

7

# 8

While it is almost always possible to obtain complete closure of the dura, this should be avoided if it appears likely to be tight and to strangulate the spinal cord and the remains of the neural plaque. In that situation, it is preferable to leave the dura open; this variation in technique appears to have no significant adverse effect either on the leakage of cerebrospinal fluid or on healing.

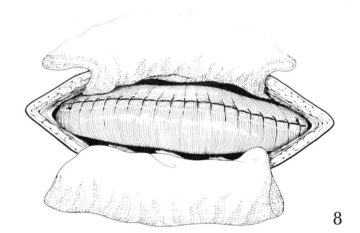

8

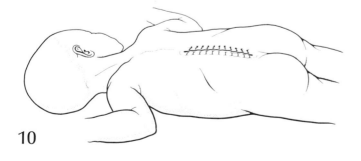

9

10

# 9 & 10

The skin is closed with interrupted sutures. If the subcutaneous fascia is reasonably well developed, a layer of subcutaneous sutures can be inserted, as these will often reduce tension on the actual cutaneous suture line. Drainage of the operative area is not necessary and should be avoided. If cerebrospinal fluid does accumulate under the wound, it is best controlled by pressure dressings and by repeated aspiration under strict sterile conditions. The skin sutures are not usually removed until after 10 days. Routine antibiotic therapy is not advocated.

# 11

Occasionally severe kyphosis in association with myelomeningocele precludes primary surgical closure, as it would be impossible to suture the skin over the spinal defect without excessive tension and the subsequent inevitable skin necrosis and infection. While the majority of such infants would, by today's standards, probably not be operated upon, this situation can be dealt with technically, and may occasionally arise if the parents insist on surgery.

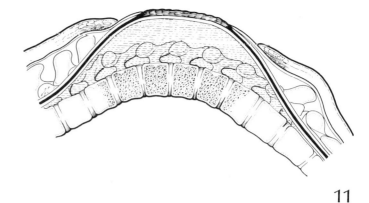

11

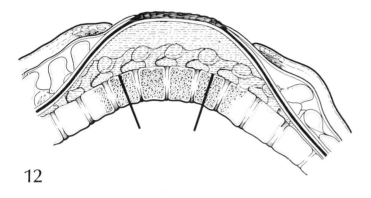

12

# 12

A double spinal osteotomy can be performed, usually by removing two or three vertebrae. It should be noted that in this situation the infant will in any event have complete paraplegia, so that damage to the spinal cord and its conducting mechanism is no problem. Indeed the entire neural plaque can be excised without increasing the existing handicap.

# 13

Following osteotomy there will be complete mobility between the upper and lower segments of the vertebral column, and wire sutures placed through adjacent vertebral bodies will straighten and stabilize the spine, correct the kyphosis, and allow a reasonably easy primary skin closure.[4] However, late recurrence of the kyphosis is not at all unusual and this type of major surgery *is no longer advocated*.

Major spinal surgery involving posterior Harrington rod or anterior Dwyer cable fusion for this group of patients is outside the scope of this chapter and is essentially an orthopaedic procedure.

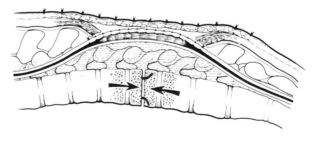

13

# Postoperative care

Following surgery, the infant should be nursed prone or in the lateral position in an incubator. The main reason for using an incubator rather than a cot postoperatively in the neonatal period is that this facilitates observation. Leakage of cerebrospinal fluid from the spinal wound is usually an indication of raised intracranial pressure and hydrocephalus, and should be treated by a ventriculoatrial or ventriculoperitoneal drainage procedure (see chapter on Hydrocephalus pages 649–658). A repeat exploration of the back incision is generally useless and carries a highly significant risk of introducing local infection which is likely to develop into ascending meningitis.

The muscle chart should be repeated prior to the infant's discharge from hospital to assess any possible damage secondary to surgery, and a routine urogram or a renal ultrasound investigation should also be performed before discharge to obtain baseline information about the likely presence of a neuropathic bladder. Recent advances in ultrasonography can provide helpful information about bladder emptying in infants with neuropathic bladder, and it is possible to estimate the volume of residual urine by this technique. Careful and prolonged follow-up by a multidisciplinary team is essential.

## GENETIC COUNSELLING

Genetic counselling and advice about the alphafetoprotein test should be offered to the parents of the myelomeningocele infant before discharge from hospital, and it is important to remember to counsel older siblings (if relevant) and other close relatives about the increased family incidence of major abnormalities of the central nervous system, of which myelomeningocele is probably one of the most important numerically.

## References

1. Sharrard, W. J. W., Zachary, R. B., Lorber, J., Bruce, A. M. (1963) A controlled trial of immediate and delayed closure of spina bifida cystica. Archives of Disease in Childhood, 38, 18–22

2. Lorber, J. (1971) Results of treatment of myelomeningocele: an analysis of 524 unselected cases, with special reference to possible selection for treatment. Developmental Medicine and Child Neurology, 13, 279–303

3. Eckstein, H. B. (1983) Myelomeningocele. In: Paediatric Neurology, E. M. Brett (ed.), pp. 385–396. Edinburgh: Churchill Livingstone

4. Eckstein, H. B., Vora, R. M. (1972) Spinal osteotomy for severe kyphosis in children with myelomeningocele. Journal of Bone and Joint Surgery, 54B, 328–333

Illustrations by Gillian Oliver

# Hydrocephalus

The late **H. B. Eckstein**  MA, MD, MChir, FRCS
Consultant Paediatric Surgeon, The Hospital for Sick Children, Great Ormond Street, London and Queen Mary's Hospital for Children, Carshalton, Surrey, UK

**L. Spitz**  MB, ChB, PhD, FRCS(Eng), FRCS(Ed), FAAP(Hon)
Nuffield Professor of Paediatric Surgery, Institute of Child Health; Consultant Paediatric Surgeon, Hospital for Sick Children, Great Ormond Street, London, UK

## Preoperative

### INTRODUCTION

Hydrocephalus, or an excess of cerebrospinal fluid within the cranial cavity, has been recognized as a major problem for a great many years. Trephine holes have been found in Egyptian mummies and innumerable fascinating and ingenious surgical procedures have been devised to relieve the condition. The multiplicity of surgical procedures used over the past 20 years demonstrates that no ideal method of treating the condition has yet been found.

## INDICATIONS FOR SURGERY

The most common cause of hydrocephalus is the Arnold–Chiari malformation, which is associated with myelomeningocele. Aqueduct stenosis, which may be congenital, is not infrequent, but birth trauma resulting in intraventricular haemorrhage and subsequent blockage of either the aqueduct or the foramina is more common. With the increasing survival rate of low-birth-weight infants, the incidence of hydrocephalus secondary to periventricular or intraventricular haemorrhage in the neonatal period is increasing.

Meningitis and ventriculitis may lead to hydrocephalus due to obstruction of the natural pathways. This was particularly common following tuberculous meningitis, which is now a relatively rare condition in developed countries.

Tumours may obstruct the cerebrospinal fluid pathway and produce hydrocephalus, but statistically, tumours of the brain rarely present with hydrocephalus.

The indication for operative intervention is progressive hydrocephalus in the infant, when the head circumference continues to increase or where there are signs of a progressive rise in intracranial pressure with related symptoms in older children.

## CLINICAL EXAMINATION

In the newborn period and in infancy the diagnosis is usually simple and straightforward. The open fontanelle may 'feel full', it may be definitely tense, or project above the normal contour of the head. Repeated measurements at weekly intervals of the head circumference will show an excessive growth rate when plotted on one of the many available head circumference charts. In severe cases, there will be typical 'sunset' appearances of the eyes caused by paralysis of the superior oblique muscle, which in turn is caused by traction on the vulnerable trochlear (IVth) nerve. Fundoscopy will show congestion of the retinal veins in early cases, and frank papilloedema in established hydrocephalus. The open or separated cranial sutures are palpable and an open lambdoid suture is virtually diagnostic of progressive hydrocephalus.

In older patients, once the sutures have started to fuse and the anterior fontanelle has closed, the clinical diagnosis becomes much more difficult and the only positive findings will be related to increased intracranial pressure. Over the age of one year, the head circumference may well remain within normal limits and can be most misleading; full radiological investigation is mandatory in any suspect patient.

## PREOPERATIVE INVESTIGATIONS

The only absolutely essential investigations in the management of hydrocephalus are culture of the cerebrospinal fluid and measurement of its protein content. Obviously, surgical interference cannot be carried out in the presence of infection, and a high protein content of the cerebrospinal fluid may render this so viscid that shunt therapy is unlikely to be successful. A skull X-ray will show widening of the suture lines and may occasionally show intracranial calcification due to tumour or toxoplasmosis. Ventriculography was previously required to display the precise anatomy and to show the site of the blockage, but in the last decade, imaging techniques have developed so much that a computerized axial tomography (CAT) scan has now become a standard investigation. It has virtually replaced ventriculography in the investigation of hydrocephalus. Likewise, there have been great advances in ultrasonography, which has none of the hazards of irradiation and enables the size of the ventricles and the thickness of the cerebral cortex to be measured easily whilst the fontanelle is still open. On occasions an artifical fontanelle (a large burr-hole) is justifiable so that ultrasonography can be used to assess progress following surgery. In the low-birth-weight baby it may give invaluable early evidence of intraventricular or periventricular haemorrhage and its sequelae. If a tumour is suspected, ventriculography may be essential. An electroencephalogram may be useful to provide baseline information on cerebral function and to identify those children who have extensive brain damage as well as hydrocephalus. A preoperative haemoglobin estimation is advisable, and it is wise for the inexperienced operator to have one unit of blood cross-matched.

# The operation

## Ventriculoatrial shunt (Holter)

### 1

The shunt consists essentially of three parts: a ventricular catheter, the length of which depends on the thickness of the cerebral cortex and the size of the lateral ventricle, the valve itself, and the distal catheter. The author uses the original A-type catheter although some prefer the C-type with the narrower tip. The valve must be tested and checked according to the manufacturers' instructions immediately before operation, to ensure that its flow rates and pressure specifications are accurate and that the valve does not reflux. Forceful syringing through the valve should be avoided as the valve mechanism is likely to be damaged.

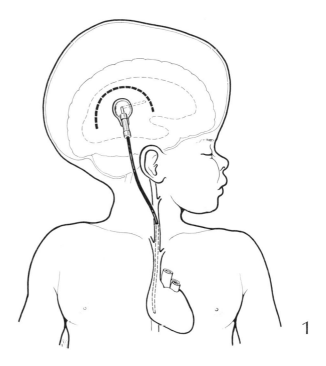

1

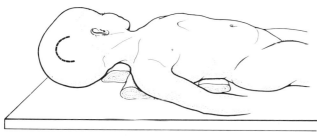

2a

### 2a

The patient is placed supine on the operating table with the head turned as far as possible to the left side. A small sandbag is placed under the neck, but excessive extension of the neck is to be avoided. The patient's head should be at the end of the operating table so that the surgeon can work from the end of the table rather than from its side. General endotracheal anaesthesia is essential and an intravenous line should be inserted in case of need. Diathermy is not essential. The patient's skin should be prepared by thorough scrubbing with chlorhexidine followed by an alcoholic iodine solution. The chest should be included in the field to be cleansed before operation, and should be covered with a sterile plastic adhesive drape. The right nipple should be visible in the operating field.

### 2b

A parietal flap incision is made over the right parietal eminence or, in an older patient, just above and behind the right ear. The periosteum is elevated with the flap and a burr-hole is made. Because of the thinness of the skull in infants with hydrocephalus, a bone nibbler is preferable to a standard brace once the skull has been perforated. The burr-hole is extended downwards as a groove for 2 cm and the groove should be wide enough to accommodate the upper part of the valve. A hole is punched through the bone at the junction of the burr-hole and the groove (a towel clip is ideal as an instrument in infants, while a drill will have to be used in older children) and a silk suture is inserted through these two holes.

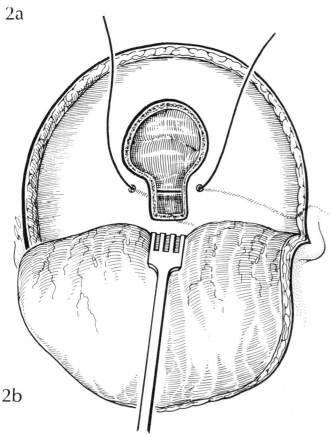

2b

## 3

A skin-crease incision is made in the neck over the right sternomastoid muscle halfway between the angle of the mandible and the medial end of the clavicle. This incision should avoid any possible damage to the external jugular vein, which may be required at a later date when the child is older. The sternomastoid muscle is split in its centre; the internal jugular vein is mobilized by blunt dissection and two ligatures are passed around it, the upper one of which is ligated. It is important not to include the vagus nerve in the ligature.

The distal catheter is now attached to the distal end of the valve and ligated to it with a silk suture. A Westminster-type trochar and cannula (without any flange) is then passed from the parietal scalp incision subcutaneously to the neck incision, taking care not to perforate either the external or the internal jugular vein. The trochar is withdrawn and the distal catheter is threaded down the cannula. The cannula is then withdrawn distally and traction on the distal catheter will pull the valve into its correct position.

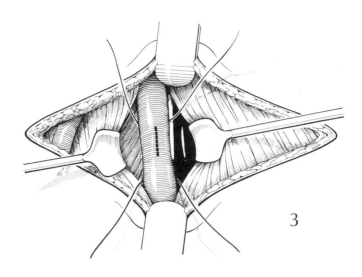

3

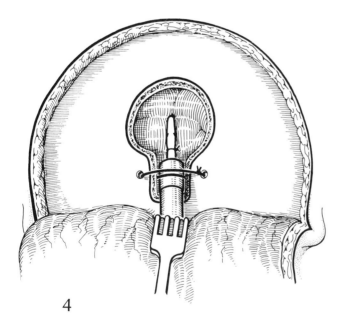

4

## 4

A 2–3 mm incision is made into the dura, avoiding any visible blood vessels and the right-angled ventricular catheter is inserted, mounted on a stilette. In practice a 5 cm catheter is usually correct. The catheter should be aimed towards the bridge of the nose. Once the ventricle is entered (cerebrospinal fluid will flow along the stilette), the stilette is withdrawn; the catheter is inserted up to the angle, and 10 ml of CSF is collected for culture. The ventricular catheter is then attached to the proximal end of the valve and secured in position with a silk ligature. The previously inserted silk suture is now tied fixing the shunt assembly to the skull. In the past 5 years, it has been our standard practice to inject 5 mg of gentamicin in 10 ml of normal saline through the ventricular catheter (after obtaining the equal volume of CSF for culture referred to above) and this procedure has dramatically reduced our incidence of shunt infection. Following surgery, gentamicin is administered intravenously or intramuscularly in the recommended dosage, according to the weight of the patient, for a five-day period. It is worth remembering that the lower limbs in these patients are usually anaesthetic, so that intramuscular injections present no major discomfort.

# 5

Most surgeons prefer to insert a Rickham reservoir between the proximal end of the valve and the ventricular catheter to facilitate later tapping of the ventricular system. In this case a straight catheter is attached to the Rickham reservoir, which in turn is attached to the proximal end of the valve through its side-arm. The disadvantage of the Rickham reservoir is that it does complicate the operative procedure to some extent and may increase the risk of shunt colonisation.

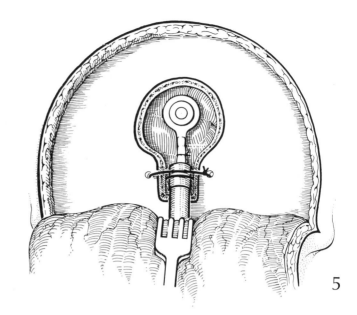

5

# 6

The proximal end of the valve should be lying comfortably in the bony groove, while the soft silastic section should be lying over the skull. Too short a groove will result in excessive projection of the metal end which may cause skin necrosis and infection, while too long a groove will allow the Silastic section of the valve to sink down so far that it cannot be easily palpated postoperatively.

At this point it is important to check that cerebrospinal fluid is escaping through the distal catheter.

The catheter is cut across at the level of the right nipple, which in infants is a reliable surface marking for the right atrium. Accurate placement of the distal catheter should be achieved with X-ray control on the operating table, or with ECG control using a saline-filled tube connected to an ECG monitor.

6

# 7

The internal jugular vein is now incised with small pointed scissors, and the previously cut distal catheter is introduced and passed along it. The distal ligature is tied sufficiently tightly to avoid haemorrhage from the vein, while at the same time ensuring that it is not so tight that it occludes the distal catheter. The valve should be pumped manually at this stage to ensure satisfactory function.

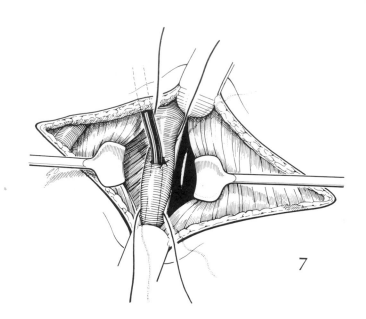

# 8

In infants over 6 months of age it is preferable to use the common facial vein as a means of entry into the vascular system, so as to leave the internal jugular vein unobstructed and patent. To achieve this exposure the neck incision should be placed slightly more posteriorly and at a slightly higher level than for the internal jugular vein, when the common facial vein can easily be identified and mobilized.

Alternatively in older children, the internal jugular vein may still be used as a means of entry, but via a small *lateral* incision which is carefully sutured with atraumatic silk and without ligating the internal jugular vein. Because of the very real prospect of future shunt revisions, the veins in the neck must be treated with great respect as they may all be required over the years to keep a shunt functioning.

# 9

The Pudenz system can be used as an alternative to the Holter system, and in practice there is probably little to choose between the two. The choice is mainly one of personal preference, and in the United Kingdom neuro-surgeons by and large tend to use the Pudenz system while paediatric surgeons seem to prefer the Holter system. The Pudenz system is slightly less bulky and the valve itself is placed in the end of the distal catheter. The major disadvantage of the Pudenz system is that it is not radio-opaque throughout but only has radio-opaque markers at the ends of the ventricular catheter and the distal catheter. The radiological diagnosis of breakages and fractures of the shunt tubing is therefore impossible.

While most shunts and valves are available in high-, medium- and low-pressure types, opening at different pressures of the cerebrospinal fluid, the author has found the low-pressure shunts eminently successful in paediatric practice, the high-pressure valves being only occasionally required in older patients with solidly fused skull bones and rather small ventricles.
Ventriculo-peritoneal shunts have become popular in recent years. They have the advantage that the numerous complications of ventriculoatrial shunts such as bacter-aemia and immune complex disease can be avoided. The insertion of a peritoneal shunt is also technically easier than a vascular shunt. On the other hand, the results of peritoneal shunts are less predictable, and blockage of the distal end by fibrin or omentum is not infrequent. The distal end of a peritoneal shunt has been known to perforate various abdominal viscera with disastrous consequences. The previously described Holter and Pudenz valves can be used satisfactorily for peritoneal shunts.

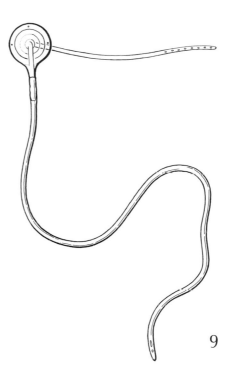

9

# 10

A special peritoneal shunt has been devised by Raimondi which has the advantage of being a single unit without any joints, ligatures or junctions, and is supplied in various lengths. The silicone tubing contains a metal spiral to prevent kinking. The proximal end of the shunt is inserted in much the same way as described for the Holter shunt. A subcutaneous channel is made between the scalp incision and the upper abdomen, and the single unit shunt tubing is pulled through. The peritoneum is opened and the distal end of the shunt is inserted into the peritoneal cavity. Ideally, the lower end of the shunt should be placed over the dome of the right lobe of the liver.

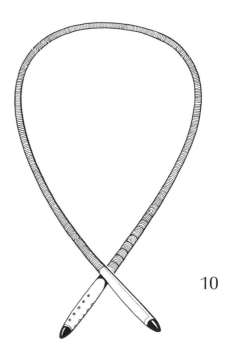

10

## 11

The peritoneal shunt lies comfortably in place, the length of the shunt system being preselected according to the size of the patient. Using the manufacturer's special introducers, only one intermediate incision (made in the neck) is necessary to pass the shunt tube from the head to the abdomen.

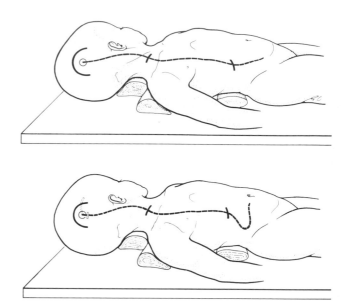

# Postoperative care

Patients with vascular shunts must have a postoperative chest X-ray to ensure the correct position of the distal catheter. If necessary the catheter may have to be lengthened, or, more frequently, shortened. A postoperative X-ray is not required with a peritoneal shunt, as the positioning of the distal end is of no great importance. Routine blood cultures should be taken postoperatively after vascular shunts to ensure that there is no bacteraemia. Antibody titres to coagulase-negative staphylococci and serial C-reactive protein levels are useful for the early detection of shunt colonization.

## COMPLICATIONS

While the shunt procedures are relatively simple and carry a minimal mortality, the complication rate is considerable and this must be fully appreciated before any such treatment is instituted.

Infection of the operative area is the result of poor surgical technique and tissue trauma. Infection following skin necrosis may result if the valve projects excessively under the infant's thin skin. In the event of infection, the entire shunt system must be removed and a new shunt will have to be inserted subsequently at another site.

## BLOCKAGE OF THE PROXIMAL CATHETER

This complication is not uncommon, especially if treatment for hydrocephalus is instituted before the ventricles are grossly enlarged. It may be caused by debris, but is more commonly the result of choroid plexus infiltrating into the ventricular catheter and obstructing it. The diagnosis is based on the symptoms and signs of progressive hydrocephalus whilst the valve remains flat or collapsed. The ventricular catheter has to be removed and replaced. If repeated occlusion of the proximal catheter occurs, it is worthwhile making a positive effort to place its tip within the anterior horn of the lateral ventricle where there is no choroid plexus. A new burr-hole placed higher and more posteriorly will be needed, but the rest of the shunt system need not be changed.

## DETACHED PROXIMAL CATHETER

The proximal catheter may become detached from the upper end of the valve because of traction secondary to growth, or possibly from trauma, or because of faulty operative technique. The shunt will cease to function and if it is still required by the patient, symptoms and signs of raised intracranial pressure will ensue. At the same time a fluid collection will develop over the upper end of the valve and emergency surgery is advocated to reconnect the proximal catheter. With a Holter system the diagnosis of a detached proximal catheter is readily confirmed by a two-plane skull X-ray.

## BLOCKAGE OF THE DISTAL CATHETER

The possibility of blockage of a peritoneal catheter has already been discussed. The atrial catheter will become blocked as the child grows; the distal catheter becomes relatively short and rises out of the right atrium into the superior vena cava. The symptoms are essentially similar to that of a blocked proximal catheter, but palpation of the valve itself may show this to feel stiff and not empty. A chest X-ray will show that the distal catheter is not in the correct place. The management of a blocked distal catheter is discussed below. The not unusual combination of partial valve failure and distal shunt obstruction can present diagnostic problems to the surgeon. If there is reflux through the upper valve cusps, the valve will appear to the examining finger to be pumping normally even in the presence of distal obstruction. Often the distal tube can be palpated and digitally compressed over the mastoid process, and this will facilitate the diagnosis. It is, however, sometimes necessary to explore a shunt on account of the patient's symptoms rather than because of the physical signs.

## VALVE FAILURE AND INFECTION

Valve failure as such is unusual, especially if the valve has been carefully checked preoperatively. If the valve does fail to empty at the correct pressure, again symptoms and signs of raised intracranial pressure will develop, and if both the proximal and distal ends of the shunt are functioning, the valve should be replaced. Infection of a shunt, almost always with coagulase-negative staphylococcus, is a relatively common complication and occurs in about 12 per cent of shunt-treated patients. A low-grade bacteraemia will result, with pyrexia, ill-health and anaemia. The spleen is usually enlarged and palpable. The diagnosis is confirmed by blood culture and by rapidly rising coagulase-negative staphylococci antibody titres, by the estimation of C-reactive protein, haemoglobin estimations, and white-cell count may also be helpful.

## SHUNT NEPHRITIS

This occurs as a result of long-standing infection in a ventriculoatrial shunt. Due to the high antibody levels and chronic antigenaemia, soluble immune complexes are deposited on the basement membrane of the renal glomeruli. The resulting inflammatory reaction gives rise to the signs of nephritis with haematuria and albuminaemia. This may progress to include oedema, hypertension, and eventually renal failure if the condition remains untreated. As shunt nephritis occurs only in long-standing infection, it can be *avoided* by early diagnosis.

## PULMONARY EMBOLI

These are surprisingly unusual, considering that a foreign body is placed within the heart. While histological evidence of pulmonary embolization is frequently found at autopsy in shunt-treated children, symptoms and signs relating to pulmonary emboli are unusual.

## CARDIAC TAMPONADE

This complication has been seen on a number of occasions when the distal catheter has perforated the heart wall and the cerebrospinal fluid has collected within the pericardium. The child will present with signs and symptoms of cardiac failure, and the chest X-ray is diagnostic of pericardial effusion. Immediate aspiration of the effusion and shortening of the distal catheter is usually curative, and the possibility of this diagnosis must be kept in mind.

## DETACHED DISTAL CATHETER

The distal catheter may become detached from the lower end of the valve, usually because of growth. The shunt will then no longer function; such detachment may be a chance finding on a routine chest X-ray in a symptomless patient. In the absence of symptoms, no action is needed unless the distal tube has passed through the right ventricle into the pulmonary artery. If necessary, such catheters can be extracted by cardiac catheterization, and thoracotomy is seldom indicated. In the event of shunt infection combined with a detached distal catheter, it is essential to remove the catheter surgically. If signs and symptoms of raised intracranial pressure should develop, further shunting procedures will be necessary and a peritoneal shunt would be preferable to a vascular one.

# Management of complications

## INFECTION

The management of obvious surgical infection following shunt insertion has already been discussed, and must involve the complete removal of the shunt and subsequent replacement. The much more frequent infection of the interior of the shunt, usually with coagulase-negative staphylococcus presents a different problem, which may develop months or even years after shunt insertion. Once shunt infection is established, antibiotic therapy, although useful in the short term, is most unlikely to be successful in sterilizing the shunt system. In our experience, immediate shunt replacement has proved to be satisfactory as a method of management and permits use of the same jugular vein. The total shunt system is removed, gentamicin is injected intravenously, and after an interval of about 20 min, a new shunt system can be inserted using the same burr-hole and the same internal jugular vein. Postoperative gentamicin is continued for 1 week.

If this procedure fails to cure the infection, the shunt will have to be removed and the patient will have to be left without a shunt for 1 or 2 weeks before inserting a new one at a different site. If symptoms of raised intracranial pressure develop, intermittent ventricular taps through one of the pre-existing burr-holes should be performed and repeated (usually once or twice in 24 hours).

Continuous external drainage of cerebrospinal fluid should be avoided if possible as this procedure carries a real risk of secondary infection, but specially designed and pre-sterilized drainage systems for this situation are now commercially available. This alternative method of management of infected shunts is to remove the shunt, to institute a competent sterile external drain (e.g. Codman or Dow Corning), and to administer intraventricular vancomycin 20 mg daily together with intravenous rifampicin (15 mg/kg per day to a maximum of 600 mg/day). In the majority of cases all evidence of infection will have disappeared by the 4th or 5th day. Reshunting, if necessary, should be carried out on the last day of antibiotic treatment. This method is suitable in all cases where the infecting organism is susceptible, and ensures success at the first attempt in most cases, along with a shorter period of external drainage.

## BLOCKAGE OF THE DISTAL CATHETER

This complication will arise in most patients sooner or later, as the child grows. In practice, however, a significant number of children seem to manage without a ventriculoatrial or other shunt by the time such blockage occurs. In the absence of signs or symptoms the blockage can be ignored. It is almost invariably associated with growth, which pulls the catheter up into the superior vena cava. If blockage of the distal catheter does occur and symptoms of raised intracranial pressure develop, the shunt will have to be revised. It may be possible to recannulate the internal jugular vein by passing dilators or, failing that, the right external jugular vein may be available and adequate to introduce the distal catheter. Alternatively, the left internal or external jugular veins may have to be used as a means of access to the right atrium. Although this procedure is technically straightforward, a radiological check at the time of operation is essential to ensure that the catheter has gone down to the right atrium and not into one of the subclavian veins!

If all neck veins have been used, it is technically possible to introduce the distal catheter through the azygos vein, or by a direct cardiotomy either into the right atrium itself or through the right atrial appendix. Both these procedures require a full thoracotomy, but present no insuperable difficulties. Alternatively, the distal catheter can be placed into the right pleural cavity; such a ventriculopleural shunt sometimes works for many years without any trouble. As another alternative, the distal catheter can be placed into the peritoneal cavity, as has been described earlier in this section.

In the author's experience of some 800 shunt-treated patients over a 20-year period, there has to date been only a single child in whom further shunt surgery was impossible as all available means of shunt placement had been used.

## LONG-TERM PROBLEMS AND PROGNOSIS

Since the management of hydrocephalus by the use of ventriculoatrial and other shunts, using the methods of Pudenz and Heyer, and Spitz and Holter, were introduced in the country only in 1958, it is impossible to give a long-term prognosis in excess of some 25 years. It would appear, however, that the results of shunt treatment are essentially satisfactory even if shunt revisions are not infrequently required. Undoubtedly a number of older patients with severe hydrocephalus and a cerebral mantle of less than 1 cm have developed into perfectly normal teenagers, have passed through a normal school education and would seem suitable for University education. Other patients, often with less severe hydrocephalus, have been more disappointing and have shown obvious evidence of mental retardation and spasticity on a long-term follow-up. Since the majority of our patients with hydrocephalus have had associated myelomeningocele with partial or complete paraplegia and incontinence of urine and faeces, it is extremely difficult to assess the end result. Even so, a significant proportion of those with multiple handicaps and hydrocephalus are suitable for further training and are likely to lead a totally independent life.

## Further reading

Bayston R. (1987) CSF shunt infections by coagulase-negative staphylococci Zebtralblatt für Bakteriologie, Mikrobiologie und Hygiene (Suppl.), 133–142, Gustav Fischer Verlag, Stuttgart

Bayston, R. (1985) Hydrocephalus shunt infections and their treatment. Journal of Antimicrobial Chemotherapy 15, 259–261

Bayston, R., Swinden, J. (1979) The aetiology and prevention of shunt nephritis. Zeitschrift für Kinderchirurgie und Grenzgebiete. 28, 377–384

Bayston, R., Spitz, L. (1977) Infective and cystic causes of malfunction of ventriculoperitoneal shunts for hydrocephalus. Zeitschrift für Kinderchirurgie und Grenzgebiete. 22, 419–424

# Spinal dysraphism

**D. N. Grant** FRCS
Consultant Neurosurgeon, National Hospital for Nervous Diseases, London; The Hospital for Sick Children, Great Ormond Street, London, UK

## Preoperative

### Definition

The term spinal dysraphism, if strictly used, applies to all disorders arising from abnormal development of the dorsal midline region of the embryo. By common usage, and for the purpose of this chapter, myelomeningocele is not included. The remaining more occult forms of dysraphism are lipoma of the conus medullaris, dermoid cyst and dermal sinus, thickening of the filum terminale, neurenteric cyst and diastematomyelia.

### Presentation

This may occur at any time between birth and adulthood. Visible or palpable midline abnormalities raise the suspicion of dysraphism. These include congenital scars often with surrounding telangiectatic skin, dermal pits or sinuses, overgrowth of hair which may be so profuse as to justify the term faun's tail, and subcutaneous lipomas. With very few exceptions there is underlying spina bifida, and the defects in the spinal canal may be palpable. Associated with the abnormalities of the spinal cord there may be maldevelopment of the lower extremities. This may take the form of unilateral or bilateral talipes or differences in length or girth of the legs. Difficulty in achieving bladder or bowel control, or loss of established control, may be a presenting feature. These deficits are usually relatively mild in early life in contrast to the severe abnormalities associated with myelomeningocele.

### Investigation

Plain radiographs of the spine usually show spina bifida which commonly involves several segments. The clefts between the laminae are usually asymmetrical or oblique. Spinous processes and laminae may be represented by grossly abnormal, partially fused plates of bone. Diastematomyelia may be recognized if a bony spur is visible between the halves of the spinal cord. The spinal canal is widened and there is a narrow disc space. Widening of the canal may also be produced by a lipoma or dermoid cyst.

Myelography is the definitive investigation, using the water-soluble contrast material metrizamide, which is injected either cisternally, by lateral cervical puncture, or by lumbar puncture. In children this procedure requires a general anaesthetic. Computerized tomography is used increasingly either to complement myelography or to replace it. Because of the incidence of associated urogenital abnormalities, intravenous pyelography and micturating cystourethrography should be included in the preliminary investigations.

### Indications

The essential feature common to the various dysraphic abnormalities is tethering of the spinal cord. The normal filum and nerve roots allow free movement of the spinal cord and conus during activity. It is postulated that repeated minor trauma transmitted by traction to the cord over a period of years can result in progressive neural damage which expresses itself as a worsening deficit in leg function and bowel or bladder control. Successful untethering prevents progressive spinal-cord damage from traction but is unlikely to reverse an established deficit.

It is not inevitable that deterioration will occur. Before recommending operation one must weigh up a prediction about the future behaviour of the lesion against the ability to achieve satisfactory untethering without adding to any existing neurological deficit.

The presence of a *dermal sinus* which communicates with the subarachnoid space poses an ever-present risk of meningitis or intraspinal abscess, and is an absolute indication for excision. No attempt should be made to inject contrast material into the external opening of such a sinus. A mass in the spinal canal, especially if associated with a dermal sinus, is likely to be a *dermoid cyst*. By accumulation of dermoid material, this acts as a progressive space-occupying lesion and hence warrants removal. A lipoma, on the other hand, usually grows in proportion with the patient, and space occupation is not usually a reason for interference.

Cosmetic considerations arise, particularly in relation to bulky *subcutaneous lipomas*. Some reduction can be undertaken during an untethering procedure, provided that wound healing is not jeopardized. Sometimes a purely cosmetic operation is appropriate if the risks of untethering are deemed to be too great. Such a decision should only be made after myelography.

## Anaesthesia

General anaesthesia with relaxation is required. An intravenous drip is essential as blood loss is frequently sufficient to necessitate replacement.

# The operation

### Position of patient

The patient is placed prone. Secure fixation of the endotracheal tube is vital. Use of a horse-shoe head-rest allows a relaxed neck position. Suitable sandbags are used to elevate the chest and pelvis to ensure that there is no abdominal compression. Venous congestion, the result of neglecting this manoeuvre can, by obscuring the anatomy, make a spinal operation exceedingly hazardous if not impossible.

### Incision and dissection

## 1

A midline incision is made after preparation of the skin and draping. Occasionally, if the abnormality is known to occupy only a single segment, a transverse skin incision may be cosmetically preferable. Congenital scars are excised at this stage but full-thickness skin is not sacrificed if this will lead to undue tension on closing the wound. Dermal sinus openings are included in the skin incision.

The paravertebral muscles are stripped from the underlying laminae by subperiosteal reflection. Care must be taken not to insert the periosteal elevator on the inner aspect of a bifid area. The most reliable safeguard is to be certain that the plane of dissection always has muscle laterally and bone or cartilage medially. Except in diastematomyelia, it is most unusual to find muscle within the bony defect in a bifid arch, however grotesque.

A laminectomy of the exposed arches is then carried out using a variety of bone nibblers. In babies, when the roof of the sacral canal is incompletely ossified, it may be possible to divide the roof along one side using heavy scissors and to hinge it outwards by making a greenstick fracture on the opposite side.

At this stage the dura is exposed, but the findings vary depending on the particular dysraphic lesion. It is helpful to line the wound with strips of haemostatic material such as Surgicel covered with wet Lintine to prevent the field being obscured by blood.

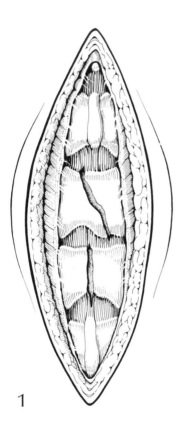

1

## Diastematomyelia

## 2

During the removal of the laminae one encounters the base of the abnormal spike of bone which passes ventrally, transfixing dura and spinal cord. The double dural tube protects the contained two half spinal cords and this should be retained intact as long as possible.

The central spike of bone is removed using progressively finer nibblers. There is often a central artery in the spike which produces tiresome bleeding with each nibble. Bone-wax is the only satisfactory method of control. It is not possible to complete the removal of the spike by extradural dissection, nor would it be possible to deal with intradural tethering bands.

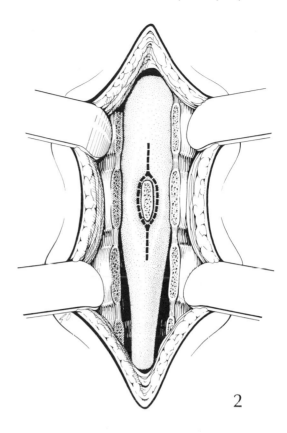

2

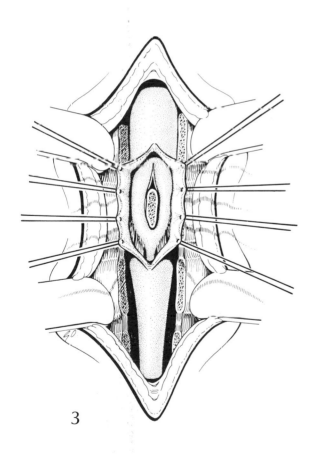

3

## 3

The dura is lifted away from the underlying spinal cord, using a fine sharp hook, and incised. The initial opening is made in the midline superiorly and this is then extended, with the cord under vision, around the central bony spike to meet in the midline inferiorly. The dural fringes are held aside with stay sutures. This reveals the two half-cords, usually with a tight commissure, applied closely to the caudal border of the spike with a wide gap superiorly.

# 4

In order to complete the removal of the spike two further manoeuvres may be helpful. Working in the split between the half-cords, the dura along the cranial border of the spike is divided in the midline and the two resulting triangular flaps retracted outwards. It is then usually possible to complete the removal of the spike down to its ventral attachment. Extradural venous bleeding is often troublesome, and should be controlled with bipolar diathermy or Surgicel.

It is occasionally possible to dislocate one or other half-cord across the midline and thus expose the residual spike in the wider gap between the half-cord and the side of the spinal canal. Working between the emerging roots, the remainder of the spike and its dural cuff are removed. It is not necessary to repair the anterior dural defect which results.

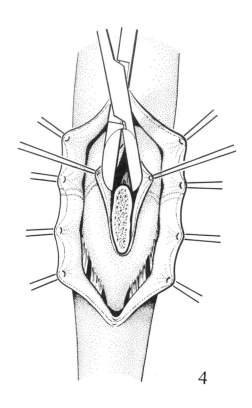

4

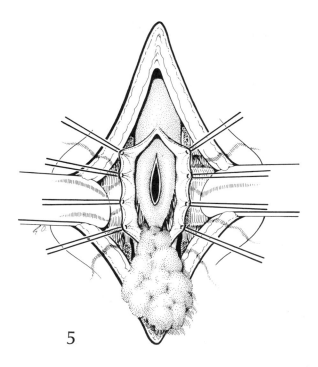

5

# 5

## Lipoma of the conus medullaris

The extradural part of such a lipoma will be encountered on completion of the laminectomy, and is often continuous with subcutaneous lipoma through the bifid area in the spinal canal. The lipoma becomes intradural through a dorsal deficiency in the dura. The dura is opened in the midline well above the emerging lipoma. The prolonged conus will then be seen merging with the intradural lipoma. The most favourable situation for untethering occurs when all the emerging nerve roots leave the spinal cord above the lipoma. In this case there is no hazard in transecting the fatty tissue. More usually, however, nerve roots are found emerging from a plane in the region where lipoma and cord fuse. Transection of the lipoma can be carried out dorsal to this plane of emergence. If nerve roots and lipoma are mingled in a less orderly fashion, it is safer to abandon the attempt to untether. If facilities for nerve stimulation or for recording evoked potentials are available the dissection of the lipoma may be less hazardous.

## Dermal sinus and dermoid cyst

On completion of the laminectomy, the situation may be somewhat similar to that encountered in dealing with a lipoma. The dermal sinus may end by becoming attached to the dura. There may be an extradural dermoid cyst which becomes continuous with dermoid intradurally through a dural hiatus. The dura should always be opened. The extradural dermoid presents no particular problem. Intradural dermoids may be small, looking like pearls among the cauda equina, and are removed without difficulty. A large dermoid may fill the spinal canal, incorporating the nerve roots in its transparent capsule.

The cyst is first opened and evacuated. The capsule is then gradually teased away from the nerve roots. Magnification is necessary. If there have been bouts of inflammation the capsule may be firmly adherent to the nerve roots, preventing total removal. Dermoid involving the conus is technically the most difficult to manage. Unless the membrane peels away without trauma it is better left *in situ*.

Occasionally a very thick-walled dermoid cyst is worth marsupializing by suturing the edges of the opened cyst to the opening in the dura. Although recurrence is likely as a result, it will to some extent be dissipated in the extradural tissues and, being excluded from the subarachnoid space, is less likely to cause troublesome arachnoiditis.

# 6

## Closure

Every attempt should be made to achieve a water-tight closure of the dura. Continuous or interrupted silk sutures are suitable. Any defect can be closed with a patch of substitute dura. Significant sites of leakage can be demonstrated by the anaesthetist carrying out a Valsalva manoeuvre. The muscle, subcutaneous tissue, and skin are then closed with layers of interrupted silk sutures. Haemostasis should be such that a drain is not necessary.

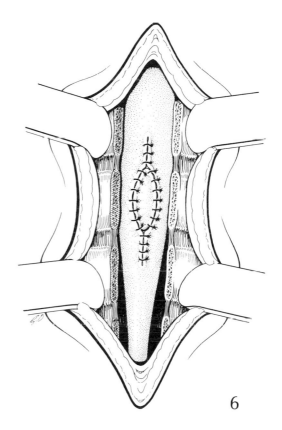

6

# Postoperative care

The patient is nursed horizontal for one week, but is allowed to turn from side to side and from prone to supine without restriction. It may be necessary to give sedation in order to maintain the horizontal position. The sutures are removed after a week and the child progressively mobilized.

## Complications

Leakage of cerebrospinal fluid is most likely to occur if dural closure has been incomplete or if mobilization has been allowed too early. It usually responds to a further period of horizontal bed rest and pressure dressing. During this time, prophylactic antibiotics are advisable. If this regime fails, it will be necessary to explore the wound in order to plug the dural leak. Usually the edges of the dura will by this time be friable and difficult to suture. A patch of muscle secured with tissue glue is often effective.

If neurological deterioration occurs, the remote possibility of a postoperative haematoma must be borne in mind. A much more probable explanation is reactionary oedema of the spinal cord and nerve roots due to the trauma of manipulation. This effect can be minimized by a short course of dexamethasone.

Urinary retention, due either to the underlying neurological abnormality or to the discomfort and enforced horizontal position may require catheterization. If this does become necessary it is often most satisfactory to leave the catheter in place until mobilization begins.

Illustrations by Gillian Oliver

# Treatment of subdural effusion

**D. N. Grant** FRCS
Consultant Neurosurgeon, National Hospital for Nervous Diseases, London; The Hospital for Sick Children, Great Ormond Street, London, UK

## Preoperative

Subdural effusion is a collection of watery fluid in the subdural space on one or both sides. It is commonly the result of preceding trauma or less often follows meningitis. The trauma may be sustained at delivery, accidentally thereafter, or, as is being increasingly recognized, by deliberate infliction. The nature of this fluid varies with the time between the trauma and the detection of the effusion. Increasing delay results in a fluid containing less obvious blood but always having an elevated protein content. The majority of patients present under the age of 6 months. The diagnosis may be established most simply by aspiration through the lateral angle of the anterior fontanelle if this is patent. If the fontanelle is closed, computerized tomography, if available, is a non-invasive means of demonstrating the effusion, but isodense effusions will not be differentiated from the brain tissue. If computerized tomography is not available, suspected subdural effusions in a child with a closed fontanelle are best shown by angiography.

Many subdural effusions may be treated conservatively provided they are asymptomatic and not causing raised intracranial pressure or progressive increase in head circumference. This applies particularly to effusions which are less than 1 cm in depth. If the effusion is causing symptoms or signs, active treatment is required. Repeated aspiration through the fontanelle at daily or twice-daily intervals until the subdural spaces are dry is possible but has several disadvantages. Repeated needling through the fontanelle, even in the most careful hands, is likely to cause further trauma with release of fresh blood into the effusion.

In spite of meticulous technique, there is a risk with repeated punctures, of introducing infection into the subdural space. If the effusion does not resolve within approximately a week, and if the fluid by then is not blood-stained, the most satisfactory procedure is subdural pleural shunting. The older operation of bilateral craniotomies with stripping of the subdural membranes is no longer thought to be necessary. Apart from having no demonstrable advantage over the simpler shunting procedure, it carried with it an appreciable morbidity and mortality.

# The operations

## 1

### TAPPING THE SUBDURAL SPACE

The baby is immobilized by wrapping in a towel, and the head is supported, face upwards, by the nurse, who uses her elbows and forearms to grip the baby's trunk and the palms of her hands to steady the baby's head. The operator works at the top of the baby's head. A wide area around the fontanelle is shaved and cleaned with cetrimide. A sharp, short bevelled needle is inserted at the lateral angle of the anterior fontanelle. The needle is passed obliquely through the skin and after advancing subcutaneously for a further millimetre, is made to penetrate the dura, which it does with a distinct sensation of 'give'. The aim is to have the puncture hole in the skin and that in the dura separated by an interval to minimize leakage. If there is a subdural collection under pressure it will emerge spontaneously. If it does not do so, the needle is rotated and finally gentle aspiration is applied with a syringe. The same procedure is carried out on the opposite side at the same time. Fluid is allowed to flow spontaneously up to a maximum of 15 ml on both sides. The removal of more fluid usually results in a sudden pallor and abnormal quietness of the baby. It is appropriate to inject 5 ml of air on both sides before withdrawing the needle. Simple anteroposterior and lateral radiographs in the brow-up and brow-down position will then reveal the extent of the subdural effusions.

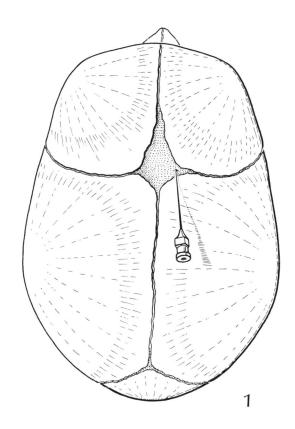

1

### SUBDURAL PLEURAL SHUNT

#### Anaesthesia

General anaesthesia using an endotracheal tube is required. The tube must be securely fixed. Should it become dislodged while the baby is draped in the face-down position, it could be disastrous. An intravenous cannula is necessary.

#### Procedure

## 2

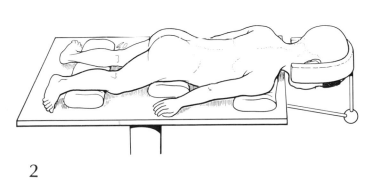

2

The baby is positioned face down with the head supported in a 'horse-shoe'. The shoulders and pelvis are raised on sandbags to lift the abdomen clear of the table. Care must be taken to protect the eyes from pressure and from drying.

Bilateral standard posterior parietal burr holes are made. The dura is opened on both sides in a cruciate fashion. The subdural membrane may be opened at the same time or separately. Subdural fluid may emerge spontaneously, but if not, the brain should be depressed with a flat instrument until one is certain that the subdural space has been entered.

# 3

Two lengths of silicone rubber tubing with additional side holes cut in the terminal 2 cm are then passed forwards into the subdural space for the measured distance required to take them approximately to the coronal suture. The catheters are anchored with a single silk suture through the pericranium.

An oblique incision is then made at the medial border of the scapula. The underlying muscle layers are split in the direction of their fibres until the pleura is exposed in a convenient intercostal space. A subcutaneous tunnel is now made to connect the burr hole wounds with the chest incision, using, if need be, an intermediate skin incision. Through this tunnel the rubber catheters are withdrawn from the scalp incision into the chest incision.

The anaesthetist now deflates the lung and a small nick is made in the pleura. The two tubes are amputated to a length of about 6 cm, additional side holes are cut in their terminal 2 cm and the tubes are passed into the pleural cavity. There is no need to attempt to close the pleura. The muscle layers are then approximated around the catheters, but before making the wound air-tight the anaesthetist is asked to inflate the lung to expel all the air from the pleural cavity. The closure of the wounds is then completed in layers with silk sutures.

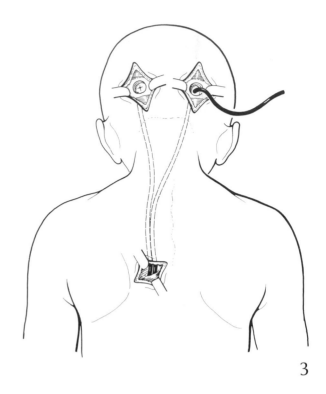

3

## Postoperative care and complications

After 24 hours the baby may be nursed in the sitting position to encourage fluid to pass down into the chest. The respiratory rate invariably rises, but this may be due to discomfort of the chest incision as much as to accumulation of fluid in the chest.

A check radiograph is taken at 24 hours. Very occasionally there may be sufficient pleural effusion to necessitate tapping of the pleural cavity. Infection in relation to catheters usually demands their removal.

The sutures are removed after 5 days.

Only if there is doubt about the efficacy of the drainage need the subdural taps be repeated. The baby is ready for discharge about a week after the operation. The tubes are only thought to function for 2 or 3 weeks but it is preferable to allow the child to recover fully and readmit at an arbitrary time such as 3 or 6 months later for removal of the tubes. If they are not removed they can cause a rather unsightly contracted cicatrix in the neck. Before their removal a check radiograph is well worthwhile, because the tubes may migrate and one may be mistakenly palpating the scar and not the tube.

Illustrations by Kevin Marks

# Trigger thumb

**J. A. Fixsen**  MChir, FRCS
Consultant Orthopaedic Surgeon, Hospital for Sick Children, Great Ormond Street, London, UK

## Introduction

'Trigger thumb', 'snapping thumb' or stenosing tenovaginitis of the flexor pollicis longus is a not uncommon cause of flexion deformity of the interphalangeal joint of the thumb in children. The condition is frequently misdiagnosed as a fracture, dislocation or congenital anomaly. In children, unlike in adults, the condition rarely occurs in the fingers, and the thumb rarely 'snaps' or 'triggers' to become locked in the flexed position. The condition can occur at any age but is most commonly found in the first 4 years of life. Spontaneous recovery does occur in childhood. It is estimated that at least 30 per cent of those noted at or soon after birth resolve spontaneously[1], and about 12 per cent of those noticed after 6 months of age

will also resolve. In children under 4 years of age, delaying the operation does not appear to lead to residual contracture at the interphalangeal joint.

Surgical release is recommended if spontaneous recovery has not occurred in 6–12 months and if the child is over 4 years of age. Clinically the interphalangeal joint is fixed in 20–50° of flexion. There is a palpable nodule in the flexor pollicis longus tendon at the level of the first metacarpal head. This is so hard that it is often mistaken for a bony lump or exostosis. The nodule can be felt to move with the tendon when the interphalangeal joint is flexed and extended, but rarely can the interphalangeal joint be snapped straight.

# The operation

This should be performed in theatre with good lighting. The use of a tourniquet to obtain a bloodless field is essential. A general anaesthetic should be used in children.

## 1

### The incision

A short transverse incision is made just proximal to the flexor crease at the base of the thumb. Great care should be taken at the radial end of the incision, as the digital nerve lies just under the skin immediately adjacent to the flexor tendon.

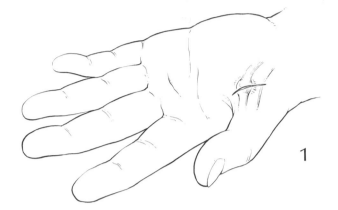

## 2 & 3

### Exposure of nodule and splitting of tendon sheath

The nodule and tendon sheath are exposed. The tendon sheath is split longitudinally with a scalpel or scissors over sufficient length to allow the tendon and nodule to move freely when the interphalangeal joint is put through a full range of flexion and extension. No attempt is made to remove the nodule or reduce it in size. Some surgeons prefer to excise a portion of the tendon sheath to ensure that there is no chance of the sheath healing back over the tendon and the constriction recurring.

The tourniquet is removed and haemostasis is obtained. The skin is then closed. No subcutaneous sutures are necessary. A self-absorbing suture such as Dexon can be used in the skin to obviate the necessity of suture removal – a procedure most children seem to dread. A cotton wool and crêpe pressure bandage is applied. In small children this should be firmly strapped in place to prevent inadvertent removal and contamination of the wound.

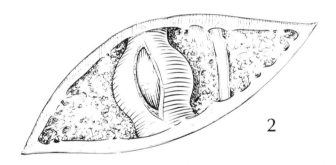

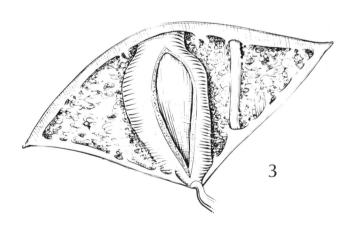

# Postoperative care

Postoperatively the arm and hand may be rested in a sling for a few days. The dressing and sutures can be removed at 7–10 days.

*Reference*

1. Dinham, J. M., Meggitt, B. F. (1974) Trigger thumbs in children: a review of the natural history and indications for treatment in 105 patients. Journal of Bone and Joint Surgery, 74B, 153–155

# Syndactyly

**David M. Evans** FRCS
Consultant Plastic Surgeon, Department of Plastic Surgery, Wexham Park Hospital, Slough, Berkshire, UK

## Introduction

Syndactyly is defined as a failure of separation of adjacent digits of the hand or foot. When the involved digits are otherwise normal and the connection consists of a skin web, the condition is simple syndactyly. Complicated syndactyly involves digits which are abnormal in other ways and the connection may extend to other tissues – neurovascular or musculoskeletal.

The inheritance of syndactyly is of a variable polygenic type, and is dominant[1]. Certain generalized syndromes which include syndactyly have a predictable pattern of inheritance – acrocephalosyndactyly (Apert's syndrome) is inherited as an autosomal dominant and the oro-facial-digital syndrome as an X-linked dominant trait.

Syndactyly accounts for approximately one-third of all congenital hand malformations.

Apart from the broad classification of syndactyly into simple and complicated, there are other varieties to consider. The classification of malformations of the hand is complex and confusing and there is considerable overlap between recognized groups. For example, the cleft hand deformity usually involves syndactyly of other digits of the same or opposite hand, and Miura[2] suggests that the two conditions are manifestations of the same process and should not be classified separately. The varieties of syndactyly are as follows.

1. Symbrachydactyly – short webbed digits: fingertips and nails present.
2. Acrosyndactyly – distal webbing with fenestration proximally (associated with ring constriction syndrome).
3. Acrocephalosyndactyly (Apert's syndrome) – severely disorganized complicated syndactyly of four limbs with major craniofacial abnormality and retardation.
4. Oligosyndactyly – syndactyly with other digits missing.
5. Syndactyly with polydactyly.
6. Syndactyly with cleft hand.
7. Poland's syndactyly – small hand and arm with syndactyly, hypoplasia of the ipsilateral breast and absence of the sternocostal head of pectoralis major.

## Indications and contraindications

Correction of syndactyly may be indicated:

1. to improve function;
2. to allow unimpeded growth; or
3. to improve appearance.

Not all of the indications are present in any one case and the decision to operate should only be made after careful consideration of any contraindications. These include:

1. general factors such as associated abnormalities, e.g. of the heart; and
2. local considerations – on occasion two fused digits may share neurovascular or musculosketal structures without which they cannot survive or function separately as independent digits.

Both function and growth of syndactylized digits will be affected if the digits are of unequal length and the corresponding joints are at different levels. This is particularly evident where the thumb and index finger are joined, and here the absence of an opposable digit and lack of the first web space are strong indications for separation.

Timing of separation is based on the same considerations. Syndactyly which prevents function or growth must be separated early and it is advisable to restore function to a syndactylized thumb in infancy. Simple syndactyly of equal digits may be carried out at any suitable age but operation within the first few years prevents the child's awareness of deformity.

Simple syndactyly of the toes is of no functional importance and should not be divided in childhood, as a graft failure could lead to scar contracture with difficulties in growth, gait or footwear. Occasionally a teenager or adult requests separation, in which case surgery is reasonable.

## Principles of surgical technique

In many cases surgery is undertaken for aesthetic reasons and it is vital that as well as satisfying these requirements no deterioration in function is produced through subsequent scar contracture or through loss of use in digits which cannot lead an independent existence. Where there was a functional indication for surgery this must be met in all aspects; it is usually found that functional and aesthetic considerations are closely linked and where one is satisfied, the other will be also.

The factor most likely to lead to contracture and impaired growth is the presence of a longitudinal scar, particularly on the volar aspect of the finger. To avoid this, steep zig-zag incisions must be used. There is always a skin deficiency and the best use must be made of local flap skin to line the base of the new cleft and to provide continuity of flap skin around each finger at strategic points to break the line of skin grafts. This should be done only with oblique or transverse scars. Skin replacement should be accurate, using full-thickness free skin grafts by choice, as these have less tendency to contract and a greater capacity for growth than split skin. A high incidence of graft take and skin flap survival should be assured by accurately planning, delicate tissue handling, haemostasis and effective postoperative splintage.

Where more than one web space is affected, it is widely held that the operation should not be carried out on both sides of the same digit at one sitting. This is certainly true in complicated syndactyly and the possibility of absence of the digital artery is a strong reason for following this advice. However, simple syndactyly of completely normal digits can be separated in neighbouring clefts provided that the presence of all neurovascular bundles is confirmed at an early stage.

# The operations

## SIMPLE SYNDACTYLY

# 1

Separation is carried out under tourniquet. The incisions are carefully planned. The base of the cleft is lined with a large dorsal flap and a smaller triangular volar flap. The dorsal flap is based at the level of the knuckle prominence and the volar flap at the proximal digital crease. The incision is continued distally in a zig-zag so that steeply pointed flaps are raised on the volar and dorsal aspects. It is important to raise only the tips of these flaps – there is no gain from undermining the base of the flap from the finger to which it will remain attached.

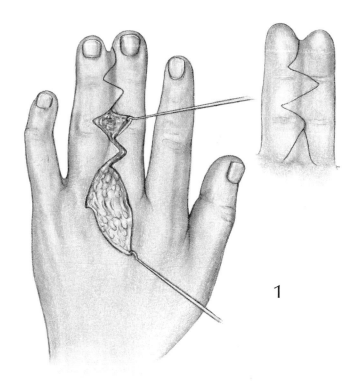

1

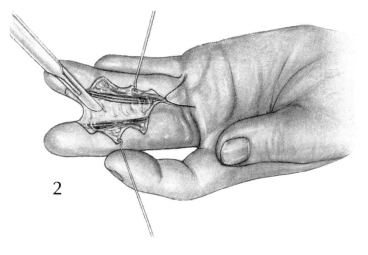

2

# 2

Separation of the soft tissues in the web is completed under direct vision, preserving the neurovascular bundle to each finger. If there is a common digital nerve it should be split into components for each finger, using magnification. If a common digital artery extends into the web, one branch has to be sacrificed, selecting the branch to the finger which is most likely to have an alternative arterial supply.

## 3

The proximal volar and dorsal flaps are sutured to each other in the base of the cleft, overlapping as far as possible but without tension. Suture material of 6/0 Vicryl is suitable for this operation in children. The remaining triangular flaps are interdigitated as far as possible and they should be designed to fit together accurately. A loose syndactyly may give sufficient skin to close the distal areas completely, but when the fingers have been closely united, only the tips or the flaps will overlap, leaving bridges of flap skin to separate the grafts. Any longitudinal skin edges should be incised so that a tuck of skin graft will break the line. A transverse incision of palmar skin may also be required to release tension in a finger that has been held flexed because of syndactyly with a shorter digit. It is unusual for further joint release to be needed in the child unless there is an associated congenital abnormality of the joint.

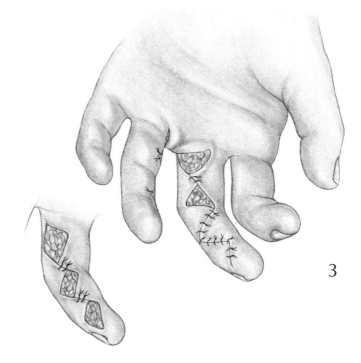

3

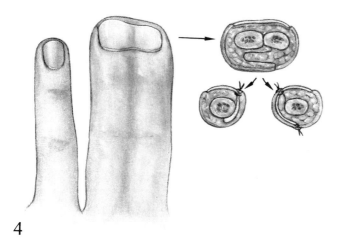

4

## 4

When there is inadequate soft tissue cover on the adjacent side of the distal phalanx, suggested by a common wide nail with no palpable movement between the two fingertips, the soft tissue can be shared by raising a thin skin flap for one finger and a subcutaneous fat flap to cover the bone on the other. A skin graft is then applied to the surface of the fat flap.

## 5

Accurate patterns are made of the raw areas between the skin flaps, and each one is numbered and orientated. The tourniquet is released and the raw surfaces wrapped in saline gauze while the skin grafts are prepared.

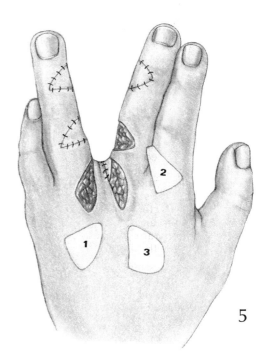

5

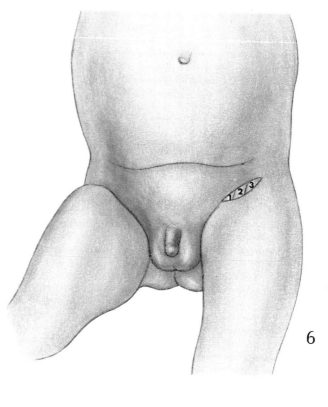

## 6

The patterns are placed in the groin crease to form an ellipse, lateral to the line of later pubic hair growth, and each shape is marked round with a scalpel.

6

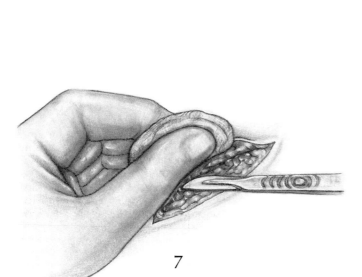

7

## 7

The skin is raised by sharp dissection at the plane between dermis and subcutaneous fat. As long as there is no more than a trace of subcutaneous tissue on the graft, it should not require further thinning.

## 8

The groin wound is closed directly with minimal undermining. Haemostasis in the hand is completed with bipolar diathermy and the viability of the skin flaps checked. If any are pale, sutures should be removed to relax tension on the affected area. The grafts are sutured accurately in place, with care to avoid gaps or overlapping. Very gentle handling of grafts and skin edges is important, avoiding any crushing with forceps.

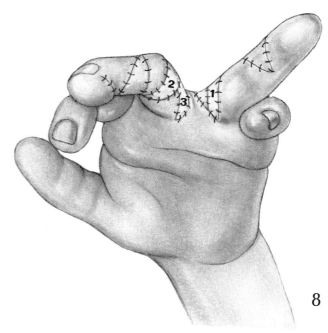

8

# 9 & 10

Occasionally a minor syndactyly involving the ring finger requires division to allow wearing of a ring. Here it is advisable to provide complete coverage of the ring finger with a volar flap taken from the base of the middle finger and a dorsal web flap.

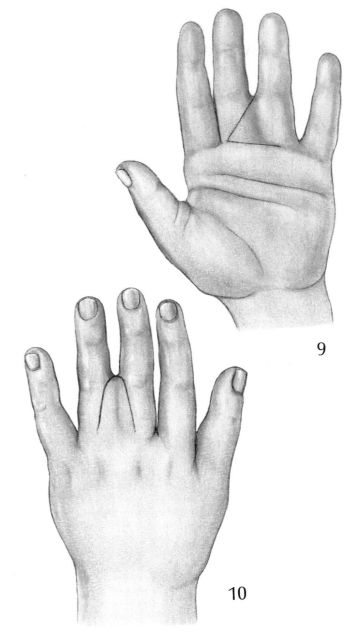

9

10

# 11

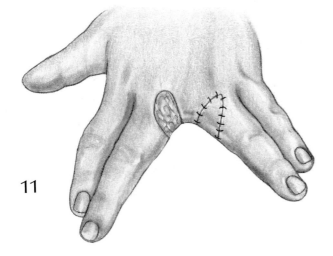

11

This leaves a larger defect for grafting on the middle finger.

## COMPLICATED SYNDACTYLY

# 12

Syndactyly of the first web space is usually associated with short fingers. Because this web space has to be wider to allow independent thumb function, a larger skin flap is required to fill the space.

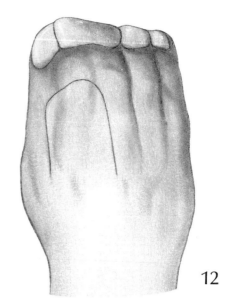

12

# 13

A much larger proportion of the sides of the digits requires grafting after this flap has been used to line the web. A full web space release may be necessary with adductor release, which may need to be maintained with a temporary Kirschner wire across the web space. In some cases a rotation osteotomy of the first metacarpal will have to be added to this procedure to restore opposition.

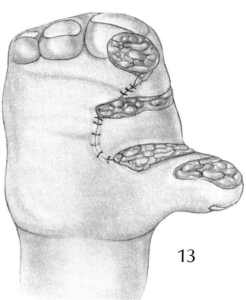

13

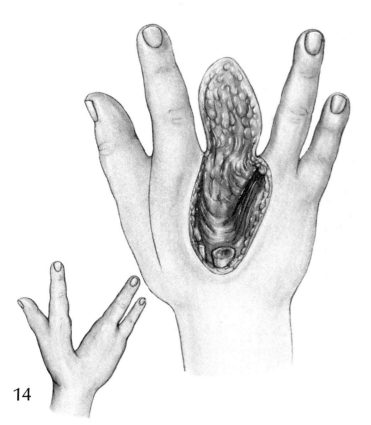

14

# 14

When correcting a cleft hand deformity it is important to use the spare skin from the cleft to line the first web space which is usually syndactylized, so the two deformities should be tackled together. The middle finger is usually absent and the abnormal cleft splits the hand in the line of the third metacarpal. The remnant of this bone should be removed except for the base, and the second metacarpal divided at the same level and transferred ulnarwards to fill the space and bring the index finger into correct relationship with the ring finger.

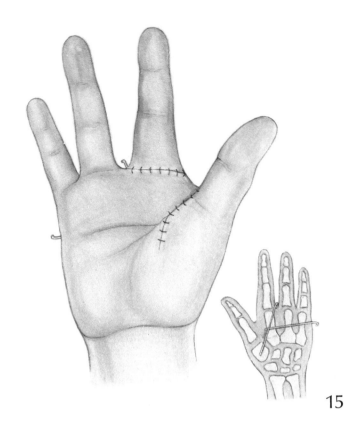

## 15

This position is held with Kirschner wires and a reconstructed deep metacarpal ligament. The skin of the cleft is raised as a palmar-based flap and has to be dissected carefully into the palm at a deep level, preserving neurovascular bundles, to allow it to move radially into the opened first web space.

15

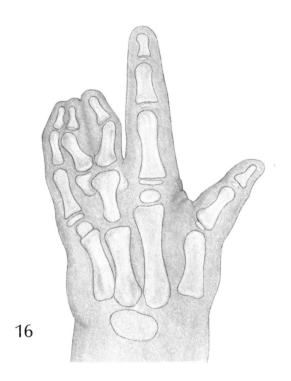

16

## 16

Some cases of complicated syndactyly require sound judgement when planning treatment. Where digits are interdependent for blood supply or movement it is often wise to resist pressure to separate them. Difficulties may also be encountered when there is polydactyly of one of the joined digits. In this example the ulnar distal half of the central digit is closely involved with a neighbouring ulnar digit. Removal would leave an unstable proximal interphalangeal joint to reconstruct with very poor prospects for motor function in the central digit. Such a case is better untreated.

As with all congenital malformations of the hand, no two cases are identical, and careful consideration is needed to find the correct treatment for each deformity.

## *Dressing*

The wounds are covered with a layer of Vaseline gauze and the cleft packed with plain absorbent gauze. The rest of the hand is wrapped, separating the other web spaces, and an above-elbow plaster of Paris splint applied. Time spent in dressing the hand firmly will ensure immobilization of the skin grafts and their survival. Flat slabs of plaster placed on the dorsal and palmar sides give a stable dressing and avoid the danger of a complete plaster cast.

## **Postoperative management**

The dressings need not be disturbed for 7–10 days provided there are no signs of infection or bleeding, but if the child is troubled by the hand or develops a pyrexia the hand should be inspected. Full-thickness grafts frequently blister and require further dressings until they heal. As soon as the wounds are dry and healed the hand may be left open and the child allowed to start using it. Children regain function well without help in most cases but any tendency for a finger or web space to contract should be immediately overcome by splintage, and refusal to use a finger or hand requires careful re-education, preferably by the child's mother.

## **Complications**

Loss of grafts may be due to haematoma or infection. As soon as this is recognized frequent dressings should start and the defect should be regrafted with split skin at the earliest opportunity. If healing by second intention is allowed a contracted scar is inevitable.

If a scar contracture does develop it should be released early to avoid secondary joint changes. A Z-plasty release is indicated but the Z-flaps will need to be supplemented with further skin grafts.

The disaster of digital ischaemia might follow ill-advised division of a digital artery in the absence of other supply to that finger, but care will avoid this occurrence.

## *References*

1. Wynne-Davies, R. (1971) Genetics and malformations of the hand. The Hand, 3, 184–192

2. Miura, T. (1976) Syndactyly and split hand. Hand, 8, 125–130

3. Buck-Gramcko, D. (1972) Operative treatment of congenital malformations of the hand. The Hand, 4, 33–36

# Polydactyly

**David M. Evans**  FRCS
Consultant Plastic Surgeon, Department of Plastic Surgery, Wexham Park Hospital, Slough, Berkshire, UK

## Introduction

Duplication of the fingers or toes occurs less frequently than syndactyly. In the hand, two-thirds of cases affected have duplication of the thumb (preaxial polydactyly), and postaxial polydactyly is more frequent than central polydactyly. In postaxial polydactyly a greater part is played by inheritance, which may be dominant. The anomaly is common in people of West African origin. Preaxial polydactyly can be produced in rat hindlimbs by intraperitoneal cytosine arabinoside on day 11 of gestation, and Nogami and Oohira[1] have demonstrated ectodermal over-growth as a result of this. Central polydactyly is more frequently associated with reduction malformations (e.g. cleft hand) and with syndactyly. Syndromes featuring polydactyly include Ellis-van Creveld syndrome (short limbs and cardiac anomalies, autosomal recessive); trisomy-13 (midline facial cleft); and Laurence-Moon-Biedl syndrome (retinitis pigmentosa, obesity and mental retardation, autosomal recessive).

In its mildest form polydactyly consists of a small rudiment attached by a narrow stalk of skin and blood vessels. Better developed supernumerary digits are connected either at a joint or the shaft of the bone, and the digit to which they are attached may or may not be abnormal. In some cases, particularly where the thumb is involved, it is difficult to decide which digit is normal and which supernumerary. More than one extra digit may be present, and complex forms occur in which conflicting distal and proximal relationships make a supernumerary digit appear to arise skeletally from one digit ray yet be syndactyl to another.

Surgical removal of extra digits is usually aimed at restoring normal appearance, and great care is needed to ensure that function and growth are not disturbed. In many respects the surgery demands no more than a carefully performed amputation, and this account will concentrate on those aspects requiring special consideration.

# The operations

## 1

The floppy rudimentary digit with a stalk should be accurately removed under operating theatre conditions. The traditional ligature around the stalk leaves a bump in the scar which requires revision later. It is possible to excise the digit under local anaesthesia in the neonate, as the needle prick is quickly forgotten and the baby is easy to hold. This is unsuitable in older babies, for whom general anaesthesia is required.

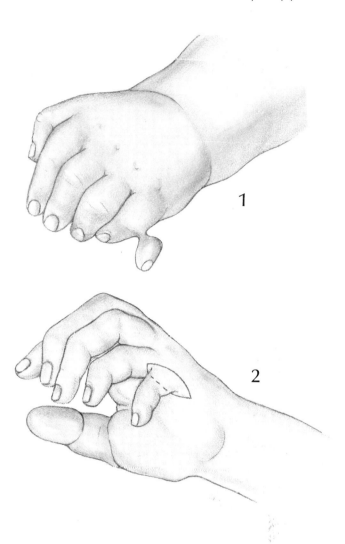

## 2

More completely formed pre- or postaxial digits are removed under general anaesthesia with a tourniquet. A racket incision is used leaving more skin on the palmar aspect to carry the scar dorsally. It is wise to leave excess skin with the initial incision, which can be trimmed when the wound is closed. The feeding vessels are ligated and digital nerves cut short and touched with diathermy to prevent neuroma formation.

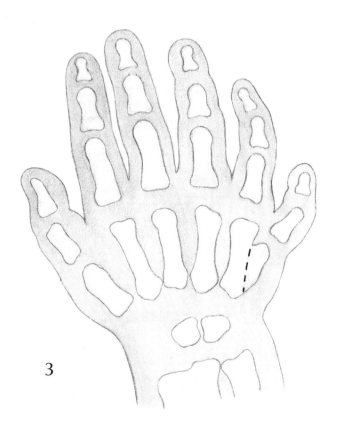

## 3

When the accessory digit arises from the shaft of the neighbouring metacarpal or phalanx the bone should be trimmed to leave a smooth shaft. A small bump left behind may grow into a prominent swelling. If an epiphysis is close it must not be damaged.

# 4

If the junction is placed at a joint, removal of the abnormal component may leave an unstable joint. The articular surface of the remaining proximal component will be shaped to accommodate both the phalanges with which it articulates and excision of one leaves the joint wide open on that side. The excess joint surface is removed and the joint aligned by a closing wedge osteotomy. The wedge of bone outlined is cut with a sharp osteotome and the gap closed. This is possible in the thumb, which has a proximal metacarpal epiphysis, but not in the fingers.

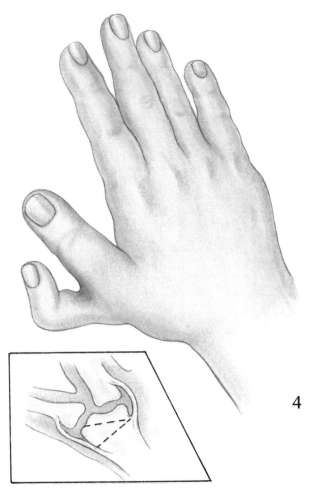

4

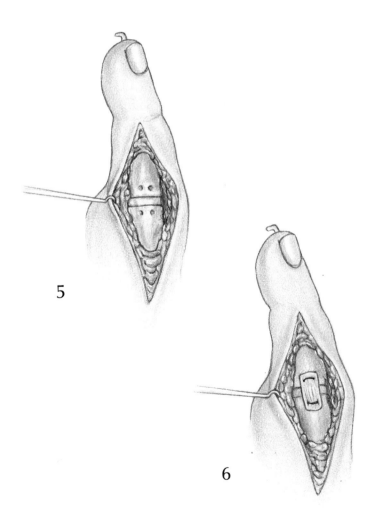

5

6

# 5 & 6

The joint should be stabilized and the osteotomy held with a longitudinal Kirschner wire. Permanent stability requires the construction of a new collateral ligament, and the extensor tendon on the removed digit provides tissue for this purpose. The ligament must be firmly fixed under tension, which is best achieved by suturing through drill holes in the bone adjacent to the joint.

# 7

In the type of case shown in *Illustration 4* there is no difficulty in choosing which of the two thumbs should be removed. When they are more equal in size and shape the decision requires some thought and should be based on observation of the hand in use and consideration of the suitability of the skeletal and motor components. When one of a more equal pair of thumbs is removed, eccentric pull of the long flexor and extensor tendons may cause gradual deviation of the interphalangeal joint towards the previously removed digit, sometimes with corresponding metacarpophalangeal angulation in the other direction. Miura[2] has demonstrated the radially placed insertion of flexor pollicis longus as a cause of this deformity and has also incriminated scar contracture as a secondary factor. This problem should be avoided by exploring the distal end of the flexor tendon at the time of primary treatment in such cases and reinserting it in the axial line of the thumb.

The incision is continued obliquely across the pulp of the thumb, preserving the neurovascular bundle. The radially placed tendon of flexor pollicis longus is divided at its insertion and reattached in the axial line of the distal phalanx by passing a suture holding the tendon through a drill hole emerging on the thumb nail. The suture is then tied firmly over a button.

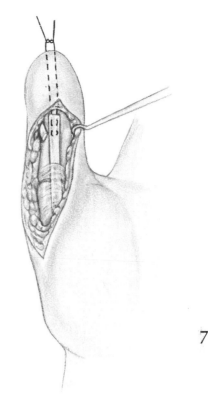

7

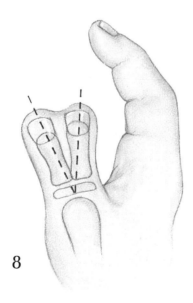

8

# 8

Terminal duplication of the thumb in equal parts may be corrected by the Bilhaut technique[3,4]. The central half of each component is removed and the two outer halves accurately approximated. The nails are avulsed and soft tissues divided with a scalpel, leaving exactly half the requirement for the whole thumb on each side. The phalangeal components are split longitudinally with a sharp osteotome so that the apex of the two cuts reaches the proximal limit of duplication. Care should be taken to avoid tissue separation in each half.

## 9

The two halves are swung together and the hemiphalanges wired together. It is important that the epiphyseal lines meet accurately so that growth occurs symmetrically. The soft tissues are repaired with meticulous alignment of the germinal and supporting matrix of the nail, using fine absorbable suture material (6/0 Dexon or catgut). In this way the inevitable ridge in the nail is minimized.

This method has been used to correct duplication extending more proximally and involving slightly unequal digits, but the technique is extremely difficult and prone to failure as even the slightest malalignment at joint level leads to stiffness and growth problems. In these circumstances it is usually wise to construct a thumb using the better half of the two digits.

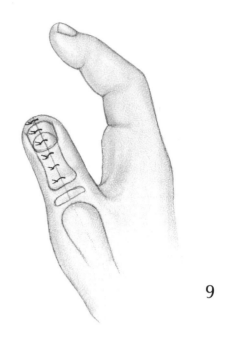

**9**

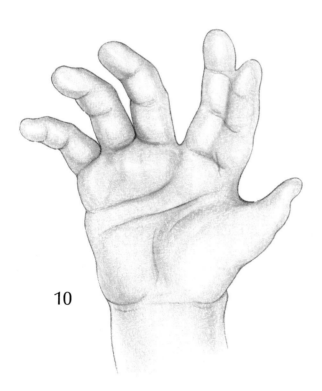

**10**

## 10

Occasionally advantage may be taken of a supernumerary digit to reconstruct another deficient digit. The example shown is typical of central polydactyly, showing the association with syndactyly of the duplicated index finger and partial amputation of the thumb. The stump of the thumb has no soft tissue cover and the duplicated radial half of the index finger can be pollicized.

## 11

The redundant index finger is dissected with a neurovascular bundle intact and freed from the enclosed skeleton, which is discarded except for the distal phalanx to provide nail support and the distal joint if it is suitable for preservation.

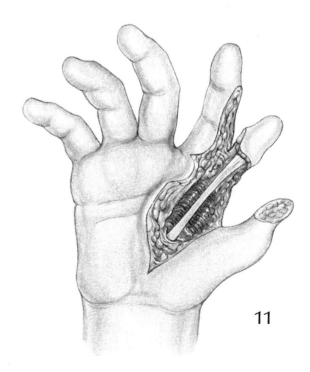

**11**

# 12

The neurovascular bundle and flexor apparatus are re-routed to the thumb and the digit is placed over the denuded proximal phalangeal stump with local rearrangement of skin. The new thumb tip is held in place with a longitudinal Kirschner wire.

When planning treatment of these complex deformities it is not possible to apply stereotyped procedures, and an imaginative approach may reveal opportunities such as those described.

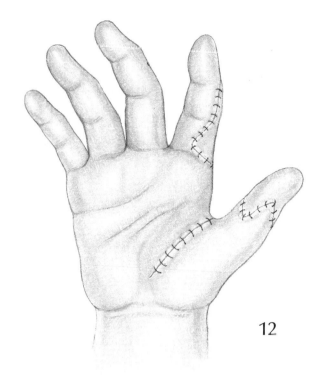

12

# Postoperative management

The hand is immobilized in an above-elbow plaster of Paris splint for 1–3 weeks depending on which structures have been repaired and need protection. The use of fine absorbable suture material (6/0) simplifies subsequent dressings.

## References

1. Nogami, H., Oohira, A. (1980) Experimental study on pathogenesis of polydactyly of the thumb. Journal of Hand Surgery, 5, 443–450

2. Miura, T. (1977) An appropriate treatment for postoperative Z-formed deformity of the duplicated thumb. Journal of Hand Surgery, 2, 380–386

3. Bilhaut, Dr. (1890) Guérison d'un pouce bifide par un nouveau procédé opératoire. Congrès Français de Chirurgie (4 Session 1889), 4, 576–580

4. Hartrampf, C. R., Vasconez, L. O., Mathes, S. (1974) Construction of one good thumb from both parts of a congenitally bifid thumb. Plastic and Reconstructive Surgery, 54, 148–152

# Ring constriction syndrome

**David M. Evans** FRCS
Consultant Plastic Surgeon, Department of Plastic Surgery, Wexham Park Hospital, Slough, Berkshire, UK

## Introduction

Of all congenital malformations the ring constriction syndrome is among the most difficult to explain and a heated debate on the subject has continued for more than a century.

The syndrome embraces a group of abnormalities which occur in a variety of combinations, mainly affecting the limbs and rarely the trunk and head. Patterson[1] classified the varieties as follows:

1. Simple ring constriction.
2. Ring constriction with distal deformity and/or lymph-oedema.
3. Ring constriction with distal fusion.
4. Intrauterine amputation.

Any of these deformities may be associated with amniotic bands, and the frequency with which these are seen increases when the infant is examined early. Amniotic bands may connect the affected area of the fetus to the amnion, in which case it is thought that the malformation will have occurred at a time when the two were closely associated; or amniotic bands may connect one part of the fetus to another, which may represent adhesion of two ulcerated parts, the adhesion gradually stretching to form a band. Montgomery[2] suggested that the amniotic bands were the cause of the ring constriction, and Denis Browne[3] espoused this view, adding a further suggestion that holes in the amnion through which the digit or limb protruded could also be a cause. In favour of the amniotic band school are the occasional reports of spontaneous reattachment of completely severed digits to another ring constriction; the occurrence of grooves which appear to run to an intrauterine amputation site; and a case described by Turner[4] of a lower limb ring constriction, the distal segment blue on delivery but soon recovering, with a saccular diverticulum in the placenta in which the affected limb fitted exactly with the narrow neck of the sac in the groove on the leg. In favour of the theory proposed by Streeter in 1930[5] – that the ring constriction represents a localized failure of development of subcutaneous tissue – are the histological similarity of the ring to a normal palmar skin crease, with a normal skin surface; deficient subcutaneous tissue and no scarring; the interruption of superficial but not deep blood vessels; the association with other unrelated malformations; and the great rarity of spiral lesions which might be expected to be commoner if a band were wrapped around the limb. It may be that different mechanisms can lead to a similar lesion in different circumstances.

Surgical correction of a ring constriction may be aimed at preventing or alleviating distal lymphoedema, separation of an associated distal fusion or removal of an unsightly groove for the sake of appearance. Where intrauterine amputation of digits has occurred there may be opportunities to improve the function potential of the hand by transfer of finger stumps from one position to another, deepening of web spaces or free toe transfer.

# The operation

A ring constriction may be found anywhere on the limbs, the commonest sites being around digits and around the forearm or leg below the knee. They are frequently multiple. When the aim of treatment is to alleviate or prevent distal lymphoedema it should be carried out as soon as the problem is recognized; otherwise surgery can be carried out at any time suitable to the patient. The operation is performed under general or regional anaesthesia depending on the age of the patient, and exsanguination of the limb with a tourniquet allows a dry field for dissection.

## 1

The skin lining the groove is excised and closed with Z-plasties to prevent secondary constriction due to the contraction of a circular scar. On fingers and toes it is often unnecessary to excise the volar section of the ring as it has the appearance of a palmar crease. In the case illustrated two Z-plasties have been designed on the dorsolateral aspects of the finger.

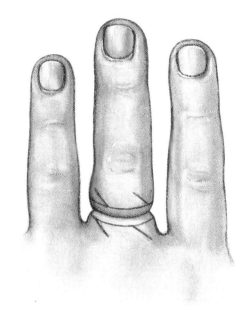

1

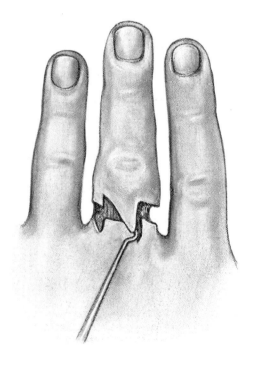

2

## 2

Each triangular flap should have a 60° angle and a side length of 6–8 mm. It is wise to cut one flap first and transpose it to determine the position of the second flap.

# 3

The flaps are transposed and the wound closed with 6/0 Vicryl.

When a ring constriction is excised higher up the limb, it is usually safe to excise the whole circumference of the ring with three Z-plasties. However, if a very deep groove is associated with questionable distal circulation only two-thirds of the circumference should be removed at one time. The triangular flaps should be correspondingly larger, with sides between one-quarter and one-third of the diameter of the limb at that point.

Two rings close together present a special problem and need to be excised in stages as the intervening bridge of skin cannot supply flaps for Z-plasties on both sides at the same time.

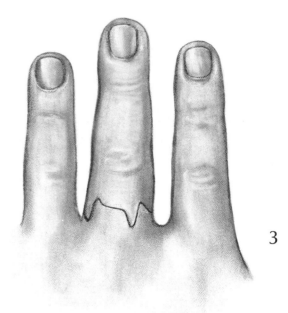

3

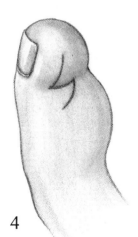

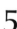

4

# 4

Ring constrictions are sometimes found close to the fingertip. This leaves a rounded bobble of tactile pulp skin which should be preserved if possible to maintain a useful padded fingertip. Usually a single Z-plasty will do this, taking the distal limb across the spherical tip.

If there is gross lymphoedema distal to the ring, it may be helpful to control this initially with a pressure garment. After excision of the ring and Z-plasty the external pressure should be continued.

Ring constriction of the lower limb may be associated with talipes equinovarus, which should receive appropriate treatment after the ring has been excised.

# 5

Distal fusion of digits is separated in the same way as any other syndactyly, except that the proximal window or fistula between the digits provides useful skin in the web space and proximal flaps for web lining may not be needed. Separation of the digits can be combined with correction of the ring.

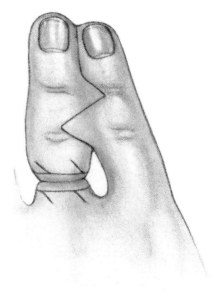

5

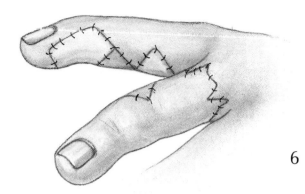

6

# 6

Despite the presence of an intact web, there may be a need for Wolfe grafts taken from the groin to complete the skin cover between the fingers (*see* chapter on 'Syndactyly', pp. 678–683).

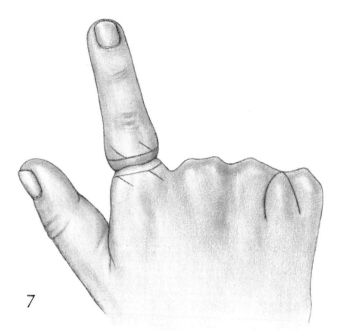

7

# 7

Occasionally there is a place for deepening of webs beyond their normal limit where several neighbouring digits are missing. Again this is achieved in the same way as syndactyly separation, with a flap lining in the proximal angle and full-thickness skin grafts on the sides of the fingers.

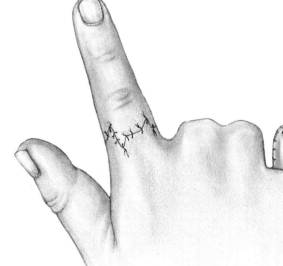

8

# 8

The web can be taken back to the level of the base of the proximal phalanx, allowing free movement of a proximal phalangeal remnant. This can be repeated for neighbouring digits.

## 9

There may be a place for transfer of a finger stump to lengthen another congenitally amputated digit, usually the thumb. Every affected hand has a different pattern of deformity and the design of reconstruction has to be tailored to meet the demands of the deformity as it exists. An index stump at web level provides useful lengthening of a thumb absent from metacarpophalangeal joint level and the widened thumb web will actually improve function provided a suitable middle finger can form a pinch grip with the reconstructed thumb. Skin incisions are designed to allow access to the index neurovascular bundles and the second metacarpal, keeping all the over-lying stump skin and the anterior and posterior flaps on the index finger. A staggered incision runs on to the thumb stump.

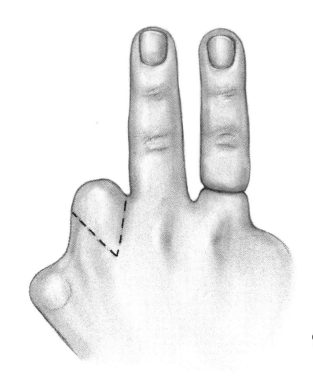

9

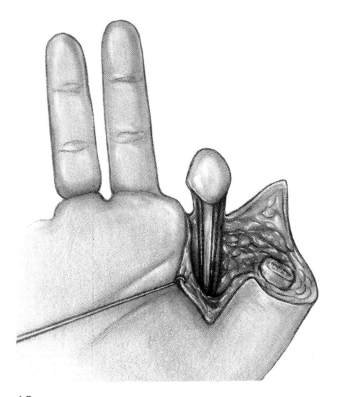

10

## 10

The neurovascular bundles are dissected out and the radial digital artery to the middle finger is divided. The metacarpal shaft is divided at the appropriate level and the remaining structures are mobilized to allow the index stump to move across the thumb.

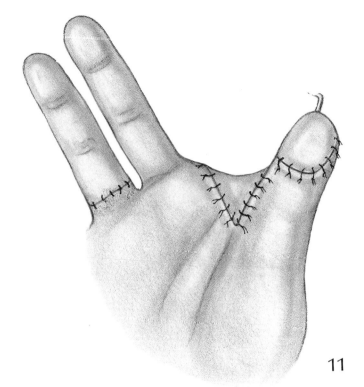

## 11

Skeletal fixation is achieved with a Kirschner wire. The remaining second metacarpal shaft is resected and the tourniquet released to check distal circulation and allow haemostasis. The skin is trimmed to allow closure, maintaining the depth and span of the thumb web.

11

# Postoperative care

Immobilization in a non-constricting plaster of Paris splint, extending above the elbow, is maintained for 1–3 weeks, depending on the procedure carried out. Thereafter the child is allowed to use the hand in play when healing is complete; no other physiotherapy should be required.

## References

1. Patterson, T. J. S. (1961) Congenital ring constrictions. British Journal of Plastic Surgery, 14, 1–31

2. Montgomery, W. F. (1832) Observations on the spontaneous amputation of the limbs of the foetus in utero with an attempt to explain the occasional cause of its production. Dublin Journal of Medical and Chemical Science, 1, 140–144

3. Browne, D. (1957) The pathology of congenital ring constrictions. Archives of Disease in Childhood, 32, 517–519

4. Turner, E. J. (1960) Intra-uterine constriction band. Journal of Paediatrics, 57, 890–891

5. Streeter, G. L. (1930) Focal deficiencies in fetal tissues and their relation to intra-uterine amputation. Contributions to Embryology, 22, 1–44

Illustrations by Kevin Marks

# Popliteal cysts

**J. A. Fixsen** MChir, FRCS
Consultant Orthopaedic Surgeon, Hospital for Sick Children, Great Ormond Street, London, UK

## Introduction

Popliteal cysts in children are common in the first decade, with a maximal incidence around the age of 6 years. They present as a cystic swelling which transilluminates and arises between the medial head of the gastrocnemius and the semitendinosus and semimembranosus tendons[1]. They are more common in boys and a traumatic origin has been suggested[2].

Unlike such cysts in adults, they are very rarely associated with intra-articular pathology. There is a rapid fall in incidence after the first decade, suggesting a high spontaneous recovery rate[2], and this is supported by Dinham[3], who showed a 73 per cent spontaneous disappearance rate over a mean period of 20 months. Surgery is indicated only if there is serious doubt about the nature of the lesion, if it persists and causes pressure symptoms or if the parents are unduly anxious about it. It is important to remember that there is a considerable risk of recurrence after surgery (42 per cent in the series reported by Dinham).

# The operation

It is essential for accurate dissection and removal of the cyst to carry out the operation under general anaesthesia with a tourniquet. The patient lies prone. A curving longitudinal incision centred over the cyst is made. A transverse incision with vertical extensions at each end is preferred by some surgeons.

# 1 & 2

## Exposure and removal of cyst

The deep fascia is divided and the cyst is exposed and carefully dissected out from the surrounding structures. It lies between the semitendinosus and semimembranous tendons medially and the medial head of the gastrocnemius laterally. The wall of the cyst is intimately attached to these structures and sharp dissection is necessary to remove it adequately. If possible, the cyst should be kept intact during the procedure.

The majority of cysts communicate with the cavity of the knee joint through an opening in the posterior capsule which remains after removal of the cyst. As intra-articular pathology is so rare in children, it is not necessary to enlarge this opening to inspect the intra-articular structures unless pathology is suspected. The opening is sutured with chromic catgut. The tourniquet is removed and haemostasis obtained. The wound is closed in layers suturing the deep fascia and skin. Care should be taken with the skin sutures to avoid an ugly scar. A subcuticular Dexon (polyglycolic acid) suture can be used, as this is self-absorbing and gives a good cosmetic result.

A firm cotton wool and crêpe bandage is applied. The patient is mobilized with crutches and allowed home as soon as he is comfortable. The procedure is commonly carried out as a day case. Skin sutures are removed at 10–14 days when the wound is healed and full use of the knee is then encouraged.

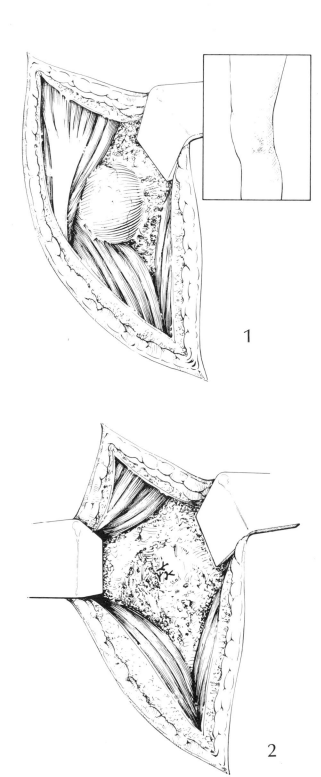

1

2

## References

1. Wilson, P. D., Eyre-Brook, A. L. and Francis, J. D. (1938) A clinical and anatomical study of the semimembranosus bursa in relation to popliteal cyst. Journal of Bone and Joint Surgery, 20, 963–984

2. Gristina, A. G. and Wilson, P. D. (1964) Popliteal cysts in adults and children. A review of 90 cases. Archives of Surgery, 88, 357–363

3. Dinham, J. M. (1975) Popliteal cysts in children: the case against surgery. Journal of Bone and Joint Surgery, 57B, 69–71

# Management of life-threatening injuries in children

**J. Alex Haller, Jr.** MD
Robert Garret Professor of Surgery, Department of Pediatric Surgery, Johns Hopkins Hospital, Baltimore, Maryland, USA

In the past two years several guidelines have been proposed for a comprehensive system of emergency medical care for children, and for the first time specific standards of care for critically injured children have been formulated[1]. The American Academy of Pediatrics' new Provisional Committee on Emergency Medicine has been charged with the responsibility of developing national standards of emergency care for children and is currently at work on what promises to be a landmark document.

In Maryland we have had a functioning statewide system for the management of life-threatening injuries in children for the past 10 years. This chapter describes the organization and current status of the Maryland system, which, with certain modifications, could serve as a model for use in other regions.

The establishment of regional trauma centres in the USA has been responsible for the development of better standards of care based on sound clinical and laboratory research. This has improved not only the acute care of patients, with more aggressive initial resuscitation, but to some extent also the long-term care and ultimate outcome. Furthermore, as a result of centralizing emergency care facilities, systems of transportation from the scene of the accident to the appropriate centre as well as continuing intensive care within the centre have also improved[2]. This systems approach is still evolving but the model is accepted and preliminary evidence clearly shows improved standards of care for this complicated 'disease' called trauma.

## Overview of trauma in children

Although much progress has been made in regionalized care for adult accident victims, the special problems of care of the severely injured child have not been adequately identified and emphasized[3]. Until the last few years there has been no clear voice for specialized care of children with major injuries.

In the USA more than 50 per cent of all deaths in children aged 1–14 years occur as a result of major trauma, compared to approximately 8 per cent (1 death in 12) from injuries in the total general population. The situation is similar in all industrialized nations of the world. Trauma in children is by far the leading cause of death[4].

Crippling injuries to children and the resulting need for rehabilitation make great demands on our health care system. The expenditure of resources and personnel, and the economic costs of lost work potential in an injured child, are enormous when compared with those in adults with similar injuries. This is due not only to the long-term rehabilitation required but also to the continued professional support needed to help with the child's subsequent growth and development. The problems of adjustment to severe disability, and the child's image of himself as an incomplete individual, may be overwhelming to him unless highly trained professionals participate in the process of recovery. It has been estimated that in the USA more than 100 000 children are seriously crippled by accidents each year and that more than 2 000 000 may be temporarily incapacitated by their injuries[5]. The need for immediate resuscitation as well as long-term rehabilitation will put further strains on our overburdened health care system unless we can find new and more effective ways of accident prevention and become more aggressive in acute care management in order to decrease the need for long-term rehabilitation.

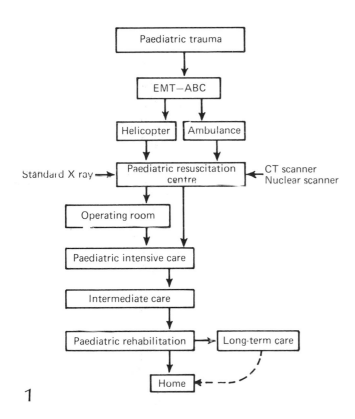

1

EMT-ABC = Emergency Medical Technician–Airways, Breathing, Circulation

# 1

# The Maryland model

Based on the Maryland experience, a regionalized system of trauma management for children includes the following components.

## Communication system

Two-way radio communication with the emergency medical technicians at the scene of the accident allows contact with a physician, who can then give instant advice, and with medical specialists in nearby hospitals to determine the destination of the individual patient.

## Transport system

An efficient transport system is an integral part of the regional trauma centre concept. It should include a police helicopter service linked by radio to an emergency medical relay centre which functions as the communication centre for the system. Transportation is arranged through the relay centre, which also passes on information about the appropriate specialty facility to which the patient should be taken.

## First responders at accident site

All emergency medical technicians must have received specialized training in the care of newborn infants and children from medical specialists such as neonatologists, paediatric surgeons and anaesthetists. They are then qualified to begin intravenous treatment of small infants and to intubate babies and young children if this is indicated. Their training must be part of a continuing training programme for emergency medical technicians within the regional system.

## Resuscitation centre

A resuscitation unit is a basic component of any regional paediatric trauma centre. After communication from the scene of the accident the child is brought by appropriate transportation to the emergency room where it is met by a team of paediatric resuscitation and paediatric surgery specialists who are trained in initial management of life-threatening injuries.

The resuscitation unit should be designed specifically for children, with miniature intubation equipment (including tracheostomy tubes) and other specialized equipment such as central venous pressure lines for children. The resuscitation team should be led either by a senior resident in paediatric surgery or by a staff paediatric surgeon working closely with well-trained paediatric emergency medicine staff. Available on call within minutes must be key paediatric surgical specialists such as paediatric neurosurgeons and paediatric orthopaedic surgeons. X-ray equipment must be immediately available in the unit for both the initial diagnostic studies and subsequent special films. It is important to emphasize that all children with major injuries are resuscitated by paediatricians and paediatric surgeons all of whom are part of the paediatric trauma team.

After emergency stabilization, appropriate diagnostic tests and specialty consultations, the child may go directly to the operating room or be admitted to a paediatric intensive care unit.

## Paediatric intensive care

Paediatric intensive care units should also be centralized. All patient stations should be equipped with multiple channel monitoring equipment and ventilators, and be staffed for the immediate detection of cardiopulmonary arrest, for resuscitation and for continuing post-trauma management. Other equipment may include a mass spectrometer, cardiac output computers, blood gas analysers, ionized calcium analysers, and γ-cameras for determination of cardiac output and similar clinical research studies. A small blood gas laboratory within the unit is ideal for immediate blood gas determination.

## Additional facilities

Three important additional facilities are needed for a fully comprehensive regional centre for the care of children with major trauma. These are (1) an intermediate care unit under the direction of paediatric neurologists; (2) a paediatric subacute rehabilitation unit under the direction of a paediatric physiotherapist; and (3) an intermediate and long-term care unit for children who need continued rehabilitation and nursing.

### Neurology-neurosurgery intermediate care unit

The intermediate care unit is directed by a paediatric neurosurgeon and a paediatric neurologist both of whom have a special interest in the care of children with head injuries. It provides a direct continuation of the intensive care of children with severe brain injuries, including continued monitoring of neurological recovery when constant monitoring and intracranial bolt measurements are no longer required[6]. Within this unit paediatric rehabilitation begins and the interplay of the paediatric physiotherapist becomes an increasingly important component of patient management.

Preliminary evidence from our experience strongly suggests that children with major head injuries producing coma lasting longer than 24 hours have a greatly improved recovery rate over that reported in the literature[7]. Only 9 per cent of the surviving children have a residual intellectual or motor deficit while 88 per cent of the survivors over 2 years of age make a good recovery without major measurable motor or intellectual deficits. It remains to be seen whether these preliminary findings reflect continuing trends but they are certainly encouraging[8].

### Paediatric rehabilitation

This is an important component of comprehensive patient care. We have a specially designed eight-bed unit which allows inpatient care and parent participation in continuing subacute and intermediate rehabilitation programmes and evaluation. This not only improves day-to-day patient care but also provides an opportunity for studying the emotional and physical responses to rehabilitation and for designing new protocols for early rehabilitation.

### Long-term rehabilitation and management

This may be carried out in the trauma centre itself or, as in our case, in an affiliated children's specialty hospital committed to the intermediate and long-term care of children with residual neurological and physical problems following major injuries. The unit should be under full time supervision by a paediatrician and ideally all physician members of the paediatric trauma centre should be on its consultative staff, taking part in frequent interdisciplinary discussions and presentations.

# Discussion

Results from the regional trauma centre for children in the state of Maryland clearly show that a *systems approach* to the management of life-threatening injuries improves standards of patient care. In 1975 only 61 children were admitted to our unit with major trauma. In 1985 this number had risen to more than 300, with a mortality of 7 per cent. Equally importantly, the trauma centre is a focus for an integrated interdisciplinary approach to the management of multiple organ injuries in children. From this centre has come the first trauma registry for children[9] and a recent opportunity to evaluate several of the new anatomical indices of injury severity both in adults and children[10,11,12]. Material from the clinical evaluation of patients is available for in-service discussion and this, together with regular peer review, helps to identify better management as well as to assess the cost effectiveness of this very expensive form of emergency care.

Our experience of the last 10 years suggests that the concept of a regional paediatric trauma centre is sound and that such centres may well act as a stimulus for concentrated paediatric trauma research. The system ensures excellent initial management at the scene of the accident and rapid transport under the care of specially trained emergency medical technicians to a designated trauma centre for children.

The preliminary stimulus for the development of regional trauma centres for children have been the special and unusual problems associated with childhood injuries[13]. A child may be affected quite differently to an adult by the same type of injury. For example, the loss of a small amount of blood, while of no consequence in an adult, assumes dramatic importance in a young child when we consider his tiny blood volume. Transfusions of large quantities of refrigerated bank blood and bottled fluids may lead to rapid loss of body heat and cause dangerously low temperatures in small infants. Such heat losses are of much less consequence in adults. Congenital abnormalities, especially congenital heart defects, are more likely to be present in a child and may complicate the treatment of his injuries.

Blunt impact accidents are responsible for the majority of serious injuries in children, accounting for approximately 80–90 per cent of multiple injuries in this age group. External evidence of internal damage may then be absent or misleading and result in serious delay of proper treatment. Evaluation and precise diagnosis are most difficult in children with head injuries. A child's head is injured more often than an adult's, possibly because it is relatively large and more poorly supported by his weaker neck muscles. Associated unconsciousness greatly increases the difficulty of evaluating generalized trauma in children[14]. Since most young children are incapable of describing and localizing their pain and other symptoms accurately, evaluation demands great patience and insight of the examining physician, as well as an ability to establish a trusting relationship with a child. The physician must rely almost entirely on objective findings under these conditions[15].

Serious injuries may have disastrous effects on the emotional well-being of young children. The terror of being separated from familiar faces is greatly magnified if the child is brought into the usual impersonal environment of a busy adult emergency room. Serious emotional disturbances may develop even after minor injuries if the child is treated in what must seem to him intimidating surroundings by physicians and nurses who are not aware of the special needs of children. Too little attention has been given to this important aspect of emergency care.

Successful management of life-threatening injuries in children requires a basic understanding of the differences between adult and childhood trauma, and experience in evaluation and initial resuscitation of young children. We believe that using an organizational framework based on a separate trauma unit for children has led to better teamwork and more efficient management of multiple injuries. Rapid, careful evaluation and sequential correction of altered physiology remain the backbone of successful therapy in children. The unique metabolic demands and miniature anatomical relationships, especially of a small child, present the physician with a special challenge and great responsibility. Rewards for successful management, however, are high; for the younger the injured child the greater is our total investment in his welfare and his future.

## References

1. Ramenofsky, M. L., Morse, T. S. (1982) Standards of care for the critically injured pediatric patient. Journal of Trauma, 22, 921–933

2. American College of Surgeons Committee on Trauma (1980) Field categorization of trauma patients and hospital trauma index. Bulletin of the American College of Surgeons, 65(2). 28–33

3. Haller, J. A. Jr. (1983) Pediatric trauma: the no. 1 killer of children. Journal of the American Medical Association, 249, 47

4. Haller, J. A. Jr. (1970) Problems in children's trauma. Journal of Trauma, 10, 269–271

5. Mayer, T., Walker, M. L., Johnson, D. G., Matlak, M. E. (1981) Causes of morbidity and mortality in severe pediatric trauma. Journal of the American Medical Association, 245, 719–721

6. Bruce, D. A., Schut, L., Bruno, L. A., Wood, J. H., Sutton, L. N. (1978) Outcome following severe head injuries in children. Journal of Neurosurgery, 48, 687–688

7. Mahoney, W. J., D'Souza, B. J., Haller, J. A. Jr., Roger, M. C., Epstein, M. H., Freeman, J. M. (1983) Long-term outcome of children with severe head trauma and prolonged coma. Pediatrics 71, 756–762

8. Mayer, T., Walker, M. L., Shasha, I. Matlak, M., Johnson, D. G. (1981) Effect of multiple trauma on outcome of pediatric patients with neurologic injuries. Child's Brain, 8, 189–197

9. Haller, J. A. Jr., Signer, R. D., Golladay, E. S., Shaker, I. J., White, J. J. (1976) Use of trauma registry in the management of children with life-threatening injuries. Journal of Pediatric Surgery, 11, 381–390

10. Baker, S. P., O'Neill, B., Haddon, W., Long, W. B. (1974) The injury severity score. A method for describing patients with multiple injuries and evaluating emergency care. Journal of Trauma, 14, 187–196

11. Baker, S. P., O'Neill, B. (1976) The injury severity score: An update. Journal of Trauma, 16, 882–885

12. Mayer, T., Matlak, M. E., Johnson, D. G., Walker, M. L. (1980) The modified injury severity scale in pediatric multiple trauma patients. Journal of Pediatric Surgery, 15, 719–726

13. Haller, J. A. Jr. (1979) An overview of emergency care for children with major injuries. Collected Papers in Emergency Services and Traumatology, R. A. Cowley (ed.), p. 264. Baltimore

14. Becker, D., Miller, J. D., Ward, J. D., Greenberg, R. P., Young, H. F., Sakalas, R. (1977) The outcome from severe head injury with early diagnosis and intensive management. Journal of Neurosurgery, 47, 491–502

15. Haller, J. A. Jr. (1973) Newer concepts in emergency care of children with major injuries. Maryland State Medical Journal, 22, 65–68

# Index